T0299002

Behavioral Emergencies for the Emergency Physician

Behavioral Emergencies for the Emergency Physician

Editor-in-Chief

Leslie S. Zun, MD, MBA

Mount Sinai Hospital, Chicago; Rosalind Franklin University of Medicine and Science/The Chicago Medical School, North Chicago, Illinois, USA

Associate Editors

Lara G. Chepenik, MD, PhD

Yale University School of Medicine, New Haven, Connecticut, USA

Mary Nan S. Mallory, MD

University of Louisville School of Medicine, Louisville, Kentucky, USA

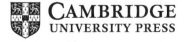

CAMBRIDGE
UNIVERSITY PRESS

CAMBRIDGE
UNIVERSITY PRESS

University Printing House, Cambridge CB2 8BS, United Kingdom

One Liberty Plaza, 20th Floor, New York, NY 10006, USA

477 Williamstown Road, Port Melbourne, VIC 3207, Australia

4843/24, 2nd Floor, Ansari Road, Daryaganj, Delhi - 110002, India

79 Anson Road, #06-04/06, Singapore 079906

Cambridge University Press is part of the University of Cambridge.

It furthers the University's mission by disseminating knowledge in the pursuit of education, learning and research at the highest international levels of excellence.

www.cambridge.org
Information on this title: www.cambridge.org/9781107018488

© Cambridge University Press 2013

This publication is in copyright. Subject to statutory exception and to the provisions of relevant collective licensing agreements, no reproduction of any part may take place without the written permission of Cambridge University Press.

First published 2013
Reprinted 2016

A catalogue record for this publication is available from the British Library

Library of Congress Cataloging in Publication data
Behavioral emergencies for the emergency physician / editor-in-chief,
Leslie S. Zun ; assistant editors, Lara Gayle Chepenik,
Mary Nan S. Mallory.
    p.   ;   cm.
Includes bibliographical references and index.
ISBN 978-1-107-01848-8 (pbk.)
I. Zun, Leslie S.   II. Chepenik, Lara Gayle.   III. Mallory,MaryNan S.
[DNLM: 1. Emergency Services, Psychiatric.   2. Mental
Disorders – diagnosis.   3. Mental Disorders – therapy.   WM 401]
616.89′025–dc23

                                                        2012024805

ISBN 978-1-107-01848-8 Paperback

Cambridge University Press has no responsibility for the persistence or accuracy of URLs for external or third-party internet websites referred to in this publication, and does not guarantee that any content on such websites is, or will remain, accurate or appropriate.

....

Every effort has been made in preparing this book to provide accurate and up-to-date information which is in accord with accepted standards and practice at the time of publication. Although case histories are drawn from actual cases, every effort has been made to disguise the identities of the individuals involved. Nevertheless, the authors, editors and publishers can make no warranties that the information contained herein is totally free from error, not least because clinical standards are constantly changing through research and regulation. The authors, editors and publishers therefore disclaim all liability for direct or consequential damages resulting from the use of material contained in this book. Readers are strongly advised to pay careful attention to information provided by the manufacturer of any drugs or equipment that they plan to use.

Contents

Contributors

James Ahn, MD
Assistant Professor, Section of Emergency Medicine, University of Chicago, University of Chicago Medical Center, Chicago, Illinois, USA.

Eric L. Anderson, MD
Assistant Professor, Department of Psychiatry and Behavioral Sciences, Johns Hopkins Hospital, Baltimore, Maryland, USA

Annette L. Beautrais, PhD
Senior Research Fellow, The University of Auckland, Faculty of Medical and Health Sciences,
Department of Surgery, South Auckland Clinical School, Auckland, New Zealand. Conflicts of interest: none.

Dennis Beedle, MD
Acting Clinical Director, Division of Mental Health, Illinois, Department of Human Services, Chicago, Illinois

Jon S. Berlin, MD
Associate Clinical Professor, Psychiatry & Emergency Medicine, Medical College of Wisconsin, Milwaukee, Wisconsin, USA. Conflicts of interest: none.

Benjamin L. Bregman, MD
Department of Psychiatry and Behavioral Sciences, and Department of Emergency Medicine, The George Washington University Medical Center, Washington, DC, USA

Peter Brown, MA
Executive Director, Institute for Behavioral Healthcare Improvement, Castleton, New York, USA

Suzie Bruch, MD, FAPA
Attending Physician, Department of Psychiatry, Alameda County Medical Center, Oakland, California, USA

Jonathan Busko, MD
Medical Director, Maine EMS Region 4, Eastern Maine Medical Center, Bangor, Maine, USA

Stuart Buttlaire, PhD, MBA
Regional Director of Inpatient Psychiatry & Continuum of Care, Kaiser The Permanent Medical Group, Oakland, California, USA

Laurie Byrne, MD
Associate Professor, Saint Louis University School of Medicine, Department of Surgery/Division of Emergency Medicine, St. Louis, Missouri, USA

Gerald Carroll, MD
Resident, Department of Emergency Medicine, Temple University School of Medicine, Philadelphia, Pennsylvania, USA

Valerie A. Carroll, PA-C
Physician Assistant, University of Wisconsin Hospital and Clinics, Madison, Wisconsin

Margaret Cashman, MD, FAASM
Clinical Assistant Professor, Department of Psychiatry and Behavioral Sciences, University of Washington School of Medicine; Attending Psychiatrist, Psychiatric Emergency Services, Harborview Medical Center, Seattle, Washington, USA

Joseph R. Check, MD
Department of Psychiatry, Yale University School of Medicine; Department of Psychiatry, The Hospital of St Raphael, New Haven, Connecticut, USA.
Conflicts of interest: none.

Lara G. Chepenik, MD, PhD
Assistant Professor, Department of Psychiatry, Yale University School of Medicine, New Haven CT, and Department of Psychiatry, Veterans Affairs Connecticut Healthcare System, West Haven, CT, USA

Robert N. Cuyler, PhD
President Clinical Psychology Consultants Ltd, LLP, Houston, Texas, USA

Preeti Dalawari, MD
Assistant Professor, Saint Louis University School of Medicine, Department of Surgery/Division of Emergency Medicine, St. Louis, Missouri, USA

Suzanne Dooley-Hash, MD
Assistant Professor, Department of Emergency Medicine, University of Michigan; Medical Director, The Center for Eating Disorders, Ann Arbor, Michigan, USA

William R. Dubin, MD
Professor and Chair, Department of Psychiatry, Temple University School of Medicine, Philadelphia, Pennsylvania, USA

Mila L. Felder, MD, MS
Attending Physician, Advocate Christ Hospital and Hope Medical Center; Associate Professor, University of Illinois at Chicago School of Medicine, Department of Emergency Medicine, Chicago, Illinois, USA

Avrim B. Fishkind, MD
Chief Medical Officer, JSA Health Telepsychiatry, LLC, Houston, Texas, USA

Reginald I. Gaylord, MD
Department of Emergency Medicine, University of Chicago, Chicago, Illinois, USA

Rachel Lipson Glick, MD
Clinical Professor, Department of Psychiatry, University of Michigan Medical School; Medical Director, Psychiatric Emergency Services, University of Michigan Health System, Ann Arbor, Michigan, USA. Conflicts of interest: none.

Travis Grace, MD
University of Nevada School of Medicine, Department of Emergency Medicine, Las Vegas, Nevada, USA

Clare Gray, MD, FRCPC
Division Chief, Community Based Psychiatry Services, Children's Hospital of Eastern Ontario; Associate Professor, Department of Psychiatry, University of Ottawa, Ontario, Canada. Conflicts of interest: none.

Anita Hart, MD
Clinical Instructor, Department of Internal Medicine, University of Michigan Health System, Ann Arbor, Michigan, USA

Ross A. Heller, MD
Associate Professor of Surgery, Division of Emergency Medicine, St. Louis University School of Medicine, St. Louis, Missouri, USA. Conflicts of interest: none.

Amanda E. Horn, MD
Assistant Professor and Assistant Residency Director, Department of Emergency Medicine, Temple University School of Medicine, Philadelphia, Pennsylvania, USA

David S. Howes, MD
Professor of Medicine and Pediatrics, Program Director Emeritus, Section of Emergency Medicine, University of Chicago, Chicago, Illinois, USA

David C. Hsu, MD
Resident Physician, Department of Psychiatry and Behavioral Sciences, Department of Internal Medicine, University of California, Davis Health System, Sacramento, California, USA. Dr. Hsu does not serve as the PI on any industry supported research projects.

Andy Jagoda, MD
Professor of Emergency Medicine, Mount Sinai School of Medicine, New York, New York, USA

Margaret Judd, LMSW, ACSW
Clinical Social Worker, Emergency Department Mental Health, Ann Arbor Veterans Affairs Medical Center, Ann Arbor, Michigan, USA

John Kahler, MD
Clinical Assistant Professor, Department of Emergency Medicine, University of Michigan Health System, Ann Arbor, Michigan, USA

Daryl Knox, MD
Medical Director, Comprehensive Psychiatry Emergency Program, Mental Health and Mental Retardation Authority of Harris County, Houston, Texas, USA

Gregory Luke Larkin, MD, MSPH, FACEP
The Lion Foundation Chair of Emergency Medicine, The University of Auckland, Faculty of Medical and Health Sciences, Department of Surgery, South Auckland Clinical School, Auckland, New Zealand. Conflicts of interest: none.

Patricia Lee, MD
Department of Emergency Medicine, Advocate Illinois Masonic Medical Center; Department of Emergency Medicine, University of Illinois at Chicago, Chicago, Illinois, USA. Conflicts of interest: none.

Jerrold B. Leikin, MD, FACP, FACEP
Director of Medical Toxicology, Northshore University Health System – OMEGA, Glenview, Illinois, USA. See Chapter 45 for disclaimer.

Eddie Markul, MD
EMS Medical Director, Chicago North EMS System; Attending Physician, Department of Emergency

Medicine, Advocate Illinois Masonic Medical Center, Chicago, Illinois, USA, and Assistant Professor of Emergency Medicine, University of Illinois at Chicago

Marc L. Martel, MD
Associate Professor, Department of Emergency Medicine, University of Minnesota; Faculty, Department of Emergency Medicine, Hennepin County Medical Center, Minneapolis, Minnesota, USA

J. D. McCourt, MD, FACEP
Vice Chair of Clinical Affairs, Associate Professor, University of Nevada School of Medicine, Department of Emergency Medicine; Medical Director University Medical Center of Southern Nevada Adult Emergency Department, Las Vegas, Nevada, USA

MaryLynn McGuire Clarke, MS, JD
Adjunct Assistant Professor, Illinois Hospital Association, Springfield, Illinois, USA. See Chapter 45 for disclaimer.

Mark Newman, MD
Resident Physician, Department of Psychiatry, University of Michigan Medical Center, Ann Arbor, Michigan, USA

Anthony T. Ng, MD
Medical Director, Psychiatric Emergency Services, Acadia Hospital, Bangor, Maine, USA

Barbara Nightengale, MD
Department of Psychiatry, University of Pittsburgh Medical Center, Pittsburgh, Pennsylvania, USA

Kimberly Nordstrom, MD, JD
Assistant Professor, University of Colorado Denver; Psychiatric Emergency Service, Denver Health Medical Center, Denver, Colorado, USA. Conflicts of interest: none. The author does not receive any funding from pharmaceutical companies.

Jagoda Pasic, MD, PhD
Associate Professor, Medical Director, Psychiatric Emergency Services, Department of Psychiatry and Behavioral Sciences, University of Washington, Harborview Medical Center, Seattle, Washington, USA

Jennifer Peltzer-Jones, PsyD, RN
Henry Ford Health System, Department of Emergency Medicine, Detroit, Michigan, USA. Conflicts of interest: none.

Marcia A. Perry, MD
Clinical Instructor and Assistant Residency Program Director, Department of Emergency Medicine, The University of Michigan, Ann Arbor, Michigan, USA

Larry Phillips, DCSW
Program Manager, St Anthony Hospital, Oklahoma City, Oklahoma, USA

Paul Porter, MD, MBA
Assistant Professor, Department of Emergency Medicine, Warren Albert School of Medicine at Brown University, Providence, Rhode Island

Seth Powsner, MD
Professor of Psychiatry and Emergency Medicine, Yale University, New Haven, Connecticut, USA

Michael S. Pulia, MD, FAAEM, FACEP
Assistant Professor, Division of Emergency Medicine, University of Wisconsin School of Medicine and Public Health, Madison, Wisconsin

Erin Rapp, MD
ER Attending Physician, Saint Louis University School of Medicine, St Louis, Missouri, USA

Divy Ravindranath, MD, MS
Clinical Assistant Professor, Department of Psychiatry, University of Michigan Medical Center, Ann Arbor, Michigan, USA

Janet S. Richmond, MSW
Psychiatric Emergency Clinician, Boston Veterans Healthcare Systems, Boston, MA and McLean Hospital, Belmont, MA; Associate Clinical Professor of Psychiatry, Tufts University School of Medicine, Boston, USA

Silvana Riggio, MD
Professor of Psychiatry and Neurology, Mount Sinai School of Medicine, New York, New York, USA

Harvey L. Ruben, MD, MPH
Clinical Professor, Department of Psychiatry, Yale University School of Medicine, New Haven, CT and Department of Psychiatry, Hospital of St. Raphael, New Haven, CT, USA

Derek J. Robinson, MD, MBA, FACEP
Chief Medical Officer, Region V, Centers for Medicare and Medicaid Services;Adjunct Assistant Professor of Emergency Medicine, Northwestern University Feinberg School of Medicine, Chicago, Illinois, USA

Douglas A. Rund, MD,
Professor Emeritus, Department of Emergency Medicine, The Ohio State University, Columbus, Ohio, USA

Omeed Saghafi, MD
The Denver Health Residency in Emergency Medicine, Denver Health Medical Center, Denver, Colorado, USA

Alicia N. Sanders, MD
Instructor, Section of Emergency Medicine, University of Chicago, Chicago, Illinois, USA

Jeffrey Sankoff, MD, FACEP, FRCP(C)
Assistant Professor, University of Colorado School of Medicine, Department of Emergency Medicine, Denver, Colorado, USA

Lorin M. Scher, MD
Health Sciences Assistant Clinical Professor, Department of Psychiatry and Behavioral Sciences, University of California, Davis Health System, Sacramento, California, USA. Dr. Scher has accepted an honorarium from Lundbeck Inc. and does not serve as the PI on any industry supported research projects.

Louis Scrattish, MD
Assistant Professor, Division of Emergency Medicine, University of Wisconsin School of Medicine and Public Health, Madison, Wisconsin, USA

Richard D. Shih, MD
Associate Professor of Surgery, New Jersey Medical School; Residency Program Director, Department of Emergency Medicine, Morristown Memorial Hospital, Morristown, New Jersey, USA

Maureen Slade, MS, APRN, BC
Director of Medicine and Psychiatry, Northwestern Memorial Hospital, Chicago, Illinois, USA. See Chapter 45 for disclaimer.

Susan Stefan, MPhil, JD
Visiting Professor, University of Miami School of Law, Corac Cables, Florida

Victor G. Stiebel, MD
Department of Psychosomatic and Emergency Medicine, University of Pittsburgh Medical Center, Pittsburgh, Pennsylvania, USA

Deborah Taber, RN, MS
Administrative Director, Department of Psychiatry and Behavioral Sciences, Evanston Northwestern Healthcare, Evanston, Illinois, USA. See Chapter 45 for disclaimer.

Vaishal Tolia, MD, MPH
Assistant Professor, Department of Emergency Medicine, Department of Internal Medicine, UC San Diego Health System, San Diego, California, USA

Gary M. Vilke, MD
Professor of Clinical Medicine, Department of Emergency Medicine, UC San Diego Health System, San Diego, California, USA

Alvin Wang, DO
Assistant Professor, Department of Emergency Medicine, Temple University School of Medicine, Philadelphia, Pennsylvania, USA

Michael A. Ward, MD
Emergency Resident Physician, Section of Emergency Medicine, University of Chicago, University of Chicago Medical Center, Chicago, Illinois, USA. Conflicts of interest: none.

Joseph Weber, MD
EMS Medical Director, Chicago West EMS System; Department of Emergency Medicine, Stroger Cook County Hospital; Assistant Professor of Emergency Medicine, Rush Medical College, Chicago, Illinois, USA

Michael P. Wilson, PhD, MD
Department of Emergency Medicine Behavioral Emergencies Research Lab, UC San Diego Health System, San Diego, California, USA

James L. Young, MD
Assistant Professor, Clinical Psychiatry, The Ohio State University, Columbus, Ohio, USA

Scott L. Zeller, MD
Chief, Psychiatric Emergency Services, Alameda County Medical Center, Oakland, California, USA. Conflicts of interest: none.

Preface

Patients frequently present to emergency settings with psychiatric complaints. Numerous factors have contributed to the steady increase in the number of patients using emergency for behavioral emergencies. These factors include reduction in inpatient psychiatric beds; limited, if any, insurance coverage for psychiatric patients; and diminished community resources for these patients. This increase in the number of patients seen in emergency departments (EDs) has put an additional burden on an already stressed healthcare system.

Care of patients with behavioral emergencies may be provided in several settings, including emergency departments, psychiatric emergency service (PES) centers, urgent care centers, primary care clinics, walk-in clinics, and mental health clinics. Although many of these settings employ specially trained personnel, the care of the psychiatric patient in the emergency department may be compromised by the lack of specialty consultants. The ability of emergency physicians to consult with psychiatrists can vary from full-time availability to little or none. However, expertise in management of behavioral emergencies is just one of several proficiencies expected of emergency care providers, regardless of their training or access to specialty consultants. This textbook is designed, primarily, to assist emergency physicians in providing care for psychiatric patients in the approximately 4500 emergency departments across the country. However, it is also intended to provide an authoritative and informative source for practitioners in the hundreds or so psychiatric emergency services (PESs) and other settings where behavioral emergencies are encountered.

There a few other texts on behavioral emergencies but most are authored by psychiatrists, primarily for psychiatrists. Behavioral Emergencies for the Emergency Physician is designed to enhance emergency physicians' knowledge and understanding of patients who present to the emergency department with behavioral emergencies.

Treatment of emergency psychiatric patients often demands the collaboration of emergency physicians, psychiatrists, psychologists, mental health workers, and social workers. This book reflects a similar level of multi-disciplinary collaboration as its authors have expertise in emergency medicine, psychiatry, social work, psychology, and legal fields. Although providers in many fields may find this book useful, it is designed for emergency physicians, residents, and allied health personnel who frequently collaborate in the ED.

This text may also be used as a reference for these providers while the patient is in the emergency setting, as a textbook for residents in emergency medicine, as a review for practicing emergency physicians, and as an adjunct for other care providers. It is a potential backbone for a course in emergency psychiatry, rotation in behavioral emergencies, or certification process for healthcare providers.

The breadth of this textbook is designed to cover topics related to the evaluation and treatment of patients who might present to emergency departments with behavioral emergencies. The book is divided into six sections to accommodate all the relevant topics: Evaluation, diagnoses, treatment, special issues, and management. The chapters run the gamut from basic topics such as medical clearance, psychosis, and treatment of agitation to advanced topics such as triage, psychiatric illness in pregnancy, and research in emergency psychiatry. The breadth of topics enables the reader to use the text as an easy reference for specific questions related to behavioral emergencies, and also provides expert advice on the most recent approaches to patient evaluation and treatment.

I want to acknowledge the dedication of the authors who have contributed to the excellence of this book. This textbook would not have been be possible without the outstanding editing performed by the associate editors, Lara Chepenik and Mary Nan Mallory, who worked tirelessly to review all of the chapters.

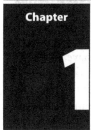

Chapter

1

The magnitude of the problem of psychiatric illness presenting in the emergency department

Gregory Luke Larkin and Annette L. Beautrais

Introduction

Mental illness is ubiquitous and increasingly recognized as a growing problem throughout the world [1]. The purpose of this chapter is to describe the magnitude of the problem of mental illness, both globally and in terms of specific mental health-related visits encountered in emergency department (ED) settings. While emergency departments may not be the optimal location to manage the growing burden of mental illness, they are often the only 24/7 port in the storm for the preponderance of patients in crisis.

Global burden

By the year 2020, psychiatric disorders are projected to rank second only to cardiovascular illness with regard to both years of potential life lost (YPLL) due to premature mortality and the years of productive life lost due to disability (also known as disability adjusted life years, DALYs) [1]. The escalation of mental illness is attributed to an increase in psychosocial and environmental stressors in many parts of the world combined with the epiphenomenon of mental illnesses becoming less stigmatized in many cultures. Indeed, a substantial increase in measured prevalence comes less from new biological challenges and much more from an increase in diagnoses; the latter diagnostic contagion has been generated in part by the proliferation of clinical psychologists, the widespread availability of structured diagnostic tools, and a populist penchant to pathologize symptoms formerly regarded as non-psychiatric.

Prevalence

Diagnostic trends notwithstanding, the worldwide prevalence of mental illness remains profound. The growing extent of the problem has been well described in the psychiatric epidemiologic studies of the World Health Organization's (WHO) World Mental Health Surveys conducted in 28 countries [2]. The WHO's cross-national comparisons show a globally high prevalence of major Diagnostic and Statistical Manual of Mental Disorders, 4th Edition (DSM-IV) mental disorders (anxiety disorders, mood disorders, impulse control disorders, substance use disorders) with 25th–75th percentiles (interquartile range,

IQR) ranging from 18.1% to 36.1%. These WHO-sponsored studies also reveal cross-nationally consistent findings of early ages at onset, high comorbidity, significant chronicity, widespread unmet treatment needs, significant delays between illness onset and treatment, and inadequate frequency and quality of treatment.

The World Mental Health Surveys found that lifetime prevalence of major DSM-IV mental disorders was highest in the United States with almost half (47.4%) the population having a lifetime risk of at least one mental illness [3]. The 12-month prevalence estimate for any disorder varied widely, and was also highest in the United States (24.6%) but lowest in Beijing (4.3%) [4]. All four major classes of DSM-IV disorders were important components of overall prevalence. Anxiety disorders (IQR, 9.9–16.7%) and mood disorders (IQR, 9.8–15.8%) were the most prevalent lifetime illnesses. Impulse control disorders (IQR, 3.1–5.7%), and substance use disorders (IQR, 4.8–9.6%) were generally less prevalent in global samples, despite their relatively high frequency among emergency department patients in North America.

Extent of mental illness across the life cycle

Most mental disorders begin early in life and often have a chronic, fulminating course. They have much earlier ages-of-onset than most chronic non-psychiatric disorders. In the U.S. sample of the World Mental Health Survey, approximately 50% of psychiatric disorders existed by age 14, and 75% by age 24 [5]. Very early age of onset occurs for some anxiety disorders, notably, phobias, and separation anxiety disorder (SAD), with median age of onset in the range 7–14 years. Early onsets are also typical for the externalizing disorders, with 80% of all lifetime attention-deficit/hyperactivity disorder beginning in the age range 4–11 and the clear majority of oppositional-defiant disorder and conduct disorder beginning between ages 5 and 15. Serious mental illnesses such as schizophrenia typically first manifest in the late teenage years or early adulthood, typically in the range of 15–35 years of age.

Adult onsets are seen for the other common anxiety disorders (panic disorder, generalized anxiety disorder, and post-traumatic stress disorder), with median onset in the age range

Behavioral Emergencies for the Emergency Physician, ed. Leslie S. Zun, Lara G. Chepenik, and Mary Nan S. Mallory. Published by Cambridge University Press. © Cambridge University Press 2013.

25–50 years old. Mood disorders have a similar age of onset to the later-onset anxiety disorders, increasing linearly from the early teens until late middle age and then declining. The median age of onset for mood disorders ranges from 25 to 45. Substance use disorders also begin in young adulthood with a median age of onset ranging from 20 to 35 years [5]. The age of onset for the dementias is generally late in older adulthood. Alzheimer's disease is typically first seen in those over 65 years of age.

Social and physical health impacts

Data from both the WHO World Mental Health Surveys and the WHO Global Burden of Disease Study show that mental disorders impose enormous personal and economic costs. These enduring costs arise in part from the combination of early onset, high prevalence, high disability, and chronicity of these disorders [2]. Early-onset mental disorders are associated with a wide array of adverse outcomes over the life course including lowered educational attainment, early marriage, marital instability, and low occupational and financial status [2]. In addition, and particularly relevant to emergency medicine, early-onset mental disorders increase risk of onset and persistence of a wide range of physical disorders including heart disease, asthma, diabetes mellitus, arthritis, chronic back pain, and chronic headache [6,7]. Adult onset mood, substance, and anxiety disorders are also associated with significant role impairment and are often comorbid with physical illnesses.

Economic burden: United States

In any given year an estimated one in four (26.2%) of the United States population has a diagnosable mental or substance use disorder [8]. Of those with a disorder, 22% are classified as serious, 37% as moderate, and 40% as mild. To address this burden, the total U.S. national health expenditure for mental health services has increased exponentially during the last two decades, from $33 million in 1986 to $100 million in 2003 [9].

Most of the World Mental Health Survey research undertaken to calculate the magnitude of the short-term societal burden of mental disorders has been done in the United States [10,11]. These studies count costs in terms of healthcare expenditures, impaired functioning, and premature mortality, and reveal an overwhelming financial burden. The annual total societal costs of anxiety disorders in the United States over the decade of the 1990s, for example, exceeded $42 billion, and the economic cost of depression in 2000 was estimated at $83 billion.

Further analyses suggest that one third of all the days lost from work or home responsibilities associated with chronic-recurrent health problems in the U.S. population are due to mental disorders, totaling billions of days of lost functioning per year in the U.S. population [12]. In addition, analyses of the impact of specific disorders found that 6.4% of U.S. workers reported an episode of major depressive disorder in the prior year, resulting in an average of over 5 weeks of lost work productivity and costing employers over $36 billion.

Changes in mental healthcare infrastructure

The burden of escalating numbers of mental health patients has been exacerbated, in the United States and worldwide, by changes in mental health infrastructure that have resulted in reduced resources and restricted access to mental health care. In the United States, psychiatric inpatient facilities have been closed, numbers of psychiatrists have declined, and numbers of both state hospital psychiatric beds and psychiatric beds in general have decreased. The number of mental health organizations in the United States have contracted, from 3512 in 1986 to 891 in 2004; the total number of psychiatric beds has fallen by 20% from 267,613 in 1986 to 212,231 in 2004; the number of psychiatric beds in state and county mental hospitals has halved, from 119,033 in 1986 to 57,034 in 2004; the number of beds per 100,000 civilian population decreased from 111.7 in 1986 to 71.2 in 2004 [9].

These striking reductions in psychiatric resources have been accompanied by reduced lengths of stay, moves to treat people in the community, increased costs of general practitioner visits, and an unfavorable reimbursement regime. Having no place else to go, patients with severe and chronic psychiatric illnesses, as well as those with acute mental illnesses, and those in severe psychological distress, have been forced to seek care at emergency departments (EDs) – the only healthcare facilities that cannot legally turn them away [13].

Overall emergency department visits

In 2008, there were almost 124 million visits to U.S. EDs, 41.4 visits for every 100 persons in the United States [14]. From 1996 to 2006, the annual number of ED visits increased from 90 to 119 million, an increase of 32%, representing an average increase of approximately 3 million (3.2%) visits every year [15]. However, as the number of visits has increased, the number of EDs has decreased, from 4019 in 1996 to 3833 in 2006, and this trend shows no sign of declining [16]. The joint effect of increasing visit rates and declining EDs is that the annual number of visits per ED has increased. The overall ED usage rate has increased by approximately 20% resulting in serious overcrowding. Mental health patients have played an increasing role in this ED oversubscription and we describe this below.

Increased mental health visits to emergency departments

An increasing fraction of annual ED visits are for mental health presentations [17]. Indeed, while overall use of U.S. ED services increased by 8% from 1992 to 2001, the number of documented mental health-related visits increased at an even faster rate – by 38%. For the past two decades mental disorders have been the fastest growing component of emergency medical practice, while psychiatric services have diminished. While, each year, almost one in three adults in the non-institutionalized community has a diagnosable mental or addictive disorder, this figure climbs to at least 40% among ED patients. In 2006, the

National Center for Health Statistics (NCHS) reported that 4.7 million patients presented to American EDs with a primary psychiatric diagnosis. However, this number does not include codes for psychiatric reason for visit, comorbid mental health issues, substance-related visits, and the many patients in whom psychiatric reasons for visit are secondary; hence, NCHS numbers are a gross underestimate.

The Emergency Medical Treatment and Active Labor Act (EMTALA) legislation and mental health insurance exclusions, as well as changes in the mental health infrastructure, mean that EDs have become the default option for urgent and acute contact for many psychiatric patients, including high severity patients and those who are suicidal. For some, the ED is their sole source of health care [18]. While many of those who present to EDs with mental health problems are uninsured, underinsured, homeless, and of racial and ethnic minorities who have no easy access to health care, the largest increase in mental health visits in the past decade comes from those who are insured [17]. As states reduce mental healthcare expenditure and the U.S. healthcare system becomes inaccessible to an increasing fraction of the American population, the 38% increase in ED psychiatric visits observed between 1992 and 2001 will likely rise still further.

As a result of these trends, emergency medicine is being forced to assume a growing responsibility for providing both primary and acute mental health care. Paradoxically, however, while ED visits increase every year, both the number of general and psychiatric EDs are declining, often because overcrowding generates high costs, rendering EDs uneconomic businesses. While there are approximately 3,800 general EDs in the United States, of which only 146 have specialized psychiatric emergency units, these resources are diminishing, even as patient visits increase [American Association for Emergency Psychiatry, personal communication, 2009].

The epidemiology of mental health visits to emergency departments

Emergency department use for psychiatric reasons has expanded over the past two decades and now accounts for more than 5% of all U.S. emergency department visits by adults [19]. Despite these recent trends, which have resulted in record-breaking numbers of patients seeking emergency services nationwide, there have been few methodologically and diagnostically sound, and nationally comprehensive studies, of the epidemiology of mental health-related emergency visits in the United States.

The most comprehensive study used National Hospital Ambulatory Medical Care Survey (NHAMCS) data which included all potentially relevant diagnostic fields, including psychiatric reason-for-visit codes, DSM-based ICD diagnoses, Supplementary Classification of Factors Influencing Health Status and Contact with Health Services (V codes), and external cause-of-injury codes (E codes) for all appropriate mental health-related disorders [17]. This study found that, from 1992 to 2001, a total of 53 million visits to U.S. EDs were made primarily for mental health–related reasons. Of these, an estimated 17 million visits were for a mental health-related primary complaint (that is, as conveyed to the clinician by the patient), but many more involved a psychiatric diagnosis (that is, the assessment of the patient's condition by the clinician). Among the estimated 53 million mental health-related visits overall, the most common diagnoses were substance-related disorders (30%), mood disorders (23%), and anxiety disorders (21%). Psychoses constituted 10% and suicide attempts 7% of all documented mental health-related visits. These five major subgroups accounted for 79% of all mental health-related visits.

The remaining visits included all other Diagnostic and Statistical Manual of Mental Disorders (DSM) diagnostic codes and reason-for-visit codes referable to other psychological and mental disorders. Rates of these miscellaneous mental health-related visits increased significantly over the decade. Rates of presentation to EDs for the most serious mental health problem (suicidal behavior) increased almost 50% from 1992 to 2001. As well as suicidal behavior, increased rates of visits were significant for all of the most prevalent disorders (mood, substance use, and anxiety disorders). However, rates of psychoses-related visits remained stable over this period.

Specific mental disorders

The goal of the following section is to describe the magnitude of the problem of ED presentations for specific mental disorders. The most prevalent conditions are highlighted. While the prevalence and illness burden of each condition are worthy of discussion, prevalence data are not available for all mental illnesses, particularly those that are less common.

Anxiety disorders

Anxiety disorders are the most common psychiatric disorders in the general population. The findings of many studies suggest that as many as one in four ED patients screen positive for anxiety disorders [20]. Many patients with anxiety disorders visit emergency departments, either to seek help for the anxiety symptoms explicitly, or because they have physical symptoms related to anxiety. While anxiety symptoms rarely constitute a life-threatening emergency, severe anxiety is a common presenting problem in emergency department patients, consuming many resources. Specific anxiety disorders include:

- Anxiety due to a general medical condition
- Substance-induced anxiety disorder
- Generalized anxiety disorder
- Panic disorder
- Acute stress disorder
- Post-traumatic stress disorder (PTSD)
- Adjustment disorder with anxious features
- Obsessive-compulsive disorder (OCD)
- Social phobia, also referred to as social anxiety disorder
- Specific phobia, also referred to as simple phobia.

Anxiety disorders affect one in five (18.1%) of the U.S. adult population each year [8]. Of these cases, 22.8% (4.2% of the total adult population) are classified as "severe" [21]. The mean age of onset of anxiety disorders is 11 years, and these disorders are more common in females than males, and less common in non-Hispanic Blacks and in Hispanics than in non-Hispanic Whites.

Despite the high prevalence rates of the anxiety disorders, they are often under-recognized and undertreated clinical problems in the general population, and in primary care. Of all cases each year, only one third (36.9%) receive treatment and for only one third of those, (12.7% of those with the disorder), is the treatment effective or adequate [22]. Anxiety disorders have a strong comorbidity with depression, and the risk of suicidal behavior in anxiety disorders is often under estimated.

Anxiety-related presentations accounted for 16% of emergency department mental health visits from 1992 to 2001, increasing from 4.9% to 6.3% of all emergency department visits across the decade [23]. This growth may reflect a rise in anxiety-related emergency department care-seeking, an increase in anxiety awareness among patients and practitioners, or both. Of all mental health visits to the ED, anxiety disorders are the least likely to result in admission, with an overall hospitalization rate of 20%.

Panic disorder

The estimated lifetime prevalence of panic disorder in the U.S. adult population is 4.7% [24,25]. Twelve-month prevalence is estimated at 2.7%. The lifetime prevalence of panic disorder is twice as high among females (6.2%) than males (3.1%). Twelve-month prevalence is 3.8% for females, and 1.6% for males. The age of onset for panic disorder is typically is the early to mid-twenties, and panic disorder is seen most commonly in people aged 15–24 years [26]. However, these population estimates may not reflect the characteristics of panic disorder patients seen in emergency room settings. For example, it has been found that panic patients in an ED were older and more likely to be male than patients seen in psychiatric clinics. One study found ED panic patients were also significantly more likely to be on Medicare and less likely to be uninsured [27].

Patients with panic disorder have high rates of use of both ED services and 911 emergency services, as well as high rates of ED recidivism. Panic patients seek emergency care not only because of the sudden, severe, and frightening onset of symptoms, but also because anxiety disorders often occur in association with somatic complaints: the direction of association is unclear but is likely to be bidirectional.

A series of ED studies has focused on patients who present with chest pain [27]. Chest pain is the most common reason for ED presentation for over 65 year olds, and the second most common reason for those aged 15 to 64 years, accounting in 2008 for 4.7 million ED visits [9]. Studies of ED chest pain patients consistently report that panic disorder can be diagnosed in two thirds of all patients presenting to an ED with medically unexplained chest pain. In several studies, the vast majority (98%) of ED patients with panic disorder were undiagnosed. These patients often receive costly cardiac workups to exclude coronary artery disease, yet they are seldom, if ever, screened for panic disorder [28].

Underdiagnosis of panic disorder is unfortunate, not only because identification of these patients might reduce their economic burden in the ED by avoiding unnecessary and expensive investigative tests, and minimizing rates of medical care usage, use of 911 services, and overall ED use, but also because effective pharmacological and psychotherapeutic treatments are available. Untreated, panic patients tend to develop depression, agoraphobia, alcohol and substance abuse problems, and impaired social and occupational functioning. Panic disorder is also associated with elevated risk of suicidal behavior. Although only 60% of people with panic disorder seek care, 32% of these patients present to EDs, rendering EDs an appropriate site for detection of panic disorder [28].

Post-traumatic stress disorder (PTSD)

While the nosology of post-traumatic stress disorder in still being debated, the estimated lifetime prevalence of PTSD among adult Americans is 6.8% [8,21]. The 12-month PTSD prevalence estimate is 3.5%. PTSD is significantly more common in women than men; the lifetime prevalence of PTSD among men is 3.6% and among women, 9.7%. The 12-month prevalence is 1.8% among men and 5.2% among women.

PTSD is often unrecognized in the general population, as well as in emergency departments which are routine reception zones for trauma and disaster victims. Emergency departments receive many patients who have experienced mass-casualty events, natural disasters, serious accidents, assault or abuse, sudden and major deaths, as well as deep emotional losses that put them at risk of PTSD.

Generalized anxiety disorder

The lifetime prevalence of generalized anxiety disorder (GAD) is estimated at 5.7% [8,21,24]. The 12-month prevalence is 2.7%. The lifetime prevalence of generalized anxiety disorder is estimated to be 7.1% in females and 4.2% among males. Past year prevalence is 3.4% among females and 1.9% in males. Generalized anxiety disorder rarely occurs in isolation from other psychiatric disorders, with an estimated 90% of people with GAD meeting criteria for another psychiatric disorder over the course of their lifetime. The most common comorbid illnesses are depression, alcohol abuse, and other anxiety disorders. In the emergency department, GAD is likely to be a secondary diagnosis to both these comorbid mental disorders as well as to physical illnesses.

Phobic disorders

Lifetime estimates suggest 12.5% of the adult U.S. population has a specific phobia [8, 21]. In any year, 1 in every 10 adults reports having a specific phobia. The lifetime prevalence is estimated at 15.8% in females and 8.9% in males. While phobias are the most prevalent anxiety disorders they are much less likely to be the reason for ED presentations than panic disorder, PTSD, and GAD.

Mood disorders

After anxiety disorders, mood disorders are the second most common psychiatric disorder in the general population, occurring in 10% of the U.S. adult population each year [8,21,29]. Of these cases, 45% (4.3% of the total population) are classified as severe. The mean age of onset is 30 years, and women are 50% more likely than men to suffer a mood disorder during their lifetime. Non-Hispanic Blacks and Hispanics are less likely than non-Hispanic Whites to experience a mood disorder during their lifetime.

Mood disorders are the most expensive mental illness in the general population because they are frequently undiagnosed, underdiagnosed, or misdiagnosed, and, even if detected, often inadequately treated. Each year, half of those in the general population with a mood disorder receive treatment and for 40% (20% of those with any mood disorder) this treatment is minimally adequate [22].

The economic burden of depression in the general population is derived not only from the healthcare costs of inadequate diagnosis and treatment, but also from workplace absenteeism and loss of productivity, lost earnings due to premature death, the costs incurred by social agencies including law enforcement, the justice system, and shelters, as well as personal costs in terms of reduced quality of life.

After substance use disorders, mood disorders (including major depressive disorder, bipolar disorder, and dysthymia) are the most common mental illness seen in the emergency department, accounting for 17% of U.S. ED visits for mental health-related reasons from 1992 to 2001 [18].

Major depression

Each year 6.7% of U.S. adults suffer a major depressive disorder (MDD) [8,21]. Of these, one third (2% of all the U.S. adult population) are classified as severe. The mean age of onset is 32 years. Women are 70% more likely than males to have a major depressive disorder during their lifetime, and MDD is 40% less common in non-Hispanic Blacks than non-Hispanic Whites. Of all those with MDD each year, only half receive treatment and of those receiving treatment, 38% (20% of those with the disorder) are receiving minimally adequate treatment.

Untreated, depression imposes a severe economic burden, resulting largely from inadequate diagnosis and treatment. In the majority (50% to 60%) of those with depression, the disorder is not accurately diagnosed [30]. Wells and colleagues found that depressed medically ill patients have significantly more pain and functional impairment than matched patients having chronic medical conditions alone [31]. Only advanced coronary artery disease accounts for more bed disability days (defined as days during which a person stayed in bed for more than half a day because of illness or injury) than depression, and only arthritis causes more pain. In terms of impaired physical functioning and ability to work, to function socially, and to care for home and family, depression is more disabling than hypertension, diabetes, arthritis, gastrointestinal, or back pain problems. Depressed patients have high rates of medical usage for a range of somatic complaints including headaches, backaches, gastrointestinal disorders, weakness, lethargy, fatigue, and insomnia. They are frequent users of emergency departments, using such services three to five times more than non-depressed patients [32].

However, depression is often neither detected nor even inquired about in emergency department settings [33]. A study of 476 ED patients in four U.S. hospitals found that, when screened for symptoms of depression, one third were positive [34]. While symptoms of depression do not necessarily equate with standardized diagnoses of depression, these results suggest that depression in ED patients may be approximately six times higher than in general population samples.

Depression is often comorbid with anxiety disorders, other mental disorders, and somatic complaints. It may be obscured in ED presentations by these other concerns unless explicit screening for depression is undertaken. However, if ED screening for depression is implemented, then there is a need to develop a range of ED-based interventions to either provide ED-delivered interventions or to link all those who screen positive for depression to appropriate services external to the ED, and furthermore, to ensure that no-one falls through gaps between ED and outpatient services.

Bipolar disorder

Bipolar disorder is a chronic mood disorder that causes significant economic burden to patients, families, and society [8,21,35]. The 12-month prevalence of bipolar disorder in the U.S. adult population is 2.6%. The majority of these cases (83%) are classified as severe. Half of those with the disorder receive treatment each year, and of those, 40% receive minimally adequate treatment.

Bipolar disorder is characterized by recurrent manic or hypomanic, and depressive, episodes that cause functional impairment and reduce quality of life [36]. At least 25% to 50% of patients with bipolar disorder also attempt suicide [37]. Bipolar patients may present to the ED in either depressed or manic states; some will have attempted suicide. There are few studies of the epidemiology of bipolar disorder visits to the ED, but one small study found that almost 7% of ED patients screened positive for bipolar disorder, considerably higher than population estimates of 1.3% [38].

Dysthymic disorder

Dysthymic disorder, or dysthymia, is characterized by long-term (2 years or longer) symptoms that may not be severe enough to be disabling but can prevent normal functioning or feeling well. People with dysthymia may also experience one or more episodes of major depression during their lifetime [8,21]. The lifetime prevalence of dysthymic disorder is estimated to be 2.5% [8,21]. The 12-month prevalence is 1.5%. Lifetime estimates are 3.1% among females and 1.8% in males. Twelve-month estimates are 1.9% among females and 1.0% in males. Dysthymia may underlie many ED visits, but it is frequently undetected and many outpatients with dysthymia may be receiving inadequate treatment.

Suicidal behavior

While suicidal behavior is not a DSM-IV disorder, it is anticipated to be part of DSM-V. Suicidal behavior is closely associated with most mental disorders, and is the most common and arguably the most serious psychiatric emergency presentation to the ED. Suicide ideation and suicide attempts are strongly linked to death by suicide and predict further suicidal behavior [39]. The lifetime prevalence of suicide ideation is 9% and the lifetime prevalence of suicide attempt is 3%. Twelve-month prevalence rates of suicide ideation, plans, and attempts are, respectively, 2%, 0.6%, and 0.3% for developed countries [40].

Suicide attempts accounted for approximately 2.5 million (5.9%) injury-related U.S. ED visits in 2006, and the rate of presentation for suicide-related visits to U.S. EDs increased by 47% during the decade from 1992 to 2001. Yet these figures underestimate the prevalence of suicide-related visits to the ED. A study by Claassen and Larkin (2005), for example, found that a significant fraction of those who present to EDs for non-mental health reasons often have occult or silent suicide ideation (estimated at 8–12%) [41].

Three clusters of ED patients can be identified as being at risk of suicidal ideation and behavior: (i) Those who present to ED with suicidal ideation or threats, or following suicide attempts; (ii) Those who present with the mental health problems with which suicide is associated; (iii) Those who present with specific physical problems but who have occult or silent suicide risk [42,43].

Almost all mental disorders have an increased risk of suicide apart from mental retardation and dementia [44]. Approximately 90% of individuals who attempt or commit suicide meet diagnostic criteria for a mental disorder, most commonly mood disorder, substance use disorders, psychoses, and personality disorders. However, both the mental disorders with which suicide is associated and suicidal ideation are frequently under-recognized and under treated in ED settings.

Those who make suicide attempts also present to ED services for a range of medical problems and have increased risks of homicide, accidents, disease, and premature death in general [45]. Patients who present to the ED with suicide ideation (without attempt) also have risks of returning to the ED with further ideation or with suicide attempts which are as high as those who present with attempts [46].

EDs have an unmatched burden of responsibility for suicidal patients. EDs are thoroughfares for a range of endophenotypes at high risk of suicidal behavior, including not only those with frank or occult suicidal behavior but also: young people; males;

prisoners; gun-owners; homeless; psychiatrically ill; binge drinkers, illicit drug users, and substance abusers; older adults; victims of abuse, trauma, and assault; perpetrators of crime, assault, and violence; substance-abusing youth; violent youth; youth with conduct disorder and those in foster and welfare care; patients with severe, chronic mental disorders, including those with depression; psychosis, and personality disorders; older adults with physical health problems, persistent pain, disability, and/or depression; adults and young adults with degenerative illnesses. Given that emergency departments are in frequent contact with suicidal patients, EDs represent underutilized sites for suicide prevention [41]. Potentially, EDs are sites that could identify and engage at-risk patients into accessible outpatient care management and suicide prevention programs.

Substance use disorders

One person in three in the U.S. population has a lifetime substance use disorder, and lifetime risk is higher among males (41.8%) than females (29.6%) [8,21]. The 12-month prevalence is 13.4%, again higher in males (15.4%) than females (11.6%).

Substance abuse is the most common mental health reason for ED presentations. Primary diagnosis of substance abuse was responsible for 30% of psychiatric-related emergency department visits in the U.S. from 1992 to 2001, and for approximately 8% of total ED visits over that time [17]. Substance abuse is often comorbid with other mental disorders, including mood and anxiety disorders in particular. Patients with comorbid major psychiatric diagnoses and substance abuse diagnoses are overrepresented in those who are frequent recidivists to EDs.

Substance abuse is also commonly involved in injury-related ED presentations including violence, falls, drownings, motor vehicle crashes, and suicide attempts. Substance misuse is also associated with hazardous and costly social consequences including driving under the influence of alcohol or drugs, arrest, and violent behavior.

Alcohol abuse or dependence

In 2000, 16.2% of deaths and 13.2% of disability-adjusted life years (DALYs) from injuries, globally, were estimated to be attributed to alcohol. The lifetime prevalence of alcohol abuse or dependence in the U.S. population is estimated to be 13.2% [8,21]. The 12-month estimate is 3.1%. Lifetime prevalence is estimated at 19.6% among males and 7.5% among females. The 12-month estimates are 4.5% among males and 1.8% among females.

Alcohol-related visits impose a significant burden on emergency departments. Because patients often withhold information about their drinking habits and drinking history, the role of alcohol in ED visits is likely underestimated. Nevertheless alcohol abuse is often implicated in ED visits for violence and injury. Half of all drug abuse/misuse visits made to EDs by individuals under 20 years old involve alcohol.

Drug abuse or dependence

An estimated 8% of the U.S. adult population has a lifetime drug abuse or dependence disorder [8,21]. The 12-month estimate is 1.4%. Lifetime estimates are 11.6% among males and 4.8% among females. The 12-month estimates are 2.2% for males and 0.7% for females. Drug-related ED visits include those made for drug abuse and misuse, suicide attempts, adverse reactions, and accidental ingestions. Drug abuse also spawned increased violence during the crack cocaine epidemic of the 1990s, and substance abuse and dependence remains a central reason for visiting the ED for many patients.

Schizophrenia and other psychotic disorders

Schizophrenia spectrum diagnoses account for approximately two thirds of all psychotic disorders. The estimated lifetime prevalence of schizophrenia in the U.S. adult population is 1.1% [8,21]. Twelve-month healthcare use is estimated at 60%.

Schizophrenia is a serious mental illness with high economic and social costs for families and for society. The overall U.S. 2002 cost of schizophrenia was estimated to be $62.7 billion, with $22.8 billion excess direct healthcare cost ($7.0 billion outpatient, $5.0 billion drugs, $2.8 billion inpatient, and $8.0 billion long-term care) [47].

A population-based study of ED mental health visits, using NHAMCS data, found that psychosis-related ED visits accounted for approximately 10% of all mental health ED visits during the decade from 1992 to 2001 [48]. Notably, while overall mental health-related ED visits increased by more than a third over this time, and rates of ED visits for other major mental health problems including suicidal behavior, substance use disorders, mood disorders, and anxiety disorders all increased, the rate of psychosis-related ED visits per capita did not change. This stability may reflect the results of recent substantial investment in early intervention and intensive case management for the seriously mentally ill.

Some patients with schizophrenia may present to EDs in a psychotic crisis that requires immediate management, and may not have been diagnosed with psychiatric illness previously. They often present diagnostic dilemmas involving organic versus psychiatric etiology and primary psychotic versus affective disorder diagnosis. Treatment may be complicated further by the presence of alcohol or drug intoxication. Previously diagnosed patients with serious mental illness may also present to the ED with a complication of treatment (e.g., adverse effects of medication) or a psychotic crisis which may arise from gaps in treatment or socioeconomic challenges engendered by serious mental illness (e.g., poverty, homelessness, social isolation, failure of support systems).

Eating disorders

Both obesity and the fear of obesity are on the rise. The lifetime prevalence of anorexia nervosa is 0.6% of the U.S. adult population; only one third of anorexia nervosa patients receive treatment [8,21]. Similarly, the lifetime prevalence of bulimia nervosa is 0.6%; 43.2% receive treatment. The 12-month prevalence is bulimia is 0.3%, and only 15.6% receive treatment over that year.

Binge eating is much more common, with a lifetime prevalence of 28%, of whom 43.6% receive treatment. The 12-month prevalence of binge eating is 1.2% of U.S. adults, of whom 28% receive treatment [49]. As many as 5% of young women exhibit symptoms of anorexia but do not meet full diagnostic criteria, and some studies show disordered eating behavior in 13% of adolescent girls in the United States.

Patients with anorexia nervosa may present to the ED with extreme weight loss, food refusal, dehydration, electrolyte abnormalities, weakness, acute abdominal pain, or shock. They are frequent users of the emergency department, and may often present at the urging of family members or friends and may often deny their disorder and their malnutrition. Major depression and dysthymic disorder have been reported in up to 50% of patients with anorexia nervosa, and these patients have an elevated risk of suicide.

Impulse control disorders

An estimated 1 in 4 of the U.S. adult population has one of the impulse control disorders (oppositional defiant disorder, conduct disorder, attention-deficit/hyperactivity disorder, or intermittent explosive disorder) [8,21]. The 12-month estimate is 10.5%. Lifetime estimates are higher for males (28.6%) than females (21.6%). Twelve-month estimates are 11.7% for males and 9.3% for females. These disorders are likely associated with ED presentations for violence and injury, and with high rates of medical usage, but are rarely assessed in the ED setting.

Personality (Axis II) disorders

Almost 1 in 10 of the adult U.S. population is estimated to have an Axis II personality disorder in any year [8,21]. People with personality disorders have high rates of comorbid mental disorders, including anxiety disorders, mood disorders, impulse control disorders, and substance abuse or dependence and may present to the ED with these mental illnesses. Although DSM-IV defines 10 categories of personality disorder, population prevalence and ED visit data are lacking for most classifications, but are available for the most common disorders: borderline personality disorder and antisocial personality disorder.

Borderline personality disorder (BPD) is a personality disorder seen frequently in EDs, and BPD patients are high users of ED services, and of psychiatric services. The 12-month prevalence of borderline personality disorder is estimated to be 1.6%, of whom 42.4% receive treatment. From 10% to 20% of all psychiatric patients are diagnosed with this disorder, which is approximately three times more common in women than men.

The major feature of BPD patients is that they are emotionally unstable and chaotic. They are often also impulsive and frequently self-harming. They tend to present to the ED in emotional crisis, and/or having made a suicide attempt or gesture by overdose or cutting their wrists in response to some emotional stressor. The majority (approximately 75%) of borderline personality disordered patients attempt suicide or display self-mutilating behaviors like cutting or burning. The risk of suicide is approximately 10%.

Antisocial personality disorder (ASPD) is a condition in which an individual chronically manipulates others and violates their rights, disregarding their feelings without remorse. ASPD is more common in males than females and ASPD is often comorbid with substance abuse disorders, depression, anxiety disorders, attention-deficit/hyperactivity disorder, and legal problems. Patients with ASPD may be high users of ED services, and may present to the ED with comorbid psychiatric conditions, but also with substance abuse, injury- or violence-related problems. While the 12-month prevalence of ASPD in the general population is only 1%, it is likely to be much higher in the ED population.

Miscellaneous/occult mental health disorders

The prevalence and ED burden of many less common mental disorders remain unknown. Studies conducted by our laboratory and by others on the prevalence of occult, unmeasured, and often unrecognized mental disorders suggest that large segments of the ED patient population have relatively severe comorbid mental health problems in addition to other somatic maladies. These relatively undercounted mental health conditions include delirium, dementia and amnestic and other cognitive disorders, somatoform disorders, dissociative disorders, conversion disorders and factitious disorders. While many of these disorders, such as the somatoform and factitious disorders, are counted among the so-called "ER frequent fliers," they are also seen in patients with asthma, diabetes, malignancies, and other nonpsychiatric health conditions. A significant proportion of ED patients with abdominal pain, chest pain, back pain, and headache are not ultimately diagnosed with somatic diseases that account for their typical symptoms. However, taking a better accounting of patients with somatoform and factitious disorders would be a first step toward

targeting those who frequently use and sometimes misuse or abuse ED services.

Most mental health patients do not abuse ED services, however, and many ED patients suffer silently from occult and comorbid mental illnesses, resulting in significant diagnostic and treatment delays at the local level, as well as a systematic epidemiologic undercounting of mental health-related ED visits on the global level. Efforts to screen more aggressively for mental illness would certainly improve psychoepidemiologic estimates of the prevalence and true magnitude of the mental health problem. Uncovering more comorbid psychopathology may also benefit patients. However, many emergency departments and psychiatric services are currently too oversubscribed and under-resourced to adequately manage those currently suffering in silence.

Conclusion

This chapter outlined the psychoepidemiology of mental illness, both in global terms and in terms of the reigning acute care system in most developed countries: emergency departments. Decreased stigmatization, enhanced legitimization, and increased public and clinical recognition of mental illness have led to significant, record-breaking, global increases in the point prevalence and incidence of mental illness in the general population. These population increases in mental illnesses have, in turn, increased the census of mentally unwell emergency department patients in need of care at the local level.

Paradoxically, psychiatric patient population expansion has developed during a time of ED overcrowding and sharp reductions in both the total number of EDs and psychiatric beds in many communities. In addition, the willingness of mental health providers to make new DSM diagnoses appears to be out of step with either a systemic unwillingness or a provider inability to provide acute psychiatric and crisis care. Gaps in crisis care and the overall lack of affordable, 24/7 access to cost-effective mental healthcare services has fostered continued and increasing reliance on ED services. Unchecked, the growing tidal wave of mental health patients in need of care can be expected to rise significantly, flooding EDs throughout the world for the foreseeable future.

References

1. Kessler RC, Aguilar-Gaxiola S, Alonso J, et al. The global burden of mental disorders: an update from the WHO World Mental Health (WMH) surveys. *Epidemiol Psichiatr Soc* 2009;**18**:23–33.

2. Kessler RC, Ustun TB. (Eds.). *The WHO World Mental Health Surveys: Global Perspectives on the Epidemiology of Mental Disorders.* New York: Cambridge University Press; 2008.

3. Kessler RC, Berglund P, Demler O, Jin R, Walters EE. Lifetime prevalence and age-of-onset distributions of DSM-IV disorders in the National Comorbidity Survey Replication. *Arch Gen Psychiatry* 2005;**62**:593–602.

4. Demyttenaere K, Bruffaerts R, Posada-Villa J, et al. Prevalence, severity, and unmet need for treatment of mental disorders in the

World Health Organization World Mental Health Surveys. *JAMA* 2004;**291**:2581–90.

5. Kessler RC, Angermeyer M, Anthony JC, et al. Lifetime prevalence and age-of-onset distributions of mental disorders in the World Health Organization's World Mental Health Survey Initiative. *World Psychiatry* 2007;**6**:168–76.

6. Scott KM, Von Korff M, Angermeyer MC, et al. Association of childhood adversities and early-onset mental disorders with adult-onset chronic physical conditions. *Arch Gen Psychiatry* 2011;**68**:838–44.

7. Ormel J, Von Korff M, Burger H, et al. Mental disorders among persons with heart disease – results from World Mental Health surveys. *Gen Hosp Psychiatry* 2007;**29**:325–34.

8. Kessler RC, Chiu WT, Demler O, Merikangas KR, Walters EE. Prevalence, severity, and comorbidity of 12-month DSM-IV disorders in the National Comorbidity Survey Replication. *Arch Gen Psychiatry* 2005;**62**:617–27.

9. National Center for Health Statistics. *Health, United States, 2010: With Special Feature on Death and Dying.* Hyattsville, MD; National Center for Health Statistics; 2011.

10. Greenberg PE, Birnbaum HG. The economic burden of depression in the US: societal and patient perspectives. *Expert Opin Pharmacother* 2005;**6**:369–76.

11. Greenberg PE, Sisitsky T, Kessler RC, et al. The economic burden of anxiety disorders in the 1990s. *J Clin Psychiatry* 1999;**60**:427–35.

12. Alonso J, Petukhova M, Vilagut G, et al. Days out of role due to common physical and mental conditions: results from the WHO World Mental Health surveys. *Mol Psychiatry* 2011;**16**:1234–46.

13. Fields WW, Asplin BR, Larkin GL, et al. The Emergency Medical Treatment and Labor Act as a federal health care safety net program. *Acad Emerg Med* 2001;**8**:1064–9.

14. Center for Disease Control. *National Hospital Ambulatory Medical Care Survey: 2008 Emergency Department Summary Tables.* Atlanta, GA: Center for Disease Control; 2011.

15. Pitts SR, Niska RW, Xu J, Burt CW. National Hospital Ambulatory Medical Care Survey: 2006 emergency department summary. *Natl Health Stat Report* 2008;**7**:1–38.

16. American Hospital Association. Trend watch chart book 2006.

17. Larkin GL, Claassen CA, Emond JA, Pelletier AJ, Camargo CA. Trends in U.S. emergency department visits for

mental health conditions, 1992 to 2001. *Psychiatr Serv* 2005;**56**:671–7.

18. Regier DA, Narrow WE, Rae DS, et al. The de facto US mental and addictive disorders service system. Epidemiologic catchment area prospective 1-year prevalence rates of disorders and services. *Arch Gen Psychiatry* 1993;**50**:85–94.

19. Merrick EL, Perloff J, Tompkins CP. Emergency department utilization patterns for Medicare beneficiaries with serious mental disorders. *Psychiatr Serv* 2010;**61**:628–31.

20. Schriger DL, Gibbons PS, Langone CA, Lee S, Altshuler LL. Enabling the diagnosis of occult psychiatric illness in the emergency department: a randomized, controlled trial of the computerized, self-administered PRIME-MD diagnostic system. *Ann Emerg Med* 2001;**37**:132–40.

21. Kessler RC, Berglund P, Demler O, et al. Lifetime prevalence and age-of-onset distributions of DSM-IV disorders in the National Comorbidity Survey Replication. *Arch Gen Psychiatry* 2005;**62**:593–602.

22. Wang PS, Lane M, Olfson M, et al. Twelve-month use of mental health services in the United States: results from the National Comorbidity Survey Replication. *Arch Gen Psychiatry* 2005;**62**:629–40.

23. Smith RP, Larkin GL, Southwick SM. Trends in U.S. emergency department visits for anxiety-related mental health conditions, 1992–2001. *J Clin Psychiatry* 2008;**69**:286–94.

24. Kessler RC, Wang PS. The descriptive epidemiology of commonly occurring mental disorders in the United States. *Annu Rev Public Health* 2008;**29**:115–29.

25. Kessler RC, Ruscio AM, Shear K, Wittchen HU. Epidemiology of anxiety disorders. *Curr Top Behav Neurosci* 2010;**2**:21–35.

26. Kessler RC, Amminger GP, Aguilar-Gaxiola S, et al. Age of onset of mental disorders: a review of recent literature. *Curr Opin Psychiatry* 2007;**20**:359–64.

27. Katerndahl DA. Chest pain and its importance in patients with panic disorder: an updated literature review. *Prim Care Companion J Clin Psychiatry* 2008;**10**:376–83.

28. Coley KC, Saul MI, Seybert AL. Economic burden of not recognizing panic disorder in the emergency department. *J Emerg Med* 2009;**36**:3–7.

29. Kessler RC, Berglund P, Demler O, et al. The epidemiology of major depressive disorder: results from the National Comorbidity Survey Replication (NCS-R). *JAMA* 2003;**289**:3095–105.

30. Greenberg PE, Stiglin LE, Finkelstein SN, Berndt ER. The economic burden of depression in 1990. *J Clin Psychiatry* 1993;**54**:405–18.

31. Wells KB, Stewart A, Hays RD, et al. The functioning and well-being of depressed patients. Results from the Medical Outcomes Study. *JAMA* 1989;**262**:914–19.

32. Katon W, Sullivan MD. Depression and chronic medical illness. *J Clin Psychiatry* 1990;**51**(Suppl):3–11; discussion 2–4.

33. Harman JS, Scholle SH, Edlund MJ. Emergency department visits for depression in the United States. *Psychiatr Serv* 2004;**55**:937–9.

34. Boudreaux ED, Clark S, Camargo CA Jr. Mood disorder screening among adult emergency department patients: a multicenter study of prevalence, associations and interest in treatment. *Gen Hosp Psychiatry* 2008;**30**:4–13.

35. Kessler RC, Rubinow DR, Holmes C, Abelson JM, Zhao S. The epidemiology of DSM-III-R bipolar I disorder in a general population survey. *Psychol Med* 1997;**27**:1079–89.

36. Kessler RC, Akiskal HS, Ames M, et al. Considering the costs of bipolar depression. *Behav Health* 2007;**27**:45–7.

37. Jamison KR. Suicide and bipolar disorder. *J Clin Psychiatry* 2000;**61** (Suppl 9):47–51.

38. Boudreaux ED, Cagande C, Kilgannon JH, Clark S, Camargo CA. Bipolar disorder screening among adult patients in an urban emergency department setting. *Primary Care Companion J Clin Psychiatry* 2006;**8**:348–51.

39. Institute of Medicine. *Reducing Suicide: A National Imperative.* Goldsmith SK, Pellmar TC, Kleinman AM, Bunny WE, (Eds.). Washington, DC: National Academies Press; 2002.

40. Borges G, Nock MK, Haro Abad JM, et al. Twelve-month prevalence of and risk factors for suicide attempts in the

World Health Organization World Mental Health Surveys. *J Clin Psychiatry* 2010;**71**:1617–28.

41. Claassen CA, Larkin GL. Occult suicidality in an emergency department population. *Br J Psychiatry* 2005;**186**:352–3.

42. Larkin GL, Smith RP, Beautrais AL. Trends in US emergency department visits for suicide attempts, 1992–2001. *Crisis* 2008;**29**:73–80.

43. Larkin GL, Beautrais AL. Emergency departments are underutilized sites for suicide prevention. *Crisis* 2010;**31**:1–6.

44. Harris EC, Barraclough B. Suicide as an outcome for mental disorders. *Br J Psychiatry* 1997;**170**:205–28.

45. Beautrais AL. Further suicidal behavior among medically serious suicide attempters. *Suicide Life Threat Behav* 2004;**34**:1–11.

46. Larkin GL, Beautrais AL, Gibb SJ, Laing S. The epidemiology of presentations for suicidal ideation to the Emergency Department. *Acad Emerg Med* 2008;**15**: S208–9.

47. Wu EQ, Birnbaum HG, Shi L, et al. The economic burden of schizophrenia in the United States in 2002. *J Clin Psychiatry* 2005;**66**:1122–9.

48. Pandya A, Larkin G, Randles R, Beautrais A, Smith RP. Epidemiological trends in psychosis-related Emergency Department visits in the United States, 1992–2001. *Schizophr Res* 2009;**110**:28–32.

49. Hudson JI, Hiripi E, Pope HG Jr., Kessler RC. The prevalence and correlates of eating disorders in the National Comorbidity Survey Replication. *Biol Psychiatry* 2007;**61**:348–58.

Delivery models of emergency psychiatric care

Scott L. Zeller

Introduction

Mental health crises account for a substantial percentage of urgent medical presentations, with more than three million psychiatrically diagnosed patient encounters in U.S. emergency departments (EDs) annually [1]. In response to this considerable demand, diverse models of specialized Emergency Psychiatry services have evolved – ranging from solo consultants in medical EDs all the way up to large, comprehensive crisis mental health facilities. This chapter will discuss the goals, designs, benefits, and shortcomings of these varied delivery models of emergency mental health care.

Development of psychiatry in emergency settings

Emergency psychiatric services became a necessity after the advent of de-institutionalization in the middle part of the 20th century, which led to a large increase in persons with severe and persistent mental illnesses living outside of long-term hospitals. Community-based psychiatric systems were at times insufficient to meet all the needs of this formerly institutionalized population, and there were unanticipated difficulties in access to regular care and appropriate housing [2]. As a result, individuals were at heightened risk to suffer exacerbations of their illnesses, and – often having little or no alternatives – they frequently presented to emergency settings seeking mental health attention [3].

To assist with these acute patients, crisis intervention programs began to be developed; over time, these expanded to become essential and oft-utilized components of community-based treatment. By 1995, one report indicated more than 135,000 emergency psychiatric assessments occurred annually in New York State alone [4]. Between 1992 and 2001, there were 53 million mental health-related ED visits in the United States, jumping from 4.9% to 6.3% of all ED visits, and moving from 17.1 to 23.6 visits per 1000 U.S. population during this period [5].

These burgeoning numbers brought many clinicians into crisis intervention work, and an entire subspecialty of Emergency Psychiatry began to be cultivated [6]. Not unlike the advancement of Emergency Medicine to its own circumscribed division of medicine, Emergency Psychiatry progressed to a defined, full-fledged paradigm of acute mental health care, with targeted goals across a wide variety of treatment locations.

Goals of psychiatric care in varied emergency settings

Emergency Psychiatry today is practiced in several different sites and configurations. These wide-ranging designs are unified by an approach based on several fundamental goals:

- Exclude medical etiologies for symptoms
- Rapid stabilization of the acute crisis
- Avoid coercion
- Treat in the least restrictive setting
- Form a therapeutic alliance
- Appropriate disposition and aftercare plan [7].

Organizations address each of these goals based upon their location, staffing, patient population, and availability of community services. This leads to the unique format of individual Emergency Psychiatry programs.

Exclude medical etiologies for symptoms

Because many medical conditions can present with symptoms that appear similar to endogenous psychoses, mania, or other acute psychiatric states, it is essential that medical etiologies be ruled out before commencing psychiatric treatment. A significant number of patients who present to emergency settings with apparent psychiatric disorders have acute medical illnesses either co-existing or at the root of their symptoms [8]; failure to recognize these conditions can lead to serious morbidity [9,10]. For example, a mistaken diagnosis of psychosis in a patient suffering from an intracranial bleed, thyroid storm, or toxic delirium can place a patient at serious, perhaps life-threatening, risk. Even commonplace medical issues in psychiatric patients, such as diabetes, hypertension, and alcohol withdrawal, can have severe sequelae if not properly addressed.

At the very least, psychiatric emergency programs need to have access to patient evaluations by a qualified medical professional, along with the measurement of vital signs, before commencement of psychiatric treatment.

Behavioral Emergencies for the Emergency Physician, ed. Leslie S. Zun, Lara G. Chepenik, and Mary Nan S. Mallory. Published by Cambridge University Press. © Cambridge University Press 2013.

Rapid stabilization of the acute crisis

Once a patient's medical stability has been ensured, emergency psychiatry programs need to focus on prompt stabilization of the acute crisis. Every effort should be made to ensure safety and prevent danger to self and others, while simultaneously working to alleviate the patient's suffering. This includes timely triage and defined levels of staff observation based on the degree of acuity.

Avoid coercion, treat in the least restrictive setting, form a therapeutic alliance

Practitioners in the emergency setting are often the first contact a patient will have with mental health care. A bad experience during this initial mental health contact may lead to long-term problems in which consumers might fear, distrust, or dislike psychiatrists and other providers. Such issues might interfere with the consumer's desire to obtain help, continue in treatment, or willingness to take medications. During the early phases of psychiatric illnesses, even brief interactions can have enduring implications for a patient's long-term wellness.

In realizing this, it is extremely important that crisis professionals work with patients in a supportive and compassionate manner, creating with the patient what is known as a *therapeutic alliance*. A therapeutic alliance might be most simply described as a collaborative relationship between a patient and a clinician. Rather than the mental health professional acting excessively authoritative or giving the patient orders, a therapeutic alliance should instead involve clinicians' attempts to bond and empathize with patients, and treat them as partners. This can lead to a working relationship with shared responsibility for achieving treatment goals in the acute setting, and often results in better outcomes. Results of studies have shown that the greater the quality of the early therapeutic alliance, the lower the possibility of a patient becoming violent during psychiatric hospitalizations [11].

Working with a therapeutic alliance mindset also means avoiding *coercion* – the use of force or threats to make patients do things against their will. In Emergency Psychiatry, this includes the administration of oral medications willingly by means of informed consent, as opposed to forcible injections; verbal de-escalation of agitated individuals to calmness, instead of imposing physical restraints; and little or no infringement on a patient's rights when possible. Treating in the least restrictive level of care is another means of avoiding coercion.

The more restrictive the level of care, the more there is a propensity for a coercive experience, and thus less opportunity for a therapeutic alliance. Examples of levels of mental health care from most to least restrictive include: physical restraints and/or seclusion rooms, locked clinical settings and involuntary inpatient units, then voluntary, unlocked facilities. The least restrictive settings are outpatient clinics where patients are free to come and go as they wish. Most individuals will do best in the appropriate level of care which is least restrictive; thus avoiding hospital admissions, when possible, can be quite advantageous for patients.

Appropriate disposition and aftercare plan

In Emergency Psychiatry, the duties of the mental health professional are not complete merely with cessation of the presenting crisis. It is strongly recommended that a patient be provided with an appropriate care plan for post-discharge. This includes appointments (when possible) with outpatient providers, referral to mental health clinics and/or substance abuse treatment programs, and instructions about what to do if crisis symptoms recur. Frequently, assistance with housing may be a part of the aftercare plan, as might be coordination of arrangements with loved ones or caregivers.

Appropriate aftercare planning can be of substantial benefit to the long-term stability of patients and help prevent recidivism. Individuals who do not have an outpatient appointment after discharge may be two times more likely to be psychiatrically hospitalized in a year than patients who went to at least one outpatient appointment [12].

Models of emergency psychiatry delivery

A colleague is known to lecture "*once you've seen one psychiatric emergency department, you've seen one psychiatric emergency department.*" Indeed, this is true – virtually every program doing crisis psychiatry has its own quirks and adaptations to local needs in an attempt to meet the goals of emergency psychiatric treatment. However, although there are numerous hybrid or idiosyncratic versions, generally emergency psychiatry programs in fixed settings fall into one of three basic models:

1. The psychiatric consultant who sees patients in the medical ED;
2. A separate section of the medical ED dedicated to mental health patients, with specially trained and dedicated staff; and
3. The stand-alone Psychiatric Emergency Service (PES), a facility separate from a medical ED that is solely for treatment of acute mental health patients.

Factors such as the total numbers of psychiatric patients seen, the geographic catchment area of the emergency setting, the availability of psychiatrists and other mental health professionals, local philosophy of mental health treatment and mental health laws, and economic constraints all play a role in determining which model is implemented. Frequently, as the quantity of patient contacts change, a system may convert from one model into another.

Psychiatric consultant in a medical emergency department

A mental health professional consultant working with patients in a general medical ED is likely the most omnipresent model in the United States. Typically, a patient with mental health complaints will initially be triaged alongside medical emergency patients and will be evaluated by an emergency medicine physician before any psychiatric interventions. If the treating physician deems it necessary, a request will be made for a psychiatric consultation.

A consultant will then be summoned to evaluate the patient, frequently from another location in the hospital or offsite. After arrival, the consultant will offer opinions on psychiatric treatment and recommend if inpatient admission is indicated. Medication prescriptions and decisions on disposition remain the province of the attending emergency medicine physician.

Pros and cons

This model can have many advantages, especially for an ED whose census of mental health consumers is relatively low and arrivals are sporadic. With no separate infrastructure for psychiatric patients needed, it is the lowest-cost and easiest to implement paradigm in a medical ED. Because all patients are primarily evaluated by an emergency medicine physician, physical concerns are assessed and organic causes of psychiatric symptoms can be ruled out before mental health consultation. Comorbid medical issues may also be addressed, in addition to psychiatric complaints. Because the mental health patients are treated in the same setting as all patients in the ED, a person seeking psychiatric assistance may appear to be no different from any other individual in the waiting room. Presenting to the general medical ED might be less worrisome for those who might fear the stigma of presenting to a recognizable psychiatric facility.

However, there are many potential disadvantages to the model as well, especially regarding timeliness and access to treatment. Definitive diagnosis and therapeutic interventions must usually await the consultant's arrival, which may take hours or even days in some circumstances, during which time the patient may be receiving little or no treatment [13]. Once present, the consultant's decision is typically restricted to the choice either to recommend admission for psychiatric hospitalization or discharge. The consultant will usually make a one-time, "snapshot" assessment, without the ability to engage a patient in treatment, or to observe the patient over time to see if improvement or decline in status might change the disposition plans.

The physical setting of the medical ED itself – with the noise, commotion, and presence of other patients who might be in severe pain or in the midst of disturbing life-saving interventions – may not be the most supportive or healing environment for those in mental health crisis. There may also be easy access to dangerous instruments or equipment that might be unsafe around highly suicidal or self-injurious patients. Because of the hazards in these surroundings and staffing issues that can limit direct observation, too often psychiatric patients in general EDs are unnecessarily placed in restraints or isolation solely as a safeguard, which can further injure an already fragile patient's mental state.

Furthermore, many ED staff may be undertrained or unfamiliar with mental illness; some may even be disdainful of the mentally ill (whom they do not see as "real" emergencies). This may lead, especially in busy EDs, to staff callousness and disregard for psychiatric patients, resulting in poorer care and less attention to patient needs. In overloaded EDs, psychiatric patients might be seen as inappropriately occupying premium bed space, and may thus be shuffled around the unit as "more important" patients arrive. They may also be targeted for premature discharge in an effort to make space available.

In this consultant model, those in mental health crisis who have been determined to require hospitalization might face a substantial stay in the ED while awaiting the location or availability of an inpatient bed. This unfortunate situation in which patients might not be receiving much, if any, treatment, and instead might just be waiting on a stretcher for extended periods, is referred to as *boarding* [14].

Boarding of psychiatric patients in medical EDs has been documented as a major issue in the United States. In a 2008 survey of ED medical directors done by the American College of Emergency Physicians, 90% of the respondents indicated that psychiatric patients were boarded at their hospital every week, with more than 55% indicating that it occurred either daily or multiple times per week. Sixty-two percent reported that there were no psychiatric services involved with patient care while patients were being boarded in their ED [15].

Types of mental health consultants in the ED

Optimally, psychiatrists with extensive experience in acute care psychiatry and psychosomatic medicine will perform mental health consultations in the ED. However, in many systems the consultants are psychologists, social workers, or licensed marriage/family therapists. Some facilities even employ psychiatric technicians or other practitioners with less than Master's level training to perform consultations, although this use of less clinically qualified personnel has been described as an "insufficient" level of care for those in psychiatric crisis [16].

Consultants who are therapists with limited medical expertise tend to be less costly, and in many cases can do exemplary work for patients, especially for individuals needing crisis counseling or assistance with access to services. However, non-psychiatrist consultants are unable to recommend psychopharmacologic treatments and are likely not qualified to rule out medical conditions such as delirium or metabolic abnormalities in their diagnoses. Also, such consultants might at times be seen as "lesser authorities" by some emergency medicine physicians, who may thus feel justified in exerting undue influence on the consultant toward certain dispositions. This can even happen with the common practice of using psychiatry residents to do ED psychiatric consults, because the physicians-in-training may be understandably anxious about countermanding an ED attending-level physician's opinion.

Indeed, reliance upon lower-qualified consultants might lead to inappropriate admissions, when a less-restrictive level of care may have been indicated instead. Studies have demonstrated that the less experienced the evaluator, the more likely it is that inpatient treatment will be recommended [17].

Some EDs' mental health consultation is provided by a visiting team from an area inpatient psychiatric facility. The impartiality of decisions by such teams may come into question because such teams' employers stand to benefit financially by increased admissions.

A growing means of providing psychiatric consultation in the ED has been through the use of telemedicine, in which a consultant interviews a patient and provides recommendations to the emergency medicine staff from a remote site by means of video teleconferencing. As this nascent technique continues to develop, it promises to increase access to, and timeliness of, psychiatric consultation. Telemedicine has been found to be safe and effective in its limited use to date, with satisfaction reported both from ED staff and the individuals receiving treatment [18].

Dedicated mental health wing of medical emergency department

In this model, a separate section of a general medical ED is allocated specifically for individuals requiring acute psychiatric care. The space is typically situated in a delineated area that may be less boisterous and more calming than the general ED environment, and is commonly staffed by nurses with specialized training in mental health. There may be social workers or therapists stationed in the unit. Psychiatrists are also in close contact and frequently onsite, although their primary worksite may be elsewhere.

Pros and cons

The designated wing may allow for a more therapeutic environment for individuals in crisis and, thus, avoid some of the pitfalls such as the disruptive clamor and dangerous nearby equipment that may confront a psychiatric patient in the general ED. The presence of staff skilled in treating mental illness enhances the likelihood of forming therapeutic alliances with patients and avoiding the disparagement that psychiatric patients may sometimes receive in general emergency beds. However, because its location is still within the ED proper, patients can also receive medical examinations from an emergency medicine physician as part of their evaluation. Additionally, because of the separate setting dedicated to mental health, there may be less urgency to move patients out in exchange for other types of emergency patients, and therefore permit time for medications and interventions to have effect before disposition decisions.

Because the model does allow for longer stays for psychiatric care, there may be more frequent opportunities for psychiatrists or other mental health clinicians to assess the patients. In a larger general hospital, especially one with an onsite psychiatric inpatient unit, a psychiatrist from the consultation/liaison or inpatient service might regularly "round" on patients in the crisis wing, doing re-evaluations and adjusting medications where indicated. As such, treatment plans can change over time, as can disposition options.

However, this model also has its potential drawbacks. The distribution of patients to a separate space permits their marginalization and potential stigma as "different" or "crazy"; some facilities have even been known to use the questionable practice of dressing crisis patients in different colored gowns (e.g., bright red) from the general population to clearly identify them as psychiatric patients. Unfortunately, sometimes the only characteristic differentiating the mental health wing from the medical section is locked doors or security guards, which may make it an even more coercive and less therapeutic environment than the general ED.

Given the limited space of many EDs, there may be demands to place overflow non-psychiatric patients into the mental health wing, or to float wing staff away to other ED duties on especially busy days. Despite the potential for onsite care, too often these sections are used as mere holding areas with little actual psychiatric treatment, and are mostly seen as a means of diverting patients out of the main ED while they await dispositions.

The psychiatric emergency services (PES) model

The PES is typically a stand-alone unit dedicated solely to the treatment of individuals in mental health crisis. Such facilities can either be locked or unlocked, or they might include both locked and unlocked areas. They may be located within a hospital's campus or in a separate structure in the community. Ideally, when located on the hospital grounds, PES facilities are situated near the medical ED [19].

PES programs come in many shapes, sizes, and abbreviations. They are also known as Comprehensive Psychiatric Emergency Programs (CPEP), Emergency Treatment Services (ETS) and Crisis Stabilization Units (CSU), among other names. In addition, their design can vary from units providing solely crisis intervention to extensive programs housing mobile crisis teams, outpatient clinics, and day treatment centers [20]. Some wide-ranging PES programs have been described as comparable for psychiatric care to a Level 1 Trauma facility for emergency medical care [21].

Pros and cons

A typical PES is staffed around the clock with psychiatric nurses and other mental health professionals, and psychiatrists are either onsite or readily available. With such staffing, diagnosis and treatment can proceed far more promptly than in the models that await a consultant's arrival. Once in a PES, a patient's psychiatric treatment can begin without delay, with the potential for patients to stabilize quickly [22].

In the "consultant in the ED" and "dedicated wing in the ED" designs, emergency psychiatry is most often practiced in a method described as the "Triage Model," which features "rapid evaluation, containment, and referral" [23]. In this model, the main task is to determine whether to psychiatrically hospitalize the patient or discharge the patient from the ED, based on the patient's presenting condition. In contrast, a typical PES follows the "Treatment Model," where, in addition to Triage Model capability, many patients can also be stabilized onsite [24]. This is possible because many PES have extended observation capability (see below), allowing them to commence treatment and to follow patients for up to 24 hours, in some circumstances even longer. This can often be sufficient time for many patients to stabilize, and thus avoid inpatient hospitalization.

Stabilization within a PES rather than an unnecessary inpatient stay is beneficial to the patient: a prompt, focused intervention can lead more quickly to a less restrictive level of care, while avoiding unsettling transfers and treatment redundancy. It is also advantageous to the mental health system by lowering costs while preserving inpatient bed availability. A PES with extended observation capacity can dramatically lower inpatient admission rates over a program using the Triage Model: one study revealed a comparative difference in admission rates of 52% for the Triage Model compared with just 36% for the extended observation model [25].

A PES also can be quite valuable for reducing congestion in area medical EDs, allowing psychiatric patients to be transferred for their evaluations and treatment, rather than waiting for consultants to arrive or for an inpatient bed to become available. In addition, many PES programs can accept ambulances, police deliveries, and self-referrals directly, permitting crisis patients to avoid medical EDs altogether.

In an era when concern about overcrowding in medical emergency facilities has been at the forefront [26], establishment of geographically logical PES locations for urgent mental health care has been growing in appreciation as a potential solution. In the 2008 survey of ED medical directors by the American College of Emergency Physicians, 81% agreed that regional, dedicated emergency psychiatric facilities would be an improvement over their current systems [15]. Patients receiving treatment also support this idea; one survey of psychiatric consumers reported that a majority had unpleasant experiences in medical emergency facilities and would prefer treatment in a specialized PES location [27].

The chief disadvantage of PES is that they are much more expensive than the other models, because of the high costs of 24/7 staffing and maintenance of a separate physical plant. For these reasons, a PES usually only makes fiscal sense to facilities or communities with relatively large numbers of acute psychiatric patient visits per month. Although the trigger point is debatable based on community standards, availability of outpatient treatment alternatives and the scope of services delivered, it has been suggested that a stand-alone PES becomes warranted when local emergency department mental health visits exceed 3,000 per year [28].

Another major obstacle for creation of a PES is finding or allocating sufficient space for its mere existence. Moving to a separate facility requires enough square footage to house a substantial number of patients, many of whom might be there for considerable hours and thus require appropriate sleep space, washrooms, and storage for their belongings. In addition, there needs to be adequate room for all the clinical staff, security, and administration to work onsite.

A third key complication for a stand-alone PES can be difficulty in finding enough dedicated personnel to maintain services around the clock. Even well-established PES programs often face a constant uphill battle to ensure appropriate staffing levels, especially in the middle of the night and on weekends.

PES programs that are physically remote from medical EDs can also face significant challenges. Limited ability to do complete medical history and physical examinations – especially if psychiatrists are the sole physicians available – might lead to missed medical issues or somatic causes of psychiatric symptoms. There may be difficulty in obtaining prompt laboratory testing and other diagnostic tools. The outside PES may also be seen as such an attractive, "quick" disposition by referring medical facilities that they might be tempted to do only cursory and inadequate medical clearances before transport.

Structure and design of PES programs

A stand-alone PES program is typically designed to accept urgent patients directly from the community and by means of transfers from other hospitals, and, therefore, will have an entrance specifically for ambulance and peace officer arrivals. In this case, a separate entrance for voluntary patients, visitors, and families is best (when possible) to permit confidentiality and privacy for the more acutely ill individuals.

Within the PES proper, there is usually: a triage area for initial evaluations; a locked area for involuntary patients and those individuals needing a higher level of security; an unlocked area for patients arriving voluntarily, family meetings, and visitors; interview rooms; an office for physical examinations; sleep rooms or dormitories for patients; a large nursing station, which is optimally centrally located; isolation rooms with restraint capabilities; and office/charting areas. The physical plant of emergency psychiatric units is discussed in more detail in a separate chapter.

Extended observation

Most PES facilities have the capability to do *extended observation*, where patients are continuously monitored for up to 24–72 hours (based on local regulations), in an attempt to preclude inpatient admissions. In some programs, the extended observation patients are housed in the general PES milieu, while others have entirely separate units with assigned beds specifically for this population. In both cases, those under treatment are still considered to be outpatients.

Extended observation allows for focused treatment of those disease states that might quickly resolve to sub-acute status, and thus permit a patient's discharge to a lower level of care in a relatively short period of time while avoiding an unnecessary inpatient stay. Such conditions might include: acute substance intoxication or withdrawal states; mild exacerbations of chronic symptoms of psychosis, such as auditory hallucinations or paranoia; acute stress or suicidal ideation in those with personality disorders; and contingent suicidality.

Treatment models in the PES

Similar to the diversity in program styles of crisis psychiatry, it seems that no two PES facilities are identical with staffing patterns either. However, the two most common designs appear to be the *primary therapist model* and the *medical model*. In the *primary therapist model*, a newly arrived patient will be triaged and assigned to a "primary therapist," most commonly a Master's level social worker, psychotherapist or nurse, who is responsible for the initial interview with a patient and subsequent organization of information gathering and care. In contrast, the *medical model* has a similar blueprint to a medical ED, with physicians as designated team leaders for each patient's care.

The primary therapist model works best in a setting where many of the patients are in need of individual attention and counseling more than medications (e.g., individuals with suicidal ideation or adjustment issues). By using several clinicians as primary therapists, the model allows for the provision of care for multiple patients while limiting the need for psychiatrist involvement. However, the primary therapist model can also lead to unnecessary duplication of labor and delays, as the physician legally responsible for the patient will often need to redo much of the evaluation. Patients can feel frustrated by having to repeat the details of their presentation to several different clinicians, and can afterward be unsure about who to turn to for updates on their status.

In settings with a larger census or more high-acuity patients, the medical model may be the most efficient, and surprisingly cost effective, even though psychiatrists are usually higher paid than Master's level therapists. Having psychiatrists doing both the medical and psychosocial evaluation can streamline care and "eliminate the middleman," as the physician can direct treatment, order medications, and make disposition decisions personally, thus doing the work that might be done by several persons in the primary therapist model. Negative aspects to the medical model can include the possibility of overtaxed psychiatrists, who have so many duties that they are unable to spend significant time with patients – especially those who may be most in need of supportive counseling and an unhurried, sympathetic ear.

EMTALA

Stand-alone psychiatric EDs, especially those affiliated with medical centers, almost always will meet the definition of a "dedicated emergency department" under U.S. Federal Emergency Medical Treatment and Active Labor Act (EMTALA) guidelines [29]. As such, a PES is required to perform a Medical Screening Examination on any individual presenting to their facility requesting care (whether medical or psychiatric), regardless of cost, and, if an Emergency Medical Condition exists, stabilize that individual within their capacity and capability.

EMTALA recognizes psychiatric infirmity where a patient has become a danger to self or a danger to others as an Emergency Medical Condition [29]. Thus, a patient considered to be in such a state in a PES (or any "dedicated emergency department") must have their psychiatric symptoms stabilized to the point they no longer pose an acute risk of danger to self or others, or be admitted to an inpatient hospital.

Of note, EMTALA does recognize that specialized emergency programs such as a PES do not have the capability to treat the most severe emergency medical conditions onsite (e.g., a cardiac arrest). If a medical screening examination at a PES finds a patient in such an emergency situation, EMTALA allows for immediate transfer to a higher level of care that has the capability of treating that condition, even if the only means of obtaining that transfer is by calling for emergency medical services (e.g., 911 in the United States or 999 in the United Kingdom).

Alternative crisis treatment modalities

Psychiatric urgent care/voluntary crisis centers

Voluntary crisis programs can provide drop-in urgent care for patients willingly seeking treatment. This can be very beneficial for patients, who can avoid the stigma of asking for psychiatric help in a general medical facility, as well as circumventing the long waits, disturbing hubbub, and locked doors frequently found in standard emergency settings. People in search of such interventions as counseling or medication refills might find a voluntary crisis center a viable option, and thus avoid the ED. Indeed, some programs are opened in concert with an area PES, to provide a voluntary alternative and to reduce PES overcrowding [30].

Typically, voluntary crisis centers do not accept patients on involuntary psychiatric detention or those who are acutely dangerous and unable to control their actions. Unfortunately, as helpful as offering both can be, most communities do not have the funding or patient population to justify both a PES and a voluntary crisis center.

Mobile crisis teams

The concept of a mobile crisis team is used across the United States, but can have a wide range of definitions and service responsibilities [31]. Some systems use mobile crisis teams as the visiting consultants (in the psychiatric consultant model described earlier) for mental health evaluations in medical EDs, while others use teams hand-in-hand with area police to intervene in homes and the community when psychiatric disturbances may arise. Often, teams are based in a PES, and are used for such undertakings as outreach to the community, and follow-up for patients recently discharged from acute treatment. Typically, crisis teams can provide assessment, supportive interventions, counseling, and referrals, but will not administer or prescribe medications on location.

Acute diversion units

A more novel and increasingly popular modality for treating urgent psychiatric crises is known as the Acute Diversion Unit or ADU. These units tend to be community-based, cost-effective, more comfortable alternatives to hospitalization, with typical capacities of 10–20 patients and lengths of stay less than 2 weeks [32]. Most commonly, good candidates for these programs are patients who would benefit from hospitalization, yet are willing to engage in treatment and are not considered to be at the level of dangerousness, confusion, or medical infirmity to require locked hospital care. Most often ADUs require an initial screening and referral from an ED or PES, but some are also designed to accept direct presentations from case managers and mobile crisis teams.

Conclusion

The dramatic rise in the number of urgent mental health crises over the past half-century has fostered the development of an entire subspecialty of Emergency Psychiatry. While many acute patients receive emergency psychiatric evaluations by consultants in the general ED, alternative specialized treatment services have been established successfully in numerous locations. In all of the models used, Emergency Psychiatry interventions can be invaluable to medical systems by providing timely, compassionate, and effective care for patients in crisis.

References

1. McCaig LF, Burt CW. *National Hospital Ambulatory Medical Care Survey: 2002 Emergency Department Summary. Advance Data from Vital and Health Statistics; no 340.* Hyattsville, MD: National Center for Health Statistics. 2004. http://www.cdc.gov/nchs/data/ad/ad340.pdf. (Accessed August 21, 2011).

2. Talbott JA. Deinstitutionalization: avoiding the disasters of the past. 1979. *Psychiatr Serv* 2004;**55**:1112–15.

3. Huffine CL, Craig TJ. Social factors in the utilization of an urban psychiatric emergency service. *Arch Gen Psychiatry* 1974;**30**:249–55.

4. Dawes SS, Bloniarz PA, Mumpower JL, et al. *Supporting Psychiatric Assessments in Emergency Rooms* (CTG Project Report 95-2). Albany, NY: Center for Technology in Government, University at Albany, SUNY; 1995. http://www.ctg.albany.edu/publications/reports/supp_psych_assess/supp_psych_assess.pdf. (Accessed September 5, 2011).

5. Larkin GL, Claassen CA, Emond JA, Pelletier AJ, Camargo CA. Trends in U.S. emergency department visits for mental health conditions, 1992 to 2001. *Psychiatr Serv* 2005;**56**:671–7.

6. Wellin E, Slesinger DP, Hollister CD. Psychiatric emergency services: evolution, adaptation and proliferation. *Soc Sci Med* 1987;**24**: 475–82.

7. Zeller SL. Treatment of psychiatric patients in emergency settings. *Prim Psychiatry* 2010;**17**:35–41.

8. Carlson RJ, Nayar N, Sur M. Physical disorders among emergency psychiatry patients. *Can J Psychiatry* 1981;**26**:65–7.

9. Hall RC, Popkin MK, Devaud RA, Faillace LA, Stickney SK. Physical illness presenting as psychiatric disease. *Arch Gen Psychiatry* 1978;**35**:1315–20.

10. Hall RC, Gardner ER, Popkin MK, Lecann AF,Stickney SK. Unrecognized physical illness prompting psychiatric admission: a prospective study. *Am J Psychiatry* 1981;**138**:629–35.

11. Beauford JE, McNiel DE, Binder RL. Utility of the initial therapeutic alliance in evaluating psychiatric patients' risk of violence. *Am J Psychiatry* 1997;**154**:1272–6.

12. Nelson EA, Maruish ME, Axler JL. Effects of discharge planning and compliance with outpatient appointments on readmission rates. *Psychiatr Serv* 2000;**51**:885–9.

13. Hoot NR, Aronsky D. Systematic review of emergency department crowding: causes, effects, and solutions. *Ann Emerg Med* 2008;**52**:126–36.

14. Ding R, McCarthy ML, Desmond JS, et al. Characterizing waiting room time, treatment time, and boarding time in the emergency department using quantile regression. *Acad Emerg Med* 2010;**17**:813–23.

15. American College of Emergency Physicians (ACEP). *ACEP Psychiatric and Substance Abuse Survey 2008.* http://www.acep.org/uploadedFiles/ACEP/Advocacy/federal_issues/PsychiatricBoardingSummary.pdf. (Accessed September 24, 2011).

16. Fishkind AB, Berlin JS. Structure and function of psychiatric emergency services. In: Glick RL, Berlin JS, Fishkind AB, Zeller SL, (Eds.). *Emergency Psychiatry: Principles and Practice.* Philadelphia, PA: Wolters Kluwer Health/Lippincott Williams & Wilkins; 2008: 9–23.

17. Flaherty JA, Fichtner CG. Impact of emergency psychiatry training on residents' decisions to hospitalize patients. *Acad Med* 1992;**67**:585–6.

18. Yellowlees P, Burke MM, Marks SL, Hilty DM, Shore JH. Emergency telepsychiatry. *J Telemed Telecare* 2008;**14**:277–81.

19. Allen MH, Forster P, Zealberg J, Currier G. *APA Task Force on Psychiatric Emergency Services Report and Recommendations Regarding Psychiatric Emergency and Crisis Services.* Washington DC: American Psychiatric Association; 2002. http://www.psych.org/lib_archives/archives/tfr200201.pdf. (Accessed September 24, 2011).

20. Lee TS, Renaud EF, Hills OF. Emergency psychiatry: an emergency treatment hub-and-spoke model for psychiatric emergency services. *Psychiatr Serv* 2003;**54**:1590–1, 1594.

21. Allen MH. Level 1 psychiatric emergency services. The tools of the crisis sector. *Psychiatr Clin North Am* 1999;**22**:713–34, vii.

22. Woo BK, Chan VT, Ghobrial N, Sevilla CC. Comparison of two models for delivery of services in psychiatric emergencies. *Gen Hosp Psychiatry* 2007;**29**:489–91.

23. Gerson S, Bassuk E. Psychiatric emergencies: an overview. *Am J Psychiatry* 1980;**137**:1–11.

24. Allen MH. Definitive treatment in the psychiatric emergency service. *Psychiatr Q* 1996;**67**:247–62.

25. Gillig PM, Hillard JR, Bell J, et al. The psychiatric emergency service holding area: effect on utilization of inpatient resources. *Am J Psychiatry* 1989;**146**:369–72.

26. Trzeciak S, Rivers EP. Emergency department overcrowding in the United States: an emerging threat to patient safety and public health. *Emerg Med J* 2003;**20**:402–5.

27. Allen MH, Carpenter D, Sheets JL, Miccio S, Ross R. What do consumers say they want and need during a psychiatric emergency? *J Psychiatr Pract* 2003;**9**:39–58.

28. Allen MH, Currier GW. Medical assessment in the psychiatric emergency service. *New Dir Ment Health Serv* 1999;**82**:21–8.

29. Department of Health and Human Services. Centers for Medicare and Medicaid Services (CMS) Manual System. Appendix V. *Emergency Medical Treatment and Labor Act (EMTALA) Interpretive Guidelines.* 2010. Available at: www.cms.hhs.gov/ manuals/downloads/ som107ap_v_emerg.pdf (Accessed September 18, 2011).

30. Hennessy-Fiske MLA. County opens mental health urgent care center near Olive View. *Los Angeles Times.* 2011. http://latimesblogs.latimes.com/ lanow/2011/08/mental-health-urgent- care-olive-view-opened.html. (Accessed September 21, 2011).

31. Geller JL, Fisher WH, McDermeit M. A national survey of mobile crisis services and their evaluation. *Psychiatr Serv* 1995;**46**:893–7.

32. Patel RM. Crisis residential settings. In: Glick RL, Berlin JS, Fishkind AB, Zeller SL, (Eds.). *Emergency Psychiatry: Principles and Practice.* Philadelphia, PA: Wolters Kluwer Health/Lippincott Williams & Wilkins; 2008: 393–412.

The medical clearance process for psychiatric patients presenting acutely to the emergency department

Vaishal Tolia and Michael P. Wilson

Introduction

Mental health-related visits to emergency departments are common [1–3]. More than ever, emergency departments have become burdened with longer wait times, overcrowding, and complex patient safety issues. Patients with primary psychiatric complaints, numbering approximately 53 million from 1992 to 2001 in the United States, now constitute 6% of all ED visits [1]. This rise in mental health visits corresponds to a 38% increase [4]. Frequently, there is an inherent challenge or even fear in dealing with these patients and their presumed psychiatric emergency, such that the medical aspects of psychiatric care are overshadowed to arrange a rapid disposition. Sigmund Freud once noted famously "when I treat a psychoneurotic, for instance, hysterical patient ... I am compelled to find explanations for the first symptoms of the malady, which have long since disappeared, as well as for those existing symptoms which have brought the patient to me; and I find a former problem easier to solve than the more exigent one of today" [5].

Although Freud's words are by now a century old, the search for the medical causes of existing psychiatric problems is still common today. This screening, usually performed by emergency physicians, has become known as "medical clearance." This process of medical screening is enigmatic and, at best, an imperfect science. The discrimination and depth of this screening, such as which patients require extensive workup and which laboratory tests are most useful, is controversial. Even the goals of screening, such as whether to identify all possible medical causes of psychiatric illness or simply to identify medical conditions that either contribute or supersede the psychiatric emergency, are often disagreed upon by specialists in psychiatry and emergency medicine.

Furthermore, the term "medical clearance" itself is controversial and often misinterpreted. In general, emergency department screening is not designed to evaluate all possible coexisting illnesses. Thus, some authors have argued that there is no such entity such as being completely "medically clear" from the emergency department, preferring instead to use the terms "focused medical assessment," "medically stable," or simply listing the screening procedures performed in a discharge summary [6–8].

Areas of consensus

Despite the controversy surrounding this process, both research and expert consensus agree upon important principles of the medical screening process. First, regardless of the details of the screening, the millions of emergency department patients who make a mental health-related visit deserve, at a minimum, an adequate history, and adequate physical exam, and measurement of vital signs. Second, emergency physicians are obligated to discover organic conditions that may be the cause for new psychiatric symptoms. These signs and symptoms, often referred to as "medical mimics" but more appropriately characterized as a delirium state, may be missed by initial evaluators, particularly in the elderly [9]. Third, emergency physicians should seek to identify and treat life-threatening medical conditions that, of course, would supersede the psychiatric emergency. Even medical urgencies are best identified before psychiatric admission, as most psychiatric facilities are neither equipped with the resources or have appropriately trained staff to treat these conditions [10]. Failure to identify these conditions can lead to dangerously bad outcomes for the patient [8]. Fourth, guidelines and protocols may help streamline the medical screening process in the emergency department (ED) [11–13].

This chapter serves to introduce and describe the process of medical evaluation, also termed medical screening, of the psychiatric patient in the emergency department. The term "screening" is deliberate, as "medically clear" is often too ambiguous and suggests a detailed history, physical exam, laboratory testing, and time frame beyond the purpose of an ED visit. The diagnosis of medical mimics is discussed first, along with the utility of both the patient history and physical exam and laboratory evaluations. The second half of the chapter discusses the use of standard screening algorithms, which have been shown in several studies to decrease testing costs for emergency department patients undergoing medical screening. Although there are no uniform guidelines for this process, attention to detail while minimizing resource over-usage, all while providing the best care for the individual patient, will likely yield the best outcome for both the patient and the institution.

Behavioral Emergencies for the Emergency Physician, ed. Leslie S. Zun, Lara G. Chepenik, and Mary Nan S. Mallory. Published by Cambridge University Press. © Cambridge University Press 2013.

Medical mimics

Ralph Waldo Emerson once said "every man is a borrower and a mimic, life is theatrical, and literature a quotation" [14]. Although Emerson was not referring to the medical mimicry of psychiatric conditions, he might as well have been. The evaluation that an emergency physician conducts is an extremely important and, albeit, limited chance for the patient to be treated for a medical condition that may be causing their symptoms.

The role of the history and physical exam in recognizing medical mimics

Although the often taught truism is that a thorough history and physical exam (H&P) is the key to making a diagnosis, the ability of the H&P to discover disease during medical screening is controversial. In part, this is because the important elements of the H&P have not yet been quantified. In a 1994 study, Henneman and colleagues analyzed the standard medical evaluation of 100 consecutive adult emergency department patients with new psychiatric symptoms [15]. Although 63 of these 100 patients were noted to have an organic etiology for their symptoms, the H&P was only significant in 33/63 patients. The authors therefore recommended performing additional laboratory evaluations along with the H&P. Unfortunately, neither the quality of the H&P performed nor the most revealing portion of the H&P for these patients were analyzed.

Other authors have noted that mental status changes (i.e., disorientation) are often associated with medical causes of psychiatric illness. However, this is surprisingly difficult to discover on physical exam, and cases of delirium are missed anywhere from 12.5% to 75% of the time in the emergency department [9,16]. As a result, many authors have also advised formal mental status screenings as part of the standard H&P. Although a prospective randomized trial of the addition of mental status screenings alongside standard H&Ps has never been performed, the performance of these exams is nonetheless reasonable in the medical assessment of psychiatric patients, particularly for patients at highest risk, such as the elderly. Expert guidelines, such as those by the American College of Emergency Physicians, also recommend an assessment of mentation as part of medical screening in emergency departments [17]. By its very nature, symptoms of delirium wax and wane, necessitating frequent patient re-evaluation and collaboration with experienced nurse observers for diagnostic sensitivity.

The role of laboratory testing in recognizing medical mimics

There has been considerable disagreement between emergency physicians and psychiatrists on the necessity for laboratory screening, with conflicting evidence about its utility [18]. In a study by Hall and colleagues, for instance, the authors performed blood work, an ECG, an EEG, and detailed medical and neurologic exams on 100 consecutive patients admitted to an inpatient psychiatric unit [19]. The authors found that 46% of these patients had an unrecognized medical illness that caused or exacerbated their symptoms, with an additional 34% of patients having an unrelated physical illness. After medical treatment, 28 of the 46 patients had rapid clearing of their psychiatric symptoms. The authors concluded that patients should have laboratory evaluations and detailed physical exams. A 1994 study by Henneman and colleagues reached similar conclusions [15]. Finally, Schillerstrom and colleagues noted that patients who were emergently medicated for agitation were more likely to have abnormal laboratory values, and suggested that these patients were medically different than non-agitated patients [20].

Other authors, however, have found that routine laboratory evaluations are of low yield. In a 1997 study, for instance, Olshaker and colleagues retrospectively investigated 345 patients with psychiatric symptoms [21]. The sensitivity of the history, physical exam, vital signs, and laboratory testing for indicating disease were calculated as 94%, 51%, 17%, and 20%, respectively. The authors concluded that the vast majority of medical problems of psychiatric patients in the emergency department could be identified by routine H&P and vital sign measurement. In a 2000 study, Korn, Currier, and Henderson retrospectively investigated 212 patients with psychiatric complaints in the emergency department [22]. In this study, patients presenting with psychiatric complaints underwent routine testing including electrolytes, blood urea nitrogen/creatinine, complete blood count (CBC), urine and blood toxicology screens, chest x-ray, and a pregnancy test. Patients with a psychiatric history, normal physical findings, stable vital signs, and no current medical problems did not have abnormal laboratory findings. The authors concluded that routine laboratory testing was of low yield. Janiak and Atteberry also retrospectively reviewed 502 charts of psychiatric patients who received routine laboratory testing by the psychiatric service and found, with only one exception, no labs ordered routinely would have changed emergency department management [23]. A similar conclusion was reached in a prospective study of 375 patients by Amin and Wang [24].

Nonetheless, routine testing is often required for patients in the emergency department with mental-health complaints. In a 2002 survey of emergency physicians by Broderick and colleagues, for instance, 35% of respondents indicated that they were required by consultants to obtain routine tests. Many respondents believed that at least some of these tests were unnecessary, with urine toxicology screening and serum alcohol testing felt to be more necessary than blood work or an electrocardiogram (ECG) [25].

Unfortunately, it is difficult to draw firm conclusions from existing studies such as these, because none of the above studies documented the comprehensiveness of their history, physical, or mental status examinations, investigated whether the testing of high-risk groups increases the number of positive laboratory investigations, or whether inpatient treatment by the psychiatry service (as opposed to emergency department management and disposition) would have changed as a result of obtaining labs. However, based on evidence of this type, the American College of Emergency Physicians recently stated in a clinical guideline on evaluation of adult psychiatric patients that routine laboratory testing for asymptomatic, alert, cooperative patients was unnecessary [17].

The role of urine drug screens in recognizing medical mimics

As with laboratory values, the utility of routine urine drug screens has also been questioned because many psychoactive substances are not tested for in the "drugs of abuse" urine assays. Some studies, such as those by Schuckman and colleagues, have indicated self-reporting of illicit drug use is unreliable in the emergency department [26]. However, several emergency department studies have indicated that urine drug screens, even when positive, do not often change emergency department management or disposition of psychiatric patients. Schiller and colleagues, for instance, prospectively investigated 392 patients presenting to a psychiatric emergency service [27]. The researchers found 20.8% of patients who denied substance use actually had positive screens, but dispositions did not change between patients in whom a routine urine drug screen was ordered and patients in whom it was not. Similar results have been found by both Fortu and colleagues in a retrospective review of 652 charts and Eisen and colleagues in a prospective study of 133 patients [28,29].

Concerns have also been raised about the accuracy of urine drug screens. In a 2009 study, Bagoien and colleagues compared a commercially available urine drug screen against liquid chromatography/mass spectrometry analysis of the same urine samples. The standard urine drug screen was correct for all five drugs of abuse included on the panel only in 75.2% of cases, with sensitivities of 43–90%, depending on the drug of interest [30].

Based primarily on evidence of this type, the American College of Emergency Physicians stated in recent guidelines about testing of adult psychiatric patients that routine urine drug testing is unnecessary in the emergency department [17]. However, the results of these types of studies have not investigated whether or not the requirement for urine drug screen testing is influenced by the type of facility to which the patient is being transferred or whether insurers have demanded these tests to cover psychiatric hospitalization.

Tips to improve the accuracy of medical screening exams

Examine thoroughly, test selectively. Despite the conflicting evidence about routine laboratory testing, most experts agree that emergency physicians can improve their diagnostic accuracy both by selective testing of certain patient groups and by increasing their knowledge of medical mimics of psychiatric disease. Obtaining an adequate history is often the first and most important step. Although most astute clinician rely primarily on the history as the most useful information when formulating a diagnosis and care plan, missing pieces of vital information regarding the history as well as inadequate physical examinations are far too common in the evaluation of the psychiatric patient. In a study in 2000, for instance, Reeves et al. found inadequate history, physical exam, and the almost universal failure of obtaining a mental status exam in those patients in whom a medical diagnosis was missed [16]. Inadequate history & physicals were also cited by Koranyi and Potoczny as the leading contributor to missed diagnoses [31].

Search for collateral information. Incomplete H&Ps are not always the fault of the clinician; it is not uncommon for psychiatric patients to be unable to provide a clear detailed history [8]. Both delirium and underlying psychosis can make it difficult for the provider to obtain accurate information, and there may be an additional degree of fear or shame that prevents some patients from being fully forthcoming regarding their symptoms [32]. Obtaining collateral history from family, friends, other providers, and prehospital personnel is important. In addition, previous or outside medical records should be carefully reviewed. Review of the patient's medication list is also important, as this can be a significant contributor to the patient's symptoms [33,34].

Stratify risk with H&P, including mental status exam. To best identify patients with an organic cause for their psychiatric symptoms, it is important to recognize patients at the highest risk of medical illness. In general, existing studies have noted that patients with a new-onset of psychiatric symptoms have a high rate of medical illness [7,11,12,15]. However, it is reasonable to suspect a high rate of medical illness in other groups as well, such as patients with pre-existing comorbid medical conditions especially immunosuppressive disease, active substance abuse, those without regular access to health care (i.e., those from lower socioeconomic situations), or the elderly [10]. Given the difficulty of obtaining a history from agitated patients and the numerous causes of agitation, these patients may form an additional high-risk group [35].

Along with obtaining a thorough medical history, a focused yet appropriately detailed physical examination can be informative. The physical exam should always begin with an assessment of vital signs, as these are more likely to be abnormal with an underlying organic cause, but should also include an assessment of general appearance, affect, a mental status examination, and a thorough neurologic examination. The physical examination should also note evidence of encephalitis, thyroid disease, signs of liver disease, seizures, trauma, toxidromes, or withdrawal syndromes, as each can present with psychiatric symptoms [36–39].

Specifically exclude delirium. Treat its causes. The goal of the mental status exam is to exclude delirium, which is defined as any acute medical condition resulting in a state of confusion or disturbance of consciousness [39]. Delirium, which often presents within a short period since symptom onset and fluctuating change in mental status, is not a diagnosis in itself. Rather, it is a common symptom of impaired brain functioning. As such, it is often accompanied by disorientation or memory deficit. This is in contrast to patients with dementia, who often have gradual onset of symptoms without changes in consciousness.

Delirium has numerous causes which are listed in Table 3.1 [39]. Several of these conditions require prompt recognition

Table 3.1. Causes of delirium due to underlying medical conditions

- Intoxication with drugs – Many drugs implicated especially anticholinergic agents, anticonvulsants, anti-parkinsonism agents, steroids, cimetidine, opiates, sedative hypnotics. Don't forget alcohol and illicit drugs
- Withdrawal syndromes – Alcohol, sedative hypnotics, barbiturates
- Metabolic causes
- Hypoxia; hypoglycemia; hepatic, renal, or pulmonary insufficiency
- Endocrinopathies (such as hypothyroidism, hyperthyroidism, hypopituitarism, hypoparathyroidism, or hyperparathyroidism)
- Disorders of fluid and electrolyte balance
- Rare causes (such as porphyria, carcinoid syndrome)
- Infections
- Head trauma
- Epilepsy – Ictal, interictal, or postictal
- Neoplastic disease
- Vascular disorders
- Cerebrovasular (such as transient ischaemic attacks, thrombosis, embolism, migraine)
- Cardiovascular (such as myocardial infarction, cardiac failure)

Reproduced from "ABC of psychological medicine: delirium" by Brown TM and Boyle MF. Volume 325 pages 644–647, 2002, with permission from BMJ Publishing Group Ltd [39]

Table 3.2. The Brief Mental Status Exam

Questions	Score number of errors × weight
What year is it now?	(0 or 1) × 4
What month is it?	(0 or 1) × 3
Repeat this phrase after me and remember it: "John Brown, 42 Market Street, New York"	
About what time is it? (correct if within 1 hour)	(0 or 1) × 3
Count backward from 20 to 1	(0, 1, or 2) × 2
Say the months in reverse	(0, 1, or 2) × 2
Repeat the memory phrase (each underlined portion is 1 point)	(0, 1, 2, 3, 4, or 5) × 2

Final score is the sum of total errors in each box. 0–8 normal, 9–19 mildly impaired, 20–28 severely impaired.

Table 3.3. The Quick Confusion Scale

Quick Confusion Scale	Scoring
What year is it now?	2 points
What month is it?	2 points
Repeat this phrase: "John Brown, 42 Market Street, New York"	
About what time is it?	2 points
Count backward from 20 to 1	2 points
Say the months in reverse	2 points
Repeat the memory phrase	5 points

Final score is the sum of the total in each box. Impaired is <11.

and treatment, and so delirium is regarded as a potential medical emergency. Despite this, emergency physicians do overlook the recognition of delirium. In a 2010 study, Reeves et al. found that elderly patients with delirium are more likely to be admitted to psychiatric units and less likely to complete a medical assessment than patients admitted to the inpatient service [40].

Assume an organic cause in the absence of previous psychiatric history. Given the number of potentially life-threatening causes of infection and studies such as those by Henneman and colleagues [15] in which a high percentage of patients with new psychiatric symptoms were found to have medical illness, a thorough workup is advised for any patient with first-time onset of psychiatric symptoms. In addition, medical screening should include an assessment for delirium. Both The Brief Mental Status Exam and The Quick Confusion Scale (see Tables 3.2 and 3.3) have been shown to be useful in the emergency department setting [41,42]. Although each asks similar questions, scoring is different for each test. The Brief Mental Status Exam has been shown to have a sensitivity of 72% when compared against emergency physician judgment. The Quick Confusion Scale has been shown to have a sensitivity of 64% for detecting cognitive impairment when compared against the Mini-Mental State Examination.

In summary, there are several ways that clinicians can improve their diagnostic accuracy when medically screening patients with psychiatric complaints. All physicians should be aware of the numerous medical causes of psychiatric illness, and should seek to exclude these illnesses in their history and physical examination. Laboratory testing should be based on the results of an adequate history and physical exam. Clinicians should have a low threshold for a broader workup in patients in whom an adequate history and physical cannot be obtained; in patients with no prior psychiatric history; or in patients at higher risk of medical illness. As part of the physical exam, emergency physicians should obtain both an assessment of mental status and a neurologic examination; validated assessment tools can be useful. Universal routine laboratory testing is not supported, especially in patients with a known psychiatric history, a presentation consistent with that psychiatric history, normal vitals, and a normal history and physical examination.

The utility of guidelines and protocols

Given the frequent disagreement between emergency medicine and psychiatry over the scope of the medical workup, many authors have argued for the use of standard protocols that have been agreed-upon in advance by all specialties involved. One algorithm was created by Zun and colleagues in their work with the Illinois Mental Health Task Force [11,12]. This protocol is implemented by asking five binary questions.

- Does the patient have any new psychiatric condition?
- Does the patient have any history of active illness needing evaluation?
- Does the patient have any abnormal vital signs?
- Does the patient have an abnormal physical exam (unclothed)?
- Does the patient have any abnormal mental status?

If the answer to all five questions was no, the patient could be safely transferred without further evaluation. Zun and Downey then performed a retrospective chart review of all emergency department patients with psychiatric complaints who were transferred to a psychiatric facility both before and after the adoption of this protocol [11]. The total cost was $269 per patient after adoption of the protocol, but $352 before. The return rate of patients to the emergency department for further evaluation after the protocol, however, was similar.

Another screening algorithm was recently proposed by Shah and colleagues [13]. In this study, the authors retrospectively reviewed the charts of 485 patients who had been screened in the emergency department with a five-item questionnaire (stable vital signs, no prior psychiatric history, alert/oriented × 4, no evidence of acute medical problem, no visual hallucinations). Only six patients (1.2%) with a "yes" to all five questions were transferred back to the emergency department for further medical workup, and none of these patients required medical or surgical admission.

A quick glance at these two screening tools finds them remarkably similar, yet, the reported effectiveness differed. Local processes, such as coordination of care, trust between providers, wait times for subsequent psychiatric admission, facility overcrowding, and subgroup demographics may play a strong role in acceptance and accuracy of the emergency medicine evaluation process. Perhaps for these reasons, a simple medical screening algorithm has not yet been widely accepted. This is unfortunate, as medical protocols have the potential to resolve many conflicts between psychiatric receiving facilities and emergency departments. Agreed-upon protocols also maintain a high standard of care for patients, reduce the cost of testing, and provide a structured format for quality improvement activities and clinical research.

Conclusions

Emergency physicians are commonly expected to evaluate patients presenting with psychiatric symptoms. Medical screening of these patients, to stabilize medical conditions, to facilitate psychiatric evaluation, and to safely transfer them to an appropriate treatment facility, is indicated. Evidence-based limitations of these assessments should be recognized.

1. Emergency physicians should not use the phrase "medical clearance," as this suggests that the patient is medically free from all disease. Instead, this phrase should be replaced by "medical stability" or by a concise discharge note listing the screening procedures performed.
2. Emergency physicians should be aware of the medical mimics of psychiatric disease. All patients with psychiatric complaints should receive an adequate history & physical exam, including both a neurologic exam and an assessment of mental status.
3. Emergency physicians should have a low threshold to obtain laboratory testing on high-risk patients. Commonly encountered high-risk patients in the emergency department include those with a new onset of psychiatric symptoms; those with pre-existing comorbid medical conditions, especially immunosuppressive disease; the elderly; patients with active substance abuse; and patients without access to health care (i.e., those from lower socioeconomic situations). Agitated patients may also be an additional under-recognized high-risk group.
4. Psychiatry services should recognize the indications and limits of routine testing. In particular, laboratory testing does not reveal significant disease in young patients with known psychiatric disease who have normal vitals, a normal H&P, and a presentation consistent with their psychiatric illness.
5. Prospectively developed protocols that are collaboratively derived by emergency medicine and psychiatry specialists can decrease the amount of testing while preserving a high level of care.

As the number of visits to emergency departments increase, the number of screenings of psychiatric patients by emergency physician will continue to increase. A systematic approach, focused medical assessment, and appropriate laboratory testing guided by the history and physical examination followed by clear communication between providers will achieve a high quality of care, control costs, and guide improvement activities. Further research may help refine the medical screening process even further, by identifying the most sensitive and specific parts of the history and physical exam, by determining the groups at highest risk for medical disease, and validating the most efficient medical screening protocols.

References

1. Larkin GL, Claassen CA, Emond JA, Pelletier AJ, Camargo CA. Trends in U.S. Emergency Department Visits for Mental Health Conditions, 1992–2001. *Psychiatr Serv* 2005;**56**:671–7.

2. Wilson MP, Zeller SL. Introduction: reconsidering psychiatry in the emergency department. *J Emerg Med* [Epub ahead of print].

3. Vilke GM, Wilson MP. Agitation: what every emergency physician should know. *Emerg Med Rep* 2009;**30**:233–44.

4. Pitts SR, Niska RW, Xu J, Burt CW. National hospital ambulatory medical care survey: 2006 emergency department summary. *Natl Health Stat Rep* 2008;**7**:1–38.

5. Freud S, Brill AA, (Eds.). *The Basic Writings of Sigmund Freud*. New York: New York Modern Library; 1938:973.

6. Tintinalli JE, Peacock FW, Wright MA. Emergency medical evaluation of psychiatric patients. *Ann Emerg Med* 1994;**23**:859–62.

7. Zun LS. Evidence based evaluation of psychiatric patients. *J Emerg Med* 2005;**28**:35–9.

8. Sood TR, Mcstay CM. Evaluation of the psychiatric patient. *Emerg Med Clin North Am* 2009;**27**:669–83.

9. Han JH, Zimmerman EE, Cutler N, et al. Delirium in an older emergency department patients: recognition, risk factors, and psychomotor subtypes. *Acad Emerg Med* 2009;**16**:193–200.

10. Gregory RJ, Nihalani ND, Rodriguez E. Medical Screening in the Emergency Department for Psychiatric admissions: a procedural analysis. *Gen Hosp Psychiatry* 2004;**26**:405–10.

11. Zun LS, Downey L. Application of a medical clearance protocol. *Prim Psychiatry* 2007;**14**:47–51.

12. Downey LA, Zun LS, Gonzales SJ. Utilization of emergency department by psychiatric patients. *Prim Psychiatry* 2009;**16**:60–4.

13. Shah SJ, Fiorito M, McNamara RM. A screening tool to medically clear psychiatric patients in the emergency department. *J Emerg Med* [Epub ahead of print].

14. Emerson RW. *Society and Solitude.* Boston: Houghton, Osgood, and Company. Available at: http://books.google.com/ (Accessed November 1, 2011).

15. Henneman PL, Mendoza R, Lewis RJ. Prospective evaluation of emergency department medical clearance. *Ann Emerg Med* 1994;**4**:672–7.

16. Reeves RR, Pendarvis RJ, Kimble R. Unrecognized medical emergencies admitted to psychiatric units. *Am J Emerg Med* 2000;**18**:390–3.

17. Lukens TW, Wolf SJ, Edlow JA, et al. Clinical policy: critical issues in the diagnosis and management of the adult psychiatric patient in the emergency department. *Ann Emerg Med* 2006;**47**:79–99.

18. Zun LS, Hernandez R, Thompson R, Downey L. Comparison of EPs' and psychiatrists' laboratory assessment of psychiatric patients. *Am J Emerg Med* 2004;**22**:175–80.

19. Hall RCW, Gardner ER, Popkin MK, Lecann AF, Stickney SA. Unrecognized physical illness prompting psychiatric admission: a prospective study. *Am J Psychiatry* 1981;**5**:629–35.

20. Schillerstrom TL, Schillerstrom JE, Taylor SE. Laboratory findings in emergently medicated psychiatric patients. *Gen Hosp Psychiatry* 2004;**26**:411–14.

21. Olshaker JS, Browne B, Jerrard D, et al. Medical clearance and screening of psychiatric patients in the emergency department. *Acad Emerg Med* 1997;**2**:124–8.

22. Korn CS, Currier GW, Henderson SO. "Medical clearance" of psychiatric patients without medical complaints in the emergency department. *J Emerg Med* 2000;**2**:173–6.

23. Janiak BD, Atteberry S. Medical clearance of the psychiatric patient in the emergency department. *J Emerg Med* [Epub ahead of print].

24. Amin M, Wang J. Routine laboratory testing to evaluate for medical illness in psychiatric patients in the emergency department is largely unrevealing. *West J Emerg Med* 2009;**2**:97–100.

25. Broderick KB, Lerner EB, McCort JD, et al. Emergency physician practices and requirements regarding the medical screening examination of the psychiatric patients. *Acad Emerg Med* 2002;**9**:88–92.

26. Schuckman H, Hazelett S, Powell C, Steer S. A validation of self-reported substance use with biochemical testing among patients presenting to the emergency department seeking treatment for backache, headache, and toothache. *Subst Use Misuse* 2008;**43**:589–95.

27. Schiller MJ, Shumway M, Batki SL. Utility of routine drug screening in a psychiatric emergency setting. *Psychiatr Serv* 2000;**51**:474–8.

28. Fortu JM, Kim IK, Cooper A, et al. Psychiatric patients in the pediatric emergency department undergoing routine urine toxicology screens for medical clearance: results and use. *Pediatr Emerg Care* 2009;**25**:387–92.

29. Eisen JS, Sivilotti MLA, Boyd KU, et al. Screening urine for drugs of abuse in the emergency department: do test results affect physician's patient care decisions? *CJEM* 2004;**6**:104–11.

30. Bagoien G, Morken G, Zahlsen K, Aamo T, Spigset O. Evaluation of a urine on-site drugs of abuse screening test in patients admitted to a psychiatric emergency unit. *J Clin Psychopharmacol* 2009;**29**:248–54.

31. Koranyi EK, Potoczny WM. Physical illnesses underlying psychiatric symptoms. *Psychother Psychosom* 1992;**58**:155–60.

32. Kalogerakis MG. Emergency evaluation of adolescents. *Hosp Community Psychiatry* 1992;**43**:617–21.

33. Gardner ER, Hall RCW. Psychiatric symptoms produced by over-the-counter drugs. *Psychosomatics* 1982;**23**:186–90.

34. Blanda MP. Pharmacologic issues in geriatric emergency medicine. *Emerg Med Clin North Am* 2006;**24**:449–65.

35. Nordstrom K, Zun LS, Wilson MP, et al. Medical evaluation and triage of the agitated patient: consensus statement of the American Association for Emergency Psychiatry Project BETA medical evaluation workgroup. *West J Emerg Med* 2012;**13**:3–10.

36. Hall RCW, Popkin MK, DeVaul R, et al. Psychiatric manifestations of Hashimoto's thyroiditis. *Psychosomatics* 1982;**4**:337–42.

37. Talbot-Stern JK, Green T, Royle TJ. Psychiatric manifestations of systemic illness. *Emerg Med Clin North Am* 2000;**18**:199–209.

38. Pitzele HZ, Tolia VM. Twenty per hour: altered mental state due to ethanol abuse and withdrawal. *Emerg Med Clin North Am* 2010;**28**:683–705.

39. Brown TM, Boyle MF. ABC of psychological medicine: delirium. *BMJ* 2002;**325**:644–7.

40. Reeves RR, Parker JD, Burke RS, et al. Inappropriate psychiatric admission on elderly patients with unrecognized delirium. *South Med J* 2010;**103**:111–15.

41. Kaufman DM, Zun LS. A quantifiable, brief mental status examination for emergency patients. *J Emerg Med* 1995;**13**:449–56.

42. Stair TO, Morrissey J, Jaradeh I, Zhou TX, Goldstein JN. Validation of the quick confusion scale for mental status screening in the emergency department. *Intern Emerg Med* 2007;**2**:130–2.

Advanced interviewing techniques for psychiatric patients in the emergency department

Jon S. Berlin

Introduction

The three core psychiatric competencies within the province of emergency medicine involve medical clearance, danger to self, and danger to others. Our purpose here is to demonstrate that, even within these narrow confines, it is crucial to talk to the patient in a meaningful way and possible to gain access to guarded but very revealing personal information briefly and effectively. This chapter is written with an awareness of the greater than usual resistance that many emergency patients exhibit and the less than usual time there is in which to see them. This material is intended for both emergency medicine practitioners and mental health specialists working in the emergency setting.

Broadly speaking, psychiatric evaluation is an iterative, three-part process that includes the gathering of data, the synthesis of data into an assessment, and the development of a plan that addresses the problems and questions outlined in the assessment. In the emergency setting, data often accumulates quickly from multiple sources: the police, the old chart, family informants and so forth. The psychiatric interview is the way to obtain the all-important history from the patient himself and to begin establishing the clinician–patient relationship and collaboration. Basic interview skills involve putting the person at ease, establishing rapport, and asking a series of questions in a semi-structured interview format that encourages him or her to speak freely but also with increasing specificity. The interviewer must be a good listener yet also directive enough to cover the important areas in a reasonable amount of time. The basic interview concludes with the interviewer and patient trying to reach some agreement about the problems to be addressed and the approaches used. In emergency practice, a patient's pressing clinical need or the demands of many patients at once may make it necessary to start out with a quick cycle of data collection, synthesis, and intervention. This may be followed by one or more subsequent cycles, but the initial interview may perforce be very brief. Advanced interview skills have been developed to search out the most valid information from the patient about the highest priority issues of risk in a very focused manner.

Time is one of the main limiting factors in the emergency department (ED), and conducting a comprehensive psychiatric evaluation on persons with mental health issues is impractical. In most quarters, a truncated assessment focusing mainly on mental status and history of present illness has taken its place. On occasion, even that may be unnecessary. Some very high-risk psychiatric cases can be managed using a standard medical model. For example, if an individual presents to the ED for a serious suicide attempt, one may need simply to treat the medical problem, order suicide precautions, and admit the patient to the hospital. However, most cases are not so straightforward. There are persons with roughly an equal number of risk factors and protective factors for harm to self or others, rendering the assessment of acuity and risk to be intermediate. There are also individuals with signs and symptoms pertinent to risk that are incomplete or inconsistent. Quite unlike the ideal short-term psychotherapy patient, the ED patient may be resistant to giving a history, unable to put his thoughts and feelings easily into words, resistant to treatment, or unmotivated. He may also have a hidden agenda, such as avoiding or securing hospitalization or medication. In these cases, the degree of risk may be frustratingly indeterminate.

From a theoretical standpoint, I will be describing a contemporary interview technique developed over the last fifteen years at the busy Milwaukee County Psychiatric Crisis Service that takes into account the special circumstances of emergency practice. First reported in a chapter I wrote with Jon Gudeman in 2007 and published in 2008 [1], it draws upon and adapts mainstream principles of psychodynamic psychiatry [2–4], short-term psychotherapy [5–7], motivational interviewing [8], and trauma informed care [9]. While not useful in all cases, it does extend one's ability to engage difficult individuals that had previously been considered out of reach. Our approach in this chapter will be to tie general principles closely to clinical material to offer practical suggestions for what a clinician might actually say and do.

Given the ease with which a person can minimize or exaggerate the severity of his condition, and the conscious and unconscious difficulties he may have expressing or allowing access to sensitive material, the existence of occult risk is quite

Behavioral Emergencies for the Emergency Physician, ed. Leslie S. Zun, Lara G. Chepenik, and Mary Nan S. Mallory. Published by Cambridge University Press. © Cambridge University Press 2013.

important to appreciate. In the cases that follow, mental content that clarifies ambiguous assessments and reveals actual risk is waiting to be uncovered.

In accord with conventional usage, by "occult" we are referring to danger that is "not revealed . . . not easily apprehended or understood . . . [and] not manifest or detectable by clinical methods alone" [10], i.e., not by rudimentary clinical methods. In our context, occult danger can also refer to danger that is *less* than it appears, as well as danger that is more than it appears. The true degree of risk is like an iceberg, partially visible and partially below the surface. In psychoanalytic metapsychology, from a topographical point of view, it is sometimes the case that the mental status content we seek is not consciously withheld, but in the person's preconscious [11]. It is something that he is not currently aware of, but that with help he can bring to mind. In keeping with Shea's classic work, the interview technique focuses on drawing out the patient to obtain the most reliable and authentic self-report possible [12]. However, whereas his approach is circumspect and systematic, ours is perhaps somewhat more time-sensitive, active and ready to exploit openings.

Faced with cases that fail both these slower and faster approaches, we have developed the ability to assess risk in other ways: obtaining collateral history from reliable sources; having multiple observers observe a person discreetly in the emergency arena over a longer period of time; and weighing identified risk factors and protective factors to arrive at an actuarial-model best estimate. All three of these avenues are useful and essential. They may be used in conjunction with a clinical interview, and they may be key. But they do have potential drawbacks. First, prematurely checking collateral history may make a patient feel discounted and dissuade him from engaging him in a genuine doctor–patient relationship. This jeopardizes one of the two most important protective factors (the other being social support) that give us confidence in referring an individual with risk factors to a level of care outside of the hospital [13]. Second, extending a person's stay can be problematic for the individual and the emergency environment. Third, an exclusive use of the actuarial approach ignores one of the most singular discoveries in the entire history of psychiatry, that the natural propensity for resistance and emotional guarding is frequently accompanied by the desire to speak and be understood [14]. (The word "resistance" is used in the technical sense, referring to the patient's "mental processes, fantasies, memories, reactions, and mechanisms that serve to defend against the progress of the analytic process – both its deepening and its emotional impact".) [15]. As we shall see, when approached in the right way, some patients will tell us exactly how high their risk is, making assessment methods not based on a good interview seem inorganic and convoluted by comparison. To use an analogy derived from Greek mythology, giving up too soon on an interview is like letting go of Proteus before he answers the question.

This chapter does not take up the subject of agitation and verbal de-escalation. Such cases involve overt acuity, and the interview skills required are somewhat different. The need to engage is the same, but the ability to help someone regain self-control is a special topic in its own right, and this text addresses it in a separate chapter. The types of cases we are describing may involve individuals who are involuntary or distressed, but they are calm enough to engage in a conversation. It is not a minor point that a probing psychiatric examination is only possible if the examiner has paid sufficient attention to stabilizing measures, such as physical comfort, medication as needed, and the containing influences of respect, rapport, active listening, attunement, and the desire to establish a useful and collaborative doctor–patient relationship [16,17]. Premature probing can cause a seemingly controlled person to erupt. It should also be appreciated that a patient must be medically stable, and that delirium, dementia, and extreme intoxication states are contraindications to an uncovering type of approach.

Case 1: Engagement and psychological guarding of occult medical acuity

We begin our discussion with a composite case illustrating a man's alarming resistance to his underlying medical acuity, and to his physician. The medical condition can be diagnosed by routine history and physical examination, but it is termed occult because the patient's psychological defenses are protean, and exceptional finesse and focus are required to overcome them. The guarding of medical acuity and its management become a useful metaphor for the case of occult psychiatric acuity that follows.

"Mr. Flood" was a 75-year-old man in the ED with a presenting complaint of vague abdominal pain. After waiting in an exam room for nearly 2 hours, he went to the nursing station saying if no one was going to see him he was ready to leave. A second-year emergency medicine resident overheard him and put down the chart of another patient she was about to see. She introduced herself, apologized for the long wait, and asked him to accompany her back to the exam room. Scanning his triage note as they walked, she gathered he had talked about calling his family doctor for 3 months, but his wife had suddenly insisted that he go to the ED with her this morning.

He was a smoker with a 60-year pack history and a family history of atherosclerosis, but no significant medical history of his own. His vital signs were normal. His only medications were a baby aspirin, a statin, and iron. He had no mental health history. The triage nurse noted no acute distress. She had assigned him a routine priority level, and until this moment, he appeared to have been waiting patiently. His wife had been with him for most of the time, but a few minutes earlier, an unexpected cell phone call had compelled her to leave the bedside to pick up their granddaughter who had taken ill at school.

Putting down the chart, the resident turned to Mr. Flood and gave him her full, undivided attention. His complexion was a little pale, and his hair and mustache were dyed black with white roots showing. He studied her too: good-looking, light on her feet, probably late twenties.

She started out with the history of present illness. He had been thinking about seeing his personal physician for several months. What happened to make his wife urge him to be seen here today? Mr. Flood shrugged his shoulders and began to speak, but just then, the resident's cell phone rang. She put her head down, told the caller she would call back, and looked up again. The resident apologized for the interruption and asked Mr. Flood please to finish what he was about to say. He said no, he had tickets to a baseball game that afternoon. He was taking his grandson who was in morning kindergarten, and he couldn't be late. He stepped down off the examining table and reached for his clothes, briefly exposing his buttocks. He took out his wallet and showed her a picture of a boy in a Little League uniform. The doctor again said she was sorry for his long wait, but promised to work quickly. She turned off her cell phone, adding that his wife may be quite alarmed if she learned he had left without being seen.

Mr. Flood stood there, thinking. He said that the game's starting pitcher had just come up from the minor leagues and probably wasn't very good. The resident thought about this comment, and then said, "Jeez, first you get stuck with a rookie pitcher, then you get stuck with me, a rookie doctor. This just isn't your day, is it?" He was amused and sat down again on the examining table. He supposed he could be a little late. She repeated the "Why now?" question. Why had his wife insisted he come to the ED today? He didn't know. She persisted. Had there been any change in his symptoms? Reluctantly, he admitted to having told his wife that morning that he had been awakened in the middle of the night by unusual pulsating sensations in his abdomen. At first, he wasn't sure if he was imagining things, but last night the feeling was unmistakable. He had felt this same symptom again in the ED just before he left the exam room and approached the nursing station to complain. He looked worried.

The resident pressed on and told Mr. Flood to lie down on the exam table. She put a blanket over the lower half of his body, pulled up his gown and leaned over him slightly. He looked inside her white coat at her delicate collarbone and figure. He said she shouldn't take this the wrong way, but her scrubs were very becoming on her. She could have been a model. She stiffened and leaned away from him. He also noted, disapprovingly, the tattoo of a small rose at the base of her neck. He said that, years ago, when he was in the Navy, when a woman had a tattoo, it meant she was a real professional. The resident froze and stood motionless. Her face turned pink. Fifteen long seconds passed. Then she relaxed and smiled and said, "Ah, yes, well, I am so glad to see that your hormones are still working. You must make your wife very happy. That's excellent. However, right now I really need to get a little peak at that belly of yours." She put on her stethoscope and auscultated. Abdominal bruits. Her first. She then asked him to point to where it seemed most uncomfortable. She examined the other areas first and found the abdomen to be soft and non-tender, but upon deeper palpation thought she appreciated a vertical, mid-line mass. She finished the rest of the exam quickly and sat down.

She wasn't certain, she said, but his condition appeared to be very serious. He needed a vascular surgery consult, imaging studies, lab work, and, more than likely, admission to the hospital. Mr. Flood was attentive and somber, but then said, no, he couldn't disappoint his grandson. He would return to the hospital this evening after the game.

The resident was alarmed. He couldn't leave. If what she suspected was true, his aorta had ballooned out and could rupture at any minute. He could die. Mr. Flood seemed unfazed. Of course he would get the problem taken care of, but he had waited this long, he could wait a little longer. She asked what would his wife say? He said she'd lived with him for forty years, she was used to him. The resident then asked what he thought would happen with his grandson were the aneurysm to rupture at the baseball game? Would a little boy be safe in the commotion of a medical emergency with thousands of strangers around? This stopped Mr. Flood. He had not considered this. His grandson came first. His head sunk down and he inhaled suddenly with his fist pressed against his mouth. Eyes closed, he nodded slowly and agreed to accept her recommendations.

Discussion

Note how the chief complaint in this case was forthcoming but the acute precipitant, the "why now" in the history of present illness, and the key physical finding, were not. Guarding and resisting the most troubling aspects of a problem is very typical. Mr. Flood used a variety of defenses. Having already avoided his primary care physician, tried to leave the ED without being seen, and tried to leave again when the resident took a phone call, he then insulted her by exposing himself, devalued her with an unconscious comparison to a barely competent baseball player, and stunned her with a crude sexual overture right at the point of palpation.

The erotic behavior was a desperate attempt to sabotage the physical exam, turn the tables on a woman in a position of power and authority, and restore a failing sense of physical integrity. Fortunately, the doctor's emotional maturity and poise enabled her to recover quickly from the humiliation and graciously acknowledge Mr. Flood's virility enough for him to submit to the exam. She clearly had a gift for hearing unconscious communication about underlying fear and anxiety [18] and for responding non-defensively and non-punitively. Interestingly, her correct interpretations of the rookie and the prostitute comments transformed his devaluation of her into respect and admiration. This may have made her even more attractive to him, but her grace under fire established a working relationship and made him willing to cooperate.

With hindsight, the resident's empathy and management did lapse briefly in making too quick a transition from the history to the physical. Ideally, when she saw the worried look on Mr. Flood's face as he confessed to the pulsating sensation, she might have said he looked concerned and seen if he needed a moment to talk about it. Had she not pressed on at this point, he might not have had to become quite so obstructive when she had him on the table. But it did not become a major issue. She intuitively appreciated that her direct approach was being experienced as a frontal attack and provoking a response that verged on emotional trauma. She was able to let her probing be forcibly suspended without losing sight of her ultimate objective. He regained his perspective that she was his physician, not his enemy.

The resident used motivational interviewing technique in handling the threat to sign out against medical advice. When Mr. Flood refused her recommendations, she first began to argue with him. She then caught herself and encouraged him to think about what was most important to him in life – not to her – and how his actions were not consistent with it. Mr. Flood was torn between facing and not facing medical risk, but he never became an overtly involuntary patient. That morning, he did not have to tell his wife about the new symptom, but he did. He did not have to stay in the ED, but he did. He couldn't face the fear himself, but he accepted his wife's pressure and his doctor's persistence. Initially, he tried to assert his male dominance and the remnants of his flagging invincibility. The resident appealed to his better self: that of being a proud grandfather and protector of his adored grandson.

Intrusions into the care environment exacerbated Mr. Flood's reluctance to become a patient. Not only did the resident have to deal with his and her own normal anxieties, she also had to tune out the "noise" of personal technology and the ED setting to create a brief protective bubble for diagnosis and treatment [19]. It is easy to forget that EDs are as demanding and stressful in their own way on the consumer as they are on the practitioner. Long waits, uncomfortable conditions, confusing policies, lack of privacy, frequent interruptions, intermediate diagnoses, temporizing treatment measures, and referrals to mutable community or hospital resources are legion. It is the practitioner's responsibility to adapt her technique to the impact of these stresses on the patient as best she can. For example, a doctor may need to leave his or her cell phone on for a very important call – perhaps a return call from a specialist – but it is prudent to advise the patient ahead of time that there may be an interruption. On hectic days, it may be helpful to say, "I know this is important and I'd like to give it my undivided attention. This is difficult to do in an ER, but let's do the best we can." Give the person a chance to vent any negatives about the visit thus far. Mental health patients may have valid complaints and just want them acknowledged. They can be quite reasonable. They can wait to discuss despair and suicidal feelings if they see an emergency resuscitation in progress. Perhaps the greatest intrusion to overcome is the experience that psychiatric patients have of feeling shunted aside in favor of the medical patient [20]. One of the goals of this textbook is to address this problem.

Case 2: Occult danger to others and the underlying crisis state of mind

Now let us consider a case with a primary psychiatric diagnosis where an assessment of risk by a physician assistant (PA) is indeterminate, but an attending physician's brief, focused interview elicits the acute precipitant and accurately identifies the underlying crisis state of mind.

"Ms. Ruger" was a 45-year-old woman who presented to an inner city ED Monday morning before eight o'clock with a request to be started on medicine for auditory hallucinations. A PA worked her up and reported the following story to his supervising attending: She has come in voluntarily, but mainly because her family had pressured her all weekend to get help. She cannot be more specific about their concerns. They did not accompany her, and she would prefer that they not be contacted. Her history is that she has heard voices since her late teens and is finally tired of them. She has always resisted the idea of psychiatric treatment in the past, but she is ready now. She has come to an ED because of its convenience, not because her problem is an emergency. Medical history and physical are unremarkable. She is in good health and on no medication. Point-of-care urine drug screen and urine pregnancy test are negative. She is a recovering alcoholic. Although the story is not one of first-break psychosis, it sounded as though it could be a first presentation, and a thorough medical workup has been done. Everything, including head CT, is negative.

Legal history is significant for her having gone to prison in her twenties for stabbing and almost mortally wounding her boyfriend. In a separate incident, she also went to jail a few years ago for domestic violence. Family history is very positive for having had an uncle who was diagnosed with schizophrenia. He was incarcerated for murder and ultimately committed suicide in prison.

On mental status exam, she presents as neat and clean in a hotel maid's uniform. She is alert and oriented, and her cognitive functions are intact. She is somewhat distant but calm and cooperative. Her thought process is linear and logical. Her affect is a little flat but her mood is fine. She is not depressed or elated and has no ideas of hurting herself or others. Her voices are quieter when her mind is occupied with something, such as today's visit. They are more pronounced when she is alone and quiet, like when she goes to bed at night. Generally, she hears several voices talking among themselves. They tend to use vulgar language. The voices sometimes address her directly. They tell her people are out to get her, but do not command her to harm anyone or herself. She can barely hear them now.

The PA's diagnostic impressions are functional psychosis, probably schizophrenia, alcoholism in remission, and some antisocial traits. He wants the psychiatry service to see her, but they cannot come until the afternoon, and she has to be at work by eleven o'clock and is pressed for time. She has some historical risk factors for harm to others, and her long-term risk might be high, but she denies homicidal ideation. Her protective factors include employment, a supportive family, and her interest in treatment now. In his opinion, her acute risk is low, and there is nothing to justify detaining her involuntarily. He can give her a 2-week supply of antipsychotic medication with one refill and an appointment at a mental health clinic in 4 weeks.

The supervising attending listened carefully. The case made him uncomfortable. What was really the acute precipitant for today's visit? Why was this woman suddenly interested in taking medicine after avoiding it for years? Why was her family suddenly so insistent that she be seen? Had something happened? He also wondered about her psychiatric illness. How could it be this serious yet go for decades without treatment? Was there more to the story? Was the crime for which she went to prison connected with her illness? Regardless, the history of felony assault alone gave pause, especially because of the more recent problem with domestic violence. Also, he wondered, why would she even reveal this history at all? On some level, was she feeling a pull to disclose more of her risk than she had consciously intended, and was the revelation of her uncle's murder history and suicide an unconscious reference to her own dangerous potential? In the attending's opinion, Ms. Ruger's signs and symptoms were insufficient and inconsistent. Her acute risk was not low. It was indeterminate.

He decided to conduct a brief, focused exam. He instructed the nurses he was not to be interrupted for 10 minutes. He turned off his cell phone and tuned out the ED, then introduced himself as he entered the room and pulled the curtain closed. He commended Ms. Ruger for seeking help, briefly recapped the history he had heard, and asked how her visit has gone so far. She complained that people who had arrived at the ED after her were called from the waiting room first. He apologized and said he really wanted to help her. In particular, he needed her to help him understand what had made her decide to seek help at this particular time in her life. She had been hearing voices for years. What led to her decision to come in just now?

She said she was just tired of the voices, and her family wanted her to get help. He tried another approach. What was it like, what was it really like, he wanted to know, to hear these voices day in, day out? It must be difficult to talk about, but some part of her must have wanted to discuss it or she would not have come in today. Here he was trying to get at the underlying crisis state of mind that prompted her to take this remarkable step. Ms. Ruger hesitated for a moment, and then replied hotly that the voices were really irritating. They were getting on her nerves. She blurted out that she was not even sure that they were hallucinations at all. Her family said they were all in her head, but she thought that people in her building were putting them there. Asked to elaborate, she said that people were spying on her in her apartment with invisible cameras. It was the same individuals that were planting the voices in her head. He asked how she knew there were cameras. She explained she knew because they were so perfectly hidden that there was no evidence of them. How did she feel about them? Was she frightened? No, she said, not frightened, but angry. Furthermore, she thought she knew exactly who these people were.

He asked if she knew why they were doing this to her and what was she thinking about doing about it? She did not know what they had against her, but she wanted to confront them, and she was afraid of getting attacked when she did. Last Friday,

she had approached a cousin she knew was a drug dealer to borrow one of his guns to defend herself. The cousin had denied her request and reported the incident to her mother. Her mother told the rest of the family, and everyone had been pestering and worrying about her all weekend. They wanted her to see a doctor about taking medicine, but she wasn't sure how medicine could stop the conspiracy. The physician said medicine was still a good idea. It would at least help her to cope with the stress and feel better. She hesitated. She had to be at work soon. He promised to order a low medium dose and check back with her in a little while. He decided on 1 mg of meltable risperidone. She consented reluctantly.

He stepped out of the room, surprised at what he had learned in just a few minutes. The gun, the paranoia, and the specific targets of her anger that were in her building were very serious risk factors, even more so considering the past history of violence. In addition, both of her main protective factors were flawed: her family was concerned but not enough to come in with her or keep her within sight at all times; and she had asked for medicine but had obvious doubts about it. Her engagement in treatment was ambivalent at best. She seemed trusting enough to have come into the ED, but how certain could he be that she would follow-up? After the antipsychotic medication he ordered had time to help her calm down, he would have to tell her that her condition was far more serious than she appreciated. He would say he was sorry, but she could not leave. If she insisted on it, he would explain how concerned he was about her ending up back in prison for shooting someone that might turn out to be completely innocent. Regardless, given her ambivalence, he would initiate a mental health hold and request the social worker to arrange psychiatric hospitalization.

A half hour later, Ms. Ruger was more relaxed but no less delusional. As expected, she was unhappy with the disposition, but, apparently understanding that the doctor was trying to act in her best interest, she did not incorporate him into her paranoid delusion, and she did not escalate. Following admission, the family informed staff that the week before, Ms. Ruger had been brandishing a knife in the hallways of her apartment building, accusing people of persecuting her. She must have known she was in crisis.

Discussion

Cases as striking as this are uncommon, but, except for some changed identifiers, it unfolded as described, and it demonstrates several key points:

1. Latent or occult risk of harm to self and others must always be considered, and routine-screening questions about dangerousness can be ineffective. They are without question necessary when patient volume is high. But a more reliable approach is to find out how life is going and pursue in earnest the history of present illness, the acute precipitant, and the underlying state of mind that led to the visit. Why is the person here now? Is there danger? Is there an underlying *crisis* state of mind?

2. A focused investigation does not always require a long interview. This one took less than 10 minutes. Rigorously screening out distractions and asking about the ED experience thus far facilitates the process of "locking in" to the patient and maximizing engagement. The more protected the interaction, the more tightly it is focused, the briefer it can be. After talking with Ms. Ruger, it was still unclear why she had decompensated at this particular point in her life. Answers to that question would require more investigation, and it was one more reason to admit her to the hospital before releasing her.

3. When hearing about paranoia, one wants to know, what is that like for you? Does it make you angry, does it make you wonder if life is worth living, or have you found a way to live with it? Three different responses to a paranoid world view (hopelessness, rage, or acceptance), and three different implications for risk. (Note: "How do you feel about that?" was once a good question, but overuse has made it more suitable now for comic relief.)

4. In most cases, the sooner psychiatric patients are seen, the better. Their psychiatric acuity and their motivation to engage and open up are in a state of dynamic tension as they sit in the waiting room. Moreover, mental illness has a biological basis, and it can insidiously deteriorate. When Ms. Ruger and Mr. Flood feel paid attention to, they are more willing to divulge crucial information. Guarding is less if an individual is seen before he "shuts down" or "acts up."

5. In all cases, expect resistance, guarding, and encoding of uncomfortable emotions and urges. Psychiatric patients who come to EDs are often action-oriented individuals to whom talking does not come easily. They may have what Sifneos refers to as "alexithymia." [7], a lack of words for feelings. When they have a painful feeling state, they are likely to resort to a drastic behavior that causes someone to bring them in. This behavior is usually called the chief complaint. But the real chief complaint is the underlying crisis state of mind, and when we ask them to describe it, we are asking them to do something that does not at all come naturally. Expect that people will need emotional support and direction doing something seemingly as simple as giving a clear history of present illness.

6. In keeping with the recommendation to stabilize before exploring, it is a good idea to fulfill appropriate patient requests for antipsychotic medication near the beginning of the interview. In general, one might prescribe medication when an assessment is completed. However, there are exceptions, and antipsychotic medicine is the main one. Outside of locked criminal settings, neuroleptics are practically never abused, and, if one is indicated and asked for or accepted voluntarily, administering it early on facilitates a more searching examination. It serves as a test dose that allows for titration or change to another agent during the ED visit. It facilitates symptom relief and crisis resolution. It is a gauge of a person's motivation for treatment. It also mitigates a patient's negative reaction to a disposition decision that he or she believes is adverse, and it is unlikely to be taken voluntarily once the patient is angry and disappointed.

7. Finally, it is interesting to note the similarity between Ms. Ruger's paranoid delusion of being monitored and her clinical need of being monitored. The two types of monitoring could not be more different. But opposites often coexist in the unconscious, and psychosis often has psychological meaning. From a psychodynamic perspective, we would postulate that Ms. Ruger's fear reflected an unconscious wish. As her actions at home and in the ED demonstrated, she had a wish for closer social contact and therapeutic attention, and she evidently had preserved a modicum of capacity for believing that they could be helpful. Without consciously thinking it through, it is this part of Ms. Ruger with which the emergency attending intuitively made every effort to form an alliance. Longer term, it is this alliance that will hopefully turn Ms. Ruger from an acute patient into an outpatient. With the rapidly shrinking availability of hospitalization, the emergency practitioner should always remind himself or herself that it is successful outpatient treatment that ultimately reduces emergency department recidivism.

Case 3: Interview skills mitigate imperfect working conditions

The emergency department environment is often sub-optimal for mental health cases, making interview skill all the more necessary. One patient who was sent to a jail's crisis observation area expressed both the therapeutic shortcomings of that setting and the positive response to clinical acumen rather elegantly.

Mr. X was an African-American veteran who had been having trouble adjusting to civilian life upon his return from Vietnam. He was arrested for disturbing the peace and expressed suicidal ideation during the booking process. He was therefore transferred to the psychiatric observation area where he spontaneously talked about his personal problems in depth with the psychiatric nurses that were there. His level of engagement was high and his suicidal ideation resolved quickly. That evening, he was informed that he would likely be discharged from the observation area, as well as released from jail, the following day. In rounds the next morning, he looked somewhat glum and told the psychiatrist he had dreamt about being back in Vietnam. The dream was very short. He was walking through the jungle and came across a ghastly site of a corpse that was disemboweled and strung up in a tree.

His doctor anticipated a report of resurgent suicidal ideation. He also began to think about adding a traumatic stress disorder diagnosis. But then he asked himself why Mr. X might have had this particular dream at this particular time. Attending to the vicissitudes of their here-and-now doctor–patient relationship, he wondered aloud if the dream was about Mr. X's experience with treatment on the observation unit, that he had spilled his guts and now was being left hanging.

He half-expected this interpretation to be dismissed, but in fact Mr. X was surprised and infrigued. He had only been dimly aware of such feelings and brushed them aside. The dream was a clue that the painful affect was much stronger than he appreciated, and the interpretation of the dream brought his feelings out into the open. It felt good to be understood on a deeper level by another person. His depressed mood lifted completely. The interaction helped the psychiatrist to double check the suicide assessment and confirm that acute risk was not high.

Regarding aftercare arrangements, it would have been preferable if the psychiatrist or one of the crisis staff saw patients in an outpatient clinic and had some time to offer him. Such things are difficult to arrange. Nonetheless, the insight made this gentleman think that a good therapist could help him to understand himself better, and when he left he was eager to begin therapy on an outpatient basis.

Dream interpretation is quite uncommon in emergency settings. But hearing unconscious communication need not be. Mr. X's use of the jungle war metaphor is similar to Mr. Flood's use of the rookie metaphor, and both were easily interpreted by keeping in mind that patients are constantly thinking about issues of safety versus danger in their relationship with their treating professional. In Mr. Flood's case, the danger was having a relatively inexperienced doctor for a serious medical condition, and, in Mr. X's case, it was forming a satisfying bond with a health professional that had to end abruptly. Both patients had a need to conceal their uncomfortable feelings from themselves, both expressed these feelings indirectly without realizing it, and both could accept the translation of the encoded expression without difficulty. Identifying the underlying interpersonal problem strengthened the therapeutic bond and facilitated a better assessment. From the standpoint of trauma informed care, in all three of the cases discussed (the two men and Ms. Ruger), sensitive handling prevented the doctor–patient interactions from becoming traumatic.

Lewis offers the interesting perspective that breaches in important relationships may be inevitable and that the process of creating and repairing the breach may be essential to intrapsychic healing and growth [21]. From this standpoint, a protective factor against risk is strengthened. Nonetheless, it is sobering to contemplate what kind of impression Mr. X would have been left with had he been dismissed from the observation area without his disguised negative reaction being addressed. Good technique salvaged this case, yet one must wonder how often this dynamic of connecting and disconnecting complicates ED visits and ED boarding in particular, and

how often it goes unrecognized. The objective of this chapter, to add to the emergency practitioner's psychiatric skill set, should not draw attention away from the equally important, longer-term goal of reducing psychiatric visits to emergency departments in the first place.

Conclusion

There are other difficult scenarios we could discuss, such as patients with risk factors for suicide that exaggerate or minimize their risk [1]. There is also the enormous challenge of interacting effectively with a psychiatric patient boarding in the ED. The key is to think of it as an imperfect treatment situation. Regardless of the scenario, however, the same concepts and techniques apply. Active listening, engagement, appreciating the defensive function of resistance, sensing the fear of trauma, hearing unconscious communication, stabilizing before probing, searching for occult acuity, mitigating crisis, motivational interviewing, and helping a patient express himself with words not action, all promote the ultimate agenda of turning an acute patient into an outpatient.

In the clinical practice of psychiatry, it cannot be emphasized strongly enough the importance of creating a bond, whether it is for a one-time intervention or a longer course of treatment. There is an interesting parallel between the gradual decision of the action-oriented, emergency medicine practitioner to handle complex mental health cases and the gradual process that a mental health sufferer often goes through accepting that he or she has a problem requiring professional help. The circumspect path that each individual takes to the establishment of a doctor–patient relationship is a complementary undertaking that gives both sides of the equation something in common. The hesitation one feels in approaching a case should sensitize him or her to the hesitation that an individual has in becoming a patient and sharing private thoughts.

Interviewing ability typically improves over a lifetime, profiting by practice, personal growth, and evolving concepts of the psychiatric interview. It is unfortunate that mental health clinicians with the most advanced technique are rarely found working in emergency settings. Healthcare reform may one day, in the uncertain future, make their presence less necessary. However, as cases such as that of Mr. Flood's demonstrate, psychiatric acumen will always be of medical value to the emergency medicine practitioner. Hopefully, cases such as those of Ms. Ruger and Mr. X demonstrate to mental health specialists how needed their knowledge and skill are in the ED and how they might tailor their technique to its unique characteristics.

For further study, the interested reader is referred to seminal works that bear reading and re-reading, such as *The Practical Art of Suicide Assessment* [12] and *The Psychiatric Interview in Clinical Practice*, both first (1971) and second edition (2006) [22,23].

References

1. Berlin JS, Gudeman J. Interviewing for acuity and the acute precipitant. In: Glick RL, Berlin JS, Fishkind A, Zeller SL, (Eds.). *Emergency Psychiatry: Principles & Practice.* Philadelphia: Lippincott Williams & Wilkins; 2008;93–106.

2. Gabbard GO. *Psychodynamic Psychiatry in Clinical Practice* (4th Edition). Washington, DC: American Psychiatric Publishing, Inc; 2005.

3. Doctor R. Psychodynamic lessons in risk assessment and management. *Adv Psychiatr Treat* 2004;**10**:267–76.

4. Rosenberg RC, Sulkowicz KJ. Psychosocial interventions in the psychiatric emergency service: a skills approach. In: Allen MH, (Ed.). *Emergency Psychiatry.* Washington, DC: American Psychiatric Publishing, Inc; 2002.

5. Castelnuovo-Tedesco P. *The Twenty-minute Hour: A Guide to Brief Psychotherapy for the Physician.* Washington, DC: American Psychiatric Publishing, Inc; 1986.

6. Davanloo H. *Intensive Short-term Psychotherapy with Highly Resistant Patients. I. Handling Resistance. Unlocking the Unconscious: Selected Papers of Habib Davanloo, MD.* New York: Wiley; 1995.

7. Sifneos PE. Alexithymia: past and present. *Am J Psychiatry* 1996;**153** (Suppl):137–42.

8. Rollnick S, Miller WR, Butler CC. *Motivational Interviewing in Health Care: Helping Patients Change Behavior.* New York: Guilford Press; 2007.

9. http://www.samhsa.gov/nctic/trauma.asp National Center for Trauma Informed Care. (Accessed December 28, 2011).

10. *Merriam-Webster On-Line Dictionary*, http://www.merriamwebster.com/dictionary/latent (Accessed December 28, 2011).

11. Freud S. *New Introductory Lectures on Psychoanalysis.* Standard Edition. XXII. London: Hogarth Press; 1953: 70–2.

12. Shea SC. *The Practical Art of Suicide Assessment.* Hoboken, NJ: John Wiley & Sons, Inc; 2002.

13. Bengelsdorf H, Levy LE, Emerson RL, et al. A crisis triage rating scale: brief dispositional assessment of patients at risk for hospitalization. *J Nerv Ment Dis* 1984;**172**:424–30.

14. Freud S. *The Interpretation of Dreams, 1900.* Standard Edition. IV–V. London: Hogarth Press; 1953: 1–627.

15. Samberg E, Marcus ER. Process, resistance, and interpretation. In: Person ES, Cooper AM, Gabbard GO, (Eds.). *Textbook of Psychoanalysis.* Washington, DC: American Psychiatric Publishing, Inc; 2005.

16. Stone L. *The Psychoanalytic Situation: An Examination of its Development and Essential Nature.* Madison, CN: International Universities Press, Inc; 1961.

17. Winnicott DW. *The Maturational Process and the Facilitating Environment.* London: Hogarth Press; 1965.

18. Langs R. *Understanding Unconscious Communication. Workbooks for Psychotherapists,* (Volume I). Emerson, NJ: Newconcept Press, Inc; 1985.

19. Buckley LM. Critical moments – doctors and patients. *N Engl J Med* 2011;**365**:1270–1.

20. Stefan S. *Emergency Department Treatment of the Psychiatric Patient.* New York: Oxford University Press; 2006.

21. Lewis JM. Repairing the bond in important relationships: a dynamic for personality maturation. *Am J Psychiatry* 2000;**157**:1375–8.

22. MacKinnon RA, Michels R. *The Psychiatric Interview in Clinical Practice.* Philadelphia: WB Saunders Co; 1971.

23. MacKinnon RA, Michels R, Buckley PJ. *The Psychiatric Interview in Clinical Practice,* (2nd Edition). Washington, DC: American Psychiatric Publishing, Inc; 2006.

Chapter 5

Use of routine alcohol and drug testing for psychiatric patients in the emergency department

Ross A. Heller and Erin Rapp

Introduction

Emergency physicians and psychiatrists across the country share the burden for the patients presenting to emergency departments with acute psychiatric symptoms and other behavioral emergencies in increasing numbers. Collaboration between clinicians is key to a successful systems-based approach for these sometimes fairly straightforward, and yet sometimes very complex, patients. Psychiatric consultants vary in their requests and expectations for "medical clearance" screening tests before their interview with the patient. The medical literature is full of articles describing what a "medical clearance" physical exam should include. Most emergency physicians (EPs) would agree that a thorough history and physical exam, including a complete neurologic exam, is necessary for clearance; however, the need for laboratory testing is not as clearly outlined or discussed.

Practices vary considerably making it challenging for EPs to decide what is needed for the safe, quality care of these patients without excessive or useless testing. There is evidence both for and against laboratory testing, to include toxicological screening; and various professional societies have varying clinical policies on the topic. By reviewing these policies, the current literature as well as reference texts, this chapter will outline a practical and useful approach to assist clinicians in the rational use of serum and urine drug tests and alcohol measurements as they relate to a psychiatric patient's "medical clearance" exam.

Reasons for drug testing

The number of patients with medical problems that caused and/or contributed to the psychiatric conditions varies considerably among reports in the medical literature. Numbers have been reported as high as 92%. Newly diagnosed medical conditions, medication overdose, drug and alcohol intoxication/withdrawal, infection, central nervous system disease, metabolic conditions, and cardiopulmonary diseases are the most common underlying causes for psychiatric symptoms [1–5]. Based on the high reported incidence of underlying medical explanations for patients' psychiatric symptoms,

laboratory testing is indicated for some patients, particularly patients in which a thorough history and physical exam is limited or impossible, and in the case of new psychiatric complaints. In these instances, drug and alcohol testing can also prove beneficial [6].

In U.S. emergency departments, routine urine drug screens typically identify amphetamines, benzodiazepines, cocaine, cannabis, methadone, opiates, phencyclidine (PCP), and tricyclic antidepressants (TCAs). This urine immunoassay can be completed in 30 minutes. (Serum ethanol, TCA, and other quantitative serum drug levels that may be useful in some patients, such as acetaminophen, aspirin, carbamazepine, depakote, and lithium, are also usually available to the emergency physician and are resulted in most hospital labs in about 1 hour.)

Caution should be used when interpreting urine drug screens. Numerous drugs cross-react with the assays in variable ways from manufacturer to manufacturer, causing false positives. Many drugs within the same class do not react, leading to false negatives. In addition, the findings of the rapid drug screen are only qualitative and do not relay the time of ingestion or amount consumed. Results must be interpreted with a discerning eye and if questions arise, further testing may be required. (See Table 5.1.) These limitations give rise to questions as to the necessity for doing these tests for psychiatric patients presenting to the emergency department.

Any EP can confirm that intoxication and substance abuse can acutely alter patients' behavior, their ability to provide a complete history, and confound the physical examination. Numerous examples of acute psychosis due to drug intoxication are described in the medical literature. Amphetamine toxicity can present with visual hallucinations, as mania, or excited delirium with psychiatric and adrenergic symptoms lasting several hours. Similar but shorter-lived symptoms are seen with cocaine use. PCP is chemically related to ketamine and low doses can result in acute paranoid psychosis with elevated pulse and blood pressure. Neurotoxicity (i.e., reversible psychosis) due to marijuana is a relatively new phenomenon likely due to the recent surge in tetrahydrocannabinol (THC) concentration of marijuana available on the market today.

Behavioral Emergencies for the Emergency Physician, ed. Leslie S. Zun, Lara G. Chepenik, and Mary Nan S. Mallory. Published by Cambridge University Press. © Cambridge University Press 2013.

Table 5.1. Common causes of false +/− on the standard urine drug screen

	False +	False −
Amphetamine	Ephedrine, pseudoephedrine, chloroquine, chlorpromazine	Methylene dioxy methamphetamine ("ecstasy")
PCP	Doxylamine, diphenhydramine, venlafaxine, dextromethorphan, ketamine	
Opiate	Poppy seeds	Hydrocodone, oxycodone, methadone, fentanyl
Benzodiazepine	Oxaprozin, sertraline	Clonazepam, lorazepam
TCA	Cyproheptadine, carbamazepine, thioridazine, chlorpromazine, cyclobenzaprine, quetiapine, diphenhydramine, promethazine, hydroxyzine, cetirizine	
Methadone	Verapamil, diphenhydramine, doxylamine, quetiapine, thioridazine	

Henneman et al. studied 100 patients who presented to their ED with new psychiatric symptoms. All patients had extensive labs, computed tomography brain scans (with the exception of 18 patients who had positive drug screens and resolution of the symptoms), and lumbar punctures if febrile. Results showed 63 had a medical disease, 30 of which were toxicological in nature [4]. While this study had a small enrollment, it is one of the few of its kind that studies patients with new psychiatric symptoms. Currently, the American College of Emergency Physicians (ACEP) recommends basing diagnostic studies on vital signs and your history and physical examination [7]. Special consideration needs to be given to the patients presenting to the emergency department with a first-time episode of psychiatric symptoms or complaints and in particular those patients with difficult examinations or incomplete histories. In these patients, drug and alcohol testing can be invaluable in determining whether the patient's symptoms are due to organic illness or a functional disorder.

In addition to causing behavioral changes, substance abuse, and acute intoxication can confound patients' underlying psychiatric illnesses. One of the most difficult aspects of the focused medical assessment is determining when a patient is not only medically stable but also has the cognitive status suitable for the psychiatric interview. Drug and alcohol testing may help the EP determine whether behavior is likely caused by acute intoxication versus a medical condition versus an acute exacerbation of psychiatric illness as well as guide the timing of reassessments and a reliable mental status examination.

Reasons against drug testing

The current American College of Emergency Physicians' (ACEP) clinical policy on the evaluation of psychiatric patients presenting to the emergency department cites numerous literature sources concluding that laboratory testing is often unnecessary and is often inaccurate [7]. In addition, positive urine drug test results often do not affect outcome or patient disposition. Let's examine these points further.

Korn et al. concluded that patients with primary psychiatric complaints with a negative physical exam and history do not need ancillary testing in the ED after 212 such patients were evaluated with comprehensive lab tests and none were positive [8]. Olshaker et al. found that medical and substance abuse problems could be identified by initial vital signs together with a history and physical exam. Their data suggest that lab and toxicological screens are of low yield [9]. Nice et al. showed that physical examination relating to a drug's toxidrome can detect >80% of acute intoxications, thus eliminating use of drug testing [10].

Rockett et al. studied the validity of declared drug and alcohol use when compared to their toxicological screens. They found that use of eight targeted substances was self-declared in 44% of females and identified in the toxicological screens of 56% of their female test population. In males, 61% reported substance use while 69% of the male test group tested positive for the targeted substances [11]. Perrone et al. also studied the validity of self-reporting drug use when compared with urine drug testing and found that "drug testing alone was never significantly better than the patients' own history." History alone detected substance use in 57% of their patient cohort and drug screening alone detected substance use in 62% [12]. Olshaker et al. found that the reliability of patient self-reported drug use had a sensitivity of 92% and specificity of 91%, while reliability of self-reported alcohol use was 96% sensitive and 87% specific [13].

Schiller et al. found that the results of urine drug tests did not affect disposition or the subsequent length of inpatient stays. Of notice, this study showed that clinicians were extremely accurate in their suspicions of drug use, failing to detect drug use using their clinical gestalt, history, and physical exam in only 10% of patients [14].

Urine drug screening is qualitative and a positive screen may reflect use during the past several days to weeks; thus, results may not account for the current symptoms of the patient. Cocaine detection time is 4–6 days, PCP 1–2 weeks, amphetamines 1–2 weeks, opiates 1 week, marijuana 5 days to 3 weeks. In addition, urine drug screens have numerous interactions with other medications and foods. Antihistamines, venlafaxine, dextromethorphan, and ketamine can result in positive PCP screens. Poppy seeds contain a trace amount of morphine; therefore, ingestion of them can result in a positive opiate urine immunoassay usually within 48 hours of ingestion.

False positives in methadone immunoassays have occurred with verapamil, diphenhydramine, doxylamine, quetiapine, and certain psychotropic drugs [15].

Lastly, each patient's level of cognition should be assessed on an individual basis. Patients regularly abusing alcohol or substances such as benzodiazepines and narcotics may exhibit tolerance. Quantitative serum alcohol levels may not correlate with a patient's degree of intoxication and ability to cooperate with examinations and interviews [16].

Conclusions

When a patient is hemodynamically stable and can provide a history and cooperate with a physical exam and all are consistent with their presentation, routine drug and alcohol testing can be avoided. This should help to alleviate many of the time and financial restraints that reflexive testing creates. ACEP guidelines support the concept that, if the patient is awake, alert and cooperative, routine drug testing does not change ED management. Nonetheless, circumstances exist in which the urine and serum drug and alcohol tests are of use. Rationally applying clinical experience and the available literature to date, laboratory and toxicological testing is indicated for patients with behavioral presentations to the emergency department who are unable to give a thorough history, who are uncooperative with the physical examination, and/or who present with a new psychiatric complaint.

References

1. Bunce DF, Jones LR, Badger LW, Jones SE. Medical illness in psychiatric patients: barriers to diagnosis and treatment. *Southern Med J* 1982;**75**:941–4.

2. Hall RC, Gardner ER, Stickney SK, LeCann AF, Popkin MK. Physical illness manifesting as psychiatric disease. *Arch Gen Psychiatry* 1980;**37**:989–95.

3. Koranyi EK. Morbidity and rate of undiagnosed physical illnesses in a psychiatric clinic population. *Arch Gen Psychiatry* 1979;**36**:414–19.

4. Henneman PL, Mendoza R, Lewis RJ. Prospective evaluation of emergency department medical clearance. *Ann Emerg Med* 1994;**24**:672–7.

5. Hall RC, Gardner ER, Popkin MK, et al. Unrecognized physical illness prompting psychiatric admission: a prospective study. *Am J Psychiatry* 1981;**138**:629–35.

6. Allen MH, Currier GW, Hughes DH, et al. The expert consensus guideline series. Treatment of behavioral emergencies. *Postgrad Med* 2001;S1–88.

7. Lukens TW, Wolf SW, Edlow JA, et al. Clinical policy: critical issues in the diagnosis and management of the adult psychiatric patient in the emergency department. *Ann Emerg Med* 2006;**47**:79–99.

8. Korn CS, Currier GW, Henderson SO. Medical clearance of psychiatric patients without medical complaints in the emergency department. *J Emerg Med* 2000;**18**:173–6.

9. Olshaker JS, Browne B, Jerrard DA, Prendergast H, Stair TO. Medical clearance and screening of psychiatric patients in the emergency department. *Acad Emerg Med* 1997;**4**:124–8.

10. Nice A, Leikin JB, Maturen A, et al. Toxidrome recognition to improve efficiency of emergency urine drug screens. *Ann Emerg Med* 1988;**17**:676–80.

11. Rockett IR, Putnam SL, Jia H, Smith GS. Declared and undeclared substance use among emergency department patients: a population-based study. *Addiction* 2006;**101**:706–12.

12. Perrone J, De Roos F, Jayaraman S, Judd E. Drug screening versus history in detection of substance use in ED psychiatric patients. *Am J Emerg Med* 2001;**19**:49–51.

13. Olshaker JS, Browne B, Jerrard DA, et al. Medical clearance and screening of psychiatric patients in the emergency department. *Acad Emerg Med* 1997;**4**:124–8.

14. Schiller MJ, Shumway M, Batki SL. Utility of routine drug screening in a psychiatric emergency setting. *Psychiatr Serv* 2000;**51**:474–8.

15. Leikin JB. Clinical interpretation of drug testing. *Prim Psychiatry* 2010;**17**:23–7.

16. Emembolu FN, Zun LS. Medical clearance in the emergency department: is testing indicated? *Prim Psychiatry* 2010;**17**:29–34.

Drug intoxication in the emergency department

Jagoda Pasic and Margaret Cashman

Introduction

Substance use is highly prevalent among patients presenting to emergency departments (EDs). According to the Substance Abuse and Mental Health Services Administration (SAMHSA), in 2009, there were approximately 2.1 million drug abuse-related ED visits nationwide [1]. Twenty-seven percent of these visits involved nonmedical use of pharmaceuticals, including prescription drugs, over-the-counter (OTC) medications, and dietary supplements; 21% involved illicit drugs alone; and 14% involved a combination of alcohol with other drugs. Using the same database, one finds that one million visits involved illicit drugs, either alone or in combination with other types of drugs. The most common illicit drugs were: cocaine (422,896 ED visits), marijuana (376,467 ED visits), and heroin (213,118 ED visits). Amphetamine- and methamphetamine-related visits accounted for 93,562 ED visits. Another one million ED visits involved the nonmedical use of pharmaceuticals. Most frequently, these visits involved use of opiate/opioid analgesics such as oxycodone, hydrocodone, and methadone. The largest pharmaceutical increase from 2004 to 2009 was observed for oxycodone (242%).

The majority of drug-related ED visits were made by patients 21 and older (81%). Rates of cocaine are highest among individuals in the 35–44 age group. There are limited data on ethnic differences in substance use. Some studies have reported that African-Americans are more likely to use cocaine than Caucasians [2], while Caucasians are more likely to use methamphetamine than African-Americans [3].

Existing studies typically address substance use in global terms and rarely elaborate on whether a patient presented in ED in a state of intoxication or withdrawal. According to one study, 32% of patients presented in the Psychiatric Emergency Service (PES) in a state of acute alcohol or drug intoxication and 17% had a primary diagnosis of substance abuse or dependence [4]. This study also reported that these patients consumed considerable time and resources, as 64% of the patients were suicidal and 26% were hospitalized.

Psychiatric comorbidity

Substance use complicates differential diagnosis of the ED patient, as substance use can mimic a variety of psychiatric syndromes. For example, in the patient who presents with psychotic symptoms and who recently has used an illicit drug, often it is unclear whether the psychosis is a direct consequence of the substance, or whether the patient has a primary psychotic disorder that coincides with drug use. One study that addressed this issue reported that, in as many as 25% of patients who presented with psychotic symptoms, the PES clinicians attributed psychotic symptoms to a primary psychotic disorder that later was determined to be a substance-induced psychosis. The potential consequences of misdiagnosing psychosis in ED or PES are several-fold: unnecessary hospitalization, inappropriate use of antipsychotics, lack of appropriate follow-up, and inattention to substance use treatment [5].

Substance use is highly prevalent among patients with psychiatric disorders and often drug or alcohol use contributes to frequent ED use. Patients with comorbid psychiatric and substance use disorders have up to 5.6 times greater use of the ED services [6].

Alcohol and substance use disorders are associated with suicide risk [7]. Individuals with a substance use disorder are approximately 6 times more likely to report a lifetime suicide attempt than those without a substance use disorder. One study found particularly high suicidality among cocaine users who presented to a large urban PES [8]. Another study evaluated the relationship of alcohol and drug use and severity of suicidality in patients who were admitted through an urban PES to an acute psychiatric inpatient unit. In the most severely suicidal group, 56% had substance use or dependence [9]. Particularly vulnerable groups for the effects of alcohol and substances include youth (age 12 to 17) and veterans. A recent study showed that veterans with a substance use disorder are approximately 2.3 times more likely to die by suicide than those who are not substance users [10].

There is a strong link between depression and suicidality in individuals with comorbid mood and substance use disorders [11]. Yoon and colleagues [12] reviewed the effect of comorbid

Behavioral Emergencies for the Emergency Physician, ed. Leslie S. Zun, Lara G. Chepenik, and Mary Nan S. Mallory. Published by Cambridge University Press. © Cambridge University Press 2013.

alcohol and drug use disorders (substance use disorders) on premature death in unipolar and bipolar people in the United States. The presence of a comorbid substance use disorder was associated with higher risk for suicide and other unnatural death and also with younger age at time of death in people with unipolar or bipolar mood disorder.

The current conventions in diagnosing comorbid psychiatric disorder and substance use disorder are as follows:

1. Don't list "substance-induced psychosis" or "substance-induced mood disorder" as additional diagnoses when the substance use exacerbates the symptoms of an already-established psychiatric disorder. Simply list the substance use disorder and the psychiatric disorder which was worsened.
2. Examine and contrast the onset of psychiatric symptoms with onset of substance use, as well as examining whether symptoms seem to persist to a robust degree even when the patient is abstinent from the substance, in determining whether to attribute a psychiatric syndrome to the substance use.
3. Most substances of abuse are associated with syndromes which persist even with prolonged abstinence. These syndromes are relatively uncommon, however.

Medical comorbidity

Chronic drug and/or alcohol use significantly increases the likelihood that a person will use an ED for medical treatment [13]. Chronic substance use has deleterious effects on the general health of drug users. For example, injection heroin users are more vulnerable to HIV, hepatitis B and C, abscess at injection sites, avascular necrosis of bone, endocarditis, and renal insufficiency. Cocaine use has been associated with stroke, acute myocardial infarction, dysrhythmias, aortic dissection, seizures, and respiratory problems. Methamphetamine use has been associated with acute renal failure due to rhabdomyolysis.

Service utilization

Substance use disorders are highly prevalent among patients presenting in ED, accounting for 22% of all ED visits [14]. Unintentional poisoning from opiate prescription drugs is a rising problem. According to a Washington State Department of Health report, poisoning death rates have increased by 395% (from 2.1 to 11.3 per 100,000) from 1990 to 2006 and opiate use and misuse seem to be driving this increase [15]. Center for Disease Control and Prevention (CDC) visits to the ED to obtain opioid analgesics for nonmedical uses increased 111% (from 144,600 to 305,900 visits per year) from 2004 to 2008 [16].

Brief interventions

The ED provides a unique opportunity to engage patients about their drug use. Screening, Brief Intervention, Referral to Treatment (SBIRT) was initiated by the SAMHSA in EDs across the United States to identify individuals at risk for drug abuse and provide a brief intervention. The SBIRT programs report a reduction in illicit drug and alcohol abuse six months after the screening. The hope is that the ongoing SBIRT programs will positively impact the progression of addiction and associated medical consequence of drug use, and lower adverse social and healthcare consequences [17].

Drugs of abuse and intoxication

Alcohol

Prevalence and community impact

Alcohol intoxication is the most prevalent of the substance intoxications encountered in the ED. Alcohol use led to over four million ED visits in the single year 2003, according to McCaig and Burt [18]. According to the CDC's Alcohol-Related Disease Impact (ARDI) tool, excessive drinking led annually to 79,646 deaths and 2.3 million years of life lost, in the United States over the years 2001–2005 [19]. Pattern analysis by Stahre et al. [20] suggests that binge drinking accounted for over half of those deaths and two thirds of the years of life lost to excessive drinking.

Binge drinking can be harmful without the drinker being alcohol-dependent. In fact, the majority of binge drinkers are not alcohol-dependent. *Binge drinking* (defined as intake of at least 5 drinks on one occasion for men and at least 4 drinks on one occasion for women) and *heavy drinking* (defined as daily intake of more than 2 drinks for men and more than 1 drink for women) are considered *excessive drinking* [21].

Compared with patients presenting to primary care settings, ED patients are more likely to be drinking alcohol to an excessive and harmful level [22]. Under-age drinking (age 12–20) is a significant factor in ED visits: alcohol caused one third of all substance-related ED visits in that age group [23]. Finally, 36.7% of the 463,000 hospital discharges in 2007 which listed an alcohol-related disorder for the principal (first-listed) condition cited alcoholic psychosis as the principal diagnosis [24].

Management

When a patient presents with suspected alcohol intoxication as part of the clinical presentation, it makes sense to check the BAL (blood alcohol level) early in the evaluation process. If the patient refuses a blood draw, a urine alcohol level is a less accurate but modestly useful method of estimating blood alcohol. The breath alcohol level appears to be less accurate as serum blood alcohol increases, so it is probably unsuitable for ED use [25]. It is important to ask the patient when he or she last drank. A person who drank a large amount just before entering the ED may have sequestered alcohol in the stomach and the BAL will continue to rise as he or she absorbs the bolus. It is also important to ask the patient about any illicit drug use and how recently the substance was used. Note that a highly tolerant individual can appear only modestly impaired at a BAL that would render the alcohol-naive individual unconscious.

Blood alcohol levels will decline at a rate determined by such factors as liver volume, liver health, ethnicity, gender, and whether or not the patient is tolerant to alcohol. Non-tolerant individuals metabolize more slowly than alcohol-tolerant individuals, and women metabolize more slowly than men if their level of tolerance is equal. Individuals with impaired hepatic function will metabolize more slowly. A rate of 0.015–0.02 g/dL per hour is a fair estimate overall of non-tolerant individuals' capacity for metabolizing alcohol. A tolerant individual may metabolize at a rate closer to 0.04 g/dL per hour. Knowing the likely rate, one can estimate how long it will take before the patient is "ready to be seen" for a mental health interview. Emergency physicians and psychiatrists take varying approaches to the timing of a mental health interview for the patient intoxicated with alcohol. No single standard exists, however, the patient should, at a minimum, be clinically assessable. Some follow more objective BAL cut-offs that correlate with established legal limits for driving and that vary by state. In some instances, for legal purposes a BAL of 0 may needed before the interview is completed.

Intoxicated patients may be brought to the ED for assessment after expressing suicidal or, less frequently, homicidal impulses and/or intent, causing disturbance in the community, or unconsciousness. The mental health exam should be completed once the patient is decisional. Suicidal or homicidal ideation may be disavowed once the patient is sober. If the patient continues to endorse suicidal or homicidal ideation after sobering, the patient should be assessed and managed accordingly.

Physical findings in the chronically over-drinking individual include conjunctival injection; abnormal skin vascularization, evident on face and neck; tongue tremor; hand tremor; hepatomegaly. Laboratory findings may include high mean red cell volume (MCV) on the complete blood count; elevated serum aspartate amino transferase (AAT); and elevated serum gamma-glutamyl transferase (GGT). The serum carbohydrate-deficient transferrin (CDT) assay also is sensitive to heavy drinking and is not affected by comorbid liver disease.

If the patient shows up-gaze paresis along with confusion, one should be concerned particularly with acute thiamine deficiency-associated Wernicke's encephalopathy. In such a situation, thiamine should be administered immediately (100 mg IV or IM) and supplemented daily with oral 100-mg doses for at least 3 days. One needs to keep in mind that high utilizers of the ED services in a state of alcohol intoxication may end up receiving high doses of thiamine, and exhibit sign of thiamine intoxication such as dysrhythmia, hypotension, headache, weakness, and seizures.

One should also keep in mind the possibility for an alcohol-intoxicated patient to have suffered a traumatic brain injury, typically from falling, before arriving at the ED. The resulting confusion could be mistaken for simple intoxication. Alcoholic psychosis may recur during subsequent episodes of alcohol intoxication. If the patient experiences a sub-acute or chronic psychosis, management with an antipsychotic medication is indicated. The assessment and management of alcohol withdrawal states in the ED is covered elsewhere in this text.

As we noted above, the ED is a critical platform for engaging alcohol-affected patients in alcohol use screening, brief intervention, and referral (SBIRT). The sobered patient can be evaluated using principles derived from motivational enhancement interviewing. The ED visit provides an excellent opportunity for brief interventions in a potentially teachable moment, focused on preparing the patient for reassessing his or her substance use and its more harmful effects. Brief interventions in the ED can lead to a reduction in harmful substance use, and this is supported by a wide body of clinical research evidence (e.g., Walton et al. [26]). Referral to more specialized treatment services, when appropriate, is another key service the ED can provide. Resources for alcohol screening and brief intervention training are available at the SAMHSA website, http://www.samhsa.gov/.

Opiates

Unless opioid intoxication occurs in the context of accidental or intentional overdose, patients rarely come to the ED in a state of opioid intoxication *per se*. Opioid abusers, however, are more likely to seek ED services in the state of opioid withdrawal. Individuals who abuse opioids typically receive medical attention because of medical complications of drug use, withdrawal, or overdose. Opioid intoxication is suspected when a patient has pupillary constriction and symptoms of slurred speech, drowsiness, and impaired attention and memory. Opioid overdose is a medical emergency and patients with the triad of symptoms – pinpoint pupils, respiratory depression, and altered sensorium/coma, warrant emergency administration of naloxone (i.v., i.m., s.q.) The usual initial dose is 0.4 to 2 mg. If the desired degree of counteraction and improvement in respiratory function is not obtained it may be repeated at 2- to 3-minute intervals. Opioid withdrawal, in contrast, is rarely fatal, but the comfort of the patient may be helped by appropriate use of an opiate withdrawal regimen.

Prescription opiate use has become increasingly prevalent among patients presenting in ED and the most commonly abused drugs include hydromorphone (Dilaudid), hydrocodone (in Vicodin), oxycodone (Oxycontin, and in Percocet) oxymorphone (Opana), although methadone also is commonly abused.

Sedative hypnotics

Benzodiazepines

Benzodiazepines are sedative, hypnotic, and anxiolytic agents that are typically referred to by drug uses as "downers".

According to the Drug Abuse Warning Network (DAWN) report, drug-related ED involving benzodiazepines increased by 41% from 1995 to 2002, and alprazolam (Xanax^{TM}) and clonazepam (Klonopin^{TM}) were the most frequently reported as the drugs of abuse [27]. While opiates most often are associated with accidental overdose, benzodiazepines are the most frequently ingested prescription medications in suicide attempts.

The symptoms of benzodiazepine intoxication are similar to alcohol intoxication and they include altered level of consciousness, drowsiness, confusion, impaired judgment, slow and slurred speech, incoordination, ataxia. Severe intoxication/overdose can lead to coma, respiratory depression, and death. Benzodiazepine overdose patients are typically managed in ED with supportive care such as maintenance of adequate ventilation and hydration. In contrast to the role in iatrogenic over-sedation, caution is advised regarding the utility of flumazenil, the benzodiazepine antidote, in a chronic user, as it may precipitate withdrawal symptoms, including seizures.

Benzodiazepine withdrawal is a serious medical emergency due to risk of seizures, peripheral nervous system and electrolyte instability (due to profuse diaphoresis), and acute anxiety syndrome with restlessness and insomnia. Patients with acute anxiety due to benzodiazepine withdrawal are often seen and managed in the psychiatric emergency service.

Barbiturates

Barbiturates are used to treat various seizure disorders. They are classified based on their duration of action: ultra-short acting, short acting, intermediate acting, and long acting. Barbiturate intoxication causes various CNS depression symptoms that are similar to alcohol and benzodiazepine intoxication including nystagmus, vertigo, slurred speech, lethargy, confusion, ataxia, and respiratory depression. Severe overdose may result in coma, shock, apnea, and hypothermia. In combination with alcohol or other CNS depressants, barbiturates have additive CNS and respiratory depression effects.

Barbiturate withdrawal is life threatening, with signs and symptoms developing within 24 hours. Patients may present to the ED with insomnia, restlessness, and severe anxiety.

Gamma-hydroxybutyrate (GHB)

GHB is known as a dietary supplement that gained popularity as a "club drug" in late 1990s and early 2000s. Sporadically, GHB is a drug of abuse leading to an ED visit. GHB, also referred to as "liquid ecstasy", is a powerful CNS depressant and the effects of intoxication are profound alteration of mental status and respiratory depression. Deaths have been reported with severe GHB intoxication [28]. GHB discontinuation can lead to a significant withdrawal syndrome that is similar to sedative/hypnotic and alcohol withdrawal. With appropriate management, most patients fully recover within 6 hours. Nevertheless, the challenge lies in the recognition and detection of GHB, because routine toxicology screening does not detect this substance [29].

Stimulants

Cocaine

As noted above, cocaine is the most common illegal substance that leads to ED visits, which in 2009 accounted for 162 visits per 100,000 [1]. Cocaine is a stimulant with powerful effects on the central and peripheral nervous system which acts by blocking the reuptake of dopamine, norepinephrine, and serotonin. It also modulates the endogenous opiate system. Cocaine intoxication leads to several physical signs and symptoms, such as: hypertension, tachycardia, chest pain, myocardial infarction (MI), mydriasis, diaphoresis, delirium, stroke, and seizures. Acute cocaine intoxication may present with anxiety, agitation, paranoia, hallucinations, feeling of increased energy, alertness, intense euphoria, and decreased tiredness, appetite and sleep.

Cocaine may be smoked, inhaled, injected, and orally ingested. The onset, peak, and duration of cocaine's effects vary depending on the route of administration (see Table 6.1). The fastest absorption and the peak effect are after inhalation. Repeated cocaine users may use it as frequently as every 10 minutes, may binge with it for as long as 7 days, and may use as much as 10 grams per day.

Chest pain due to cardiac ischemia is the most frequent cocaine-related medical event for which patients seek treatment in inner-city EDs [30]. The most frequently occurring cardiac complications of cocaine are syncope, angina pectoris, and MI. In some instances, the outcome is acute cardiac death. The typical patient with cardiac-related MI is a young man without cardiovascular risk factors other than smoking. The relative risk of MI is elevated 24 times within 60 minutes after cocaine use, and the incidence of MI is approximately 6% [31]. There have been recent reports of fever and severe agranulocytosis, associated with cocaine which had been adulterated with levamisole [32].

Psychiatric symptoms are prominent in cocaine intoxication and accounted for approximately 30% of cocaine-related presentations compared to 16% and 17% for cardiopulmonary and neurologic symptoms, respectively. Suicidal intent was the most common psychiatric reason for presentation [33]. Psychiatric manifestations of cocaine intoxication include anxiety, agitation, euphoria, and intense paranoia, while depression and suicidal thoughts often accompany acute cocaine withdrawal. Excessive tearfulness has been described as a distinct

Table 6.1. Cocaine: onset of effects, peak effects, and duration of euphoria by route of administration

Route	Onset	Peak effect (min)	Duration (min)
Inhalation	7 sec	1–5	20
Intravenous	15 sec	3–5	20–30
Nasal	3 min	15	45–90
Oral	10 min	60	60

sign of cocaine-induced depression in patients presenting in a busy urban PES [34].

A typical patient with cocaine-related psychiatric symptoms presents to the ED in the early morning hours after a binge, in a state of high adrenergic dysregulation, dysphoric and suicidal, with injected conjunctiva, asking for food and promptly falling asleep. Disposition of such patients may be a challenge due to their suicidality [35].

The treatment of cocaine intoxication is determined by the presenting symptoms. Chest pain warrants a medical workup for cardiac complications. Such patients often receive hydration and benzodiazepine or other sedating agents to reduce anxiety. In patients who are severely agitated or intensely paranoid, treatment with oral or intramuscular antipsychotic medication may be needed.

Methamphetamine

While in the early 2000s, there was a nation-wide methamphetamine epidemic, according to recent reports, ED visits involving methamphetamine have been on the decline. In 2004, methamphetamine use accounted for 8.2% of all ED visits that involved drugs, and in 2008 this dropped to 3.3% [1]. Although overall methamphetamine use has decreased nationally, it remains a serious health concern.

Like cocaine, methamphetamine exerts powerful stimulant effects on the brain, but the effects last longer than after cocaine use, giving rise to more pronounced medical and psychiatric symptoms. Methamphetamine intoxication can lead to serious medical consequences including hypertension, arrhythmias, MI, stroke, acute renal failure due to rhabdomyolysis, seizure, delirium, and death. Psychiatric consequences include: psychosis; mania-like symptoms; severe agitation; and violence. Psychosis is the most common presenting symptom (80%) in patients who are seen in PES. These patients were most often Caucasians (75%) referred by police, with an extended duration of stay in ED [3]. By clinical observation, patients most often present in a state that has been described by the term "tweaking," a state of high arousal, agitation, and uncontrollable movements, with prominent dysphoria, hallucinations, and paranoia.

Due to their extreme agitation, patients with methamphetamine intoxication often are treated with sedating agents (benzodiazepines), alone or in combination with antipsychotic agents. There are regional differences that dictate the usage of physical restraints and involuntary administration of medications in methamphetamine-intoxicated patients. However, it is important to keep in mind that such patients are highly distressed and are fairly likely to accept medications voluntarily, particularly if the medication is offered in a rapidly dissolvable form such as olanzapine (Zydis^{TM}) or risperidone (M-Tab^{TM}) [3]. As in treating cocaine-intoxicated patients in the ED, methamphetamine-intoxicated patients may need intravenous rehydration to correct electrolyte imbalance and acute renal insufficiency.

Ecstasy (3,4-methylenedioxymethamphetamine – MDMA)

Ecstasy is known as a "club drug" and typically it is used by young individuals in parties, raves, and clubs. A recent survey of ED admissions in Israel reported that most admissions happened at night (68%), half of them on weekends (52%) and 44% of use occurred in the context of clubs and parties [36]. Although ecstasy accounts for only approximately 1–4% of all drug-related ED visits, according to the DAWN's latest report, ecstasy-related ED visits increased by 100% from 2004 to 2009 [37].

Ecstasy is a powerful indirect releaser of serotonin and a moderate releaser of dopamine. Regarded by most users as a harmless substance, the acute effects of MDMA intoxication are an increase in energy and a sense of empathy. Its psychiatric effects include blunting of the senses, confusion, lack of judgment, depression, anxiety, anger, paranoia, hallucinations, and aggression. Three factors make individual responses to ecstasy quite unpredictable: (1) It is consumed orally in the form of tablets of varying potency which may be adulterated with other substances, such as ketamine or amphetamines [38]. (2) Genetic polymorphism leads to large variation in the activity of certain enzymes of the two metabolic pathways involved in breaking down ingested ecstasy: the hepatic enzyme CYP2D6 and the COMT enzyme. This means that some individuals will lack a dose–response relationship after ingesting ecstasy, so that a toxic response may not relate to the amount taken. (3) Most ecstasy users also use an array of other drugs (particularly cocaine) and alcohol and the combined substances can interact [39]. Ecstasy may also interact fatally with prescribed medications, such as antiretroviral medications (which inhibit CYP2D6), and SSRI antidepressants (leading to the serotonin syndrome).

Ecstasy intoxication can lead to serious medical complications such as hypertension, tachycardia, rhabdomyolysis with acute renal failure, and hyperthermia. Ecstasy users may present in a hyperactive delirious state. ED staff must be alert to addressing serotonin syndrome, which can be precipitated by the patient's concurrent use of stimulant drugs. Most standard urine drug screen tests have low sensitivity for MDMA, so the ecstasy level needs to be quite high to show a positive test.

"Bath salts"

Recently there has been increased attention to a new generation of designer drugs, the so-called "bath salts". These products were sold legally online under a variety of names, such as "Ivory Wave", "White Lightning" and "Vanilla Sky", but in 2011, the Drug Enforcement Agency (DEA) declared "bath salts" to be a controlled substance. Use of such products has led to an increasing number of ED visits and overdoses throughout the country. These products contain amphetamine-like substances such as methyleneoxypyrovalerone, mephedrone, and methylone. Ingesting or snorting bath salts can cause arrhythmias, chest pain, MI, hypertension, hyperthermia, seizure, stroke, aggressive and violent behavior, hallucinations, paranoia and delusions, and in extreme cases, death. Bath salts rapidly absorb after oral ingestion with intoxication peaking at 1.5 hours and lasting for 3–4 hours. Patients who are intoxicated on bath salts may require physical restraints and high doses of sedatives because of the risk of harming themselves or others. Treatment includes hydration to address emerging rhabdomyolysis and benzodiazepines to control seizures [40].

Methylphenidate

Methylphenidate is a CNS stimulant used for the treatment of attention-deficit/hyperactive disorder. The primary abusers are young individuals (<25 years of age) who obtain the drug from a friend or a classmate. Other abusers may obtain it from a fraudulent prescription or doctor shopping. According to DAWN, nonmedical use of methylphenidate accounted for an estimated 4,953 visits to the ED in 2009, which was more than twice the estimated 2,446 visits in 2004. Acute intoxication with methylphenidate results in symptoms similar to those seen with cocaine, including euphoria, delirium, confusion, paranoia, and hallucinations. Additional symptoms may include extreme anger, threats, or aggressive behavior.

Hallucinogens and dissociative agents

Phencyclidine (PCP)

Since phencyclidine entered the market in 1957 as a dissociative anesthetic, it has become a significant drug of abuse, due to its psychotropic effects. In 2008, PCP was responsible for over 37,200 emergency department visits in the U.S. It is smoked (usually in a mix with marijuana) or, less often, ingested orally. Low doses cause an acute confusional state with excited delirium lasting several hours; stimulant effects predominate. Larger doses cause nystagmus, muscle rigidity, ataxia, stereotyped movements, hypertension, hypersalivation, sweating, amnesia, and an agitated psychosis. The psychotic state induced by phencyclidine is so similar to that of schizophrenia that intermittent administration of phencyclidine has become a standard pharmacological model for schizophrenia in the laboratory.

Unfortunately, PCP is relatively easy and inexpensive to manufacture illicitly. Marijuana has replaced alcohol as the most common secondary substance of abuse in phencyclidine abusers who present for medical attention.

The PCP user is managed conservatively in the ED by keeping the patient physically safe and providing reduced stimulation. An early check for emerging rhabdomyolysis is advisable, and hydration should be maintained.

Ketamine

Ketamine, or the street named "K", "Special K", "Kitkat", "Vitamin K", is a powerful dissociative anesthetic that produces similar effects to phencyclidine but with a shorter duration. The common presenting complaints include prominent anxiety, chest pain and palpitations, and common findings include confusion, amnesia, mydriasis, bi-directional nystagmus, tachycardia, rigidity, seizures, and usually short-lived hallucinations. The most common complication of ketamine intoxication is severe agitation and rhabdomyolysis. Symptoms are typically short lived and patients most often are discharged within 5 hours of presentation [41]. Ketamine intoxication is managed with benzodiazepines to mitigate the anxiety and agitation. Lorazepam, 1–2 mg orally or IV, is the mainstay of treatment.

Lysergic acid (LSD)

LSD is not a common drug of abuse. However, its abuse is prevalent among high school students. National Institute on Drug Addiction data for 2008 revealed that 4.0% of high school seniors had used LSD at least once in their life, with 2.7% having used it within the past year.

Typically it is ingested in pill form or dissolved on a piece of paper. The signs and symptoms of intoxication develop within an hour after ingestion and include tachycardia, hypertension, hyperthermia and dilated pupils, distorted perception of time, and depersonalization. LSD is associated with the unique sensory misperception called synesthesia, whereby colors are "heard" and noises are "seen". These symptoms usually clear 8–12 hours after ingestion, although feelings of "numbness" may last for several days [42].

ED presentations typically include manifestations of the intense anxiety, such as a panic attack ("bad trip"), and can be managed with reassurance and in some instances, lorazepam or diazepam. Other presenting symptoms include delirium with hallucinations, delusions and paranoia. Occasionally, a patient may present to the ED with ongoing psychotic symptoms, long after the drug was eliminated from the system, or with the spontaneous recurrence of drug effects, known as "flashbacks". While death from an overdose of LSD is rare, ingestion of high doses carry significantly higher risk of death due to convulsions, hyperthermia, and cardiovascular collapse.

Mescaline, from the Peyote cactus, and and psilocybin/psilocin, psychoactive ingredient in Psilocybin mushrooms, are also hallucinogens. Frequency of use is really unknown because ED visits for intoxication are uncommon. The effects of intoxication are similar to LSD.

Dextromethorphan

Dextromethorphan (DXM) is a cough suppressant that is found in many over-the-counter cough and cold preparations, such as Coricidin™, Nyquil™ and Robitussin™. Some popular street names for DXM include "Tripple C", "Candy", "Dex", "Robo", "Rojo", and "Tussin". According to DAWN reports, DXM accounts for approximately 1% of all drug-related ED visits. However, the significance of DXM misuse is that 50% of such ED visits are made by youth, age 12–20 years. Structurally related to the opiate receptor antagonist codeine, its metabolite dextrorphan exhibits serotonergic activity and inhibits NMDA receptors. Its unique mechanism of action results in psychotropic effects that are similar to ketamine and phencyclidine. Neurobehavioral effects of DXM typically begin shortly after the ingestion (30–60 minutes) and persist for up to 6 hours. DXM intoxication leads to a combination of euphoric, stimulant dissociative and sedative effects, and neurological signs such as ataxia, dystonia mydriasis, nystagmus, and coma. It also causes nausea and vomiting, diaphoresis, hypertension, tachycardia, and respiratory depression. In rare instances, DXM has been associated with the development of serotonin syndrome. To address these dangers, the American Association of Poison Control Center has developed practice guidelines for the management of DXM poisoning/intoxication [43].

Inhalants

Inhalants and inhalant use disorders recently were the subject of a comprehensive review by Howard et al. [44]. Inhalants are substances that produce a psychoactive effect when their vapors are inhaled, rarely abused by any other means. These substances include **aerosols** (containing propellants and solvents), **gases** (e.g., nitrous oxide), **volatile solvents** (liquids that vaporize at room temperature, such as correction fluid, paint thinner, dry-cleaning fluids, and glues), and **nitrites**. Common household products often are a source for the first three types of inhalants. This makes the inhalants a particular problem among early- to mid-adolescents, who may not have easy access to other substances of abuse [45]. Inhalant use appears to have decreased among 8th to 12th grade students in the U.S.A. over the past 15 or more years, according to the most recent Monitoring the Future study results (Institute for Social Research, 2010). This is not, however, an invitation to complacency. In 2006–2008, nearly 7% of 12-year olds had reported using an inhalant to get high, above the rate for cigarettes and marijuana usage. In fact, only alcohol had a higher rate of use for 12-year olds [46]. The first three types of inhalants act directly on the central nervous system.

The fourth type of inhalant, the *nitrites* (e.g., amyl nitrite, isobutyl nitrite), are abused by adults and older teens, for the most part, with a goal of enhancing sexual experience. Unlike the first three types of inhalant, nitrites relax muscle and dilate blood vessels. Known as "poppers" or "snappers," abuse of nitrites is linked to unsafe sexual practices and increasing the risk of contracting and spreading hepatitis and HIV.

Inhalants enter the bloodstream rapidly and produce intoxication effects within seconds of inhalation. The common methods for using inhalants are listed in Table 6.2. The short-term effects may include initial euphoria, dizziness, impaired coordination, slurred speech, loss of inhibition, hallucinations, and delusions. Users often deal with the short duration of intoxication by inhaling repeatedly, which can lead to decreased level of consciousness and death. After repetitive use within the span of a few minutes, an inhalant user may be drowsy for several hours. Headache often accompanies repetitive inhalation.

Table 6.2. Common methods of inhalant abuse

"Sniffing" or "snorting" fumes from containers
Spraying aerosol directly into the nose or mouth
"Bagging" – sniffing or inhaling fumes from substances sprayed or deposited inside a plastic or paper bag
"Huffing" – inhaling from an inhalant-soaked rag stuffed in the mouth
Inhaling from balloons filled with nitrous oxide

From National Institute on Drug Abuse (NIDA) Research Report Series 2010. "Inhalant Abuse." *NIH Publication Number 10–3818*, revised July 2010.

Several common inhalants (butane, propane, freon, trichloroethylene, amyl nitrite, butyl nitrite) are linked to "sudden sniffing death syndrome." Chronic abuse of volatile solvents can lead to demyelination and clinical syndromes resembling multiple sclerosis. Such neurologic functions as movement, vision, hearing, and cognition can be affected. In the worst cases, dementia is the result. Hepatoxicity, cardiomyopathy, impaired immune function, lung and kidney damage all can result from inhalant abuse. In earlier stages, such damage may be partially or even completely reversible. There are concerns about prenatal exposure to inhalants, as well [47].

Cannabinoids

The increasing medicalization of marijuana has thrown a new wrinkle into our understanding of the costs and benefits of marijuana's use. As Nussbaum and colleagues [48] point out, medicalization (typically, for severe pain or severe nausea and vomiting associated with chemotherapy) often encourages regular use. Such steady use can tip the balance so that what might have been a relatively minor contributor to psychiatric problems becomes more substantial. In some patients, for example, increased marijuana use can be associated with increased impulsivity and suicidality, with or without a pre-existing depression [49].

The acute effects of marijuana intoxication such as sedation, failure to consolidate short-term memory, altered sense of time, perceptual changes, decreased coordination, and impaired executive functioning are commonly seen. There is solid evidence that patients with schizophrenia who use cannabis experience a more severe course of illness [50]. Patients with recent-onset psychosis who use cannabis regularly have more severe psychotic symptoms and more cognitive disorganization than comparable patients who do not use cannabis [51].

Cannabis dependence is associated with physiological tolerance and a physiological withdrawal syndrome. Symptoms may appear as early as a day after discontinuation and last 1 to 3 weeks. Withdrawal symptoms include craving, irritability, anger, dysphoric mood, restlessness, insomnia, and diminished appetite. Treatment relies on psychosocial therapies such as motivational interviewing, specific cognitive–behavioral therapy, and contingency management.

Further complicating our understanding of cannabinoids in the ED, synthetic cannabinoids (e.g., "Spice" products or "K2") are a rapidly emerging class of drugs of abuse [52]. Adverse effects reported with these synthetic cannabinoids are listed in Table 6.3. To date, at least 10 different plant species are being used in the manufacture of these substances, and the potency, duration of action, and potential for unexpected toxicity is variable as well. These products will not show up on current urine toxicological screens.

Conclusion

Drug intoxication is commonly involved in ED visits, and patients may present with a variety of medical and psychiatric complaints. Drug intoxication complicates clinical presentation and can lead to prolonged ED length-of-stay, deployment of resources, including the use of restraints in severe intoxication syndromes, and creates a challenge for disposition and treatment. Clinicians who work in the ED setting, both emergency medicine physicians and psychiatrists, should be familiar with the *toxidromes* of the common drugs of abuse to: (1) make an appropriate diagnosis, (2) provide emergency management, including appropriate psychiatric and substance-use assessment and administration of medications, (3) refer to a short-term treatment that may include detoxification or admission into the hospital, or (4) refer to a longer-term treatment in the community.

Table 6.3. Adverse clinical effects reported with synthetic cannabinoids

Central nervous system	Seizures
	Agitation
	Irritability
	Loss of consciousness
	Anxiety
	Confusion
	Paranoia
Cardiovascular	Tachycardia
	Hypertension
	Chest pain
	Cardiac ischemia
Metabolic	Hypokalemia
	Hyperglycemia
Gastrointestinal	Nausea
	Vomiting
Autonomic	Fever
	Mydriasis
Other	Conjunctivitis

From Seely KA, Prather PL, James LP, Moran JH. Marijuana-based drugs: innovative therapeutics or designer drugs of abuse? *Mol Interv* 2011;11:36–51.

References

1. Center for Behavioral Health Statistics and Quality. *The DAWN Report: Highlights of the 2009 Drug Abuse Warning Network (DAWN) Findings on Drug-related Emergency Department Visits.* Rockville, MD: Substance Abuse and Mental Health Services Administration, Center for Behavioral Health Statistics and Quality; 2010 December 28. Available at: http://www.oas.samhsa.gov/2k10/DAWN034/EDHighlights.htm (Accessed February 14, 2012).

2. Schiller MJ, Shumway M, Batki SL. Patterns of substance use among patients in an urban psychiatric emergency service. *Psychiatr Serv* 2000;51:113–15.

3. Pasic J, Russo J, Ries R, Roy-Byrne P. Methamphetamine users presenting to psychiatric emergency services: a case-control study. *Am J Drug Alcohol Abuse* 2007;33:675–86.

4. Breslow RE, Klinger BI, Erickson BJ. Acute intoxication and substance abuse among patients presenting to a psychiatric emergency service. *Gen Hosp Psychiatry* 2006;18:183–91.

5. Schanzer BM, First MB, Dominquez B, Hosin DS, Caton CIM. Diagnosing psychotic disorders in the emergency department in the context of substance use. *Psychiatr Serv* 2006;57:1468–73.

6. Curran GM, Sullivan G, Williams K, et al. The association of psychiatric comorbidity and use of the emergency department among persons with substance use disorders: an observational cohort study. *BMC Emerg Med* 2008;8:17.

7. Wilcox HC, Conner KR, Caine ED. Association of alcohol and drug use disorders: an empirical review of cohort studies. *Drug Alcohol Depend* 2008;76 (Suppl):S11–9.

8. Garlow SJ, Purlselle D, D'Orio B. Cocaine use disorders and suicidal ideation. *Drug Alcohol Depend* 2003;70:101–4.

9. Ries RK, Yuodelis-Flores C, Roy-Byrne P, Nilssen O, Russo J. Addiction and suicidal behavior in acute psychiatric inpatients. *Compr Psychiatry* 2009;50:93–9.

10. Ilgen MA, Bohnert AS, Ignacio RV, et al. Psychiatric diagnosis and risk of suicide in veterans. *Arch Gen Psychiatry* 2010;67:1152–8.

11. Conner KR, Pinquart M, Gamble SA. Meta-analysis of depression and substance use among individuals with alcohol use disorder. *J Subst Abuse Treat* 2009;37:127–37.

12. Yoon YC, Chiung M, Yi H, Moss HB. Effect of comorbid alcohol and drug use disorders on premature death among unipolar and bipolar disorder decedents in the United States, 1999 to 2006. *Compr Psychiatry* 2011;52:453–64.

13. McGeary KA, French MT. Illicit drug use and emergency room utilization. *Health Serv Res* 2000;35:153–69.

14. Larkin GL, Claassen CA, Emond JA, Pelletier AJ, Camargo CA. Trends in U.S. emergency department visits for mental health conditions, 1992 to 2001. *Psychiatr Serv* 2005;56:671–7.

15. Washington State Department of Health. *Poisoning and Drug Overdose.* Olympia (WA) 2008. Available at:

http://doh.wa.gov/hsqa/emstrauma/injury/pubs/icpg/DOH530090Poison.pdf (Accessed February 14, 2012).

16. Centers for Disease Control and Prevention (CDC). Emergency department visits involving nonmedical use of selected prescription drugs – United States, 2004–2008. *Morb Mortal Wkly Rep (MMWR)* 2010;**59**:705–9.

17. Madras BK, Compton WM, Avula D, et al. Screening, brief interventions, referral to treatment (SBIRT) for illicit drug and alcohol use at multiple healthcare sites: comparison at intake and six months. *Drug Alcohol Depend* 2009;**99**:280–95.

18. McCaig LF, Burt CW. National hospital ambulatory medical care survey: 2003 emergency department summary. *Adv Data* 2005;**358**:1–38. Available at: http://www.cdc.gov/nchs/data/ad/ad358.pdf (Accessed February 14, 2012).

19. Centers for Disease Control and Prevention (CDC). *Alcohol Related Disease Impact* [Internet]. 2008 Available at: http://apps.nccd.cdc.gov/DACH_ARDI/Default.aspx (Accessed February 14, 2012).

20. Centers for Disease Control and Prevention (CDC). Alcohol-attributable deaths and years of potential life lost due to excessive alcohol use in the U.S. *Morb Mortal Wkly Rep (MMWR)* 2004;**53**:866–70.

21. National Institute of Alcohol Abuse and Alcoholism. NIAAA council approves definition of binge drinking. *NIAAA Newsletter* 2004;**3**:3. Available at: http://pubs.niaaa.nih.gov/publications/Newsletter/winter2004/Newsletter_Number3.pdf (Accessed February 14, 2012).

22. Cherpitel CJ. Drinking patterns and problems: a comparison of primary care with the emergency room. *Subst Abuse* 1999;**20**:85–95.

23. Center for Behavioral Health Statistics and Quality. *The DAWN Report: Trend in Emergency Department Visits Involving Underage Alcohol Use: 2005 to 2009.* Rockville, MD: Substance Abuse and Mental Health Services Administration, Center for Behavioral Health Statistics and Quality; 2011 September 13. Available at: www.samhsa.gov/data/2k11/WEB.../WEB_DAWN_020_HTML.pdf (Accessed February 14, 2012).

24. Chen CM, Yi H. *Surveillance Report #89: Trends in Alcohol-related Morbidity Among Short-stay Community Hospital Discharges, United States, 1979–2007.* Bethesda, MD: National Institute on Alcohol Abuse and Alcoholism; 2002. Available at: pubs.niaaa.nih.gov/publications/surveillance89/HDS07.pdf (Accessed February 14, 2012).

25. Currier GW, Trenton AJ, Walsh PG. Innovations: emergency psychiatry: relative accuracy of breath and serum alcohol readings in the psychiatric emergency service. *Psychiatr Serv* 2006;**57**:34–6.

26. Walton MA, Chermack ST, Shope JT, et al. Effects of a brief intervention for reducing violence and alcohol misuse among adolescents. *JAMA* 2010;**304**:527–35.

27. *Addiction Benzodiazepines.* SAMHSA (DAWN) Drug Abuse Reports 2009 [Internet]. 2012 January 8. Available at: http://addictionbenzodiazepines.com/samhsa-dawn-drug-abuse-reports-2009/ (Accessed February 14, 2012).

28. Galicia M, Nogue S, Miro O. Liquid ecstasy intoxication: clinical features of 505 consecutive emergency department patients. *Emerg Med J* 2011;**28**:462–6.

29. Mason PE, Kerns WP. GAMMA hydroxybutyric acid (GHB) intoxication. *Acad Emerg Med* 2002;**9**:730–9.

30. Wryobeck JM, Walton MA, Curran GM, Massey LS, Booth BM. Complexities of cocaine users presenting to the emergency department with chest pain: interactions between depression symptoms, alcohol, and race. *J Addict Med* 2007;**4**:213–21.

31. Vroegop MP, Franssen EJ, van den Voort PHJ, et al. The emergency care of cocaine intoxications. *Neth J Med* 2009;**67**:122–6.

32. Zhu NY, Legatt DF, Turner AR. Agranulocytosis after consumption of cocaine adulterated with levamisole. *Ann Intern Med* 2009;**150**:287–9.

33. Rich JA, Singer DE. Cocaine-related symptoms in patients presenting to an urban emergency department. *Ann Emerg Med* 1991;**20**:616–21.

34. Zarkowski P, Pasic J, Russo J, Roy-Byrne P. Excessive tears: a diagnostic sign for cocaine-induced mood disorder? *Compr Psychiatry* 2007;**48**:252–6.

35. Pasic J, Ries R. *Cocaine Users Presenting in Psychiatric Emergency Services.* Proceedings of the 20th U.S. Psychiatric Congress; 2007 Oct 11–14; Orlando, FL.

36. Halpern P, Moskovich J, Avrahami B, et al. Morbidity associated with MDMA (ecstasy) abuse: a survey of emergency department admissions. *Hum Exp Toxicol* 2010;**30**:259–66.

37. Center for Behavioral Health Statistics and Quality. *The DAWN Report: Emergency Department Visits Involving Ecstasy.* Rockville, MD: Substance Abuse and Mental Health Services Administration, Center for Behavioral Health Statistics and Quality; 2011 March 24. Available at: http://www.oas.samhsa.gov/2k11/DAWN027/Ecstasy.htm (Accessed February 14, 2012).

38. Parrott AC. Is ecstasy MDMA? A review of the proportion of ecstasy tablets containing MDMA, their dosage levels, and the changing perceptions of purity. *Psychopharmacology (Berl)* 2004;**173**:234–41.

39. Schifano F. A bitter pill: overview of ecstasy (MDMA, MDA) related fatalities. *Psychopharmacology (Berl)* 2004;**173**:242–8.

40. Ross EA, Watson M, Goldberger B. "Bath Salts" intoxication. *N Engl J Med* 2011;**365**:967–8.

41. Hoffman RJ. Ketamine Poisoning. In: Basow DS, (Ed.). *UpToDate.* Waltham, MA: UpToDate; 2012.

42. Passie T, Halpern JH, Stichtenoth DO, Emrich HM, Hintzen A. The pharmacology of lysergic acid diethylamide: a review. *CNS Neurosci Ther* 2008;**14**:295–314.

43. Chyka PA, Erdman AR, Manoguerra AS, et al. Dextromethorphan poisoning: an evidence-based consensus guideline for out-of-hospital management. *Clin Toxicol (Phila)* 2007;**45**:662–7.

44. Howard MO, Bowen SE, Garlan EL, Perron BE, Vaughn MG. Inhalant use and inhalant use disorders in the United States. *Addict Sci Clin Pract* 2011;**6**:18–31.

45. Garland EL, Howard MO, Vaughn MG, Perron BE. Volatile substance misuse in the United States. *Subst Use Misuse* 2011;**46**(Suppl 1):8–20.

46. Office of Applied Studies (*OAS*) *Spotlight: 12 Year Olds More Likely to Use Inhalants Than Cigarettes or Marijuana.* Rockville, MD: Substance Abuse and Mental Health

Services Administration, Office of Applied Studies; 2010 March 11 [cited 2012 February 14]. Available at: http://www.oas.samhsa.gov/2K10/inhalents/Spotlight001AdolInhalantHTML.pdf (Accessed February 14, 2012).

47. Bowen SE. Two serious and challenging medical complications associated with volatile substance misuse: sudden sniffing death and fetal solvent syndrome. *Subst Use Misuse* 2011;**46** (Suppl 1):68–72.

48. Nussbaum A, Thurstone C, Binswanger I. Medical marijuana use and suicide attempt in a patient with major depressive disorder. *Am J Psychiatry* 2011;**168**:778–81.

49. Pedersen W. Does cannabis use lead to depression and suicidal behaviors? A populations-based longitudinal study. *Acta Psychiatr Scand* 2008;**118**:395–403.

50. Foti DJ, Kotov R, Guey LT, Bromet EJ. Cannabis use and the course of schizophrenia: 10-year follow-up after first hospitalization. *Am J Psychiatry* 2010;**167**:987–93.

51. Grech A, Van Os J, Jones PB, Lewis SW, Murray RM. Cannabis use and outcome of recent onset psychosis. *Eur Psychiatry* 2005;**20**:349–53.

52. Seely KA, Prather PL, James LP, Moran JH. Marijuana-based drugs: innovative therapeutics or designer drugs of abuse? *Mol Interv* 2011;**11**:36–51.

Drug withdrawal syndromes in psychiatric patients in the emergency department

Paul Porter and Richard D. Shih

Introduction

Mental illness, drug abuse, and alcoholism extremely commonly occur together. Approximately half of all patients with psychiatric disorders have, or will have, substance abuse issues at any given time. Numerous studies have shown that concurrent substance abuse has a negative impact on mental illness. Psychiatric treatment is more difficult and patients are less compliant with therapies when drug and alcohol comorbidity exist [1–4].

The emergency physician assessing and treating a patient with a psychiatric emergency will frequently encounter patients with withdrawal syndromes [5–8]. Symptoms of withdrawal occur when a patient takes one or more substances over a period of time and then that substance is removed or decreased. The mechanisms involved in withdrawal are complex and differ depending on the agent involved.

Drug withdrawal can occur from a myriad of agents. This chapter will focus on agents that develop a recognized syndrome when the agent or a closely related agent is administered to relieve withdrawal symptoms. Agents that satisfy this definition generally affect inhibitory neurotransmission. An agent such as cocaine which causes excitation can be associated with a syndrome of lethargy and neuro-excitatory depression after discontinuation of usage. These post-usage syndromes associated with excitatory agents will not be addressed. This chapter will focus on the most common and important syndromes that meet this definition: withdrawal associated with ethanol, sedative hypnotics, gamma-hydroxybutyrate (GHB), and opioids.

Ethanol withdrawal

Alcohol dependence affects approximately 10% of the population of the United States [9]. Additionally, chronic alcoholism and psychiatric illness occur together commonly. Approximately 40% of adults diagnosed with alcoholism are given one or more psychiatric diagnoses over their lifetime [1,2,10]. Severe ethanol withdrawal can be life-threatening. However, the fatality rate for ethanol withdrawal has dropped from approximately 40% to under 5% in the past few decades with current treatment regimens.

Given its high potential mortality when untreated and the effectiveness of treatment, it is important to recognize ethanol withdrawal even when it is not the presenting complaint. Ethanol withdrawal may become manifest after a patient is admitted or boarded for a prolonged time in the Emergency Department, which can be a frequent occurrence for patients presenting with primary psychiatric complaints.

Ethanol is a central nervous system depressant. It acts by enhancing inhibitory neurotransmission (GABA) and suppressing excitatory neurotransmission (NMDA receptor). The net effect from chronic ethanol exposure leads to increased NMDA and decreased GABA receptor activity to maintain a relatively homeostatic balance of excitatory and inhibitory neurotransmission [6]. When ethanol ingestion is stopped or decreased, the receptor stimulation from ethanol is lost and the net excitation–inhibition balance favors excitation. The clinical manifestations of this excitation can be mild to severe, and include increased autonomic sympathetic signs and symptoms, seizures, hallucinations, and altered mental status.

Alcohol withdrawal occurs in the setting of alcohol dependence, which typically takes a minimum of 3 months of chronic ethanol ingestion or significant binge drinking for approximately 1 week. Withdrawal symptoms can occur without the complete cessation of drinking by decreasing the amount or frequency of alcohol consumption.

Clinically, ethanol withdrawal manifests as increased autonomic symptoms, alcohol withdrawal hallucinosis, alcohol withdrawal seizures, and delirium tremens. All of these manifestations can occur by themselves, but typically occur together. Because of the degree of overlap, some authors simply group symptoms into minor or major ethanol withdrawal.

Increased autonomic symptoms, commonly referred to as "the shakes," typically occur 6–36 hours after cessation of ethanol consumption. Symptoms may last between 2 to 7 days and include hypertension, tachycardia, anorexia, anxiety, hyperreflexia, insomnia, nausea, and tremors.

Alcohol withdrawal hallucinosis is typically seen approximately 24 hours after the last ethanol drink. Hallucinations are primarily visual and persecutory. The hallucinations are transient with global cognition unimpaired.

Alcohol withdrawal seizures are also commonly known as "rum fits." The seizures typically occur 8–48 hours after the cessation of ethanol consumption. These seizures are generally

Behavioral Emergencies for the Emergency Physician, ed. Leslie S. Zun, Lara G. Chepenik, and Mary Nan S. Mallory. Published by Cambridge University Press. © Cambridge University Press 2013.

tonic–clonic, not accompanied by an aura, of short duration, self-terminating, and have a brief post-ictal phase. If the seizure has not spontaneously resolved, it is generally terminated easily with benzodiazepines. Additionally, benzodiazepines have been shown to prevent their recurrence [11]. Phenytoin does not have effects at GABA or NMDA receptors and is therefore ineffective for ethanol withdrawal seizures [12,13]. It is also helpful to consider potential causes for seizure other than alcohol withdrawal as one study showed nearly 20% of patients with presumed alcohol withdrawal seizures had structural lesions in their brains [14].

Delirium tremens (DTs) is the most severe form of alcohol withdrawal. DTs typically occur 48–96 hours following the cessation of drinking and, unlike other ethanol withdrawal manifestations, are relatively rare [15]. It is difficult to predict which patients with withdrawal symptoms will go on to have DTs, although several historical features suggest a higher likelihood. These include higher levels of alcohol consumption, greater number of past withdrawal episodes, and more severe alcohol-related medical problems [15,16].

Symptoms include the autonomic symptoms tachycardia, hypertension, diaphoresis, agitation, and tremors, along with globally altered cognition and fever. With current treatment regimens, death is rare. When it occurs, it is typically due to aspiration, arrhythmia, or a comorbid condition.

Treatment

Patients with minor symptoms of alcohol withdrawal without a history of DTs and who intend to continue drinking are often discharged without receiving any specific medications. For patients who have major symptoms of withdrawal or are unable to be discharged from a hospital for medical reasons, pharmacologic treatment is initiated to alleviate symptoms and help prevent progression to seizure or DTs.

Over the past 50 years, there have been numerous studies assessing the different agents used for treating alcohol withdrawal [6,10,17–24]. Several findings have become clear. Antipsychotics are not effective therapy for treating alcohol withdrawal and should be avoided if possible [6,18–24]. This may be difficult when treating a patient with comorbid psychiatric symptoms. Another major finding is that many of the sedative-hypnotic medications are therapeutically effective. Within this class of medications, benzodiazipines appear to be superior because of ease of use, limited side effects, and beneficial pharmacologic characteristics [17,19,20,21]. Although chlordiazepoxide (Librium) was involved in many of the early studies and gained wide acceptance as an effective therapy, several other benzodiazepines may be more useful especially for treating severe symptoms. Diazepam (Valium) has a rapid time to peak effect (5–10 minutes intravenously), which allows for rapid titration to clinical symptoms. In addition, it has a long half-life (>40 hours) and has an active metabolite (desmethyldiazepam) that has an even longer half-life. This prolonged half-life and duration of action can act as an effective taper of the drug's effect, which may be useful in the treatment of withdrawal.

Alternatively, lorazepam (Ativan), another benzodiazepine, has slightly slower time to peak effect (10–20 minutes). Used for alcohol withdrawal symptoms in a titrated manner, stacked doses may be given before the full effects of dosing have been achieved. Despite this, lorazepam may be preferable in the setting of advanced liver disease where hepatic metabolism of diazepam may be a liability.

Benzodiazepines exert their beneficial effect by enhancing GABA transmission. They are titrated with a goal of reversing most of the withdrawal symptoms. Ideally, the patient will be mildly sedated and vital signs near normal. Historically, patients were administered scheduled dosages of benzodiazepines (i.e., chlordiazopoxide 50 mg every 6 hours). Additional dosages were then administered as needed. Unfortunately, the scheduled approach to medication administration often led to under- or overdosing. Several studies have shown that "symptom triggered" dosing regimens are more effective. Signs and symptoms of withdrawal are assessed using a scoring system to assess the severity of the withdrawal manifestations. The most well-studied, validated, and accepted of these tools is the Clinical Institute Withdrawal Assessment of Alcohol Scale, revised (CIWA-Ar, see Figure 7.1) [6,25–27]. This scale contains 10 clinical questions that take several minutes to complete and can be administered by a registered nurse [19]. A CIWA score of 8–10 correlates with mild alcohol withdrawal symptoms, whereas greater scores signify more severe levels. Its use in the treatment of alcohol withdrawal is analogous to an insulin sliding scale used for diabetic patients. A higher CIWA score corresponds to a higher dosage of benzodiazepine administration. The score is typically assessed hourly when initiated, then decreased or increased in frequency as a patient improves, worsens or has more severe symptoms. For mild withdrawal symptoms (CIWA score 8–10) an oral dose of diazepam (5–10 mg) or chlordiazepoxide (25–50 mg) can be administered. For more severe symptoms (CIWA score >10), an intravenous dose of diazepam (5–20 mg) or lorazepam (1–4 mg) would be appropriate [6,19]. For moderate or severe symptoms a CIWA reassessment should not wait an hour and assessment scheduling should be tailored to the patient's response to therapy.

Symptom-triggered treatment regimens are useful in most cases of withdrawal. In rare instances, clinical response using a single benzodiazipine proves insufficient, and an additional agent may need to be added [28]. Few studies address this issue. However, case studies document the success of adding a barbiturate, an alternative benzodiazepine, or propofol [29]. Additionally, these patients often manifest hypotension, need for mechanical ventilation, and ICU support [28,30]. Other adjunctive agents such as beta blockers (i.e., metopropolol) and alpha agonists (i.e., clonidine) are less clearly defined. At best, they are considered adjunctive, rather than primary, treatment for ethanol withdrawal [8,19].

CLINICAL INSTITUTE WITHDRAWAL ASSESSMENT OF ALCOHOL SCALE, REVISED (CIWA-AR)

Patient:_____ Date:_____ Time:_____
(24 hour clock, midnight = 00:00)
Pulse or heart rate, taken for one minute:_____ Blood pressure:_____
NAUSEA AND VOMITING – Ask "Do you feel sick to your stomach? Have you vomited?" Observation. 0 no
nausea and no vomiting 1 mild nausea with no vomiting
2 3 4 intermittent nausea with dry heaves 5 6 7 constant nausea, frequent dry heaves and vomiting
TREMOR – Arms extended and fingers spread apart. Observation. 0 no tremor 1 not visible, but can be felt fingertip
to fingertip
2 3 4 moderate, with patient's arms extended 5 6 7 severe, even with arms not extended
PAROXYSMAL SWEATS –Observation. 0 no sweat visible 1 barely perceptible sweating, palms moist 2
3 4 beads of sweat obvious on forehead 5 6 7 drenching sweats
ANXIETY – Ask "Do you feel nervous?" Observation. 0 no anxiety, at ease 1 mildly anxious 2
3 4 moderately anxious, or guarded, so anxiety is inferred 5 6 7 equivalent to acute panic states as seen in severe
delirium or acute schizophrenic reactions
AGITATION – Observation. 0 normal activity 1 somewhat more than normal activity 2 3 4 moderately fidgety
and restless 5 6 7 paces back and forth during most of the interview, or constantly thrashes about
TACTILE DISTURBANCES – Ask "Have you any itching, pins and needles sensations, any burning, any numbness,
or do you feel bugs crawling on or under your skin?" Observation. 0 none
1 very mild itching, pins and needles, burning or numbness 2 mild itching, pins and needles, burning or numbness 3
moderate itching, pins and needles, burning or numbness 4 moderately severe hallucinations
5 severe hallucinations 6 extremely severe hallucinations 7 continuous hallucinations
AUDITORY DISTURBANCES – Ask "Are you more aware of sounds around you? Are they harsh? Do they frighten
you? Are you hearing anything that is disturbing to you? Are you hearing things you know are not there?" Observation.
0 not present 1 very mild harshness or ability to frighten 2 mild harshness or ability to frighten 3 moderate harshness or
ability to frighten 4 moderately severe hallucinations 5 severe hallucinations 6 extremely severe hallucinations 7
continuous hallucinations
VISUAL DISTURBANCES – Ask "Does the light appear to be too bright? Is its color different? Does it hurt your
eyes? Are you seeing anything that is disturbing to you? Are you seeing things you know are not there?" Observation.
0 not present 1 very mild sensitivity 2 mild sensitivity 3 moderate sensitivity 4 moderately severe hallucinations 5
severe hallucinations 6 extremely severe hallucinations 7 continuous hallucinations
HEADACHE, FULLNESS IN HEAD – Ask "Does your head feel different? Does it feel like there is a band around
your head?" Do not rate for dizziness or lightheadedness. Otherwise, rate severity. 0 no present
1 very mild 2 mild 3 moderate 4 moderately severe 5 severe
6 very severe 7 extremely severe
ORIENTATION AND CLOUDING OF SENSORIUM –
Ask "What day is this? Where are you? Who am I?" 0 oriented and can do serial additions 1 cannot do serial additions
or is uncertain about date 2 disoriented for date by no more than 2 calendar days 3 disoriented for date by more than 2
calendar days
4 disoriented for place/or person
Total CIWA-Ar Score_____ Rater's Initials_____ Maximum Possible Score 67

The CIWA-Ar is not copyrighted and may be reproduced freely. Sullivan, J.T.; Sykora, K.; Schneiderman, J.; Naranjo, C.A.; and Sellers, E.M.
Assessment of alcohol withdrawal: The revised Clinical Institute Withdrawal Assessment for Alcohol scale (CIWA-Ar). British Journal of
Addiction 84:1353-1357, 1989.

Figure 7.1

Disposition of patients with ethanol withdrawal

Most patients with signs of alcohol withdrawal will require at least inpatient observation if the plan is the cessation of alcohol ingestion. Patients with severe symptoms or delirium tremens will require ICU management [7,31].

Sedative hypnotic drugs withdrawal

Overview

Sedative hypnotic agents such as barbiturates and benzodiazepines, like ethanol, exert their effects by means of augmentation of GABA inhibitory neurotransmission [6]. Therefore, symptoms of withdrawal from these agents are very similar to alcohol withdrawal [6,32]. These manifestations include hypertension, tachycardia, diaphoresis, agitation, tremor, hallucinations, seizures, and altered mental status. Many of these agents have very long half-lives as well as active metabolites with long half-lives [32]. In essence, these types of agents selftaper when they are discontinued. Therefore, withdrawal necessitating medical intervention is much less common than with alcohol withdrawal. For withdrawal symptoms to occur, chronic use greater than four months is usually necessary to develop symptoms. As with most withdrawal syndromes the severity of symptoms is related to the pharmacology of the specific agent, dosage, and duration of use [33]. Symptom onset can occur as quickly as 1–2 days after drug cessation, or up to 1 week with medications that have long half-lives.

Duration of symptoms is related to drug half-life and can last up to several weeks for resolution.

The principles of treatment of sedative hypnotic drug withdrawal resemble the ones for alcohol withdrawal. Benzodiazepines are generally first-line agents. However, the use of a barbiturate for withdrawal from barbiturate usage may also be reasonable. Treatment with medication, as with treating alcohol withdrawal, is aimed at light sedation and near normalization of vital signs. Once a stable dose of a particular agent has been achieved, a drug taper is performed over 2 to 3 weeks [34].

Gamma-hydroxybutyrate (GHB) withdrawal

Gamma-hydroxybutyrate (GHB) was first synthesized in the 1960s as an anesthetic agent. However, since then, it has been used as a body building supplement, narcolepsy treatment, and recreational drug of abuse [35–37]. Gamma-hydroxybutyrate is an inhibitory neurotransmitter with its own specific receptor site. When ingested as a drug of abuse, supra-physiologic levels are reached and GHB mediates its effects by means of the $GABA_2$ receptor [35–37]. This GABA receptor interaction, like ethanol and sedative hypnotics, leads to inhibition of neurotransmission and subsequent clinical effects. Gamma-hydroxybutyrate, as well as its precursors (γ-butyrolactone and 1,4-butanediol), have all been abused for their sedating and euphoric effects. Gamma-hydroxybutyrate was sold over the counter in the United States until 1990, and its precursors until 2000 [38].

Withdrawal from GHB and its precursors (γ-butyrolactone and 1,4-butanediol) are similar to alcohol withdrawal and other sedative hypnotics. However, because of GHB's short half-life (20–30 minutes) withdrawal onset is often more rapid and can occur several hours to several days after cessation of usage. Symptoms of withdrawal are similar to alcohol and sedative hypnotic withdrawal and include hypertension, tachycardia, diaphoresis, agitation, tremor, hallucinations, seizures, and altered mental status.

However, GHB withdrawal typically has more central nervous system and less sympathomimetic manifestations compared to alcohol withdrawal [36]. The reason for this difference is unclear and may be related to differing GABA receptor binding (GHB for $GABA_2$ receptors and ethanol for $GABA_1$).

Treatment is similar to that for alcohol withdrawal. However, higher doses of benzodiazepines may be necessary. This may be due to $GABA_2$ receptor activation by GHB versus $GABA_1$ binding of benzodiazepines [2]. Use of a $GABA_2$ agonist such as baclofen has been reported and may be useful as a first-line agent or in cases refractory to benzodiazepine therapy [35].

Opioid withdrawal

Opiate abuse, like alcoholism, is commonly found in the psychiatric population. In 2004, there were nearly 200,000 opioid-related Emergency Department visits in the United States [39].

Opioids act by binding to opioid receptors and inhibiting neurons to cause their pharmacologic effects. Chronic stimulation of these receptors leads to neuro-adaptive responses likely mediated through the second messenger cyclic adenosine monophosphate (cAMP), which leads to increased intrinsic excitability [6]. The net effect of these chronic adaptive changes is to negate the inhibitory effects of continued opioid receptor stimulation. With sudden cessation of opioid ingestion, decreased dosage, or administration of an opioid antagonist, excitability results from a shift in the net neuronal balance, causing opioid withdrawal symptoms.

Depending upon the opioid involved, most commonly heroin, withdrawal symptoms generally occur six to 12 hours after the last dose; onset of withdrawal from methadone can be delayed 24–72 hours. Withdrawal symptoms include influenza-like symptoms without altered mental status, nausea, vomiting, abdominal cramps, dilated pupils, diarrhea, lacrimation, myalgias, piloerection, rhinorrhea, sneezing, and yawning [6]. The piloerection appearing like a "plucked turkey" is where the common term "cold turkey" evolved from.

Opioid withdrawal is not life-threatening. However, it is very unpleasant and painful to endure. Due to cross-reactivity of the different opioids, any opioid can be administered to alleviate withdrawal symptoms [8]. Unfortunately, recurrence of the withdrawal symptoms occurs when the effects of the drug have worn off. Therefore, methadone is a common agent used in this setting due to its long half-life. However, the use of methadone for acute withdrawal in the Emergency Department is controversial. The unpleasant nature of treating opioid-abusing patients, side effects associated with methadone, and the lack of mortality associated with opioid withdrawal cause many Emergency Departments not to dispense methadone, preferring that patients seek care at detoxification centers or methadone clinics. Additionally, many authors caution against prescribing methadone to an unfamiliar patient. Methadone is sought for both recreational use and economic gain. Patients frequently present to Emergency Departments factitiously claiming to have missed a methadone dose and experiencing withdrawal symptoms. This secondary gain is often very difficult to differentiate from patients with true symptoms. In addition, respiratory depression or death has occurred when patients have manipulated Emergency Department staff into giving them an overdose of methadone [40]. The desire to do no harm by causing an unintentional overdose or contributing to a secondary market for methadone can conflict with a physician's oath to ease pain and suffering.

Outpatient methadone clinics can use dosages of methadone as high as 150 mg. However, those individuals began therapy with much lower doses, which are gradually increased as tolerance to opioids occurs. When confronted with a patient who claims to have missed their methadone clinic appointment, calling the clinic and confirming the patient's treatment plan is the ideal approach. Unfortunately, this is not always achievable. Another option is to administer a lower and temporizing dose of methadone (10 mg dose) that alleviates the majority of the withdrawal symptoms. Intramuscular administration of this dose is preferred as oral dosages may be vomited by the patient [8].

Another medication that has been used for treating opioid withdrawal is clonidine [6]. Clonidine is a centrally acting presynaptic alpha-2 agonist that suppresses central sympathetic outflow. The typical dose is 0.1–0.2 mg every 6 hours. It is generally used in patients with mild symptoms or where methadone is not available. Benzodiazepines such as diazepam or lorazepam can also be used in addition to clonidine [6,8].

Patients undergoing withdrawal are most often treated on as outpatients. Those with refractory symptoms or significant comorbidities may require hospitalization.

References

1. Kessler RC, Berglund P, Demler O, et al. Lifetime prevalence and age-of-onset distributions of DSM-IV disorders in the National Comorbidity Survey Replication. *Arch Gen Psychiatry* 2005; **62**:593–602.

2. Kavanagh DJ, Waghorn G, Jenner L, et al. Demographic and clinical correlates of comorbid drug use disorders in psychosis: multivariate analyses from an epidemiological sample.*Schizophr Res* 2004;**66**:115–24.

3. Regier DA, Farmer ME, Rae DS, et al. Comorbidity of mental disorders with alcohol and other drug abuse. Results from the Epidemiologic Catchment Area (ECA) Study. *JAMA* 1990;**264**:2511–18.

4. Sharp MJ, Getz JG. Self-process in comorbid mental illness and drug abuse. *Am J Orthopsychiatry* 1998;**68**:639–44.

5. RachBeisel J, Scott J, Dixon L. Co-occurring severe mental illness and substance use disorders: a review of recent research.*Psychiatric Serv* 1999;**50**:1427–34.

6. Kosten TR, O'Connor PG. Management of drug and alcohol withdrawal.*N Engl J Med* 2003;**348**:1786–95.

7. Jenkins DH. Substance abuse and withdrawal in the intensive care unit. *Surg Clin North Am* 2000;**80**:1033–53.

8. Olmedo R, Hoffman RS. Withdrawal syndromes. *Emerg Med Clin North Am* 2000;**18**:273–85.

9. Swift RM. Drug therapy for alcohol dependence. *N Engl J Med* 1999;**340**:1482–90.

10. Bourgeois JA, Nelson JL, Slack MB, et al. Comorbid affective disorders and personality traits in alcohol abuse inpatients at an Air Force Medical Center. *Mil Med* 1999;**164**:103–6.

11. D'Onofrio G, Rathlev NK, Ulrich AS, et al. Lorazepam for the prevention of recurrent seizures related to alcohol. *N Engl J Med* 1999;**340**:915–19.

12. Chance JF. Emergency department treatment of alcohol withdrawal seizures with phenytoin. *Ann Emerg Med* 1991;**20**:520–2.

13. Rathlev NK, D'Onofrio G, Fish SS, et al. The lack of efficacy of phenytoin in the prevention of recurrent alcohol-related seizures.*Ann Emerg Med* 1994;**23**:513–18.

14. Earnest MP, Feldman H, Marx JA, et al. Intracranial lesions shown by CT scans in 259 cases of first alcohol related seizures. *Neurology* 1988;**38**:1561–5.

15. Schuckit MA, Tipp JE, Reich T, et al. The histories of withdrawal convulsions and delirium tremens in1648 alcohol dependent subjects. *Addiction* 1995;**90**:1335–47.

16. Ferguson JA, Suelzer CJ, Eckert GJ, et al. Risk factors for delirium tremens development. *J Gen Intern Med* 1996;**11**:410–14.

17. Holbrook AM, Crowther R, Lotter A, et al. Meta-analysis of benzodiazepine use in the treatment of acute alcohol withdrawal. *CMAJ* 1999;**160**:649–55.

18. Adams F, Dernandez F, Andeson BS. Emergency pharmacotherapy of delirium in the critically ill cancer patient. *Psychosomatics* 1986;**13**:56–60.

19. Mayo-Smith MF. Pharmacological management of alcohol withdrawal: a meta-analysis and evidence-based practice guideline.*JAMA* 1997;**278**:144–51.

20. Amato L, Minozzi S, Vecchi S, et al. Benzodiazepines for alcohol withdrawal. *Cochrane Database Syst Rev* 2010;**3**: CD005063. DOI: 10.1002/14651858. CD005063.pub3.

21. Mayo-Smith, Beecher LH, Fischer TL, et al. Management of alcohol withdrawal delirium. An evidenced-based practice guideline. *Arch Intern Med* 2004;**164**:1405–12.

22. Thomas DW, Freedman DX. Treatment of the alcohol withdrawal syndrome: comparison of promazine and paraldehyde. *JAMA* 1964;**188**:244–6.

23. Chambers JF, Schultz JD. Double-blind study of three drugs in the treatment of acute alcoholic states. *Q J Stud Alcohol* 1965;**26**:10–18.

24. Sereny G, Kalant H. Comparative clinical evaluation of chlordiazepoxide and promazine in treatment of alcohol-withdrawal syndrome. *BMJ* 1965;**1**:92–7.

25. Mayo-Smith, Beecher LH, Fischer TL, et al. Management of Alcohol Withdrawal Delirium. An evidenced-based practice guideline. *Arch Intern Med* 2004;**164**:1405–12.

26. Daeppan JB, Gache P, Landry U, et al. Symptom-triggered vs. fixed-schedule doses of benzodiazepine for alcohol withdrawal: a randomized treatment trial. *Arch Intern Med* 2002;**162**:117–21.

27. Hecksel KA, Bostwick JM, Jaeger TM, Cha SS. Inappropriate use of symptom-triggered therapy for alcohol withdrawal in the general hospital. *Mayo Clin Proc* 2008;**83**:274–9.

28. Saitz R, Mayo-Smith MF, Roberts MS, et al. Individualized treatment for alcohol withdrawal: a randomized double-blind controlled trial. *JAMA* 1994;**272**:519–23.

29. Hack JB, Hoffman RS, Nelson LS. Resistant alcohol withdrawal: does an unexpectedly large sedative requirement identify these patients early? *J Med Toxicol* 2006;**2**:55–60.

30. McCowan C, Marik P. Refractory delirium tremens treated with propofol: a case series. *Crit Care Med* 2000;**28**:1781–4.

31. Nolop KB, Natow A. Unprecedented sedative requirement during delirium tremens. *Crit Care Med* 1985;**13**:246–7.

32. DeBellis R, Smith BS, Choi S, et al. Management of delirium tremens. *J Intensive Care Med* 2005;**20**:164–73.

33. Lann MA, Molina DK. A fatal case of benzodiazepine withdrawal. *Am J Forensic Med Pathol* 2009;**30**:177–9.

34. Moller HJ. Effectiveness and safety of benzodiazepines, benzodiazepine

dependence and withdrawal: myths and management. *J Clin Psychopharmacol* 1999;**19**:115–25.

35. Voshaar RC, Couvee JE, van Balkom AJ, et al. Strategies for discontinuing long-term benzodiazepine use: meta-analysis.*Br J Psychiatry* 2006;**189**:213–20.

36. LeTourneau JL, Hagg DS, Smith SM. Baclofen and gamma-hydroxybutyrate

withdrawal. *Neurocritical Care* 2008;**8**:430–3.

37. Wojtowicz JM, Yarema MC, Wax PM. Withdrawal from gamma-hydroxybutyrate, 1,4-butanediol and gamma-butyrolactone: a case report and systematic review. *Can J Emerg Med Care* 2008;**10**:69–74.

38. Perez E, Chu J, Bania T. Seven days of gamma-hydroxybutyrate (GHB) use

produces severe withdrawal.*Ann Emerg Med* 2006;**48**:219–20.

39. Palmer RB. Gamma-Butyrolactone and 1,4-butanediol: abused analogues of gamma-hydroxybutyrate. *Toxicol Rev* 2004;**23**:21–31.

40. *Drug-Related Emergency Department Visits*. DAWN Series D-28, DHHS Publication No. (SMA) 06–4143, Rockville, MD; 2006.

Chapter 8

The patient with depression in the emergency department

James L. Young and Douglas A. Rund

Introduction

Fluctuations of mood including happiness, sadness, joy, and elation are a normal part of life. Those suffering from mood disorders, however, experience extreme mood states that can impair functioning and threaten life.

Psychiatric disorders are classified by groupings of symptoms and their duration in *The Diagnostic and Statistical Manual of Mental Disorders, 4th Edition, Text Revision* (DSM-IV-TR) [1]. Mood disorders are grouped into four broad categories: depressive disorders, bipolar disorders, mood disorder due to a general medical condition, and substance-induced mood disorders. Although we have a growing database of the biological and genetic components of the mood disorders, we are not yet able to group these disorders into more precise categories on the basis of specific pathophysiology.

Patients with mood disorders are often seen in the emergency department (ED). In one recent screening study, 32% of ED patients met criteria for depression and 4% met criteria for mania [2]. In this chapter, we will provide some guidelines on the assessment and management of mood disorders in the ED setting.

Clinical features

Major depressive disorder

Major depressive disorder is characterized by one or more major depressive episodes, as defined by DSM-IV-TR criteria (Table 8.1) and a lifelong absence of manic episodes. These criteria are broadly grouped into four major categories: mood, psychomotor activity, vegetative function, and cognition [3]. A helpful mnemonic, SIG E CAPS, of the criteria for depression is shown in Table 8.2.

Mood

To meet the DSM-IV TR criteria for depressive episode, the patient must have either a depressed mood or anhedonia. Patients in a depressed state often feel profound hopelessness and helplessness. They may describe feeling sad, gloomy, dejected, unhappy, anguished, discouraged, or in low spirits. They may also experience feelings of anxiety and irritability.

Anhedonia is a decreased capacity to experience pleasure or interest in previously pleasurable or satisfying activities. Patients may have stopped doing formerly pleasurable activities entirely.

Psychomotor activity

In depression, physical activity can be either increased or decreased. Psychomotor retardation is a significant slowing of physical activity. In addition to a decreased range of movement, patients may also present with a slumped posture, creased brow, arms folded, mouth turned down, and eyes closed or downcast. Alternately, some patients may exhibit psychomotor agitation, which can manifest as irritability, fidgeting, pacing, hand wringing, rubbing of the skin, or restlessness.

Vegetative function

Vegetative symptoms include disturbances in four areas: sleep, appetite, sexual function, and energy.

Patients may complain of sleeping either too much: hypersomnia, or too little: insomnia, and may also fluctuate between these two states. Insomnia may present as difficulty falling asleep (initial insomnia), frequent awakenings throughout the night (middle insomnia), or early-morning wakening, and inability to fall back to sleep (terminal insomnia). Depressed patients with hypersomnia may report sleeping 12 to 14 or more hours a day.

Alterations in appetite and eating patterns can also occur. Patients may eat too much or too little with resulting significant weight gain or loss over a short period of time. Although patients may not regularly weigh themselves, they may notice that their clothes are becoming either too tight or too loose.

Patients with depression often complain of decreased amounts of energy and increased fatigue. This is both a primary symptom of depression and can be the result of disrupted eating and sleeping patterns.

Although not formally a DSM-IV-TR criteria, a person experiencing a depressed episode may experience a loss of interest in sexual activity or impaired sexual functioning. It should be mentioned that these problems can also be a side effect of antidepressant medications.

Behavioral Emergencies for the Emergency Physician, ed. Leslie S. Zun, Lara G. Chepenik, and Mary Nan S. Mallory. Published by Cambridge University Press. © Cambridge University Press 2013.

Table 8.1. Summary of DSM-IV-TR criteria for a major depressive episode

A. Five or more of the following symptoms present almost every day during the same 2-week period and represent a change from previous functioning; at least one of the symptoms is either (1) depressed mood or (2) loss of interest or pleasure. Note: Do not include symptoms caused by a general medical condition, and do not include mood-incongruent delusions or hallucinations.

1. Depressed mood (can be irritable mood in children and adolescents)
2. Loss of interest or pleasure in activities
3. Significant weight loss when not dieting, or weight gain or decrease, or increased appetite
4. Insomnia or hypersomnia
5. Psychomotor agitation or retardation
6. Fatigue or loss of energy
7. Feelings of worthlessness, or excessive or inappropriate guilt
8. Diminished ability to think or concentrate, or indecisiveness
9. Recurrent thoughts of death (not just fear of dying), recurrent suicidal ideation, or a suicide plan or attempt

B. Symptoms do not meet criteria for a "mixed episode"

C. Symptoms cause clinically significant distress or impairment in social, occupational, or other functioning.

D. Symptoms are not caused by direct physiologic effects of a substance (e.g., drug of abuse, medication) or a general medical condition (e.g., hypothyroidism).

E. Symptoms are not better accounted for by bereavement; after the loss of a loved one, the symptoms persist for longer than 2 months or are characterized by marked functional impairment, morbid preoccupation with worthlessness, suicidal ideation, psychotic symptoms, or psychomotor retardation.

Modified from American Psychiatric Association: *The Diagnostic and Statistical Manual of Mental Disorders, 4th ed, Text Revision*. Washington, DC: American Psychiatric Association; 2000.

Table 8.2. Mnemonic for the symptoms of depression

SIG E CAPS (prescribe energy capsules)

Sleep amount increased or decreased

Interest (anhedonia)

Guilt

Energy level decreased

Concentration decreased

Appetite increased or decreased

Psychomotor activity increased or decreased

Suicidal ideation

Cognition

Depression may also consist of impaired concentration that presents as diminished mental quickness, forgetfulness, or difficulty maintaining attention and focus. Executive functioning such as prioritization, problem solving, and planning can be impaired. In severe cases, such impairment can cause decreased ability to sufficiently care for oneself, including inability to perform basic activities of daily living such as maintaining acceptable hygiene, paying bills, and the purchase and preparation of food.

Thought content tends to be negative, including such thoughts as recurrent guilt, failure, worthlessness, and self-criticism.

Patients in a depressed episode are at increased risk for suicide. Suicidal thoughts may range from vague notions that life is not worth living to fully envisioned suicide plans with definitive intent to die. Depressed patients should be questioned about suicidal thoughts. Such questioning does not increase the likelihood of a future attempt and provides an opening for a dialog to address the patient's safety. Because patients are not often forthcoming with their thoughts on suicide, and a patient who is currently denying plan or intent may impulsively attempt suicide in the future, a thorough review of risk factors (such as prior suicide attempts, prior psychiatric hospitalizations, anxiety, hopelessness, substance abuse issues, and access to firearms) and protective factors (such as a stable support system, religious prohibitions, future goals, and family responsibilities) can inform clinical decisions regarding the level of care needed. Over 40% of patients who complete suicide have been seen in an emergency department within a year before their death, often on multiple occasions and after failed suicide attempts [4]. Partnered with psychiatric services, the emergency department can play a critical role in suicide prevention.

Patients with severe depression may have psychotic symptoms. The hallucinations and delusions that accompany depression most often are mood-congruent with themes that are consistent with the depressed mood. For example, the patient may experience hallucinations that repeat derogatory statements or insist that the patient commit suicide. The patient may report nihilistic delusions (Cotard's syndrome) such as being "already dead" or feeling like "my insides have rotted away" [5]. Mood-incongruent psychotic symptoms, such as paranoid delusions, do not reflect the mood as clearly and are less likely to occur in a depressed state.

Special considerations

Depression in the elderly

Depression is not a natural consequence of aging, and unfortunately often goes undetected in the elderly population [6]. Prevalence rates of depression are 27–30% in elderly patients presenting to the emergency department [7]. Late-life depression often leads to reduced quality of life, loss of autonomy, increased resource usage, increased burden on caregivers, and even increased mortality [8]. This patient population is also at increased risk for suicide. The elderly may have a tendency to report more somatic complaints than younger adults with depression. Depression also occurs more often in the elderly in the context of medical comorbidities. The elderly are more vulnerable to development of melancholic depression, which is characterized by early morning awakening, diurnal variation in mood, low self-esteem, and low mood reactivity [9].

Older patients with depression can also present with symptoms that suggest dementia rather than depression, such as memory loss, inattention, withdrawal from daily activities, confusion, lapses in personal hygiene, and socially inappropriate behavior. Depressive disorders in the elderly are often treatable, and therefore reversible, conditions. Distinguishing them from dementia is essential for correct diagnosis and treatment.

Children and adolescents

The essential criteria for depression in children and adolescents are the same as for adults. Pediatric depression may present differently than in adults and is often misunderstood, masked in its presentation, or simply overlooked.

Prepubertal children are more likely to have somatic complaints, psychomotor agitation, and mood-congruent hallucinations, and are less likely to have disturbances in sleep and appetite. Some children are misdiagnosed as having attention-deficit disorder, especially if symptoms involve poor concentration, listlessness, agitation, and withdrawal from daily activities [10].

Adolescents with depression may show increased oppositional behavior and substance abuse, and tend to describe more irritability than depressed mood [11]. Other characteristics include social withdrawal, increased rejection sensitivity, and a decline in school performance.

Treatment of childhood and adolescent depression most often includes psychosocial interventions and antidepressant medications. The SSRI fluoxetine is currently the only medication approved by the U.S. Food and Drug Administration (FDA) for the treatment of child and adolescent depression [12]. There is some evidence that treatment of adolescents and young adults with antidepressant medications may lead to increased suicidal ideation and this has resulted in an FDA "black box" warning. It is important that these patients be treated for depression, but also monitored closely for suicidal thoughts, especially shortly after initiation of treatment with an selective serotonin reuptake inhibitor (SSRI) [12].

Postpartum depression

"Postpartum blues," consisting of tearfulness, irritability, mood lability, and insomnia, have been reported to occur in 15–85% of women within the first 10 days after giving birth, with a peak incidence at the fifth day [13]. Postpartum blues are a risk factor for progression to postpartum depression [13]. Postpartum depression (major depressive disorder with postpartum onset) is diagnosed when the patient meets the criteria for a major depressive episode within 1 month of delivery. Risk factors for postpartum depression are a history of depression, either during or before the pregnancy, a previous episode of postpartum depression, a history of premenstrual dysphoric disorder, stressful life events, lack of social support, marital conflict, poverty, immigrant status, and young maternal age [13].

Bipolar disorders

Patients with bipolar disorders experience both manic/hypomanic and depressed episodes. There are variations in the pattern of symptom manifestation, and we conceptualize bipolar disorder as occurring on a spectrum. DSM-IV-TR divides bipolar disorder into type I, type II, cyclothymic disorder, and not otherwise specified (NOS) [1]. The presence of at least one manic episode defines bipolar I disorder. Bipolar II disorder requires evidence for a hypomanic episode and at least one major depressive episode. A hypomanic episode includes the features of a manic episode but is shorter in duration and lacks psychosis, marked impairment of function, or the need for hospitalization. Cyclothymic disorder is characterized by a life of mood swings of insufficient severity to meet criteria for either a depressive or a manic episode. Persons with this disorder may have a chaotic life characterized by frequent sub-clinical mood episodes, unstable relationships, and uneven school or work performance. Bipolar disorder NOS is a category for patients who do not meet the full criteria for type I, type II, or cyclothymia. Patients with bipolar disorder may require different forms and intensities of treatment at different stages of the illness.

Bipolar depression

The criteria for a depressed episode in bipolar disorder are identical to that for major depressive disorder. Those with bipolar depression tend to exhibit higher rates of associated psychotic symptoms, hypersomnia, and predictable fluctuations in their mood throughout the day, often referred to as diurnal variation [14]. Comparatively, those with major depressive disorder tend to have more problems with lack of self-worth, decreased energy, and lack of libido [14]. It is important, although often challenging, to make the correct diagnosis because the recommended treatments are different. Depressive episodes due to major depressive disorder are treated with antidepressants. Patients with depressive episodes due to bipolar disorder generally do not respond to antidepressants, and there is some evidence that they may cause manic symptoms or rapid mood cycling [15].

Manic episode

To meet diagnostic criteria for a manic episode the patient must have an elevated mood or excessive irritability that last greater than 2 weeks (or any amount of time should the severity of the condition warrant inpatient psychiatric hospitalization). The DSM-IV-TR criteria for a manic episode are listed in Table 8.3. A mnemonic to remember criteria for a manic episode, DIG FAST, is shown in Table 8.4. In many cases, manic patients are brought to the ED by someone else (e.g., family, police, or emergency medical services). Patients who are experiencing a manic episode may present as gregarious, humorous, and engaging. Their presentation is often labile and may suddenly switch to belligerence or irritability. The patient may display pressured, rapid, or loud speech, without pauses between thoughts or sentences, and resistance to interruption. The thought process in mania is often illogical, with loose associations and flight of ideas. An inflated self-esteem and grandiose delusions may cause the patient to be argumentative, impatient, or condescending. Grandiosity often centers on very expansive, dramatic, or universal themes such as religion or politics. Patients may also demonstrate a lack of impulse control and a profound paucity of insight. Despite obvious altered behavior and impaired judgment and impulse control, the patient may insist that there is nothing wrong, or blame problems on others.

Table 8.3. Summary of DSM-IV-TR criteria for a manic episode

A. Distinct period of abnormally and persistently elevated, expansive, or irritable mood, lasting at least 2 weeks (or any duration if hospitalization is necessary).

B. During the period of mood disturbance, three or more of the following symptoms have persisted (four, if the mood is only irritable) and have been present to a significant degree:

1. Inflated self-esteem or grandiosity
2. Decreased need for sleep (e.g., feels rested after only 3 hours of sleep)
3. More talkative than usual or pressure to keep talking
4. Flight of ideas or subjective experience that thoughts are racing
5. Distractibility (i.e., attention too easily drawn to unimportant or irrelevant external stimuli)
6. Increase in goal-directed activity (either socially, at work or school, or sexually) or psychomotor agitation
7. Excessive involvement in pleasurable activities that have a high potential for painful consequences (e.g., buying sprees, sexual indiscretions, foolish investments)

C. Symptoms do not meet criteria for a "mixed episode."

D. Mood disturbance is sufficiently severe to cause marked impairment in occupational functioning or social activities or to necessitate hospitalization to prevent harm to self or others, or psychotic features are present.

E. Symptoms are not caused by direct physiologic effects of a substance (e.g., drug of abuse, medication) or a general medical condition (e.g., hyperthyroidism).

Modified from American Psychiatric Association: *The Diagnostic and Statistical Manual of Mental Disorders, 4th ed, Text Revision.* Washington, DC: American Psychiatric Association; 2000.

Table 8.4. Mnemonic for the symptoms of mania

DIG FAST

Distractibility

Irritability

Grandiosity

Flight of ideas

Activity increased

Sleeplessness

Thoughtlessness (impulsivity, increased risk taking)

Manic patients have decreased or absent need for sleep, and typically report being awake for days. They may be involved in large projects outside of their expertise (e.g., writing a novel, editing the Bible, solving world poverty), may spend excessively (e.g., excessive shopping and purchase of frivolous items), may completely disregard consequences of actions (e.g., credit cards revoked, spend the family's resources), and may engage in other risky behaviors (e.g., sexual liaisons with strangers, risky driving). A corroborating history obtained from family or others who know of the patient's behavior may provide evidence of these behaviors. Manic patients may present to the ED as trauma patients, injured by an action reflecting the patient's grandiosity (e.g., attempting to fly), impulsivity, or belligerence (e.g., fighting, resisting arrest). A manic episode may be punctuated by abrupt periods of tearfulness and profound depression, including suicidal ideation. When depressive and manic features occur concurrently in such a manner, the disorder is termed mixed or bipolar disorder, mixed episode.

Mood disorders caused by a general medical condition

Depression and medical illness frequently co-occur and each can exacerbate the other. Patients presenting to the emergency department for any reason may have a comorbid mood disorder that could be a primary or contributing factor. Alternately, patients who present primarily for mood disorder symptoms, such as suicidal ideation, should be screened for underlying medical problems that could be playing a role. Patients with mood disorders and comorbid medical problems are at increased risk for suicide. Certain medical illnesses have a well-known association with mood disorder and some are briefly mentioned below. A more comprehensive list can be found in Table 8.5.

Cancer is often associated with depression at all stages of the illness and may be a result of distress about the diagnosis, side effects of treatment, or the pathophysiology of the cancer itself. Patients with pancreatic, head, neck, and lung cancer have a relatively high incidence of depression compared to those with lymphoma, colon, and gynecological cancers, which have relatively lower rates [16,17].

Cardiovascular diseases, such as coronary artery disease, myocardial infarction, and stroke, are also often associated with depression [18]. After a myocardial infarction, patients with depression experience a 3.5-fold increase in cardiovascular mortality compared with nondepressed patients [19]. There is a positive correlation for both manic and depressive episodes with vascular risk factors, especially later in life [20].

Patients with depression appear to be more likely to develop stroke [21], diabetes [22], and osteoporosis [23] than those who are not depressed.

Other illnesses that have higher rates of comorbid depression are systemic lupus erythematosus [24], end-stage renal disease [25], HIV/AIDS [26], and Parkinson's disease [27].

Mania caused by a general medical condition, also known as secondary mania, has also been reported in a variety of medical illnesses such as right hemispheric stroke [28] and in HIV/AIDS patients [29].

Depression related to medical conditions can differ in some respects from primary depression and responds less favorably to antidepressant medication [30]. Two significant issues arise in the assessment of patients with depression who have a serious medical illness. First, symptoms of depression can be difficult to distinguish from the symptoms and signs associated with serious medical illness (e.g., weight loss, loss of energy, slowing of activity, sleep disturbance, loss of ability to concentrate). Second, it is important to determine if mood changes associated with terminal, rapidly progressive, or painful illness should be considered appropriate adjustment and grief. Although patients with such diseases may understandably be distressed, most do not have

Table 8.5. Medical illnesses associated with onset of depression

Neurologic
  Parkinson's disease
  Stroke
  Multiple sclerosis
  Head trauma
  Sleep apnea
Neoplastic
  Pancreatic carcinoma
  Brain tumor
  Disseminated carcinomatosis
Endocrine
  Hypothyroidism
  Hyperthyroidism
  Cushing's disease
  Addison's disease
  Diabetes mellitus
Infectious
  Human immunodeficiency virus
Cardiac
  Coronary artery disease
  Myocardial infarction
Renal
  End-stage renal disease
  Renal dialysis
Connective tissue
  Lupus erythematosus
  Rheumatoid arthritis

Table 8.6. Medications that can cause depressive or manic symptoms

Depressive symptoms

  Antihypertensives
    Beta-blockers
    Captopril
    Clonidine
    Diltiazem
    Enalapril
    Nifedipine
    Prazosin
    Thiazide diuretics
  Anticonvulsants
    Phenytoin
    Topiramate
    Valproic acid
  Hormones
    Anabolic steroids
    Contraceptives
    Corticosteroids
    Thyroid hormone
  Sedative-hypnotics
    Barbiturates
    Benzodiazepines
Manic symptoms

  Psychiatric agents
    Antidepressants
  Antibiotics
    Acyclovir
    Chloroquine
    Interferon
    Isoniazid
    Norfloxacin
    Ofloxacin
    Sulfonamides
  Other agents
    Amantadine
    Bromocriptine
    Cyclobenzaprine
    Cycloserine
    Digitalis
    Disopyramide
    Levodopa
    Metoclopramide
    Nonsteroidal anti-inflammatory drugs
    Phenylpropanolamine
    Theophylline

major depressive disorder. For those who do have major depressive disorder, treatment and proper referral should be considered.

Also, patients with severe medical issues can present in a delirious state. Delirium is defined by DSM-IV-TR as disturbance in consciousness with impairment in maintenance of attention that may also involve perceptual disturbances, and can fluctuate throughout the day. Patients may present with agitation that could mimic the symptoms of a manic episode. Also, delirium can present as a withdrawal that can mimic the symptoms of a depressed episode. Delirium is most likely due to serious medical problems that need evaluation, disposition, and treatment separate from that of mood disorders.

Mood disorders caused by medications or other substances

Certain medications are associated with symptoms of mood disorders (Table 8.6). Intoxication or chronic, heavy use of alcohol, sedatives, hypnotics, anxiolytics, narcotics, and other central nervous system depressants can mimic symptoms of a major depressive episode. By contrast, stimulants such as cocaine, hallucinogens, and amphetamines can have primary effects that are similar to symptoms of a manic episode. Mood disorder symptoms can also develop during substance withdrawal. In addition, substance abuse may often result from patients' attempts to self-medicate an underlying mood disorder, further complicating assessment [31].

Diagnostic strategies

The diagnosis of a mood disorder is based on history, collateral information, and observation of the patient's behavior. Mood disorders should be suspected in patients with multiple, vague, nonspecific complaints and in patients who are frequent users of medical care. When evaluating the patient, one should focus on the presenting complaint and evaluate the possibility that drug abuse, medications, or a general medical condition may be responsible for the patient's condition.

Precipitating events (e.g., loss of a job or relationship), accompanying symptoms (e.g., hallucinations, delusions, anxiety disorder, mania), and suicidal ideation or intent should be assessed. The patient's history should be confirmed through interviews with family, friends, or eyewitnesses to the events that precipitated the ED visit. A tentative diagnosis can be established using DSM-IV-TR criteria.

Management

Emergency department stabilization

The creation of a safe and stable environment for the patient should be a first priority in management. The patient with an acute manic episode may be disruptive, refuse medical evaluation, and make repeated attempts to leave the ED. The initial step in treating such a disruptive patient is to offer assistance in reducing their agitation (placing the patient in a single room, recommending medication). At times, this approach does not work and the patient may need to be placed in seclusion or physical restraints for his or her safety, and that of others.

Initiating treatment for a mood disorder is not typically done in the ED. An exception is the acute manic episode (or possibly a severe depressive episode with psychosis) with behavior so extreme that the patient or others are threatened. Such cases may well involve significant hallucinations, delusions, and other features of psychoses. In such cases, an antipsychotic agent is often indicated. For years, clinicians have used intramuscular or oral haloperidol with or without lorazepam to calm such patients. A typical regimen for "rapid tranquilization" is an initial dose of 5 mg of haloperidol with 2 mg of lorazepam IM, and then reassessment in 30 to 45 minutes for resolution of "target" symptoms such as agitation. Another 5-mg dose is administered after 30 to 60 minutes as needed for improvement in hallucinations, delusions, agitation, or violent behavior [32]. Most patients respond after one or two doses. Some cases may require administration of medications without patient consent, typically in compliance with local laws or regulations. Benztropine (Cogentin), 1 to 2 mg po or IM, is often given initially to prevent extrapyramidal symptoms.

The "atypical" antipsychotic medicines include ziprasidone, risperidone, olanzapine, aripiprazole, and quetiapine. The atypical agents are favored because they produce few of the side effects associated with conventional antipsychotic agents, such as acute dystonia, other extrapyramidal symptoms, and sedation [32]. Oral doses should be offered first, and several agents, including risperidone, olanzapine, and aripiprazole, are available in rapidly dissolving tablet form. Three atypical agents are available for intramuscular injection: ziprasidone (Geodon), olanzapine (Zyprexa), and aripiprazole (Abilify). Ziprasidone 10 to 20 mg is effective; however, its use is limited to 40 mg per 24 hours. Olanzapine 2.5 to 10 mg is also effective, but is associated with postural hypotension, and is not recommended in combination with benzodiazepines due to risk of hypoventilation syndrome. Aripiprazole at doses of 9.75 to 15 mg seems to be the least sedating of the atypical antipsychotic medications. However, it is more likely to cause nausea and vomiting.

Suicide risk management

Admission to a safe and secure setting, such as an inpatient psychiatric ward, is generally indicated for a patient who presents to the emergency department with intention of attempting suicide and a specific suicide plan that has a high chance of lethality. Admission is generally recommended after a suicide attempt or an aborted suicide attempt. Admission should occur especially if the patient has psychotic symptoms, the attempt was nearly lethal, premeditated, or violent, and precautions were taken to avoid rescue or discovery. Admission should also be considered if the patient has limited family or social support, if they have had recent impulsive behavior, are severely agitated, demonstrate evidence of poor judgment, or have a pattern of refusal of help [33].

If suicidal ideation or a suicide attempt occurred as a response to a definitive precipitating event, consideration can be given for release from the emergency department should the patient's view of the situation change since their initial presentation. This can also be considered if the suicide plan and intent have a low risk of lethality, if the patient has a stable and supportive living environment, or if the patient is currently in treatment and able to cooperate with recommended follow-up [33].

Conclusion

Mood disorders are prevalent, especially in the medically ill population, and patients with these disorders will frequently present to the ED for evaluation. The presence of mood symptoms may indicate the presence of, or can complicate the treatment of, other medical problems. Additionally, patients with mood disorders are at higher risk for suicide. It is important to consider these issues in all patients who present to the ED.

References

1. American Psychiatric Association. *Diagnostic and Statistical Manual of Mental Disorders, 4th Edition, Text Revision*. Washington, DC: The American Psychiatric Association; 2000.

2. Boudreaux ED, Clark S, Camargo CA Jr. Mood disorder screening among adult emergency department patients: a multicenter study of prevalence, associations and interest in treatment. *Gen Hosp Psychiatry* 2008;**30**:4.

3. Akiskal HS. Mood disorders: clinical features. In: Sadock BJS, Sadock VA, Ruiz P, (Eds.). *Kaplan & Sadock's Comprehensive Textbook of Psychiatry*, (9th Edition). Philadelphia, PA: Lippincott Williams and Wilkins; 2009: 1679.

4. Cruz DD, Pearson A, Saini P, et al. Emergency department contact prior to suicide in mental health patients. *Emerg Med J* 2011;**28**:467–71.

5. Pearn J, Gardner-Thorpe C. Jules Cotard (1840–1889): his life and the unique syndrome which bears his name. *Neurology* 2002;**58**:1400–3.

6. Vink D, Aartsen MJ, Schoevers RA. Risk factors for anxiety and depression in the elderly: a review. *J Affect Disord* 2008;**106**:29–44.

7. Edwards CD, Glick R. Depression. In: Glick R, Berlin JS, Fishkind AB, Zeller SL, (Eds.). *Emergency Psychiatry: Principles and Practice*. Philadelphia: Lippincott Williams and Wilkins; 2008: 175–87.

8. Charney DS, Reynolds CF, Lewis L, et al. Depression and bipolar support alliance consensus statement on the unmet needs in diagnosis and treatment of mood disorders in late life. *Arch Gen Psychiatry* 2003;**60**:664–72.

9. Sadock BJS, Sadock VA. Geriatric psychiatry. *Kaplan & Sadock's Synopsis of Psychiatry*, (10th Edition). Philadelphia: Lippincott Williams & Williams; 2008: 1348–58.

10. Sadock BJS, Sadock VA. Mood disorders and suicide in children and adolescents. *Kaplan & Sadock's Synopsis of Psychiatry*, (10th Edition). Philadelphia: Lippincott Williams & Williams; 2008: 1258–69.

11. Bhatia SK, Bhatia SC. Childhood and adolescent depression. *Am Fam Physician* 2007;**75**:73–80.

12. AACAP Official Action. Practice parameter for the assessment and treatment of children and adolescents with depressive disorders. *J Am Acad Child Adolesc Psychiatry* 2007;**46**:1503–26.

13. Pearlstein T, Howard M, Salisbury A, Zlotniick C. Postpartum depression. *Am J Obstet Gynecol* 2009;**200**:357–64.

14. Forty L, Smith D, Jones L, et al. Clinical differences between bipolar and unipolar depression. *Br J Psychiatry* 2008;**192**:388–9.

15. Nivoli AMA, Colom F, Murru A, et al. New treatment guidelines for acute bipolar depression: a systematic review. *J Affect Disord* 2011;**129**:14–26.

16. Jia L, Jiang S, Shang Y, et al. Investigation of the incidence of pancreatic cancer-related depression and its relationship with the quality of life of patients. *Digestion* 2010;**82**:4–9.

17. Breitbart WS, Lederberg MS, Rueda-Lara MA, Alici A. Psychosomatic medicine: psycho oncology. In: Sadock BJ, Sadock VA, Ruiz P, (Eds.). *Kaplan & Sadock's Comprehensive Textbook of Psychiatry*, (9th Edition). Philadelphia: Lippincott Williams and Wilkins; 2009: 2314–53.

18. Shapiro PA, Wulsin LR. Psychosomatic medicine: cardiovascular disorders. In: Sadock BJ, Sadock VA, Ruiz P, (Eds.). *Kaplan & Sadock's Comprehensive Textbook of Psychiatry*, (9th Edition). Philadelphia: Lippincott Williams and Wilkins; 2009: 2250–63.

19. Gilbody S. Whitty P. Grimshaw J. Thomas R. Educational and organizational interventions to improve the management of depression in primary care: a systematic review. *JAMA* 2003;**289**:3145–51.

20. Subramaniam H, Dennis MS, Byrne EJ. The role of vascular risk factors in late onset bipolar disorder. *Int J Geriatr Psychiatry* 2007;**22**:733–7.

21. Pan A, Sun Q, Okereke OL, Rexrod KM, Hu FB. Depression and risk of stroke morbidity and mortalilty. *JAMA* 2011;**306**:1241–9.

22. Knol MJ, Twisk JWR, Beekman ATF, et al. Depression as a risk factor for the onset of type 2 diabetes mellitus. A meta-analysis. *Diabetologia* 2006;**49**:837–45.

23. Cizza G, Primma S, Csako G. Depression as a risk factor for osteoporosis. *Trends Endocrinol Metab* 2009;**20**:367–73.

24. Petri M, Naqibuddin M, Carson KA, et al. Depression and cognitive impairment in newly diagnosed systemic lupus erythematosis. *J Rheumatol* 2010;**37**:2032–8.

25. Agganis BT, Weiner DE, Giang LM, et al. Depression and cognitive function in maintenance hemodialysis patients. *Am J Kidney Dis* 2010;**56**:704–12.

26. Leserman J. Role of depression, stress, and trauma in HIV disease progression. *Psychosom Med* 2008;**70**:539–45.

27. Reijnders J, Ehrt U, Weber W, Aarsland D, Leentjens A. A systematic review of prevalence studies of depression in Parkinson's disease. *Mov Disord* 2008;**23**:183–9.

28. Perez DL. Catenaccio E. Epstein J. Confusion, hyperactive delirium, and secondary mania in right hemispheric strokes: a focused review of neuroanatomical correlates. *J Neurol Neurophysiol* 2011;**S1**:1–5.

29. Spiegel DR, Weller AL, Pennell K, Turner K. The successful treatment of mania due to acquired immunodeficiency syndrome using ziprasidone: a case series. *J Neuropsychiatry Clin Neurosci* 2010;**22**:111–14.

30. Popin MK. Consultation-liaison psychiatry. In: Jacobson JL, Jacobson AM, (Eds.). *Psychiatric Secrets*, (2nd Edition). Philadelphia: Hanley and Belfus; 2004: 381.

31. Bolton JM, Robinson J, Sareen J. Self-medication of mood disorders with alcohol and drugs in the National Epidemiologic Survey on Alcohol and Related Conditions. *J Affect Disord* 2008;**115**:367–75.

32. Rund DA. Ewing JD. Mitzel K. Votolato N. The use of intramuscular benzodiazepines and antipsychotic agents in the treatment of acute agitation or violence in the ED. *J Emerg Med* 2003;**31**:317–24.

33. American Psychiatric Association. *Practice Guideline for the Assessment and Treatment of Patients with Suicidal Behaviors*. 2003. Available at: http://psychiatryonline.org/guidelines.aspex (Accessed February 10, 2012).

Assessment of the suicidal patient in the emergency department

Clare Gray

Introduction

Suicidal patients account for approximately 2% of all emergency department (ED) visits [1]. Patients with suicidal ideation and suicide attempts often present to the ED for help. In addition, patients who make serious suicide attempts are brought to the ED for medical intervention and stabilization. The assessment of the suicidal patient in the ED and the determination of suicide risk is an important skill for Emergency Physicians as they need to decide on the most appropriate disposition for these patients.

Each year in the United States, approximately 650,000 patients present to emergency departments with suicidal ideation and behavior [2]. Suicide ranks eleventh among causes of death in the United States, and is the third leading cause of death (after accidents and homicides) for youth 15–24 years of age [3].

This chapter will outline the epidemiology and risk factors for suicide as this provides the busy ED physician with a good framework around which to structure the patient interview. In addition, an approach to assessing the individual patient's suicide risk will be reviewed. Finally, management and disposition alternatives for the suicidal patient will be discussed.

Epidemiology

Suicide is a major public health concern. In 2007, more than 34,000 suicides occurred in the United States. This equates to almost 100 suicides per day and an overall population rate of 11.3 suicide deaths per 100,000 people [4]. The 2009 Youth Risk Behavior Surveillance survey conducted by the Center for Disease Control in the United States revealed that 13.8% of high school students had seriously contemplated attempting suicide in the 12 months preceding the survey. Nationwide, 6.3% of students had attempted suicide at least once during the same time period and 1.9% of students had required medical attention for their suicide attempts [5]. An estimated 8 to 25 suicide attempts occur for every suicide completion. However, there are even wider variations to this ratio. Some estimate that there are approximately 100 to 200 suicide attempts for every completed suicide in youth aged 15 to 24 years old, particularly among young women. Among older adults (aged 65 and over) the ratio is much lower with approximately four suicide attempts for every completed suicide [3].

Risk factors for suicide

Knowledge about the risk factors related to suicide is important as it helps to guide the assessment of the suicidal patient in the ED. One needs to obtain information regarding the presence of any risk factors for suicide, as this will contribute to the determination of suicide risk. It is important to remember that these factors are characteristics associated with suicide; however, they are not necessarily direct causes of suicide.

Gender

Males complete suicide four times more often than females [4]; however, females attempt suicide far more often than males. Males tend to use more lethal methods such as hanging and firearms, which may help to explain this discrepancy. Females tend to use less lethal means such as overdose [6,7].

Age

Young males (15 to 24 years of age) are at higher risk of suicide as are elderly males over the age of 65 years. The suicide rate in males over the age of 85 years is approximately 47/100,000 or more than 4 times the national average [4].

Psychiatric illness

The literature has shown that approximately 90% of those who complete suicide ("suicide completers") have a diagnosable psychiatric disorder at the time of their deaths [7–9]. The most common diagnosis is major depressive episode (50%). Substance abuse is also an important risk factor with approximately 30% of suicide completers having an elevated blood alcohol level at the time of their deaths [10]. In another study examining completed suicides in young people, the most frequent psychiatric diagnoses were mood disorder (42.1%) substance-related disorders (40.8%), and disruptive behavior disorder (20.8%) [11].

However, it is important to note that it is a small percentage of patients with psychiatric illness who commit suicide. Reviews of the literature place the lifetime risk for suicide at 2 to 8% for mood disorders, 4 to 5% for schizophrenia, and 7% for alcohol dependence [12–15]. The rate of suicide in clinical samples of

Behavioral Emergencies for the Emergency Physician, ed. Leslie S. Zun, Lara G. Chepenik, and Mary Nan S. Mallory. Published by Cambridge University Press. © Cambridge University Press 2013.

patients with borderline personality disorder is approximately 5 to 10% [16].

The risk of suicide is related to the type and severity of the psychiatric illness. In psychotic illnesses, such as schizophrenia, the risk for suicide can be especially high if the patient is experiencing command hallucinations telling the patient to kill him- or herself. It is important to remember that with respect to depression, it may well be that at the time of initial improvement in the early phase of recovery from depression patients may be at increased risk of suicide. This is believed to be due, in part, to the fact that as patients recover from depression, they initially can see improvements in their energy level, appetite, concentration, motivation and sleep while their mood may remain depressed. Patients at this point in recovery still feel sad, hopeless, and suicidal but have regained the necessary energy and focus to develop and implement a suicidal plan. While this is a strongly held conviction among clinicians, there are no research data to support such beliefs—however, it is important to monitor patients for suicide risk throughout their recovery [17,18].

While psychiatric illness is usually a chronic risk factor for suicide, it is important to remember that the timing of suicidal behavior is often connected to stressful life events, especially psychosocial or environmental situations such as bereavement, divorce, job loss, threat of incarceration, humiliation, and other challenges to self-esteem and confidence that overwhelm a patient's coping skills [19,20]. Discharge following psychiatric hospitalization is also a period of high risk for suicide, especially in the first few weeks postdischarge [21].

Previous suicide attempt

If one examines suicide completers, the literature shows that a previous suicide attempt is a strong predictor of completed suicide even when controlling for the presence mood disorders [22]. An international review of studies involving suicide completers found that approximately 40% of those who died by suicide had made a previous suicide attempt [23].

However, if one examines suicide attempters, research has shown that approximately 10% of people who attempt suicide will go on to die by suicide at a future time. One review article summarizing 90 studies involving people who had made suicide attempts, found that approximately 7% (range: 5–11%) of attempters eventually completed suicide, approximately 23% had subsequent suicide attempts, and 70% had no further suicidal behavior [24]. Yet another study which followed suicide attempters found similar suicide completion rates of 4.0% at 5 years, 4.5% at 10 years, and 6.7% at 18 years [25]. There has been a more recent study that found a slightly higher suicide completion rate following suicide attempts. This was a 37-year follow-up study from Finland that showed an eventual suicide completion rate of 13% following a suicide attempt [26].

In children and adolescents who make a suicide attempt, between 25 to 66% will go on to make another attempt [27,28]. The period of greatest risk of suicide completion following a suicide attempt in a child or youth seems to be in the first 6 to 12 months following the attempt [29].

Access to firearms

The risk of suicide completion increases in patients with access to weapons, most notably firearms. Firearms are more lethal than other methods for suicide, with approximately 85% of suicide attempts with firearms being fatal [30]. A study of adolescent suicide attempters and completers found that those who died by suicide were two times more likely to have firearms in their homes [31]. More suicide completers use firearms (50.7%) than any other method. After firearms, hanging/strangulation (23.1%) and poisoning (18.8%) are the next most frequent methods used. Male suicide completers most commonly use firearms (56%) followed by hanging (24.4%), whereas female suicide completers most often use poisoning (40.8%) followed by firearms (31.9%) [32].

Marital status

Overall, single individuals who have never been married commit suicide at twice the rate of those who are married [33]. Research has consistently found that married persons are at decreased risk of suicide [34]. However, divorce appears to be more of a risk factor for men than for women. One study found that divorced or separated men were more than twice as likely to commit suicide as married men. There were no significant differences for married versus divorced or separated women in terms of suicide rate. In addition, in this particular study, there was no effect on suicide rate for being single or widowed [35]. However, another study found markedly elevated suicide rates for young widows and widowers less than 50 years of age. This study reported a 9- to 17-fold increase in suicide rate for widowed men (aged 20 to 34 years) compared to married men of the same age [36].

Chronic medical illnesses

The presence of a general medical condition can increase the risk for suicide. Studies of suicide completers have found that having a chronic medical illness is a strong predictor of completed suicide [37–39]. The exact manner by which chronic medical illnesses influence suicide attempts and completions is unclear. Hypotheses include direct effects of the medical condition on the brain leading to increased impulsivity and disinhibition such as with acute brain injuries; the development of a psychiatric illness such as depression or psychosis secondary to the medical condition; or patients finding the chronic pain or disfigurement from an illness overwhelming.

Elevated suicide rates are found in patients with neurological illnesses (seizures, multiple sclerosis, Huntington's chorea, brain injury) and cancer. In one study of patients with at least one general physical illness, 25.2% reported suicidal ideation and 8.9% reported a suicide attempt. In this same study, increased rates of suicidal ideation were found in patients with asthma and bronchitis and a 4-fold increase in suicide attempt was found for patients with asthma and cancer [39]. Another study examining elderly patients found an association between completed suicide and several common physical illnesses, including congestive heart failure, seizures, and chronic pulmonary diseases [40]. Patients with end-stage renal disease have also been found to have significantly higher rates of suicide than the general population [41]. Although the incidence of suicide among patients infected with HIV has decreased in recent years, this group continues to remain at high risk for suicide [42]. Higher incidences of suicide have been found in other conditions such as peptic ulcer disease and spinal cord injury [43,44]. Patients with physical illnesses who commit suicide usually have a comorbid psychiatric illness, most commonly depression and alcoholism [45].

Sexual orientation

Lesbian, gay, and bisexual (LGB) adolescents express higher rates of suicidal ideation and attempt suicide more frequently than their heterosexual counterparts [46]. The reasons for this increased risk among LGB youth are unclear. Increased suicidal behavior among LGB youth may be due to other risk factors such as bullying, rejection following disclosure, social isolation, or substance abuse. A study of adult male twin pairs demonstrated an increased lifetime prevalence of suicidal behaviors among male twins reporting same sex sexual orientation when compared to heterosexual male twins. This increased prevalence persisted even when results were controlled for substance abuse and depression [47].

Family history and genetics

The risk of suicide increases in patients with a family history of suicide. There is a 6-fold increase in suicide risk for patients with a first-degree relative who has committed suicide [3]. It is not clear whether this familial influence on increased suicide risk is related to the transmission of a gene for suicide or psychiatric illness, or to environmental factors such as family dysfunction, abuse, or even possibly imitation of the suicide completer. In some families, it may be that suicide is viewed as a solution for difficult problems which becomes repeated over generations.

History of childhood abuse

Child maltreatment can take many forms, including physical abuse, sexual abuse, verbal abuse, or neglect. Research has shown that adults with a previous history of maltreatment can be up to 25 times more likely to attempt suicide than adults without a history of abuse [48]. In adults with a past history of abuse, 21% to 34% report having made a suicide attempt compared to 4% to 9% of adults without a past history of abuse [3]. Sexual and physical abuse have the strongest relationship to suicide attempts. One study that examined depressed adults found those with a history of childhood sexual or physical abuse were more likely to have made a suicide attempt than those without an abuse history. This study also found that abuse

in childhood was associated with an earlier age of onset of suicidal behavior: often beginning in childhood or adolescence [49]. A history of sexual abuse also carries a very high risk of repeated suicide attempts in adolescents [50].

Other risk factors

Personal qualities such as the presence of hopelessness, impulsiveness, and high emotional reactivity are associated with a higher suicide risk [51,52]. Each of these qualities can contribute to feelings of increased distress and ultimately lead to suicide [53]. One prospective study examining almost 7000 psychiatric outpatients, found hopelessness to be an important risk factor for suicide [21].

Protective factors

Having strong social supports (family, friends) is an important protective factor in providing support, a sense of belonging and acceptance, as well as supervision for patients with suicidal ideation. Being responsible for the care of others (as in the case of pregnancy and parenting) may prevent some suicidal patients from taking action out of a sense of duty to others. Religious and cultural beliefs that discourage suicide may also serve to lower the risk of suicide [54]. One study found that people with no religious connections had significantly higher risk of attempted suicide, and more first-degree relatives who committed suicide, than those with religious affiliations. In addition, those without religious connections also had fewer moral objections to suicide and fewer reasons for living [55].

The SADPERSONS scale

When assessing suicidal patients, it can be very helpful to have a framework to help recall the risk factors for suicide. The SADPERSONS scale is one tool that is commonly used as a helpful reminder in these situations [56].

SADPERSONS scale		
S	Sex	Males are at higher risk
A	Age	<19 years old or >65 years old are at higher risk
D	Depression	Does the patient have symptoms or diagnosis of depression?
P	Previous attempt	Previous suicide attempt increases risk
E	Ethanol abuse	Substance abuse associated with higher risk
R	Rational thinking loss	Psychosis, organic brain syndromes at higher risk
S	Social supports lacking	Strong social supports can be a protective factor
O	Organized plan	Careful planning and access to means increases risk
N	No spouse	Separated, divorced, widowed, and single at higher risk
S	Sickness	Chronic medical illnesses increase risk

To score the SADPERSONS scale, each item is given a score of 1 if it is present and then the score is totalled out of 10. The table below outlines the possible actions to be taken depending on the tabulated score.

Scoring the SADPERSONS scale	
Total score	Proposed disposition
0 to 2	Discharge with follow-up
3 to 4	Provide close follow-up, consider admission
5 to 6	Strongly consider admission, depends on confidence with follow-up arrangements
7 to 10	Admit to hospital, consider involuntary admission if necessary

It is important to remember that patients don't kill themselves because of risk factors. Risk factors are determined by studying large populations and work well in providing general clues to characteristics associated with suicide but do not work as well on an individual basis. A patient can have many risk factors for suicide but never attempt suicide whereas another patient may attempt or complete suicide with very few risk factors. This may lead a clinician to question why gather information about risk factors at all. The importance of asking about risk factors is to arouse the clinician's suspicions that the patient in front of them *may* be at risk of suicide, thereby prompting the further evaluation of the individual patient's own suicidal ideation and planning [57]. It is only by assessing each individual patient's thinking and planning regarding suicide that a true appreciation of a patient's suicide risk can be determined.

The patient evaluation

The immediate medical stabilization of patients following a suicide attempt is the first priority. Only once patients are medically stable can an assessment of their suicidal risk begin. It is important for ED physicians to keep a high index of suspicion when treating patients with unexplained injuries or certain types of trauma (fall from heights, motor vehicle collisions) as these patients may have covert suicidal intentions. It is also important to ensure that patients do not have any weapons, sharps, or pills in their possession that they could use to attempt suicide in the ED. Patients should be placed in a room that has been designed to provide a safe environment, free from equipment and/or instruments that patients could use to harm themselves. These measures in addition to close observation while in the ED helps to ensure the patient's safety.

To assess the suicide risk in an individual patient, one might first consider establishing a therapeutic alliance sufficient to allow the patient to be open and honest about his or her thinking and planning with regard to suicide. In a busy ED, this is can be particularly challenging. If a patient truly believes that a clinician is interested in trying to understand and help them, then they may be more forthcoming with the important personal details needed to assess suicide risk.

In approaching the suicidal patient, the busy ED clinician might consider slowing down and appearing unrushed. Emergency physicians who take the time to sit down, make eye contact, and are empathic can be more likely to set their patients at ease. The ED clinician facilitates the interview through their sensitivity, openness, and nonjudgmental manner. It is important that the ED clinician be aware of their own feelings with regard to suicide and suicidal patients, as this may influence the outcome of the interview if a negative or frustrated atmosphere is created.

Suicidal ideation

Patients may not spontaneously volunteer information regarding their suicidal thinking and planning, but might do so when asked. Slow and gentle introduction of the topic of suicidality can help to put the patient at ease. It is suggested that clinicians begin with more general and less intrusive questions and then move to more direct and specific questions regarding thoughts and plans about suicide [58]. Asking a patient directly about suicide does not increase the suicide risk [8]. People can find it very distressing to have suicidal thoughts and are more than willing to discuss these thoughts if they are asked about them.

Below is an example of a series of questions moving from the more open-ended variety to the more direct and specific. When asking about suicidal risk, it is important to remember that clinicians should develop and use their own phrasing and terminology with which they are comfortable. Common sense suggests that this will contribute to the creation of a relaxed atmosphere where patients might feel more willing to share personal thoughts and feelings.

- Have you ever had the feeling that you didn't want to get up to greet the day?
- Have you ever had thoughts that you can't go on living?
- Do you ever think that you would be better off dead?
- Do you ever think that if you went to sleep and didn't wake up that that would be ok?
- With this much stress in your life, have you ever thought about ending your life?
- Have you ever thought of a plan to end your life?
- If yes then – Tell me about your plan
- How close have you come to implementing your plan?
- Do you have access to a (gun)?
- What has prevented you from acting on this plan?
- What stops you from killing yourself?

Assessment of the frequency, intensity, and duration of suicidal thinking may provide clues to the patient's current suicidal risk. Frequency of suicidal thinking can be obtained by asking "How often do you think about ending your life?" Using scales of 1 to 10 might be helpful in gauging the intensity of the suicidal thinking. For example, asking a patient "On a scale of 1 to 10, with 1 being no intention to follow through and 10 being definite intention to end your life, what is the likelihood that you will follow through with your suicidal plan?" can aid the clinician in estimating the degree of suicidal intent, although these measures are untested in predicting outcomes. To assess duration of suicidal thinking, clinicians can ask "For how long have you been thinking of ending your life?"

Another important area to assess is hopelessness – an overall feeling of negativity toward the future. Research has shown that hopelessness is an important risk factor for both suicide ideation and completed suicide in depressed adults [21]. When patients are without hope and cannot see any possible solutions to their problems, then they can view suicide as a solution. Asking a patient "Do you have hope that things will get better?" can provide insight into the degree of hopelessness.

The presence of future orientation is also important to assess. Asking patients about plans for the immediate future (i.e., that evening or the next day) as well as asking about long-term goals (i.e., graduation from high school, career plans) can be very helpful in determining if the patient sees themselves with a future which may indicate a lower suicidal risk. Another way of assessing future orientation is to ask the patient about his or her own particular reasons for living. Relationships or responsibilities that give a person's life meaning or a sense of purpose can be protective in terms of lessening suicidal risk [59]. In a study looking at the role of future orientation in adults with depression, results showed that being future oriented correlated with reduced current suicidal ideation [60].

Suicide attempts

The assessment of suicidal risk following a suicide attempt needs to include the collection of specific information regarding the planning and execution of the attempt as well as details about what transpired following the attempt as this information will be crucial for the determination of suicide risk. It is important to start with open-ended questions such as "What happened to bring you to the ED?" or "Can you tell me what happened today?" This allows the patient to describe the details of their attempt in their own words and can contribute to a positive therapeutic alliance. The clinician then needs to follow-up with more directed questions to gather the information required to determine ongoing suicidal risk.

Additional questions might seek to determine whether the suicide attempt was well organized, carefully considered, and planned (higher risk) or whether it was an impulsive act completed in the heat of the moment (somewhat lower but possibly more chronic risk). In assessing a suicide attempt, the lethality as well as the availability of help or potential to abort the attempt should be considered as this may provide clues to the intensity of the suicide risk in a particular patient. For example, a patient who has chosen highly lethal means (such as firearms or hanging), combined with low chance of discovery or little ability to abort the attempt, is more likely to be at higher suicidal risk than a patient who has chosen means of low lethality with high chance of being discovered or being able to abort the attempt. Finally, details regarding what happened after the attempt, including specifically how the patient came to the ED,

needs to be established as this can provide additional clues with regard to intent to die. For example, was the patient discovered unexpectedly (higher risk) or did the patient call for help immediately after the attempt (lower risk)?

In terms of lethality, the ED physician will know the objective lethality of a suicide attempt by virtue of his or her medical training. However, it is important to assess the patient's understanding of how lethal they thought their attempt was going to be, as this will indicate their level of intent to die. Clinicians should not automatically dismiss an overdose of low lethality (such as with prescription antibiotics), as patients can believe that any prescription medications are lethal in overdose. Asking the patient "What did you think taking those 5 penicillin pills would do?" can reveal the subjective lethality of the attempt.

The assessment of a suicide attempt also includes information about the availability of help or intervention from others at the time of the attempt. Patients who make suicide attempts in the company of others or in situations where there is the high likelihood of intervention are most certainly expressing a degree of distress at the time, but their level of intent to die is low. These patients may be using suicidal behavior as a means of expressing their level of distress, looking for additional support or to manipulate the behavior of others. On the other hand, patients who attempt suicide in situations where their discovery is unlikely would be considered to have a much higher intent to die. Similarly, discerning the potential for the patient to abort their suicide attempt is also important as it may give some guidance as to the intensity of the suicidal feelings and desire to die. Suicide attempts using firearms are most often fatal as this method does do not give the option of changing one's mind; however, overdosing and even potentially hanging and carbon monoxide poisoning provide time during the attempt when patients could potentially change their mind and abort the attempt.

During the assessment of a suicide attempt, it is also informative to evaluate how the patient is feeling post-attempt. Questions such as "How do you feel now that you did not kill yourself?" can reveal whether there is ongoing suicidal ideation and planning. Patients who report relief at not having killed themselves can be deemed to be at lower suicidal risk when compared to patients who are disappointed that their attempt failed. Another helpful question can be "What, if anything, do you think you have learned from this experience?" Responses to this question can help the clinician to determine whether the suicide attempt has had any influence in terms of the patient's perception of their life problems, support systems, and general value of their own life.

To summarize, below is a sampling of questions demonstrating the level of detailed questioning required in the assessment of a suicide attempt by overdose.

- What happened to bring you to the ED? (open ended)
- Can you tell me what happened today? (open ended)
- For how long were you thinking about taking the pills?
- Where did you get the pills?

- How many pills were in the bottle? How many pills did you take? What stopped you from taking all of the pills?
- How were you feeling as you took the pills?
- What was it about today that you ended up taking the pills?
- Where were you when you took the pills? Was anyone else there or were you alone?
- What did you think the pills would do to you?
- What happened after you took the pills?
- How do you feel now that you didn't kill yourself?
- Is there anything that you have learned from this experience?
- If you were feeling the same way again, what might you do differently?

Determination of risk

There is no formula for the determination of suicide risk. As outlined in this chapter, the experienced clinician first gathers information from the patient regarding general population risk factors, combines this with the information gathered with respect to the individual patient's thinking and planning regarding suicide and uses good judgment to generate an overall sense of the patient's suicide risk. While the presence of many risk factors can be cause for concern, it is the individual patient's own thinking and planning about suicide in combination with the patient's own protective factors that helps to determine the patient's unique suicide risk. Gathering collateral information from family members or friends can also be extremely helpful in the determination of suicide risk. If there is still doubt regarding a patient's level of suicide risk, ED physicians can and should consult Psychiatry.

As a guide, higher-risk patients would be those with many risk factors (those with hopelessness, poor social supports, lack of future orientation, and psychosis with command hallucinations to commit suicide), a highly lethal or carefully planned attempt, and active ongoing plans for suicide with access to means. Moderate-risk patients would be those with risk factors, but with more ambivalence regarding suicide planning, stronger social supports that can provide supervision and limit access to means, a willingness to seek treatment, and more hope that things will improve. Lower-risk patients would include those who regret their suicide attempts, have good social support, feel hopeful about the future, are more satisfied with their lives, can identify more reasons for living [61,62], and are willing to engage in outpatient care.

Key indicators of a high-risk suicidal patient

- Patient felt that their attempt would kill them
- Low chance of being found following attempt
- Ongoing suicidal ideation and planning
- Reluctant to communicate much about their feelings and the suicide attempt
- Lack of social support,
- Unwilling to accept help

Management of the suicidal patient

Once suicidal risk is determined, appropriate disposition can be arranged. This decision will depend on the degree of suicidal risk the patient presents. Patients deemed to be at high risk for suicide should be hospitalized – either voluntarily or involuntarily. For voluntary patients deemed to be at high risk for suicide, consideration should be given to the need for constant observation using a sitter. However, involuntary patients will always require constant observation to prevent elopement and ensure safety.

Decisions regarding the disposition of patients at moderate risk for suicide will depend on several factors. Clinicians need to assess the patient's ability and motivation to actively participate in the creation of a discharge plan. Plans made at the time of discharge are only useful if the patient and family follow them. To be comfortable discharging a patient at moderate risk for suicide, the clinician must be confident in the availability of follow-up services. Ideally, outpatient mental health services for a patient at moderate risk for suicide should be available promptly, preferably within a few days. If the clinician is at all concerned that follow-up will not be easily accessed, then consideration may need to be given to admit the patient to hospital until such time as the required outpatient follow-up services can be put in place.

Patients deemed to be at lower risk for suicide can be discharged with instructions to follow-up with their primary care physician and/or with a referral to outpatient mental health services.

Each discharge plan will need to be developed in consultation with the patient and family and will vary from patient to patient. The discharge plan should consist of a written statement with information about the plans for continued treatment (who, where, and when) and prescribed medications (if any). There should be a discussion with the patient and family, and documentation of their agreement to remove access to means for suicide (locking up medications, removing firearms). The patient should be provided with key contact phone numbers – including outpatient providers, crisis lines, mobile crisis teams, primary care physician, community mental health agencies, or peer-support centers. It is also important to provide the patient and family with specific instructions about the signs and symptoms that would indicate a need to return to the ED. As a final component of the discharge plan, the patient and family should always be reminded that they can return to the ED at anytime should there be a need.

Safety planning

Over the years, many clinicians have used the idea of "contracting for safety" or "no suicide contracts" when discharging patients from the ED with suicidal ideation. There is no evidence to support these approaches. To create a contract where a suicidal patient agrees not to have any more suicidal ideation may provide false reassurances of safety for clinicians and these contracts have simply not been proven to be effective [63,64]. A much more realistic approach is to create a safety plan with the suicidal patient. This plan is developed in collaboration with the patient and lists what the patient agrees to try should their suicidal ideation return or worsen. While safety plans will vary from patient to patient, components of a comprehensive safety plan would include listing the potential triggers for suicidal thinking; listing potential coping strategies that help reduce the patient's level of distress (taking a bath, going for a walk, listening to music, reading); listing social supports (family, friends) that can be relied on to offer help in times of distress; listing crisis line or mental health professional contact numbers; instructions on when to return to the ED; and how to make the home environment safe (removing firearms, having a friend or family member live short-term with patient to provide supervision).

Documentation

Careful documentation of suicide risk assessments provides an accurate and complete picture of a patient's current suicidal thinking and planning, as well as important information for the ongoing care of the patient. This documentation should include the presence of both suicidal risk factors and protective factors as well as a record of the patient's current suicidal thinking and intent. Including direct quotes from the patient, such as "I would never do anything to end my life," can also be useful. In the process of documentation, clinicians should also indicate any other sources of collateral information and link their determination of suicidal risk with the planning for disposition and future interventions for the patient.

Summary

Suicidal patients can present to the ED with a range of behaviors including suicidal thoughts, suicidal plans, and suicide attempts. The role of the ED physician is to assess the patient's suicidal risk so as to make appropriate decisions regarding the disposition of the patient. The assessment of suicidal behavior involves the collection of information regarding suicide risk factors, examination of the individual patient's current thinking and planning regarding suicide and decision making regarding disposition.

Important in the assessment of suicide risk is the development of a positive therapeutic alliance with the patient. All patients with suicidal behaviors should be approached in an empathic, sensitive, and nonjudgmental manner. The interview should proceed from more general inquiry to specific questions about suicidal thinking and planning. It is important to remember that asking a patient about suicidal thinking will not increase suicide risk.

The ability to complete a comprehensive assessment of suicidal behaviors is a crucial skill for all ED physicians. It is important to remember that most suicidal ideation is temporary. Using excellent interviewing skills, careful decision making, and comprehensive discharge planning, ED physicians are well placed to instill hope and to organize close follow-up for suicidal patients until their suicidal ideation has passed.

References

1. Baraff LJ, Janowicz N, Asarnow JR. Survey of California emergency departments about practices for management of suicidal patients and resources available for their care. *Ann Emerg Med* 2006;**48**:452–8.

2. Centers for Disease Control and Prevention, National Hospital Ambulatory Medical Care Survey: 2008 Emergency Department Summary Tables. Available at: http://www.cdc.gov/nchs/fastats/suicide.htm. (Accessed December 30, 2011).

3. Xu J, Kochanek KD, Murphy SL, et al. Deaths: final data for 2007. *National Vital Statistics Reports*: 2010;**58**:19. Available at: http://www.cdc.gov/NCHS/data/nvsr/nvsr58/nvsr58_19.pdf. (Accessed December 30, 2011).

4. National Institute of Mental Health. Available at: http://www.nimh.nih.gov/health/publications/suicide-in-the-us-statistics-and-prevention/index.shtml – CDC-Web-Tool. (Accessed February 8, 2012).

5. Youth Risk Behavior Surveillance (YRBS).2009. http://www.cdc.gov/mmwr/pdf/ss/ss5905.pdf. (Accessed September 15, 2011).

6. Miller M, Azrael D, Hemenway D. The epidemiology of case fatality rates for suicide in the northeast. *Ann Emerg Med* 2004;**43**:723–30.

7. Mann JJ. A current perspective of suicide and attempted suicide. *Ann Intern Med* 2002;**136**:302–11.

8. Hirschfeld RM, Russell JM. Assessment and treatment of suicidal patients. *N Engl J Med* 1997;**337**:910–15.

9. Moscicki EK. Epidemiology of completed and attempted suicide: toward a framework for prevention. *Clin Neurosci Res* 2001;**1**:310–23.

10. Centres for Disease Control and Prevention (CDC). Toxicology testing and results for suicide victims – 113 states, 2004. *MMWR Morb Mortal Wkly Rep* 2006;**55**:1245–8.

11. Fleischmann A, Bertolote JM, Belfer M, et al. Completed suicide and psychiatric diagnoses in young people: a critical examination of the evidence.*Am J Orthopsychiatry* 2005;**75**:676–83.

12. Bostwick JM, Pankratz VS. Affective disorders and suicide risk: a re-examination. *Am J Psychiatry* 2000;**157**:1925–32.

13. Hor K, Taylor M. Review: suicide and schizophrenia: a systematic review of rates and risk factors. *J Psychopharmacol* 2010;**24**:81–90.

14. Palmer BA, Pankratz VS, Bostwick JM. The lifetime risk of suicide in schizophrenia: a re-examination. *Arch Gen Psychiatry* 2005;**62**:247–53.

15. Inskip HM, Harris EC, Barraclough B. Lifetime risk of suicide for affective disorder, alcoholism and schizophrenia. *Br J Psychiatry* 1998;**172**:35–7.

16. Oumaya M, Friedman S, Pham A, et al. [Article in French] [Borderline personality disorder, self-mutilation and

suicide: literature review]. *Encephale* 2008;**34**:452–8.

17. American Psychiatric Association Practice guidelines for the assessment and treatment of patients with suicidal behaviors. *Am J Psychiatry* 2003;**160** (Suppl):1–60.

18. Mittal V, Brown WA, Shorter E. Are patients with depression at heightened risk of suicide as they begin to recover? *Psychiatr Serv* 2009;**60**:384–6.

19. Brent DA, Perper J, Moritz G, et al. Stressful life events, psychopathology, and adolescent suicide: a case control study. *Suicide Life Threat Behav* 1993;**23**:179–87.

20. Baca-Garcia E, Parra CP, Perez-Rodriguez MM, et al. Psychosocial stressors may be strongly associated with suicide attempts. *Stress Health* 2007;**198**:191–8.

21. Qin P, Nordentoft M. Suicide risk in relation to psychiatric hospitalization: evidence based on longitudinal registers. *Arch Gen Psychiatry* 2005;**62**:427–32.

22. Brown GK, Beck AT, Steer RA, et al. Risk factors for suicide in psychiatric outpatients: a 20-year prospective study. *J Consult Clin Psychol* 2000;**68**:371–7.

23. Cavanagh J, Carson A, Sharpe M, et al. Psychological autopsy studies of suicide: a systematic review. *Psychol Med* 2003;**33**:395–405.

24. Owens D, Horrocks J, House A. Fatal and non-fatal repetition of self-harm: systematic review. *Br J Psychiatry* 2002;**181**:193–9.

25. DeMoore GM, Robertson AR. Suicide in the 18 years after deliberate self-harm a prospective study. *Br J Psychiatry* 1996;**169**:489–94.

26. Suominen K, Isometsä E, Suokas J, et al. Completed suicide after a suicide attempt: a 37-year follow-up study. *Am J Psychiatry* 2004;**161**:563–4.

27. Stewart SE, Manion IG, Davidson S, et al. Suicidal children and adolescents with first emergency room presentations: predictors of six month outcome. *J Am Acad Child Adolesc Psychiatry* 2001;**40**:580–7.

28. Rosewater KM, Burr BH. Epidemiology, risk factors, intervention, and prevention of adolescent suicide. *Curr Opin Pediatr* 1998;**10**:338–43.

29. Hawton K, Fagg J. Suicide, and other causes of death, following attempted

suicide. *Br J Psychiatry* 1988;**152**:359–66.

30. Vyrostek SB, Annest JL, Ryan GW. Surveillance for fatal and nonfatal injuries – United States, 2001. *Morb Mortal Wkly Rep* 2004;**53**:1–57.

31. Brent DA, Perper JA, Allman CJ, et al. The presence and accessibility of firearms in the homes of adolescent suicide: a case-control study. *JAMA* 1991;**266**:2989–95.

32. Karch DL, Dahlberg LL, Patel N. Surveillance for violent deaths – national violent death reporting system, 16 States, 2007 Surveillance Summaries *MMWR Morb Mortal Wkly Rep* 2010;**59**:1–50.

33. Sadock BJ, Kaplan HI, Sadock VA. *Synopsis of Psychiatry: Behavioral Sciences/Clinical Psychiatry* (10th Edition). Philadelphia: Lippincott Williams & Wilkins; 2007.

34. Smith JC, Mercy JA, Conn JM. Marital status and the risk of suicide. *Am J Public Health* 1988;**78**:78–80.

35. Kposowa AJ. Marital status and suicide in the national longitudinal mortality study. *J Epidemiol Community Health* 2000;**54**:254–61.

36. Luoma JB, Pearson JL. Suicide and marital status in the United States, 1991–1996: is widowhood a risk factor? *Am J Public Health* 2002;**92**:1518–22.

37. Kaplan MS, McFarland BH, Huguet N, et al. Physical illness, functional limitations, and suicide risk: a population-based study. *Am J Orthopsychiatry* 2007;**77**:56–60.

38. Goodwin RD, Marusic A, Hoven CW. Suicide attempts in the United States: the role of physical illness. *Soc Sci Med* 2003;**56**:1783–8.

39. Druss B, Pincus H. Suicidal ideation and suicide attempts in general medical illnesses. *Arch Intern Med* 2000;**160**:1522–6.

40. Jurrlink DN, Herrmann N, Szalai JP, et al. Medical illness and the risk of suicide in the elderly. *Arch Intern Med* 2004;**164**:1179–84.

41. Kurella M, Kimmel PL, Young BS, et al. Suicide in the United States end-stage renal disease program. *J Am Soc Nephrol* 2005;**16**:774–81.

42. Carrico A, Johnson M, Morin SF, et al. Correlates of suicidal ideation among HIV-positive persons. *AIDS* 2007;**21**:1199–203.

43. Bahmanyar S, Sparen P, Mittendorfer Rutz E, et al. Risk of suicide among operated and non-operated patients hospitalized for peptic ulcers. *J Epidemiol Community Health* 2009;**63**:1016–21.

44. Hartkopp A, Bronnum-Hansen H, Seidenschnur AM, et al. Suicide in a spinal cord injured population: its relation to functional status. *Arch Phys Med Rehabil* 1998;**79**:1356–61.

45. Berger D. Suicide risk in the general hospital. *Psychiatr Clin Neurosci* 1995;**49**:S85–9.

46. Silenzio VM, Pena JB, Duberstein PR, et al. Sexual orientation and risk factors for suicidal ideation and suicide attempts among adolescents and young adults. *Am J Public Health* 2007;**97**:2017–19.

47. Herrell R, Goldberg J, True WR, et al. Sexual orientation and suicidality: a co-twin control study in adult men. *Arch Gen Psychiatry* 1999;**56**:867–74.

48. Santa Mina EE, Gallop RM. Childhood sexual and physical abuse and adult self-harm and suicidal behaviour: a literature review. *Can J Psychiatry* 1998;**43**:793–800.

49. Brodsky BS, Oquendo M, Ellis SP, et al. The relationship of childhood abuse to impulsivity and suicidal behavior in adults with major depression. *Am J Psychiatry* 2001;**158**:1871–7.

50. Brown J, Cohen P, Johnson JG, et al. Childhood abuse and neglect: specificity of effects on adolescent and young adult depression and suicidality. *J Am Acad Child Adolesc Psychiatry* 1999;**38**:1490–6.

51. Horesh N, Rolnick T, Iancu I, et al. Anger, impulsivity and suicide risk. *Psychother Psychosom* 1997;**66**:92–6.

52. Zouk H, Tousignant M, Seguin M, et al. Characterization of impulsivity in suicide completers: clinical, behavioral and psychosocial dimensions. *J Affect Disord* 2006;**92**:195–204.

53. Nock MK, Borges G, Bromet EJ, et al. Suicide and suicidal behavior. *Epidemiol Rev* 2008;**30**:133–54.

54. Stack S, Lester D. The effect of religion on suicide ideation. *Soc Psychiatry Psychiatr Epidemiol* 1991;**26**:168–70.

55. Dervic K, Oquendo MA, Grunebaum MF, et al. Religious affiliation and suicide attempt. *Am J Psychiatry* 2004;**161**:2303–8.

56. Patterson WM, Dohn HH, et al. Evaluation of suicidal patients, THE SAD PERSONS Scale. *Psychosomatics* 1983;**24**:343–9.

57. Shea SC. *The Practical Art of Suicide Assessment: A Guide for Mental Health Professionals and Substance Abuse Counsellors*. New York: John Wiley & Sons, Inc; 1999.

58. McDowell AK, Lineberry TW, Bostwick JM. Practical suicide-risk management for the busy primary care physician. *Mayo Clin Proc* 2011;**86**:792–800.

59. Britton PC, Duberstein PR, Conner KR, et al. Reasons for living, hopelessness, and suicide ideation among depressed adults 50 years or older. *Am J Geriatr Psychiatry* 2008;**16**:736–41.

60. Hirsch JK, Duberstein PR, Conner KR. Future orientation and suicide ideation and attempts in depressed adults ages 50 and over. *Am J Geriatr Psychiatry* 2006;**14**:752–7.

61. Malone KM, Oquendo MA, Gretchen L, et al. Protective factors against suicidal acts in major depression: reasons for living. *Am J Psychiatry* 2000;**157**:1084–8.

62. Montross LP, Zisook S, Kasckow J. Suicide among patients with schizophrenia: a consideration of risk and protective factors. *Ann Clin Psychiatry* 2005;**17**:173–82.

63. Edwards SJ, Sachmann MD. No-suicide contracts, no-suicide agreements, and no-suicide assurances: a study of their nature, utilization, perceived effectiveness, and potential to cause harm. *Crisis* 2010;**31**:290–302.

64. Kelly KT, Knudson MP. Are no-suicide contracts effective in preventing suicide in suicidal patients seen by primary care physicians? *Arch Fam Med* 2000;**9**:1119–21.

Chapter 1

The patient with somatoform disorders in the emergency department

Reginald I. Gaylord

Introduction

Patients often present to the emergency department (ED) with complaints of physical symptoms that are suggestive of organ system pathology. When a pertinent ED evaluation is completed and negative for abnormalities, it is reasonable to consider a somatoform disorder (SD) as a diagnosis. SDs consist of a group of psychiatric conditions that cause unintentional physical symptoms suggestive of a general medical condition. The presenting symptoms, however, cannot be explained entirely by a known general medical condition, the direct effects of a substance or other psychiatric disorder [1].

Appropriate use of the Diagnostic and Statistical Manual of Mental Disorders, 4th Edition, Text Revision (DSM-IV-TR) or the International Statistical Classification of Disease and Related Health Problems, 10th Revision (ICD-10) is helpful in correctly diagnosing psychiatric conditions. According to these sources, as well as the findings of other diagnostic tools more specific to evaluating SDs, approximately 10–36% of patients in the primary care setting have an SD [1–8]. This range may reflect the variation in individual practitioner application of diagnostic criteria, as well as variable use of other evaluative examinations [9].

SDs are burdensome to patients, patients' families, society, and the healthcare system as a whole. Unemployment, substance abuse, and relationship problems are common in patients with an SD. Patients with an SD may have a greater overall level of impairment or disability when compared to individuals with other general medical conditions [10]. SD patients may display behaviors that enhance or reinforce their concept of being ill, with a possible unconscious motive of enacting or fulfilling the "sick role" to get attention [11]. Patients with SDs use up to twice the medical care resources as patients without an SD, possibly contributing to an estimated $256 billion in U.S. healthcare expenditures annually [10].

SDs specifically addressed in this chapter include somatization disorder, undifferentiated somatoform disorder, conversion disorder, pain disorder, hypochondriasis, body dysmorphic disorder, and somatoform disorder not otherwise specified. There is significant overlap among the different SDs and other psychiatric illnesses such as mood, anxiety,

malingering, and factitious disorders [11–13]. The overlap of current SD diagnostic criteria and clinical characteristics has fueled much debate over the categorization of SD diagnoses in the future release of the DSM-V (2013 expected release) and ICD-11 (2015 expected release) [11,13–20].

An evaluator must keep in mind numerous ethical and medicolegal ramifications of inadequate evaluation, consultation, and treatment. Even when highly suspected, a diagnosis of an SD in the ED is usually one of exclusion. The ED practitioner should first rule out life- or limb-threatening conditions that are symptomatically similar to the varying complaints of an SD. Determining if SD symptoms are representative of an organic disease process or unintentionally fabricated may prove challenging.

Clinical characteristics

There are general similarities among the different somatoform disorders that may help guide a healthcare provider's evaluation. For example, the unintentional symptoms of SDs are often associated with psychosocial stressors [4]. The symptoms are usually disabling, and lead to functional impairment that warrants medical attention [1,2]. Patients with an SD often describe their symptoms in an imprecise or nonfactual manner, ranging from overly detailed to incredibly vague [21,22]. While evidence suggests an association between SDs and genetic, cultural and educational factors, evidence demonstrating a causal relationship is lacking [1,2].

Somatization disorder

Somatization disorder consists of a combination of multiple nonspecific physical complaints, involving several organ systems, which do not coincide with a general medical condition. Somatization disorder has an onset before the age of 30 years and has a chronic, but fluctuating, course over a period of several years [1,2,20]. Somatization disorder symptoms include a combination of pain, pseudoneurologic, gastrointestinal, and sexual symptoms. Pain symptoms must involve four different physiologic functions or anatomical sites (e.g., menstruation, extremities). There must be at least two gastrointestinal

Behavioral Emergencies for the Emergency Physician, ed. Leslie S. Zun, Lara G. Chepenik, and Mary Nan S. Mallory. Published by Cambridge University Press. © Cambridge University Press 2013.

symptoms (e.g., bloating). There must be at least one sexual or reproductive symptom other than pain (e.g., menorrhagia, ejaculatory dysfunction). Finally, there must be at least one neurologic symptom (e.g., impaired balance, seizures) [1].

The lifetime prevalence of somatization disorder in the general population varies from 0.1% to 2%, and is up to 20 times more common in women [1]. This gender difference may in part be due to childhood sexual abuse or exposure to violence [23].

Evidence demonstrates that interpersonal conflicts exacerbate somatization disorder symptoms, particularly in the setting of other psychiatric conditions such as anxiety and depression [13]. It is common for somatization disorder, depression, and anxiety to co-occur; co-diagnosis should be considered [7,13].

Undifferentiated SD

Patients with symptoms that do not fulfill somatization disorder diagnostic criteria may have *undifferentiated somatoform disorder*. Undifferentiated somatoform disorder consists of the presence of at least 6 months of one or more physical complaints of unknown etiology [1]. In comparison to somatization disorder, undifferentiated somatoform disorder has a shorter duration and involves fewer organ systems or physiologic functions [1,2].

Conversion disorder

Conversion disorder consists of unexplained symptoms or abnormalities in voluntary motor or sensory functions [1]. The ways in which voluntary motor or sensory functions are involuntarily affected typically do not correspond to known anatomic pathways or physiologic mechanisms [4]. These pseudoneurologic symptoms may correlate with the understanding a patient has of a specific medical condition [24]. Patients with little medical knowledge may present with symptoms that are less plausible, whereas patients with greater overall funds of knowledge may have symptoms that closely resemble a specific medical condition [1,24].

Acute psychosocial stressors frequently precede the onset of conversion disorder symptoms, which typically abate when the stressor is removed or addressed [1]. While the presenting symptoms of conversion disorder can be quite alarming (e.g., sudden blindness, seizures, or paralysis), patients may display a virtual lack of concern about the significance of their symptoms (*la belle indifférence*) [22]. Given the nature of the symptoms, an evaluator may consider other disease processes such as seizure disorders, stroke, multiple sclerosis, and myasthenia gravis.

Imaging modalities such as computed tomography (CT) and magnetic resonance imaging (MRI) scans are useful during evaluation. Functional MRI studies have implicated several intracranial neural pathways involved in processing and integrating information in patients with SDs. In patients with conversion disorder, limbic structures such as the amygdala and cingulate cortex, as well as nonlimbic structures such as the temporoparietal junction and primary sensorimotor cortex appear to be involved [21,25–29]. Molecular studies demonstrate possible abnormalities in cortisol levels in some patients with conversion disorder symptoms [30]. Although preliminary, this research begins to contribute objective data that might aid in future evaluation and treatment of patients with an SD.

The prevalence of conversion disorder ranges from 1 to 50/100,000 in the general population, but up to 3% in outpatient psychiatric clinics [1,24]. Individuals who are less knowledgeable about medical conditions or from lower socioeconomic groups are more likely to present with conversion disorder [21]. Conversion disorder usually affects individuals from late childhood to early adulthood [1].

Pain disorder

Pain is one of the most common complaints of patients who present to the ED. The patient's pain may be due to a variety of etiologies, some of which may be more than obvious, while others are more elusive. In patients suffering from *pain disorder*, various psychiatric factors cause or strongly contribute to the onset, severity, exacerbation, and continuation of pain for which there is often no identifiable organic etiology [1,2]. Different subtypes of pain disorder differentiate pain caused exclusively by psychiatric factors, or pain associated with both psychiatric factors in conjunction with a general medical condition [1].

Recent studies of chronic pain better describe the complexities of how chronic pain is influenced by, and in turn influences, both biologic and psychosocial factors [31]. For example, individuals with chronic pain may not engage in regular physical activity and have adverse health consequences from a sedentary lifestyle (e.g., weight gain). In turn, these health consequences may bring about further pain, as well as increase the likelihood of developing a psychiatric condition such as depression [31]. Furthermore, there is an increased likelihood that individuals with pain disorder will develop prescription analgesic or anxiolytic dependence or abuse patterns [32–35].

Hypochondriasis

Hypochondriasis is a disorder in which patients have an excessive preoccupation or fear about their health, with a particular focus on misinterpreted physical signs or symptoms [1,2]. Patients interpret normal physical signs or symptoms (often involving multiple physiologic processes) as being representative of real disease processes. Symptoms must last at least 6 months and persist despite appropriate medical evaluation and support [1]. Patient attempts to understand the authenticity, causation, and meaning of the symptoms become pathologic.

Fear of illness, accidents, criminal victimization, and death are common features observed in hypochondriasis [35,36]. There is a higher likelihood that patients suffering from hypochondriasis were exposed to victimization, illness, or death at a young age [1,35,36]. Patients may volunteer an overly detailed narrative regarding their perceptions of their health during basic evaluations. Patients often "doctor-shop" in an effort to secure "proper" care for their perceived or pending illness. This doctor-shopping often compromises the physician–patient alliance, leading to frustration on the part of both, and potentially compromising definitive evaluation and treatment [20,35].

In the general population, the prevalence of hypochondriasis ranges from 1% to 9% and is present equally in men and women [1]. Hypochondriasis usually begins in early adulthood and has a chronic, although fluctuating, course throughout a sufferer's life [35]. There are many overlapping characteristics between hypochondriasis and body dysmorphic disorder, mood and anxiety disorders; co-diagnosis should be considered [35,37,38].

Body dysmorphic disorder

Body dysmorphic disorder is characterized by the preoccupation and excessive concern about an imagined or exaggerated defect in physical appearance [1,37]. Any anatomic structure can be the subject of a patient's preoccupation, but structures frequently fixated upon include the face, hair, skin, and genitals [1,37]. Patients may isolate themselves from social interactions and even undergo surgical correction [39,40]. Ironically, studies indicate that patients who have had surgery to address their perceived defect frequently have no relief of their symptoms [37].

Present in approximately 0.7–2.3% of the population, body dysmorphic disorder may begin in childhood and persist throughout a sufferer's life [37,40]. Other conditions with overlapping clinical characteristics include eating disorders, obsessive-compulsive disorder, and social phobia [37,38].

Somatoform disorder not otherwise specified

Somatoform disorder not otherwise specified is a nonspecific category that includes conditions that do not meet the full criteria of a specific SD. These conditions may also be categorized as medically unexplained symptoms (MUS), but future categorization may further delineate the criteria required to meet specific SD diagnoses [14–19].

Perhaps the most intriguing of these disorders is *pseudocyesis* (a.k.a. false pregnancy, hysterical pregnancy), which can occur in men and women. Patients with pseudocyesis believe that they are pregnant and accordingly develop objective signs of pregnancy including gradual abdominal enlargement, breast engorgement, nausea, amenorrhea, and subjective signs of fetal movement [41,42]. The primary cause of pseudocyesis is psychiatric, although there is laboratory evidence demonstrating measurable changes in hormones involved in pregnancy [41,42].

Assessment

Emergency department evaluation

The ED is the frontline of modern medicine and is at the service of the entire population. On a daily basis, an ED practitioner is confronted with the challenge of managing the spectrum of human malady. The primary role of the ED physician is to manage life- or limb-threatening illnesses. In evaluating other illnesses, the ED physician subsequently determines appropriate outpatient or inpatient evaluation. In doing so, the ED physician should uphold the central ethic that quality emergency care is a fundamental right, and access to emergency services should be available to patients who perceive the need for emergency services [43]. Yet, this conflicts with the efficient use of time and resources demanded of an ED, particularly in the setting of progressively increasing ED patient visits, yet decreasing number of EDs [44].

There are inherent difficulties to evaluating SD patients in the ED which may contribute to both patient and physician discontent. Complex psychosocial dynamics of both the patient and evaluating healthcare providers (from triage nurse to treating ED physician) may strongly influence patient presentation, examiner evaluation, and ultimate patient outcome [20,35,44]. Patients presenting to the ED with multiple vague SD-like complaints are not often determined to have "emergent" or "urgent" medical ailments, which may result in longer ED wait-times [44]. Furthermore, the ED evaluation is frequently interactive between the clinician and patient, and action-based to maximize its efficiency. Patients may feel that they are not getting the time or attention they need, whereas the physician may feel the patient is inappropriately using ED time and resources.

By default, the ED physician evaluation is typically directed toward the management of emergent medical conditions rather than somatoform disorders. Modern ED medicine frequently allows for rapid protocol-based "rule-out" medicine that helps ensure emergent organic pathology is not present [20]. There are multiple general medical problems where a patient may have symptoms similar to SD patients (Table 10.1). An ED physician's index of suspicion is often broad. Laboratory studies that are commonly ordered include a complete blood count, complete metabolic panel, cardiac enzymes, pregnancy test, drug screen, and thyroid hormone studies. Imaging modalities frequently used include X-ray, CAT-scan, and ultrasonography. Depending on the ED resources and time constraints, additional studies such as MRI, electroencephalogram, electromyocardiogram, and cardiac stress test may be ordered in conjunction with specialist consultation. In this technologic age, perhaps the most effective evaluation and diagnostic tool is still the patient interview. An interview and physical exam with a symptom-oriented focus and heightened awareness of psychosocial stressors in patients suspected of having an SD may be very informative.

Somatoform disorder patients receive a broad spectrum of attention from different healthcare professionals. This may contribute to patient sick-role and doctor-shopping behavior in an effort to receive needed attention and potential validation of symptoms [11,20]. Reviewing old patient records and contacting the primary care physician may contribute significantly to the evaluation. In the setting of multiple negative ED and clinic evaluations, it may be pertinent to assign a frequent-visitor flag to a patient's records to optimize patient care and resource usage.

Consultation

Emergency department evaluation in conjunction with inpatient or outpatient subspecialty follow-up is critical. While being conscious to avoid reinforcement of the sick-role, the ED physician can be proactive and mediate patient follow-up with a primary care physician, psychiatrist, and other subspecialist as needed. Ironically, patients with an SD may have such frequent and extensive evaluations by different physicians that they may have an increased risk of underdiagnosis [45]. In addition, the morbidity and mortality of SD patients may be increased to dangerous medication combinations or undergoing numerous (usually nondiagnostic) medical examinations, procedures, hospitalizations, and surgeries [39,40].

Inpatient or outpatient psychiatric evaluation will likely provide the greatest benefit. An initial psychiatric evaluation in the ED (when available) might enhance future patient–physician interactions. A psychiatrist may complete a battery of tests to better understand the etiology of the psychiatric disturbance. Such tests may include the Mini-Mental Status Exam, the Personality Assessment Inventory, or the self-administered Patient Health Questionnaire [46,47]. These tests may also be re-administered throughout the course of treatment to evaluate the progress of care [46,47].

An outpatient healthcare professional may use several additional resources to enhance the care of a patient with an SD. One tool that has demonstrated benefit is a formal consultation letter [4,20]. A formal consultation letter outlining strategies of care that the patient's psychiatrist sends to the primary physician may lead to a better outcome and lower healthcare expenses [4]. In addition, consultation and treatment by a physical therapist may benefit patients, particularly in the setting of chronic pain management [20].

Management

Emergency department physicians are in a position to greatly influence the overall health outcome of a patient with a somatoform disorder, for better or worse. Discussing the results of studies, as well as tentative diagnoses and treatments is often difficult. Effectively communicating with patients in a reassuring, non-accusatory, and self-empowering manner that validates the symptoms has demonstrated effectiveness [20,48]. This may present a challenging test of a physician's patient-interaction skills given that patients may not be willing or ready to accept the information provided. An ED physician should avoid simple dismissal (rejection) or blind agreement (collusion) with patient interpretations of symptoms [20]. A critical component to an empowering explanation is to describe legitimate psychosocial or psychophysiologic mechanisms that contribute to the unintentional symptoms [20]. An ED physician can essentially explain that there is no evidence of life-threatening illness, but rather evidence of there being a well-described, yet poorly understood, condition that causes the symptoms [32].

Stronger treatment alliances with healthcare providers form if patients do not feel blamed for producing their unintentional symptoms [20,45]. A treatment alliance can start in the ED, but ideally continues with inpatient or outpatient mental healthcare professionals or other specialists. It is ideal to avoid hospitalization as this may further reinforce the sick-role of a patient. A secure outpatient treatment alliance better allows the patient to receive long-term, empathetic, safe, and cost-effective care [34,35].

Diagnosis

Assigning a diagnosis of an SD in the ED is problematic for multiple reasons. First, the diagnostic criteria for the different somatoform disorders contain much overlap among different somatoform disorders, as well as with other medical conditions. Patients may fall into the category of having medically unexplained symptoms with no clear direction or indication for further evaluation and treatment [49].

Second, the ED is an environment that does not usually provide sufficient surroundings or culture to effectively diagnose or treat an SD. Patients may benefit from evaluation and treatment in a consistent and secure outpatient environment. An accurate diagnosis of an SD may take several regularly scheduled outpatient appointments over the course of months [50]. If a patient is misdiagnosed after an insufficient evaluation, it may contribute to distrust of the healthcare providers and possibly further doctor-shopping behavior. As well, a patient who is misdiagnosed may now have a reason to perseverate on, or enact the sick-role [32,51].

Third, assigning a diagnosis of a psychiatric disorder in general (let alone in the ED), is associated with significant patient and societal stigma that has the potential to hinder further evaluation and treatment [52]. In the ED, it may be pertinent to share a diagnosis of uncertainty rather then providing a specific diagnosis to what might be causing the patient's symptoms. Psychiatric specialists may be better equipped to deliver a diagnosis of an SD than most other practitioners. Furthermore, a psychiatrist may incorporate the delivery of a diagnosis with a discussion of different treatment options.

Treatment

Once the challenge of making the correct diagnosis is complete, the challenge of figuring out successful treatment ensues. In the setting of SDs, the objective of a treatment regimen should be to decrease the severity of symptoms, psychiatric distress, disability, and healthcare burden [20]. An effective treatment regimen begins with getting patients to recognize and accept that a problem exists [20]. This is often problematic in the setting of somatoform disorders given the unintentional nature of the symptoms [35]. Treatment plans should have sequential and pre-determined realistic goals [9,49,53]. Such goals may encourage patients to focus on improving everyday functionality, or to decrease (vs. eradicate) the severity of symptoms

[9,33,49]. Treatment plans and goals are best managed through regular outpatient appointments, which decreases the likelihood that symptoms develop in order for the patient to receive clinical attention [11,20,49].

Patients should be empowered to choose between different treatment options to increase the likelihood of treatment compliance [9,20]. Finding an ideal treatment regimen may be a challenge due to various preconceived patient biases. For example, some patients may completely refuse to take medications due to dislike of pills, or fear of adverse effects [9]. Furthermore, patients may distrust the prescribing caretaker, or personally lack the desire to truly get better [9,52].

Cognitive behavioral therapy (CBT) and antidepressant medication have each demonstrated success in treating patients with SDs [4,9,52]. Other therapeutic interventions that have demonstrated success include usage of an official consultation letter, administering a collaborative care model, family therapy, and use of St. John's Wort [52]. Patients may benefit the most from using a combination of treatments.

Cognitive-based therapy

Cognitive behavioral therapy is a form of psychotherapy that has demonstrated the greatest success in the management and treatment of patients with an SD [4,9,52,54]. Cognitive behavioral therapy includes a spectrum of therapeutic strategies that may include individual therapy, group therapy, assertiveness training, desensitization, biofeedback, or progressive muscle relaxation [4,9,52,54]. Patients may be less threatened by these forms of intervention and may be more likely to use them alone or in conjunction with a healthcare practitioner or support group. There is not a specific type of CBT or timeline of use that has demonstrated the greatest benefit [4,9]. Catering the CBT regimen to the individual patient has the best results. Cognitive behavioral therapy, once acquired, is a skill set that patients can use independently [9,54].

Pharmacotherapy

Multiple pharmaceutical agents may be used in the treatment of somatoform disorders. Medications frequently used to treat both the symptoms and underlying causes of SDs include psychotherapeutic agents (e.g., antidepressants), analgesics, anxiolytics, and herbal supplements (e.g., St John's Wort) [52]. In general, prescribing analgesics and anxiolytics should be avoided due to their addictive profile and higher propensity for being misused [55]. An ED physician who is unaware of the patient's SD history may unwittingly contribute to polypharmacy or patient dependence on prescription medications.

Antidepressant medications have demonstrated the greatest success in the treatment of somatoform disorders and associated symptoms [4,54–58]. Classes of antidepressants include selective serotonin reuptake inhibitors (SSRIs) as well as tricyclic antidepressants (TCAs) [54–58]. Coincidently, these agents are also useful in treating comorbid conditions such as depression and anxiety. It may be further advantageous to combine CBT with antidepressants [52].

A physician may use multiple assessment tools to better manage patients who require opioids for treatment. Such patients typically have evidence of an organic source of pain. The tools, which are ideal for outpatient physician use, include the Screener and Opioid Assessment for Patients with Pain (SOAPP), Opioid Risk Tool (ORT), and Current Opioid Misuse Measure (COMM) [34]. Proper use of such tools may decrease inappropriate and potentially dangerous prescribing and treatment practices [59]. If the ED physician does prescribe opioids for symptom control, they should be in limited quantities.

If available, the physician should refer to electronic prescription drug registries to identify patients who are possibly misusing the prescription medications. Finding an ideal treatment regimen may be a challenge for both healthcare provider and patient. Deliberation over the ethics of prescribing powers and the potential for negative patient outcomes will likely continue to contribute to the controversy surrounding prescription analgesics and anxiolytics. Given the possibility of adverse medication side effects, the ED physician should be cautious prescribing psychiatric medications from the ED, unless done in direct conjunction with a psychiatrist who can ensure outpatient follow-up. Such measures decrease the likelihood of negative patient and societal outcomes, as well as other medicolegal ramifications [34].

Summary

Emergency department physicians should compassionately rule out life- or limb-threatening illnesses while addressing patient suffering and distress. Evaluating, diagnosing, and treating the unintentional symptoms of patients with SDs contribute to burdensome healthcare expenses. Updated diagnostic and treatment criteria in the pending release of the DSM-V and ICD-11 should aid finding more accurate diagnoses and plausible treatment options.

Table 10.1. Considerations for the differential diagnosis of somatoform disorders

Psychiatric diseases
Anxiety
Depression
Malingering
Factitious disorder
Substance abuse

General medical diseases
Coronary artery disease
Venous thromboembolism
Endocrine disorders
Systemic lupus erythematosus
Poisonings
Multiple sclerosis
Myasthenia gravis
Guillain-Barré syndrome

A diagnosis of an SD in the ED is one of exclusion. If the ED physician suspects a patient has an SD after an unremarkable ED evaluation, the ED physician should help mediate definitive evaluation and treatment. Carefully communicating evaluation results and discussing a tentative, although uncertain, diagnosis is important. Obtaining psychiatric consultation for the patient as an inpatient or outpatient is critical in improving overall outcome. An SD patient will benefit the most from regular outpatient psychiatric evaluations with implementation of CBT or antidepressant therapy.

SD patients may present repeatedly to the same ED with the similar combination of SD complaints. To optimize patient care as well as healthcare resource usage, it may be pertinent to flag the patient's chart or establish a predesignated ED treatment plan in conjunction with the primary physician or psychiatrist. Managing SDs can be a challenge. Each patient visit to the ED can be looked upon as a new opportunity to rule out causation of symptoms due to other medical problems as well as inform, convince, and empower SD patients to pursue definitive treatment.

References

1. American Psychiatric Association. *Somatoform Disorders. Diagnostic and Statistical Manual of Mental Disorders* (4th Edition). Text Revision. Washington, DC: American Psychiatric Association; 2000.

2. World Health Organization. *International Statistical Classification of Diseases and Related Health Problems: Tenth Revision. Neurotic, Stress-Related and Somatoform Disorders (F40-F48).* [http://www.who.int/classifications/icd/en/]. c2007 [Updated November 12, 2006] Available at: http://apps.who.int/classifications/apps/icd/icd10online/ (Accessed August 25, 2011).

3. Fink P, Sorensen L, Engberg M, et al. Somatization in primary care: prevalence, health care utilization and general practitioner recognition. *Psychosomatics* 1999;**40**:330–8.

4. Kroenke K. Efficacy of treatment for somatoform disorders: a review of randomized controlled trials. *Psychosom Med* 2007;**69**:889–900.

5. Spritzer RL, Williams JB, Kroenke K, et al. Utility of a new procedure for diagnosing mental disorders in primary care. *JAMA* 1994;**272**:1749–56.

6. Ormel J, Vonkorff M, Ustun TB, et al. Common mental disorders and disability across cultures. *JAMA* 1994;**272**:1741–8.

7. Kroenke K, Spitzer RL, Williams JBW. The phq-15: validity of a new measure for evaluating the severity of somatic symptoms. *Psychosom Med* 2002;**64**:258–66.

8. Kroenke K, Rosmalen JG. Symptoms, syndromes, and the value of psychiatric diagnostics in patients who have functional somatic disorders. *Med Clin North Am* 2006;**90**:603–26.

9. Looper KJ, Laurence J. Behavioral medicine approaches to somatoform disorders. *J Consult Clin Psychol* 2002;**70**:810–27.

10. Barsky AJ, Orav EJ, Bates DW. Somatization increases medical utilization and costs independent of psychiatric and medical comorbidity. *Arch Gen Psychiatry* 2005;**62**:903–10.

11. Krahn LE, Bostwick JM, Stonnington CM. Looking toward DSM-V: should factitious disorder become a subtype of somatoform disorder? *Psychosomatics* 2008;**49**:277–82.

12. Lieb R, Meinlschmidt G, Araya R. Epidemiology of the association between somatoform disorders and anxiety and depressive disorders: an update. *Psychosom Med* 2007;**69**:860–3.

13. Lowe B, Spitzer RL, Williams JB, et al. Depression, anxiety and somatization in primary care: syndrome overlap and functional impairment. *Gen Hosp Psychiatry* 2008;**30**:191–9.

14. Voight K, Nagel A, Meyer B, et al. Towards positive diagnostic criteria: a systematic review of somatoform disorder diagnoses and suggestions for future classification. *J Psychosom Res* 2010;**68**:403–14.

15. Reif W, Isaac M. Are somatoform disorders 'mental disorders'? A contribution to the current debate. *Curr Opin Psychiatry* 2007;**20**:143–6.

16. Rief W, Rojas G. Stability of somatoform symptoms – implications for classification. *Psychosomatics* 2007;**48**:277–85.

17. Kroenke K, Sharpe M, Sykes R. Revising the classification of somatoform disorders: key questions and preliminary recommendations. *Psychosomatics* 2008;**49**:362.

18. Mayou R, Kirymayer LJ, Simon G, et al. Somatoform disorders: time for a new approach in DSM-V. *Am J Psychiatry* 2005;**162**:847–55.

19. Fava GA, Fabbri S, Sirri L, et al. Psychological factors affecting medical condition: a new proposal for DSM-V. *Psychosomatics* 2007;**48**:103–11.

20. Stephenson DT, Price JR. Medically unexplained physical symptoms in emergency medicine. *Emerg Med J* 2006;**23**:595–600.

21. Feinstein A. Conversion disorder: advances in our understanding. *CMAJ* 2011;**183**:915–20.

22. Stone J, Smyth R, Carson A, et al. La belle indifférence in conversion symptoms and hysteria: systematic review. *Br J Psychiatry* 2006;**188**:204–9.

23. Eberhard-Gran M, Schei B, Eskild A. Somatic symptoms and diseases are more common in women exposed to violence. *J Gen Intern Med* 2007;**22**:1668–73.

24. Tomasson K, Kent D, Coryell W. Somatization and conversion disorders: co-morbidity and demographics at presentation. *Acta Psychiatr Scand* 1991;**84**:288–93.

25. Browning M, Fletcher P, Sharp M. Can neuroimaging help us to understand and classify somatoform disorders? A systematic and critical review. *Psychosom Med* 2011;**73**:173–84.

26. Van Beilen M, Vogt B, Leenders K. Increased activation in cingulate cortex in conversion disorder: what does it mean? *J Neurol Sci* 2010;**289**:155–8.

27. Ghaffar O, Staines R, Feinstein A. Unexplained neurologic symptoms: an fMRI study of sensory conversion disorder. *Neurology* 2006;7:2036–8.

28. Voon V, Brezing C, Gallea C, et al. Emotional stimuli and motor conversion disorder. *Brain* 2010;133:1526–36.

29. Voon V, Gallea C, Hattori N, et al. The involuntary nature of conversion disorder. *Neurology* 2010;74:223–8.

30. Tunka Z, Ergene U, Fidaner H, et al. Reevaluation of serum cortisol in conversion disorder with seizure (pseudoseizure). *Psychosomatics* 2000;41:152–3.

31. Sharpe M, Carson A. "Unexplained" somatic symptoms, functional syndromes, and somatization: do we need a paradigm shift? *Ann Intern Med* 2001;134:926–30.

32. Keefe FJ, Lumley MA, Buffington AL, et al. Changing face of pain: evolution of pain research in psychosomatic medicine. *Psychosom Med* 2002;64:921–38.

33. Marazziti D, Mungai F, Vivarelli L, Presta S, Dell'Osso B. Pain and psychiatry: a critical analysis and pharmacological review. *Clin Pract Epidemiol Ment Health* 2006;2:31.

34. Chou R, Fanciullo GJ, Fine PG, et al. Clinical guidelines for the use of chronic opioid therapy in chronic noncancer pain. *J Pain* 2009;22:113–30.

35. Abramowitz JS, Braddock AE. Hypochondriasis: conceptualization, treatment, and relationship to obsessive-compulsive disorder. *Psychiatr Clin North Am* 2006;29:503–19.

36. Barsky AJ, Ahern DK, Bailey D, et al. Hypochondriacal patients' appraisal of health and physical risks. *Am J Psychiatry* 2001;158:783–7.

37. Pavan C, Simonato P, Marini M, et al. Psychopathologic aspects of body dysmorphic disorder: a literature review. *Aesthetic Plast Surg* 2008;32:473–84.

38. Mayou R, Krmayer LJ, Simon G, et al. Somatoform disorders: time for a new approach in DSM-V. *Am J Psychiatry* 2005;162:847–55.

39. Sarwer DB, Crerand CE, Didie ER. Body dysmorphic disorder in cosmetic surgery patients. *Facial Plast Surg* 2003;19:7–18.

40. Mackley CL. Body dysmorphic disorder. *Dermatol Surg* 2005;31:553–8.

41. Small GW. Pseudocyesis: an overview. *Can J Psychiatry* 1986;31:452–7.

42. Trivedi A N, Singh S. Pseudocyesis and its modern perspective. *Aust N Z J Obstet Gynaecol* 1998;38:466–8.

43. Sama A, Chaney C, Jones CA. ACEP Policy Compendium. American College of Emergency Physicians [internet compendium]. 2011. Available at: www.acep.org/workarea/downloadasset.aspx?id=76542 (Accessed August 28, 2011).

44. Nawar EW, Niska RW, Xu J. *National Hospital Ambulatory Medical Care Survey: 2005 Emergency Department Summary.* Advance data from vital health statistics; no. 386. Hyattsville, MD: National Center for Health Statistics; 2007.

45. Epstein RM, Shields CG, Meldrum SC, et al. Physician's responses to patients' medically unexplained symptoms. *Psychosom Med* 2006;68:269–76.

46. Thompson AW, Hantke BA, Phatak V, et al. The personality assessment inventory as a tool for diagnosing psychiatric non-epileptic seizures. *Epilepsia* 2010;51:161–4.

47. Kroenke K, Spitzer RL, Williams JB, et al. The patient health questionnaire somatic, anxiety, and depressive symptoms scales: a systematic review. *Gen Hosp Psychiatry* 2010;32:345–59.

48. Salmon P, Peters S, Stanley I. Patients' perceptions of medical explanations for somatization disorders: qualitative analysis. *BMJ* 1999;318:372–6.

49. Mayou R. Medically unexplained physical symptoms. *BMJ* 1991;303:534–5.

50. McCahill ME. Somatoform and related disorders: delivery of diagnosis as first step. *Am Fam Physician* 1995;52:193–204.

51. Sumathipala A. What is the evidence for the efficacy of treatments for somatoform disorders? A critical review of previous intervention studies. *Psychosom Med* 2007;69:889–900.

52. Sirey JA, Bruce ML, Alexopoulos G S, et al. Stigma as a barrier to recovery: perceived stigma and patient-rated severity of illness as predictors of antidepressant drug adherence. *Psychiatr Serv* 2001;52:1615–20.

53. Hurwitz TA, Prichard JW. Conversion disorder and fMRI. *Neurology* 2006;67:1914–15.

54. Bleichhardt G, Timmer B, Reif W. Cognitive behavioral therapy for patients with multiple somatoform symptoms-a randomized controlled trial in tertiary care. *J Psychosom Res* 2004;56:449–54.

55. Manchikanti L, Giordano J, Boswell MV, et al. Psychological factors as predictors of opioid abuse and illicit drug use in chronic pain patients. *J Opioid Manag* 2007;3:89–100.

56. O'Malley PG, Jackson JL, Santoro J, et al. Antidepressant therapy for unexplained symptoms and symptom syndromes. *J Fam Pract* 1999;48:980–90.

57. Fallon BA. Pharmacotherapy of somatoform disorders. *J Psychosom Res* 2004;56:455–60.

58. Ipser JC, Sander C, Stein DJ. Pharmacotherapy and psychotherapy for body dysmorphic disorder. *Cochrane Database Syst Rev* 2009;1:CD005332.

59. Rosenblum A, Marsch LA, Joseph H, et al. Opioids and the treatment of chronic pain: controversies, current status, and future directions. *Exp Clin Psychopharmacol* 2008;16:405–16.

Chapter 11

The patient with anxiety disorders in the emergency department

Mila L. Felder and Marcia A. Perry

"There is no question that the problem of anxiety is a nodal point at which the most various and important questions converge, a riddle whose solution would be bound to throw a flood of light on our whole mental experience"
Sigmund Freud

Introduction

Anxiety disorders are among the most common psychiatric presentations to the emergency department (ED). One fourth of the U.S. population has a current or past history of anxiety disorder symptoms [1]. A certain level of anxiety is essential for the "fight or flight" response in stressful situations. Anxiety that surpasses a moderate and manageable threshold may become pathologic, leading to the disruption of daily life. Up to 40 million Americans over the age of 18 are affected by some form of anxiety disorder each year [1]. Anxiety disorders are also the most common reason for disability in the U.S. workforce [2]. Anxiety-related complaints are frequently linked with alcohol and substance abuse, further complicating the Emergency Physician's assessment.

Knowledge and skill in recognizing anxiety disorders will aid emergency clinicians in appropriate referral and disposition planning. The ability to differentiate anxiety symptoms and disorders from acute life-threatening conditions is paramount in providing treatment that is thorough, safe, and accurate. This can be particularly challenging when dealing with the time constraints faced in the Emergency Department, and financial limitations encountered in the un-insured and the underinsured patients.

Anxiety presentations in the ED may be classified into one of four groups [3]:

1. Primary psychiatric illness, e.g., generalized anxiety disorder
2. Response to a stress or stressful event, e.g., acute stress disorder
3. Medical illness or substance abuse mimicking anxiety symptoms, e.g., hyperthyroidism
4. Anxiety disorder comorbid with other medical or psychiatric disorder

Definition and diagnosis of various anxiety disorders

Anxiety is characterized by a state of heightened arousal. It presents with somatic symptoms, including but not limited to cardiopulmonary symptoms of tachycardia, tachypnea, and diaphoresis; gastrointestinal symptoms of nausea, vomiting, and diarrhea; and neurologic symptoms of weakness, paresthesias, and tremor. It also presents with behavioral manifestation of avoidance or repetitive checking, as well as distractibility [4]. It is associated with a state of fear, apprehension, and/ or obsession. In contrast to a normal fear and stress reaction, anxiety disorders do not have an obvious external threat or stimulus, or the threat is significantly exaggerated. Thus, anxiety disorders are considered when an extreme or unrealistic fear or worry that is associated with at least some degree of life impairment is present. There is a significant degree of comorbidity with other psychiatric disorders [5]. In the United States National Institute of Mental Health Epidemiological Catchment Area Study completed at five sites during 1980–1985, 54% of patients with generalized anxiety disorder (GAD) suffer from concomitant panic or depressive illness [7].

Anxiety disorders range in severity from common, mild phobias to chronic and disabling conditions such as GAD. The diagnoses for anxiety disorders are made based on the specific description of each syndrome. Among the spectrum of anxiety disorders, GAD is the most common. GAD first appeared in Diagnostic and Statistical Manual of Mental Disorders, 3rd Edition (DSM-III) but was also described by Freud in 1894.

The DSM-III and DSM-IV both focus on the specific symptom of worry or "apprehensive expectation for at least 6 months" (Appendix 11.1). The International Statistical Classification of Disease and Related Health Problems, 10th Revision (ICD-10)

Behavioral Emergencies for the Emergency Physician, ed. Leslie S. Zun, Lara G. Chepenik, and Mary Nan S. Mallory. Published by Cambridge University Press. © Cambridge University Press 2013.

diagnostic criterion for GAD (Appendix 11.2) includes "anxiety which is generalized and persistent and not restricted to particular or environmental circumstances, i.e., it is free floating." These and other symptoms have to be present for at least several months [6]. At least 4 of the 22 symptoms are required for the diagnosis of GAD to be made. These symptoms are further divided into:

- Autonomic symptoms
- Symptoms of chest or abdomen
- Symptoms involving mental state
- General symptoms
- Nonspecific symptoms.

Functionally, ICD-10 criteria are more relaxed than those listed in the DSM-IV. The ICD-10 definition of anxiety as generalized, persistent, and free-floating lacks the excessive focus on worry, while still presenting apprehension as one of the key symptoms of this disorder. The ICD-10 puts less emphasis on requiring a duration of at least 6 months before a diagnosis can be made. This chapter on anxiety disorders comes together at a time of active development in identification, diagnosis, and treatment of anxiety disorders. Updates for both the DSM-V and ICD-11, are expected to become effective in 2013 and 2015, respectively [7].

Initially thought to be a relatively mild disorder, GAD has since been proven to be an independent, chronic, and severe illness. It causes serious impairment in function and ability. Despite a high rate of patients seeking help with GAD, the remission rates continue to remain low.

Cause of anxiety disorders

The precise cause of anxiety and anxiety disorders has never been found, despite extensive research in the biochemical, genetic, behavioral, and cognitive fields. Multiple mechanisms for abnormal neurotransmission/neuromodulator function have been explored. Norepinephrine, adenosine, serotonin, cholecystokinin, gamma-amino butyric acid (GABA), and neurosteroids have been implicated in the development of anxiety with mixed results. Most likely, there is a component of up-regulation of anxiety through noradrenergic and serotonergic systems, and likely modulation by adenosine and GABA. The combined evidence suggests that the biochemical contribution to anxiety is multifaceted, and likely combines contributions by all of the above, and possibly more systems [8,16].

Differential diagnosis

The diseases that commonly mimic anxiety disorders include cardiovascular disorders, respiratory disorders, neurological disorders, endocrine disorders, and comorbid substance abuse, among others (Appendix 11.3).

The prevalence of anxiety disorders in patients presenting to the ED with unexplained chest pain has been difficult to establish. The Panic Screen Score (PSS) is one tool available for evaluation of ED patients presenting with unexplained chest pain which may be used to help determine prevalence as well as guide referral for further mental health evaluations [17]. Of all patients presenting to EDs across the nation for evaluation of chest pain, up to 25% of them are thought to be chest pain induced by panic disorder [5]. Emergency physicians should consider palpitations, chest pain and shortness of breath significant for cardiac diseases such as acute coronary syndrome (ACS) or dysrhythmias, or pulmonary diseases such as pulmonary embolism, acute asthma exacerbation, or COPD exacerbation. The "typical" cardiac patient present with an "elephant sitting on my chest" pain, associated with symptoms like shortness of breath, nausea, and diaphoresis [9]. Anxiety patients are more likely to present with a rapid heartbeat or vague chest pain [19].

There are several physical examination signs that should prompt a clinician to check for organic illness. Some of those include a significantly abnormal heart rate or blood pressure, low pulse oximetry readings, the presence of nystagmus, focal weakness or asymmetry, and a fluctuating level of consciousness. There is a suggestion that the following clinical facts or states may appropriately signal the onset of a panic attack:

- Fear of losing control
- Family history of anxiety problems
- Onset of symptoms between 18 and 45 years of age
- A major life event
- Or the presence or pattern of agoraphobic or avoiding behavior

Typically, cardiac monitoring and electrocardiogram identify acute dysrhythmias if symptoms are present during the ED evaluation. Additional monitoring, such as Holter or 30-day event monitoring could be considered for questionable cases. It is important to consider and evaluate the possible causes of cardiac presentations any time there is unclear history, and before attributing the patient's symptoms to anxiety. This evaluation may include serial cardiac markers, additional imaging or functional studies of the cardiopulmonary system, among others.

Hypoparathyroidism may present with muscle cramps and paresthesias seen with carpopedal spasms that can also be associated with a generalized state of anxiety. Up to 20% of patients with hypoparathyroidism present with a primary complaint of anxiety [10]. Frequently, hypoglycemic patients present with anxiety symptoms as well. Hence, a bedside blood glucose test is an easy and immediately available way to eliminate a common physiological cause of anxiety. Less common, but significantly more dramatic, is pheochromocytoma, which can present with a mask of anxiety symptoms. This rare catecholamine-producing tumor causes paroxysmal anxiety as well as headache, sweating, vomiting, and diarrhea, in addition to general vital sign abnormalities. Evaluation of these patients should include urinary catecholamine and plasma metanephrine, as well as a consultation with the endocrinology department. Checking the patients' thyroid function levels is usually a sufficient evaluation for hyperthyroidism which may also present with anxiety symptoms.

Among neurological disorders, anxiety could be associated with, or mistaken for, transient ischemic attacks. True neurological problems are likely to be overlooked if neurological symptoms resolve before the patient's arrival to the ED, leaving only apparent anxiety symptoms in their wake. Seizures, in particular temporal lobe seizures, may present with a panic attack. In chronic neurological disorders, such as multiple sclerosis, Huntington's disease, and Parkinson's disease, anxiety may accompany presentation and could perhaps be the most dramatic component or the principal finding [11].

Patients presenting with the appearance of hyperstimulation should be considered for possible prescribed or illicit substance exposure and overdose. This is especially important because of the growing identification of both ADD and ADHD and accompanying stimulant use. Furthermore, natural supplements, like caffeine, caffeine's equivalent guarana, which are used in energy drinks, or an even newer "memory supplement" named ginkgo can produce a substance-related generalized state of apprehension. This can be easily missed if it is not considered on the list of possible differential diagnoses. Psychotropic drugs can cause anxiety due to apparent use or in a state of withdrawal. Benzodiazepines (BDZs), barbiturates, and alcohol withdrawal syndromes also present with anxiety symptoms. In cases of alcohol addiction, early anxiety symptoms can appear when the level of alcohol drops below a patient's baseline. Full anxiety presentations may be seen within 48 hours of the withdrawal state. In cases of benzodiazepines and barbiturates, the presence and timing of withdrawal symptoms is directly related to the half-life of the specific medication used. This may range from severe early withdrawal symptoms of 1–2 days when associated with the use of intermediate acting barbiturates to periods as long as a week with longer acting agents such as clonazepam.

Evaluation of anxiety disorders

Admittance into an ED can be a stressful life experience. The environment surrounding emergency patient care is often wrought with various stressors and stimuli. This may contribute to the onset of an anxiety or panic attack in patients at risk for attacks. To diminish and even alleviate the environmental contribution, the design of EDs should ideally include an assessment room without bright lights and loud noises. If a psychiatric care room is not available in the department, then a family discussion area can be used. Patients presenting with a scope of anxiety complaints are often agitated and may be difficult to calm. In these situations, it is important to avoid the use of physical or chemical restraints.

The patient's family can offer invaluable clues to evaluating the patient. History taking should include both medical and psychiatric history, length of symptoms, the triggering event, symptom severity, behavioral concerns, substance abuse, and other associated concerns or recent health and environmental changes such as recent divorce or personal loss.

If any abnormality is found on physical examination, it should be addressed before or concurrently with the psychiatric evaluation. Open-ended questions in a calm, reassuring, and reserved manner help to elicit a better history of the patient's

stress and anxiety. Depending on the patient's age and other medical conditions, a thorough history and physical exam may be all that is required. This is especially true in diagnosing anxiety in young and otherwise healthy patients with normal exam findings. In contrast, older patients or those with multiple comorbidities may require more detailed testing to address their complaints and findings. Even when the isolated diagnosis of anxiety is certain, a complete physical exam with special attention to the somatic complaint helps alleviate the patient's anxiety [12].

After completing a thorough patient assessment and organic causes have been excluded through the history, physical exam, and/or diagnostic evaluation, the possibility of anxiety as the symptom cause should be addressed with the patient. Emergency physicians should then direct patients to a certified or licensed social worker or therapist for further psychiatric treatment.

Treatment of anxiety disorders

Emergency management of anxiety spectrum disorders is highly variable and is dependent on the specific patient's presentation.

The majority of anxiety conditions require a combination of psychological and pharmacological management (Appendix 11.5). In cases of panic disorders, patients almost always require pharmacotherapy. In isolated generalized anxiety disorder, the failure to diagnose appropriately is extremely common and it remains difficult to treat upon diagnosis. The poorly remitting and persistent nature of GAD makes it a condition that is likely to affect long-term quality of life, even with appropriate management. Huh et al. reviewed 36 studies on the treatment of GAD and found that "Standard benzodiazepine and antidepressant treatment for generalized anxiety disorder has been inadequate." They further concluded that "imipramine, hydroxizine, and pregabalin provided the most consistent reduction in anxiety symptoms and the highest remission rates."[18]

Pharmacologic interventions are rapidly moving to the primary use of selective serotonin reuptake inhibitors (SSRIs) in the treatment of GAD. SSRIs provide a reduced side-effect profile and less potential for abuse. In most patients improvement is not usually seen until four weeks after initiation of therapy, and the titration process may be slow and difficult for both the physician and patient. Other medications such as buspirone have been used successfully in the management of anxiety, specifically in GAD. This medication has been found to have less dependency and sedation side effects. However, its use is limited due to a slow onset of action, commonly in excess of two weeks or more. Monoamine oxidase inhibitors and tricyclic antidepressants were commonly used in the past for the anxiety group of disorders. They have been falling out of favor recently due to serious side-effect profiles as well as medication and diet interactions associated with them. Benzodiazepines are frequently used for immediate symptomatic improvement in anxiety patients. When reassurance and education alone are insufficient, emergency physicians often order Lorazepam or Alprazolam due to their very rapid symptomatic relief. These medications, however, are sedating and may cause long-term dependence and withdrawal.

Nonpharmacological approaches may include cognitive therapy, behavioral therapy, social skills coaching, counselling, and crisis intervention. Some recently proposed but less tested approaches involve hypnosis, biofeedback, and meditation. There is evidence to support both the efficacy and effectiveness of cognitive behavioral therapy (CBT) as an acute treatment for adult anxiety disorder [17]. Most times, it is sufficient to reassure the patient about the nature of their problem and educate them about resources available for continuing care. After a thorough discussion of resources and the specific follow-up plans are complete, the physician should consider discussing the involvement of the patient's support system. If the patient agrees, both family and friends may be recruited and educated on the symptoms of anxiety and the management plan. In cases where pharmacological therapy is necessary in the ED and even more rarely, upon discharge, short-acting benzodiazepines such as Lorazepam and Alprazolam can be used [15]. For cases of acute stress reaction causing anxiety, a short course of less than 7 days of 1 or 2 times per day short-acting benzodiazepine can be considered (see Appendix 11.6).

Summary

Anxiety associated disorders are common presenting complaints in the ED. Initial evaluation, stabilization, and management of these patients are expected of all emergency physicians. Physicians must strive to establish a trusting relationship with their patients to alleviate stress or unnecessary anxiety. An environment with minimal distractions or stimulation is preferred in the care of these patients, and physical restraints should be avoided if possible. Once a diagnosis of anxiety disorder has been made, a patient's source of anxiety should be addressed with both the patient and family. Patient education should focus on coping mechanisms, self-awareness, and personal independence. If further management is deemed necessary, patients should be referred to the care of a licensed psychiatric support specialist. Short-term BDZs may help to alleviate acute symptoms, but must be accompanied by appropriate education on their side effects and risks of addiction. These medications are not considered long-term management; which is often a combination of pharmacologic therapy and CBT.

Appendix 11.1 DSM-IV-TR

Criteria for generalized anxiety disorder are as follows:

A. Excessive anxiety and worry (apprehensive expectation), occurring more-days-than-not for at least 6 months, about several events or activities (such as work or school performance).

B. The person finds it difficult to control the worry.

C. The anxiety and worry are associated with three (or more) of the following six symptoms (with at least some symptoms present for more-days-than-not for the past 6 months).

1. restlessness or feeling keyed up or on edge
2. being easily fatigued
3. difficulty concentrating or mind going blank
4. irritability
5. muscle tension
6. sleep disturbance (difficulty falling or staying asleep, or restless unsatisfying sleep)

D. The focus of the anxiety and worry is not confined to features of other Axis I disorder (such as social phobia, OCD, PTSD etc.)

E. The anxiety, worry, or physical symptoms cause clinically significant distress or impairment in social, occupational, or other important areas of functioning.

F. The disturbance is not due to the direct physiological effects of a substance (e.g., a drug of abuse, a medication) or a general medical condition (e.g., hyperthyroidism), and does not occur exclusively during a mood disorder, psychotic disorder, or a pervasive developmental disorder [13].

Appendix 11.2 ICD-10 criteria

F41.1 Generalized anxiety disorder

Note: For children different criteria may be applied (see F93.80).

A. A period of at least six months with prominent tension, worry and feelings of apprehension, about every-day events and problems.

B. At least four symptoms out of the following list of items must be present, of which at least one from items (1) to (4).

Autonomic arousal symptoms

(1) Palpitations or pounding heart, or accelerated heart rate.
(2) Sweating.
(3) Trembling or shaking.
(4) Dry mouth (not due to medication or dehydration).

Symptoms concerning chest and abdomen

(5) Difficulty breathing.
(6) Feeling of choking.
(7) Chest pain or discomfort.
(8) Nausea or abdominal distress (e.g., churning in stomach).

Symptoms concerning brain and mind

(9) Feeling dizzy, unsteady, faint, or light-headed.
(10) Feelings that objects are unreal (derealization), or that one's self is distant or "not really here" (depersonalization).
(11) Fear of losing control, going crazy, or passing out.
(12) Fear of dying.

General symptoms

(13) Hot flushes or cold chills.
(14) Numbness or tingling sensations.

Symptoms of tension

(15) Muscle tension or aches and pains.
(16) Restlessness and inability to relax.

(17) Feeling keyed up, or on edge, or of mental tension.

(18) A sensation of a lump in the throat, or difficulty with swallowing.

Other non-specific symptoms

(19) Exaggerated response to minor surprises or being startled.

(20) Difficulty in concentrating, or mind going blank, because of worrying or anxiety.

(21) Persistent irritability.

(22) Difficulty getting to sleep because of worrying.

C. The disorder does not meet the criteria for panic disorder (F41.0), phobic anxiety disorders (F40.-), obsessive-compulsive disorder (F42.-) or hypochondriacal disorder (F45.2).

D. Most commonly used exclusion criteria: not sustained by a physical disorder, such as hyperthyroidism, an organic mental disorder (F0) or psychoactive substance-related disorder (F1), such as excess consumption of amphetamine-like substances, or withdrawal from benzodiazepines.

Appendix 11.3

Anxiety disorders include several well-known and researched conditions united by the presence of anxiety. The usual classification of those is defined below, as adopted from the American Psychiatric Associations' DSM-IV, and the World Health Organization's International Classification of Diseases and Related Health Problems (ICD-10).

Generalized anxiety disorder	The excessive anxiety and worry occurring more days than not for at least 6 months about several events or activities., not related to direct effects of a substance, causing clinically significant distress or impairment in functioning: ✓ Persistent, markedly inappropriate anxiety, with motor tension, autonomic hyperactivity, apprehension and vigilance. ✓ Specific sources may not be identified ✓ Lasts for months
Panic disorder (with or without agoraphobia)	Recurrent, unexplained panic attacks with at least one of the attacks followed by one of the following: ✓ persistent concern about having additional attacks ✓ worry about the implications of the attack ✓ change in behavior
Specific phobia	✓ A marked and persistent, excessive and unreasonable fear cued by the presence or anticipation of specific object. ✓ A person recognizes that the fear is excessive. ✓ The object or situation is avoided or endured with intense stress
Social phobia	✓ A marked or intense fear of social or performance situations ✓ Exposure to feared situation almost invariable evokes anxiety response
	✓ The person recognizes that fear is excessive ✓ Often fear of being observed rather than fear of situation
Obsessive-compulsive disorder	Obsession is intrusive and distressing thoughts that are not specific to a traumatic event that the person is unable to ignore. Compulsion is defined as repetitive behaviors that the person feels driven to perform in response to obsession: ✓ Thoughts and behaviors cause marked distress and are time consuming ✓ Not due to the effect of a substance
Post-traumatic stress disorder (PTSD)	✓ The person has been exposed to traumatic event ✓ The traumatic event is persistently re-experienced ✓ There is persistent avoidance of stimuli associated with trauma ✓ Persistent increased arousal not present before trauma ✓ Duration is more than 1 month (delayed in onset) ✓ Clinically significant distress and impairment in functioning caused by the disturbance
Acute stress disorder	Similar to PTSD except: ✓ Symptoms must occur within 4 weeks of event ✓ Symptoms must remit within 4 weeks of presentation

Appendix 11.4 Differential diagnosis of anxiety disorders [14]

Drug-related	
Intoxication	Anticholinergic Xanthines (caffeine, theophylline) Steroids Amphetamines, cocaine Aspirin Hallucinogens Sypathomimetic agents Tobacco
Withdrawal	Alcohols Sedative/ hypnotics Narcotics
Cardiovascular/respiratory	Hypoxia Congestive heart failure Mitral valve prolapse Pulmonary embolism Cardiac dysrhythmia Hypertension Myocardial infarction or angina
Endocrine	Carcinoid Hyperparathyroidism and hyperthyroidism Menopausal symptoms and premenstrual symptoms Pituitary disorders Cushing's syndrome Pheochromocytoma

Neurological and other disorder	Anaphylaxis Huntington's disease Multiple sclerosis Pain Ulcerative colitis Wilson's disease Epilepsy Migraine Organic brain syndrome Peptic ulcer Vestibular dysfunction

Appendix 11.5 Management plans (adopted from Fast Facts: Anxiety, Panic, and Phobias)

	Psychological	Pharmacological
Generalized anxiety disorder (GAD)	Counseling Relaxation Cognitive therapy	Benzodiazepines Antidepressants Buspirone Beta-blockers
Panic disorder	Behavioral therapy Cognitive therapy	SSRIs Benzodiazepines Tricyclic antidepressants MAO inhibitors

Agoraphobia	Behavioral therapy	As for panic disorder
Social anxiety disorder	Behavioral therapy Cognitive therapy Social skills training	SSRIs Benzodiazepines Beta-blockers MAO inhibitors
Specific phobia	Behavioral therapy Cognitive therapy	Only symptomatically
Obsessive-compulsive disorder	Behavioral therapy	SSRIs Clomipramine
Post-traumatic stress disorder	Crisis intervention Behavioral therapy Cognitive therapy	SSRIs Tricyclic antidepressants MAO inhibitors

Appendix 11.6 Evaluation and management of patients presenting to the ED with anxiety symptoms

Based on your working differential diagnosis consider the following diagnostic test:

- ECG, CXR, cardiac marker to rule out ACS
- ECG, CXR, D-dimer /chest CT to rule out pulmonary embolism

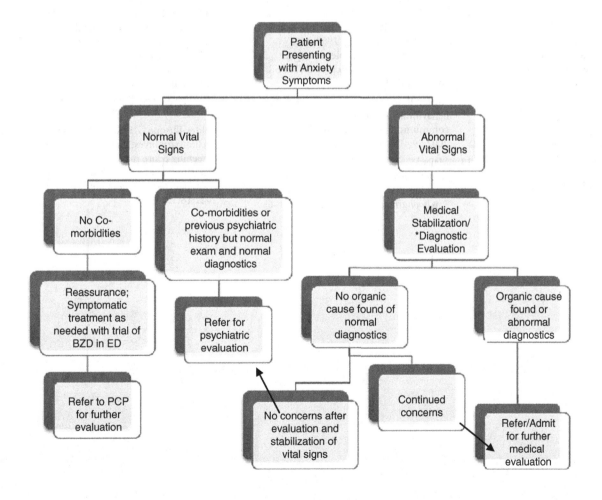

- ABG to evaluate level of hypoxia and acid base status
- Finger stick glucose to rule out hypoglycemia
- Urine drug screen (UDS), ECG, and electrolytes, to evaluate for intoxications/withdrawals
- Thyroid function test to rule out hypothyroidism
- Electrolytes, specifically calcium for suspected hypoparathyroidism.
- Urine catecholamine and plasma metanephrine for suspected pheochromocytoma.

References

1. Brawman-Mitnzer O. *Generalized Anxiety Disorder. The Psychiatric Clinics of North America*. Philadelphia: W.B. Saunders Company 2001;**24**:xi–xii.

2. Oyewumi LK, Odejide O, Kazariann SS. Psychiatric emergency services in a Canadian city: II. Clinical characteristics and patients' disposition. *Can J Psychiatry* 1992;**37**:96–9.

3. Marx J, Hockberger R, Walls R, (Eds.). *Rosen's Emergency Medicine Concepts and Clinical Practice* (7th Edition, Chapter 110). Philadelphia: Mosby/ Elsevier; 2010: 1445–51.

4. Ballenger JC, Davidson JR, Lecrubier Y, et al. Consensus statement on generalized anxiety disorder from the International Consensus Group on Depression and Anxiety. *J Clin Psychiatry* 2001;**62**:53–8.

5. Demiryoguran NS, Karcioglu O, Topacoglu H. Anxiety disorder in patients with non-specific chest pain in the emergency setting. *Emerg Med J* 2006;**23**:99–102.

6. Isberg RS. Emergency care of anxious patients. In: Bassuk EL, (Ed.). *Emergency Psychiatry: Concepts, Methods, and Practices.* New York: Plenum Press; 1984: 233–60.

7. Milner KK, Florence T, Glick RL. Mood and anxiety syndromes in emergency psychiatry. *Psychiatr Clin North Am* 1999;**22**:766–77.

8. Shelton R. Current diagnosis and treatment: psychiatry. In: Ebert M, Losen P, (Eds.). *Anxiety Disorders*, (2nd Edition, Chapt. 22). Columbus, OH: McGraw-Hill Companies; 2008: 328–41.

9. WHO. *ICD-10 Classification of Mental and Behavioral Disorders, Clinical Descriptions and Diagnostic Guidelines.* Geneva: WHO; 1992.

10. Wittchen HU, Gloster AT. Developments in the treatment and diagnosis of anxiety disorders. *Psychiatr Clin North Am* 2009;**32**:XIII–XX.

11. Inter-University Consortium for Social and Political Research. *Epidemiologic Catchment Area Study, 1980–1985 [United States]*. Available at: http://www.icpsr.umich.edu/icpsrweb/ICPSR/studies/06153.

12. Kurlan R, Como PG, Miller B, et al. The behavioral spectrum of tic disorders: a community-based study. *Neurology* 2002;**59**:414–20.

13. Maier W, Falkai P. The epidemiology of comorbidity between depression, anxiety disorders and somatic diseases. *Int Clin Psychopharmacol* 1999;**14**(Suppl 2):S1–6.

14. Sadock BJ, Sadock VA. Panic disorder and agoraphobia. In: *Kaplan and Sadock's Synopsis of Psychiatry Behavioral Sciences/ Clinical Psychiatry*, (10th Edition). Philadelphia: Lippincott Williams & Wilkins; 2007.

15. Pollard CA, Lewis LM. Managing panic attacks in emergency patients. *J Emerg Med* 1989;**7**:547–52.

16. Lader MH, Uhde TW. *Fast Facts: Anxiety, Panic, and Phobias*, (2nd Edition). Oxford, UK: Health Press Limited; May 2006.

17. Otte C. Cognitive behavioral therapy in anxiety disorders: current state of the evidence. *Dialogues Clin Neurosci* 2011;**13**:413–21.

18. Huh J, Goebert D, Takeshita J, Lu BY, Kang M. Treatment of generalized anxiety disorder: a comprehensive review of the literature for psychopharmacologic alternatives to newer antidepressants and benzodiazepines. *Prim Care Companion CNS Disord* 2011;**13**:pii.

19. Foldes-Busque G, Fleet R, Poitras J, et al. Preliminary investigation of the Panic Screening Score for emergency department patients with unexplained chest pain. *Acad Emerg Med* 2011;**18**:322–5.

Chapter 12

The patient with post-traumatic stress disorder in the emergency department

Michael S. Pulia and Janet S. Richmond

Introduction

As emergency physicians (EPs), we work in the midst of constantly evolving human drama. We also bear witness to intense events that our patients may experience as profound psychological trauma. In contrast to our extensive experience in handling acute medical crises, for most EPs, it is relatively unusual to encounter patients presenting solely for treatment of psychiatric complications from traumatizing events. Rather, it is more common for these patients to present with various somatic complaints that cannot be explained by a unifying diagnosis [1]. These patients often have residual symptoms from remote trauma and may lack awareness that their acute symptoms are due to an underlying psychiatric etiology. Although patients with mild or moderate symptoms are much more likely to visit their primary care physician, EPs play an important role in diagnosing cases among those without primary care or who manifest symptoms that mimic life-threatening pathologies such as acute coronary syndrome and stroke [2].

This chapter will highlight the two specific psychiatric manifestations of trauma as defined by the Diagnostic and Statistical Manual of Mental Disorders, 4th Edition, Text Revision (DSM-IV-TR), acute stress disorder (ASD) and its counterpart post-traumatic stress disorder (PTSD) [3]. In addition, it will discuss management strategies for patients with ASD/PTSD in the emergency department (ED) and how the EP can effectively identify the various presentations of PTSD, even when the symptoms are subthreshold for a formal diagnosis [4]. For a comprehensive discussion of normal and pathologic reactions to acute trauma and techniques to manage these patients in crisis, see Chapter 32, Trauma and loss in the emergency setting, in this text.

History

The inextricable link between traumatic events and subsequent psychopathology has been reported since antiquity, such as in Homer's account of Achilles in the *Iliad* [5], and formally recognized for well over 200 years. It was Napoleon's field surgeons documenting the psychiatric casualties of war who coined the term "nostalgia" as the first formal diagnosis for these symptoms [6]. Since the 17th century, the classification

and understanding of this pathology has changed many times (battle fatigue, soldier's heart [Da Costa's syndrome], traumatic neurosis, shell shock, Gross Stress Reaction, Buchenwald syndrome) and it continues to evolve today. From their work with combat soldiers, Grinker and Spiegel set the stage for the development of current theories of trauma, both on and off the battlefield [7].

Diagnostic criteria

Although each individual may have their own idea about what constitutes a traumatic event, the DSM-IV-TR has established a specific definition for the purposes of diagnosing ASD/PTSD. The essential requirements are that the event involves perceived or actual threat of self-harm (including death) to oneself or a loved one and that it evokes intense fear, helplessness, or horror [3]. Thus, only the most intense forms of trauma (assault, rape, combat, disasters, etc.) will satisfy these criteria. It is interesting to note that experiencing an event through the media, such as that which occurred for millions during the September 11th terrorist attacks, is specifically excluded. However, current thinking considers media exposure as a potential risk factor for the development of PTSD, particularly in vulnerable populations, such as children [8]. Furthermore, those who treat trauma survivors, even experienced clinicians, are at risk for developing secondary PTSD because of the high exposure rate [9]. Finally, there is a possibility that humiliation can be a form of trauma, because the victim's sense of personal integrity is destroyed. For further in-depth discussion on vicarious traumatization and humiliation as a form of trauma, see Chapter 32 "Trauma and loss in the emergency setting" in this text. For those clinicians working in the Veterans Affairs system or who encounter a veteran presenting with signs and symptoms of PTSD, it is critical to understand that there may not be a single identifiable event responsible for the PTSD. In fact, the cumulative nature of repeated stress and violence experienced in combat zones does meet the DSM definition of trauma.

Once having experienced a traumatic event, a diagnosis of PTSD requires that the patient must experience 1 month of distressing or disruptive symptoms in three general areas:

Behavioral Emergencies for the Emergency Physician, ed. Leslie S. Zun, Lara G. Chepenik, and Mary Nan S. Mallory. Published by Cambridge University Press. © Cambridge University Press 2013.

re-experiencing the event, avoidance of reminders, and hyperarousal [3]. Similar symptoms with onset in the first month post-trauma and lasting less than 1 month total are classified as ASD. Symptoms with delayed presentation, initial onset more than 1 month after the exposure, or those lasting longer than 1 month fall under the diagnosis of PTSD [3]. The varied list of potential symptoms for both disorders reflects the highly individualized nature of traumatic events due to factors such as mechanism, proximity, intensity, and duration. Part of the challenge for the EP is that PTSD, by definition, has many heterogenous clinical presentations. A general knowledge of the constellation of symptoms to expect during an encounter involving a patient with ASD or PTSD is critical for the EP as these symptoms often create barriers to effective patient care and can mimic other medical and psychiatric conditions.

Differential diagnosis

As EPs we are trained to focus first and foremost on life-threatening pathologies. However, in patients presenting with altered mental status, we must remind ourselves not to overlook psychiatric illness (in this case PTSD-related flashbacks) as a potential cause. A thorough history and physical should distinguish psychiatric illness from the medical conditions that commonly manifest as delirium (e.g., sepsis, metabolic derangements, intracranial injury, intoxication and withdrawal states). Failure to elucidate a history of psychiatric trauma can result in costly, unnecessary medical workups and delay proper treatment.

When evaluating a patient with avoidant behavior, insomnia, exaggerated startle response, amnesia, hallucinosis, psychomotor agitation, or autonomic instability, PTSD should again remain on the differential. As many of these symptoms can be attributed to other Axis I (e.g., panic disorder and generalized anxiety disorder) and Axis II disorders, inquiring about past or recent trauma can be critical in establishing the correct diagnosis [10]. Symptoms of avoidance and re-experiencing are unique to PTSD and should help distinguish it from related anxiety disorders. In 1999, the single greatest cause of PTSD since Vietnam was reported to be motor vehicle accidents (MVAs). Therefore, when screening for more intense forms of trauma, EPs should also assess for a recent MVA [11].

Diseases associated with psychiatric trauma

The potential for clinically relevant physiologic manifestations of psychiatric stress is clearly demonstrated by Takotsubo cardiomyopathy (TCM). This condition is often referred to as "broken heart syndrome," as in many cases it is temporally related to intense emotional strain (e.g., the death of a loved one). TCM presents as chest pain with electrocardiogram and cardiac enzyme findings which mimic ST segment elevation myocardial infarction. Cardiac catheterization reveals a characteristic left ventricular apical ballooning and absence of occlusive coronary artery disease. Although the exact pathophysiology is unknown, proposed mechanisms focus on stress-related catecholamine surges with subsequent toxicity to the left ventricle, which contains the highest concentration of sympathetic innervation [12,13]. This is just one striking example of the mind–body connection that further underscores how psychiatric distress can produce physiologic manifestations (e.g., palpitations, shortness of breath, tremor, nausea, insomnia, unexplained pain) [2]. Similar mechanisms may explain why chronic diseases such as hypertension, coronary artery disease, asthma, and chronic pain syndromes are more prevalent in persons with PTSD compared to the general population [2,14,15]. A shortened lifespan has also been observed in prisoners of war exposed to repetitive trauma, indicating a possible cumulative exposure–response relationship [16].

Presentations and recognition

Individuals with PTSD often present to the ED with a multitude of medical comorbidities and complaints, yet may not consider it relevant to report a history of trauma. Chronic PTSD may present in a myriad of ways, and the emergency clinician may initially not understand the patient's particular behavior, which might be incongruent to the situation. The patient may be hypervigilant, argumentative, unduly frightened, or resistant to aspects of the physical examination. Any unusual behavior or emotion requires the EP to consider the possibility of a past trauma which is interfering with the patient's presentation or ED course. Because the amygdala is activated during flashbacks [17,18], some patients may appear to be hallucinating or psychotic, but in reality they are experiencing a flashback. Because somatization can be a residual symptom of PTSD, when medical symptoms do not correlate with any objective physical findings or diagnostic results, investigation into past trauma is useful. For example, a patient complaining of severe abdominal pain with a negative evaluation may actually be re-experiencing a past rape unaware that this event has bypassed overt psychological symptoms and has developed into physical distress. This type of somatization syndrome is a well-known feature of PTSD [19].

Although the EP might be reluctant to ask about topics that are distressing, it is critical to inquire about past traumatic events in these situations. When screening for traumatic exposure, it is best to begin with a vague question such as "What's the worst thing that ever happened to you?"[20]. For patients reporting new or severe symptoms, it is useful to inquire about recent trauma with an open-ended question such as "Has anything stressful happened to you or your family recently?" It is the authors' experience that patients do not volunteer this relevant history without the clinician gently inquiring into a history of trauma. As avoidance is a major symptom of PTSD and discussion of a traumatic event can be embarrassing or humiliating, most patients will require some degree of prompting. There will also be a large subset of patients who are completely unaware of the link between past trauma and their acute symptoms, which may lead them to unknowingly omit a key part of their history. Careful inquiry into this topic can help

Table 12.1. Primary care PTSD screener

In your life, have you ever had any experience that was so frightening, horrible, or upsetting that, in the past month, you:

1. Have had nightmares about it or thought about it when you did not want to?
   YES / NO

2. Tried hard not to think about it or went out of your way to avoid situations that reminded you of it?
   YES / NO

3. Were constantly on guard, watchful, or easily startled?
   YES / NO

4. Felt numb or detached from others, activities, or your surroundings?
   YES / NO

Current research suggests that the results of the PC-PTSD should be considered "positive" if a patient answers "yes" to any three items.

the clinician prevent further trauma to the patient. The authors have found that a calm and matter of fact approach with open-ended questions is an effective means to obtain this sensitive history. A simple, four question PTSD screen has also been validated in the primary care setting and could be adapted for use in the ED (Table 12.1) [21,22].

Unprovoked hostile, phobic, or paranoid behavior on the part of the ED patient may be due to underlying trauma and can easily confuse the treating physician. For example, a female patient demanding to see a female physician when the complaint requires a pelvic examination may have a history of rape by a male rapist. While clearly this generalization is unfair to the male EP, it is a common manifestation of past trauma. Such behavior can leave the physician feeling shunned (a form of humiliation), unfairly characterized, frustrated, or even angry about how this request may disrupt productivity in a busy ED. Such situations are ripe for conflict, threaten to disrupt the physician–patient relationship, and may result in delayed care or missed diagnoses. For the treating physician, it is important to appreciate that the aggressive or defensive behaviors are actually an attempt to cope with fear and anxiety. If only a male physician is on duty, a female staff member (nurse or patient care technician) can be present during the encounter to help allay the patient's fears [23,24]. Acknowledging a patient's emotional state and allowing time for expression of concerns should be encouraged [25]. In severe cases, providing an anxiolytic medication to facilitate the examination can be particularly helpful.

Severe physical illness or painful procedures can also be considered traumatizing events: a cancer survivor may unconsciously connect visits to a hospital or to a physician as a memory trigger. As avoidance is a hallmark of PTSD, these medically traumatized patients may engage in treatment non-compliance through missed follow-up visits and leaving prematurely when they require inpatient medical care [19,26].

Despite the best efforts of the ED staff, certain medical encounters may result in humiliation and subsequent traumatization for a patient. The vulnerability of being unclothed, prodded, and the subject of invasive procedures can be stress provoking. Because physicians are also particularly vulnerable

to humiliation [27], this combination may increase tension in the physician–patient relationship. Physician vulnerability to humiliation is a by-product of residency training where it is often used as a motivational tool.

Subthreshold presentations and delayed onset PTSD

There is also a subset of patients who have had a history of a traumatic event and never develop the minimal diagnostic criteria for PTSD (or whose symptoms are in partial remission). These patients may demonstrate subclinical symptoms, such as exaggerated startle responses, anxiety, depression, somatization, or substance abuse [2,4]. In other circumstances, patients do not exhibit symptoms of PTSD until years after the traumatic event. A positive or negative life-cycle event (marriage, birth of a child, retirement) can trigger memories and symptoms; for others aging and the onset of a medical illness can be the precipitant [28].

Management

The first step to managing PTSD in the ED is to recognize it. A clinical presentation which does not fit cohesively with the history and physical exam raises a red flag and indicates the need for further inquiry. Once you elicit a history of traumatic exposure, the next step is to be empathic, but not pitying of the patient who may already feel humiliated by the trauma, subsequent symptoms, or the act of revealing intimate information to a stranger. Helping the patient understand the psychobiologic mechanism for their symptoms can reduce self-stigmatization and improve willingness to seek care. Educating oneself and the patient about how trauma can interfere with medical care might also help. This may increase the chance to form a comfortable physicians–patient relationship and decrease the patient's sense of shame and humiliation. As part of the care provided during an immediate post-trauma ED visit, the EP should educate the patient about symptoms they may expect in the days and weeks to follow. Emphasis should be placed on the transient nature of these symptoms in the vast majority of patients and reinforcement that they are normal responses to a very abnormal experience. Encouraging newly traumatized patients to resume their usual activities and routines will promote a return to psychological homeostasis through usage of inherent coping mechanisms. Specific follow-up instructions and a list of available resources should be provided for those who develop distressing or persistent symptoms. Routine outpatient psychotherapy for all trauma victims is not currently recommended, although several trials have demonstrated reduced rates of PTSD with early cognitive–behavioral treatment sessions. In instances when the patient likely meets the diagnostic criteria for ASD/PTSD, referral to outpatient psychiatric treatment is recommended. Such therapy may include psychopharmacology and cognitive behavioral, cognitive processing, or exposure therapy [29].

There are no prophylactic pharmacologic agents for PTSD. Selective serotonin reuptake inhibitors have shown efficacy in the management of chronic PTSD [30,31] and sertraline and paroxetine have U.S. Food and Drug Administration approval for this indication. In most practice settings, pharmacologic treatment should be initiated and managed outside of the ED by a primary care physician or mental health professional. The EP may encounter patients presenting in the immediate post-trauma period with symptoms such as intractable insomnia. In these cases, a short course (less than 2 weeks) of benzodiazepines or antihistamines to aid sleep has been recommended [18]. There is no role for long-term benzodiazepine therapy in treating ASD or PTSD [32,33].

For the vast majority of patients with PTSD, they may expect complete remission, or persistence of only mild symptoms. Only approximately 10% of patients experience chronic diagnostic symptoms [10]. One recent development for treating PTSD takes advantage of the now ubiquitous smart phones. The Department of Veterans Affairs-National Center for PTSD has recently developed the "PTSD Coach" mobile application that provides interactive tools for self-assessment and symptom management, and links to urgent care when needed [34]. It was designed as an adjunct, not replacement, for traditional mental health care. Another application of technology is virtual reality exposure therapy, which effectively reduces symptom severity [35,36].

Conclusion

Although a chief complaint of PTSD will be a rare occurrence in the ED, the lifetime prevalence of this disorder in the United States is approximately 8%, and EPs are guaranteed to encounter this psychopathology in one of its various manifestations [37]. Recognition of subtle manifestations of PTSD and usage of strategies to minimize its impact on the ED current encounter constitute essential skills for EPs. The varied nature of presentations of PTSD and a lack of efficacious therapies for this disorder in the acute care setting can make treating this chronic disorder frustrating for the EP. However, acting in a compassionate, nonjudgmental manner while ensuring the patient has ample time to "tell their story" and express concerns is often enough to successfully navigate these complex encounters.

References

1. London RT. PTSD: another great masquerader ["The Psychiatrist's Toolbox"]. *Clinical Psychiatry News* 2009;**37**:23.

2. Yehuda R. Post-traumatic stress disorder. *N Engl J Med* 2002;**346**:108–14.

3. American Psychiatric Association. *Diagnostic and Statistical Manual of Mental Disorders DSM-IV-TR*, (4th Edition). Washington, DC: American Psychiatric Publishing, Inc; 2000.

4. Marshall RD, Olfson M, Hellman F, et al. Comorbidity, impairment, and suicidality in subthreshold PTSD. *Am J Psychiatry* 2001;**158**:1467–73.

5. Shay J. Learning about combat stress from Homer's Iliad. *J Trauma Stress* 1991;**4**:561–79.

6. Jones FD, Sparacino LR, Wilcox VL, Rothberg JM, Stokes JW. War psychiatry. In: Zajtchuk R, Bellamy RF, (Eds.). *Textbook of Military Medicine*. Washington, DC: Department of the Army, Office of The Surgeon General, Borden Institute; 1995.

7. Grinker RR, Spiegel J. *Men Under Stress*. Philadelphia: Blakiston; 1945.

8. Otto MW, Henin A, Hirshfeld-Becker DR, et al. Posttraumatic stress disorder symptoms following media exposure to tragic events: impact of 9/11 on children at risk for anxiety disorders. *Anxiety Disord* 2007;**21**:888–902.

9. Figley CR. Compassion fatigue: psychotherapists chronic lack of self care. *J Clin Psychol* 2002; **58**:1433–41.

10. Sadock BJ, Sadock VA. Anxiety disorders: clinical features. In *Kaplan & Sadock's Comprehensive Textbook of Psychiatry*, (8th Edition. Chapt. 14.8). Philadelphia: Lippincott Williams and Wilkins; 2005.

11. Butler DJ, Moffic HS, Turkal NW. Post-traumatic stress reactions following motor vehicle accidents. *Am Fam Physician* 1999;**60**:524–31.

12. Khallafi H, Chacko V, Varveralis N, Elmi F. "Broken heart syndrome": catecholamine surge or aborted myocardial infarction?. *J Invasive Cardiol* 2008;**20**:9–13.

13. Dorfman TA, Iskandrian AE. Takotsubo cardiomyopathy: state-of-the-art review. *J Nucl Cardiol* 2009;**16**:122–34.

14. Boscarino JA. Posttraumatic stress disorder, exposure to combat, and lower plasma cortisol among Vietnam veterans: findings and clinical implications. *J Consul Clin Psychol* 1996;**64**:191–201.

15. Katsouyanni K, Kogevinas M, Trichopoulus M. Earthquake-related stress and cardiac mortality. *Int J Epidemiol* 1986;**15**:326.

16. Segal J, Hunter EJ, Segal Z. Universal consequences of captivity: stress reactions among divergent populations of prisoners of war and their families. *Int J Soc Sci* 1976;**28**:593–609.

17. Van der Kolk BA, McFarlane AC, Weisaeth L, (Eds.). *Traumatic Stress: The Effects of Overwhelming Experience on Mind, Body, and Society*. New York: Guilford Press; 1996.

18. Clayton NM, Nash WP. Medication management of combat and operational stress injuries in active duty service members. In: Figley CR, Nash WP, (Eds.). *Combat Stress Injury*. New York: Routledge; 2007: 219–45.

19. Herman JL. *Trauma and Recovery*. New York: Basic Books; 1997.

20. Ramaswamy S, Madaan V, Qadri F, et al. A primary care perspective of posttraumatic stress disorder for the Department of Veterans Affairs. *Prim Care Companion J Clin Psychiatry* 2005;**7**:180–7.

21. Prins A, Ouimette P, Kimerling R, et al. The primary care PTSD screen (PC-PTSD): development and operating characteristics. *Prim Care Psychiatry* 2003;**9**:9–14.

22. Prins A, Ouimette P, Kimerling R, et al. The primary care PTSD screen (PC-PTSD): corrigendum. *Prim Care Psychiatry* 2004;**9**:151.

23. Lenehan GP. A SANE way to care for rape victims. *J Emerg Nurs* 1991;**17**:1–2.

24. Ledray LE. The sexual assault resource service: a new model of care. *Minn Med* 1996;**79**:43–5.

25. Ehlers A, Clark DM. A cognitive model of post-traumatic stress disorder. *Behav Res Ther* 1999;**38**:319–45.

26. Shemesh E, Rudnick A, Kaluski E, et al. A prospective study of posttraumatic stress symptoms and nonadherence in survivors of a myocardial infarction (MI). *Gen Hosp Psychiatry* 2001;**23**:215–22.

27. Lazare A. Shame and humiliation in the medical encounter. *Arch Intern Med* 1987;**147**:1653–8.

28. Richmond JS, Beck JC. Post traumatic stress disorder in a World War II veteran. (letter). *Am J Psychiatry* 1986;**143**:1458–86.

29. U.S. Department of Veterans Affairs. *VA/DoD Clinical Practice Guidelines-Management of Traumatic Stress Disorder and Acute Stress Reaction* [Internet]. 2010. Available at: http://www.healthquality.va.gov/PTSD-FULL-2010c.pdf (Accessed September 26, 2011).

30. Davidson JR, Rothbaum BO, van der Kolk BA, Sikes CR, Farfel GM. Multicenter, double-blind comparison of sertraline and placebo in the treatment of posttraumatic stress disorder. *Arch Gen Psychiatry* 2001;**58**:485–92.

31. Connor KM, Sutherland SM, Tupler LA, Malik ML, Davidson JR. Fluoxetine in post-traumatic stress disorder: randomised, double-blind study. *Br J Psychiatry* 1999;**175**:17–22.

32. Braun P, Greenberg D, Dasberg H, Lerer B. Core symptoms of posttraumatic stress disorder unimproved by alprazolam treatment. *J Clin Psychiatry* 1990;**51**:236–8.

33. Gelpin E, Bonne O, Peri T, Brandes D, Shalev AY. Treatment of recent trauma survivors with benzodiazepines: a prospective study. *J Clin Psychiatry* 1996;**57**:390–4.

34. U.S. Department of Veterans Affairs. National Center for PTSD. *Mobile App: PTSD Coach* [Internet]. 2011 [updated July 7, 2011]. Available at: http://www.ptsd.va.gov/public/pages/ptsdcoach.asp (Accessed September 25, 2011).

35. Rothbaum BO, Hodges LF, Ready D, Graap K, Alarcon RD. Virtual reality exposure therapy for Vietnam veterans with posttraumatic stress disorder. *J Clin Psychiatry* 2001;**62**:617–22.

36. Difede J, Hoffman HG. Virtual reality exposure therapy for World Trade Center post-traumatic stress disorder: a case report. *Cyberpsychol Behav* 2002;**5**:529–35.

37. Kessler RC, Sonnega A, Bromet E, Hughes M, Nelson CB. Posttraumatic stress disorder in the National Comorbidity Survey. *Arch Gen Psychiatry* 1995;**52**:1048–60.

Chapter 13

The patient with psychosis in the emergency department

J. D. McCourt and Travis Grace

Introduction

Psychosis is an impaired perception of reality usually manifested by delusions and/or hallucinations. Other symptoms such as thought disorganization, catatonia, agitation, aggression, and impulsivity are common [1]. Emergency clinicians are often the first healthcare providers to encounter patients with psychosis, which has a lifetime prevalence of greater than 3% [2]. Multiple psychiatric and medical conditions can present as psychosis, posing many challenges to the emergency physician. The clinician must recognize subtle features that suggest a psychiatric or medical cause, assess the patient's safety risk to self and others, and provide initial treatment and disposition.

This chapter will cover the initial evaluation and management of the psychotic emergency department patient with particular emphasis on the process of separating psychiatric causes from medical causes of psychosis. The development of a differential diagnosis will be covered focusing on key elements of the history, physical exam, and ancillary tests used to determine the cause of psychosis. Special topics of interest to the emergency clinician will be discussed along with initial management recommendations and approaches to disposition of the psychotic patient.

Features of psychosis

Psychosis by definition is a state of impaired reality testing. Patients see things that are not there, hear voices that are not present, or firmly believe things for which there is strong evidence to the contrary. Hallucinations, delusions, thought disorganization, agitation, and catatonia are the most common features of psychosis.

A *hallucination* is a false perception that occurs in the waking state without a sensory stimulus to account for what is perceived [3]. For example, a person spontaneously perceives a voice talking to them without any auditory stimulus. This is to be distinguished from an illusion, in which a person receives a stimulus and incorrectly interprets it. Cataracts predispose one to visual illusions, while tinnitus can incite auditory ones. Hallucinations may be auditory, visual, olfactory, gustatory, tactile, and/or somatic in nature [3].

Auditory hallucinations are the most common type of hallucination and are frequently associated with primary psychiatric disorders. However, they can also be a manifestation of psychosis caused by medical conditions. Non-auditory hallucinations, especially visual ones, increase the likelihood of medical illness but are also seen in patients with psychiatric disorders. Olfactory and gustatory hallucinations are usually seen in relation to epilepsy, schizophrenia, or CNS tumors. Cocaine or amphetamine use is classically associated with formication, a tactile hallucination, resulting in the sensation of insects crawling on the skin. Somatic hallucinations are most commonly seen in schizophrenia or hallucinogen abuse. They manifest broadly, in such ways as falsely perceiving motion (flying, sinking) or having bodily sensations related to paranoid delusions (abdominal pain after a meal prepared by "the enemy").

Persons with schizophrenia typically experience auditory hallucinations of voices, but may experience any sort of false perception related to their delusions [3]. For instance, they could "feel their body being carried away by aliens" or "taste the poison in their food each night."

Careful questioning and examination by the clinician must be performed to confirm that the patient's misperception is truly a hallucination rather than an illusion. Macular degeneration may cause a patient to see "wavy blobs," but this is part of their organic visual disorder, not psychiatric in origin. A depressed patient may complain of hearing a phone ring but without a detailed history and physical exam, an aspirin overdose may go unrecognized. Clinicians are also encouraged to use caution when attributing complaints of pain to a somatic hallucination before a thorough history and physical exam.

Delusions constitute false beliefs that are firmly maintained despite evidence to the contrary, and are not typical of the patient's cultural or religious background. There are several types of delusions including those of persecution, grandiosity, religiosity, jealousy, love, eroticism, and somatic sensation [3]. Delusions promote major dysfunction in relationships and productivity and may be bizarre (implausible) or nonbizarre (plausible). A bizarre delusion is exemplified by, "my son was

Behavioral Emergencies for the Emergency Physician, ed. Leslie S. Zun, Lara G. Chepenik, and Mary Nan S. Mallory. Published by Cambridge University Press. © Cambridge University Press 2013.

replaced with a robotic humanoid," which could not possibly be true based on today's technology. A nonbizarre delusion might involve "the FBI is tapping my phone line," which, although very unlikely, could possibly be true [1]. There are no consistent associations linking the content of delusions to the underlying cause of psychotic illness. However, delusions of marital infidelity are quite often seen in alcoholic men, and delusions of grandeur (being a celebrity, being God, etc.) are frequently a consequence of bipolar mania [3]. Spontaneous reporting of delusions is infrequent and clinicians must specifically question about delusional thoughts in all patients suspected to be psychotic.

Disorganization of thought is a sign of severe psychosis and manifests in many ways. The tempo, fluency, logical organization, and intent of thinking may become disordered, making the interview quite challenging. Schizophrenics often display *private logic*, a detailed personal framework of thinking that justifies an odd behavior or bizarre lifestyle. In *flight of ideas*, thinking is accelerated and speech is often pressured. Goal direction is lost and the connection between ideas may become governed by external sounds or linguistic associations (rhyming, etc.). The patient may experience this as "racing thoughts [3]."

Agitation is a state of heightened anxiety and emotionality associated with increased motor activity. It often manifests with aggressive verbal or physical outbursts, posing a threat to both the patient and caregivers. Agitation may worsen with increased thought disorganization, delusions, and repetitive auditory hallucinations resulting in acts of violence commonly seen in patients with acute psychosis. Early treatment with medications is recommended to reduce the risk of violent behavior.

The *catatonic* patient appears unresponsive, and in a state that may resemble obtundation or coma. Exam reveals no sign of structural brain disease. Pupillary and motor reflexes are maintained. The eyes move concurrently as the head is turned, and the patient often resists eye opening. Posturing in seemingly uncomfortable positions may occur for prolonged periods (*catalepsy*). Patients may also express repetitive movements that can be misinterpreted as seizure activity or choreiform jerking [4].

Conditions presenting as psychosis

Multiple conditions present with psychosis, which we divide initially into organic and functional categories (Table 13.1) [1,5–7]. Psychiatric (functional) etiologies include schizophrenia spectrum disorders, bipolar mania, depression with psychotic features, and delusional disorders. Psychosis of a medical (organic) origin may be drug-induced, secondary to organic brain lesions, withdrawal, or a consequence of delirium triggered by medical illness related to infectious, metabolic, cardiopulmonary, endocrine, hepatic, and/or renal dysfunction. Emergency physicians have a primary responsibility to determine which category – organic or functional – defines a patient's psychotic episode. Common conditions that present to the emergency department with psychosis are described below.

Organic causes of psychosis

Delirium often results in psychotic thinking or behavior. It is an acute confusional state with fluctuating course in which the patient has difficulty focusing, along with disorganized thinking or altered level of consciousness. It is a reversible state of brain dysfunction without permanent changes to brain structure [8]. There are hypoactive, hyperactive, and mixed subtypes. Hypoactive delirium presents with psychomotor depression that may mimic lethargy. For this reason, emergency physicians frequently fail to recognize it [9]. The hyperactive form is often accompanied by agitation characterized by increased motor activity, which can result in traumatic injury to the patient or medical staff. In the mixed type, patients have a waxing and waning level of consciousness and may display alternating somnolence and agitation. All delirious patients are prone to perceptual disturbances such as hallucinations (often visual), delusions, and vivid dreams. Those with mixed or hyperactive forms demonstrate difficulty sleeping, emotional lability, and hyper-responsiveness to external stimuli [8,9]. The vast majority of patients present with mixed or hypoactive delirium [9].

The pathophysiology of delirium is not entirely clear, but generally results from aberrant neurotransmitter systems, especially dopaminergic circuits. Genetics may play a role. Delirium is the brain's reaction to an inflammatory response. Trauma, fever, or any other cause of inflammation can result in delirium, especially among elderly persons. Table 13.1 lists several conditions which may cause psychosis. Many of these – sepsis, UTI, other infections, hyperglycemic emergencies, hypoglycemia, electrolyte abnormalities, hypoxemia, encephalopathies, endocrine disorders, heat-related illnesses, hypothermia, and many substance-induced illnesses promote psychosis by causing delirium [1,5–7]. Delirium is particularly common and important to recognize in the elderly population, and is thus discussed further in the geriatric section of this chapter.

The patient presenting with psychotic symptoms of delirium will usually have aberrant vital signs and an abnormal physical exam along with an altered level of consciousness. These signs help distinguish patients with psychosis secondary to delirium from those with psychosis caused by psychiatric illness, as the latter often have normal vital signs, physical exam, and clear sensorium.

Excited delirium syndrome (EDS) is characterized by delirium with severe agitation, traditionally during a physical altercation involving law enforcement. Patients often have intense fear, panic, shouting, violence, and hyperactivity, and sometimes hyperthermia. Bystanders or police often describe the individual demonstrated "superhuman" strength. The syndrome is not a billable psychiatric or medical diagnosis, and there has been debate as to whether it is a well-defined medical syndrome or merely the sequelae of criminal–police altercations. Patients with EDS are at risk of death, although the mechanisms are not yet fully elucidated [10].

Most cases of EDS involve stimulant drug use; cocaine is the classic offender. It is felt that genetically predisposed cocaine

Table 13.1. Causes of psychosis

Organic		Functional
Systemic causes of delirium	Drug abuse or overdose	Psychiatric
Sepsis or severe infection (PNA, UTI, meningitis, etc)	Hallucinogens (LSD, PCP, ketamine, etc)	Schizophrenia
DKA, HHS, or hypoglycemia	Marijuana, synthetic cannabinoids	Schizoaffective disorder
Hypo- or hypernatremia	Salvia divinorum	Bipolar mania
Hypoxemia (CHF, COPD, ARDS, etc)	Sympathomimetics (cocaine, metamphetamine, MDMA, methyphenidate, etc)	Postpartum psychosis
Encephalopathy (uremic, hepatic, Wernicke's, etc)	Bath Salts	Major depression w/ psychotic features
Endocrine (thyroid, adrenal, etc)	Inhalants	Brief psychotic disorder
Anemia	Drug-induced psychosis (at therapuetic dose)	Delusional disorder
Hypo- or hyperthermia, heatstroke	Antibiotics (PCNs, MACs, FQ), antivirals (acyclovir, etc)	
Medications (benzodiazepines, diphenhydramine, etc.)	Anticonvulsants	
Organic brain disorders	Corticosteroids	
Brain tumor, abscess, metastases, etc.	Isoniazid	
Stroke	Digitalis, beta-blockers, antiarrhythmics	
Traumatic brain injury	Anticholinergics (atropine, diphenhydramine, etc.)	
Epilepsy (esp. temporal lobe epilepsy)	Antihistamines	
Multiple sclerosis	Meperidine	
CNS vasculitis (SLE, etc)	ADHD stimulants (methyphenidate, etc.)	
Normal pressure hydrocephalus	Anabolic steroids	
Meningitis, encephalitis, etc.	Substance-related syndromes	
Wilson's disease	Delirium tremens	
Dementia (Alzheimer's, Parkinson's, etc.)	Benzodiazepine withdrawal	
Neuropsychiatric porphyrias (AIP, VP, CP)	Baclofen withdrawal	
	Medication polypharmacy	
	Serotonin syndrome	

Abbreviations: PNA, pneumonia; UTI, urinary tract infection; DKA, diabetic ketoacidosis; HHS, hyperglycemic hyperosmolar state; CHF, congestive heart failure; COPD, chronic obstructive pulmonary disease; AIP, acute intermittent porphyria; VP, variegate porphyria; CP, coproporphyria; LSD, lysergic acid diethylamide; PCP, phencyclidine; MDMA, 3,4-methylenedioxymethamphetamine; PCN, penicillin; MAC, macrolides; FQ, fluoroquinolones

abusers are at greatest risk of bad outcomes. EDS-related deaths are due to respiratory arrest or cardiac dysrhythmia, and two thirds of them occur at the scene or during transport by EMS or police. Among those lucky enough to survive, disseminated intravascular coagulation, rhabdomyolysis, and acute renal failure commonly ensue [10].

There has been speculation as to whether EDS mortality is related to the use of taser products. Studies show that taser use does not cause arrhythmias or troponin elevations and is unlikely to increase mortality in EDS [11,12]. It also has been hypothesized that restraint-induced positional asphyxia caused deaths in EDS. Studies have shown, however, that even the prone maximal restraint position – the position thought most likely to be the culprit – does not result in hypoxia [13]. Still, there have not been studies on positional asphyxia in patients in an agitated hypermetabolic state, and it is possible that positional asphyxia contributes to outcomes. Chronic cocaine-induced myocardial adaptations seem to play a key role, as more than half of those who die have cardiovascular disease [10].

Management of EDS involves sedation, external cooling, IV fluids, and monitoring. In many ways, these patients represent the most severe form of agitation and thus require physical and chemical restraints. Haloperidol and lorazepam in respective doses of 5 mg IM and 2 mg IM are a reasonable first treatment choice. If hyperthermia persists after sedation and external cooling, dantrolene may be used [10].

Organic lesions of the brain can result in psychosis. Damage to the limbic system or its projections, occurring secondary to trauma, stroke, epilepsy, or brain tumor, can cause a presentation similar to that of schizophrenia [14]. The basal temporal lobes are particularly important, as evidenced by cases of temporal lobe epilepsy and herpes encephalitis presenting as psychosis [15,16]. Temporal lobe lesions (seizure, stroke) have been known to cause auditory, visual, olfactory, and gustatory hallucinations, as well as emotional and behavior disturbances [17].

Neurologic deficits (especially focal ones), seizure activity, fever, headache, depressed mental status, and vomiting are critical in differentiating the presence of a cerebral lesion from psychiatric causes of psychosis. Temporal lobe stroke may result in visual disturbances (field defects, macropsia, micropsia), aphasia, hearing deficits, vestibular disturbance, and abnormal time perception. Temporal lobe epilepsy can cause the same symptoms, often in association with clinically evident (or EEG-proven) seizure activity [17].

Brain abscess usually presents with headache, while fever is present in half of cases, and focal neurologic deficit in only approximately one third. Half of cases have signs of increased intracranial pressure such as vomiting, confusion, or obtundation. Meningitis and encephalitis can present with similar findings, but fever, neck stiffness or pain, seizure, and cranial nerve deficits are also common. Encephalitis is more likely than meningitis to produce delirium with psychiatric symptoms [18].

Dementia is frequently associated with psychosis, particularly vascular dementia and Alzheimer's disease. Studies indicate that 41% of Alzheimer's patients experience psychosis, with 36% experiencing delusions and 18% hallucinations. Visual hallucinations are more common than auditory ones, in contrast to schizophrenia. Delusions are usually simple, nonbizarre, and paranoid. They are often related to memory deficits. Patients misplace items and assume someone stole them or assume family members are imposters. Vascular dementia is even more likely than Alzheimer's to be complicated by psychotic features [19].

Various other central nervous system pathologies can promote psychosis, as listed in Table 13.1. These include multiple sclerosis, normal pressure hydrocephalus, meningitis, systemic lupus erythematosus (SLE), Wilson's disease, and porphyrias. Two disorders, SLE and Wilson's disease, are discussed in the pediatric section of this chapter because they often present before age 18.

Drug exposure and toxicity can result in acute psychosis, and sometimes a chronic psychotic disorder. Abuse of illicit substances is classically implicated with psychosis. However, some medications, taken even at therapeutic doses, can elicit psychotic symptoms, especially in children and the elderly. Common mechanisms of substance-induced psychosis include sympathomimetic stimulation, N-methyl-D-aspartate-receptor (NMDAR) antagonism, anticholinergic side effects, and withdrawal syndromes.

Sympathomimetic drugs affect the cardiovascular, neurologic, and respiratory systems, resulting in a sympathomimetic toxidrome, reflected by elevated vital signs, mydriasis, piloerection, and psychomotor agitation. Drugs in this class are vast, including cocaine, methamphetamine, and ADHD medicines

to name a few. Psychosis secondary to these agents may be complicated by severe agitation, excited delirium, and hyperthermia, which in combination with vasoconstriction, can result in cardiovascular collapse and metabolic derangements. High-dose sedation and external cooling may be life-saving.

Hallucinations can result from intoxication with LSD, psilocybin mushrooms, cannabinoids, anticholinergics, amphetamines, cocaine, and other substances [20,21]. The *hallucinogens* are a heterogeneous group of drugs ingested to alter the perception of reality. LSD, mescaline, and psilocybin all produce similar effects, including visual hallucinations, vivid dreams, and depersonalization. Auditory hallucinations are rare. Hallucinations may be horrific and may be so severe as to cause panic attacks with accompanying tachypnea and tachycardia. Marijuana can produce mild effects similar to alcohol at low doses (drowsiness and euphoria), but effects akin to LSD at higher doses [22]. Occasionally, long-term abuse of these drugs can result in prolonged psychotic states that can resemble schizophrenia. Patients can have spontaneous relapses ("flashbacks") years after use [22].

Phencyclidine (PCP), ketamine, and dextromethorphan are *N-methyl-D-aspartate-receptor (NMDAR) antagonists*. Because NMDA receptor antagonists induce a state called dissociative anesthesia, these drugs are sought for abuse. At sub-anesthetic doses, these drugs have mild stimulant effects. At higher doses, they promote dissociation and hallucinations. PCP ingestion can produce a psychotic episode lasting up to a week or more, and thus may mimic a schizophrenic relapse. [22]. Ketamine, a dissociative anesthetic biochemically related to PCP, produces short-lived perceptual changes, ideas of reference, thought disorganization, and other features prominent in schizophrenia [23].

Dextromethorphan is available in over-the-counter cough suppressants. Large amounts must be ingested to produce hallucinations. This is concerning because preparations often contain ingredients such as diphenhydramine and acetaminophen, which can cause anticholinergism and hepatotoxicity, respectively. Therefore electrocardiogram, acetaminophen level, and liver panel must be considered in patients who present with dextromethorphan-induced hallucinations [24].

Drugs with *anticholinergic* activity such as atropine, scopolamine, and diphenhydramine may produce psychotic symptoms, especially visual hallucinations. Delirium, confusion, agitation, dysarthria, and auditory hallucinations may also occur. A systemic anticholinergic toxidrome may be observed, with dry mucous membranes, flushed and warm skin, tachycardia, and mydriasis. An electrocardiogram may show a wide-complex tachydysrhythmia with a long QT interval [25].

Withdrawal from alcohol, benzodiazepines, and opioids can also produce hallucinosis [20]. Delirium tremens (DT), the most serious form of alcohol withdrawal, is commonly seen in the emergency department. It can result in profound psychotic disturbances requiring intensive inpatient medical management. DT is characterized by disorientation, delusions, vivid hallucinations (auditory and visual), tremor, agitation, and sleeplessness. Patients display tachycardia, tachypnea, hypertension, fever, mydriasis, and diaphoresis (autonomic stimulation). It usually occurs 3–5 days after the last ethanol ingestion. Unrecognized and untreated, mortality can be as high as 5–15%. Usually this is secondary to autonomic stimulation, which can result in sentinel events such as myocardial infarction [26].

Baclofen is a GABA receptor agonist used to reduce muscle spasticity in children and adults with spinal cord injuries. Children with cerebral palsy often receive the drug through an intrathecal pump system. Pump failure can result in *baclofen withdrawal*, which includes symptoms such as psychosis, muscle rigidity, hyperthermia, tachycardia, and hyper- or hypotension. Psychosis may be mild, involving only transient visual hallucinations. Profound cases can feature auditory, visual, and tactile hallucinations along with paranoid delusions and depersonalization requiring days of antipsychotic therapy. Baclofen administration is usually a sufficient treatment [27,28].

Some medications, taken even at therapeutic doses, have been reported to induce frank psychosis. Dawson and Carter (1998) reported a case of steroid-induced psychosis in an 8-year-old girl being treated for asthma exacerbation. After receiving just four 20-mg doses of oral prednisone (over 2 days), the child developed visual hallucinations of "little orange men" and spoke with pressured monosyllabic speech. She repeated the phrase "Koo Koo" and was disoriented to place and time. She had no auditory hallucinations. Her recovery was prompt, and she was fully oriented 48 hours after her last prednisone dose [29]. Psychosis is an uncommon, although well-known, side effect of corticosteroid use. However, penicillins, anticonvulsants, and many others medications may also precipitate these symptoms (see Table 13.1) [1,5–7].

In addition to the traditional drugs of abuse already mentioned, there are a few *uncommon causes of drug-induced psychosis*, which occur particularly in the adolescent age group. Abuse of salvia leaves, nutmeg, morning glory seeds, jimson weed, and angel's trumpet can produce psychosis, usually in the form of mild short-lived visual hallucinations and delusions [24,30].

Legal synthetic drug abuse is a recent cause of psychosis that is becoming more frequent. Efforts to thwart use of substances such as cocaine and marijuana have led to production of legal designer drugs [31,32]. In 2010, over-the-counter products marketed as bath salts and incense became popular legal sources of stimulants and cannabinoids, respectively. The active ingredients in these formulations often do not show up in urine drug screening (UDS) [32]. A wave of substance-induced psychotic presentations swept emergency departments in 2010 and 2011, prompting attempts at legislation of these products [31].

Synthetic cannabinoids marketed as Spice Gold, Banana Cream Nuke, and other names, are sold as incense, but are smoked to gain effects similar to marijuana (Table 13.2) [31–34]. Use is common. A study by Hu et al. in September 2011 found 8% of college students at a major university had used synthetic cannabinoids [32]. These drugs are cannabinoid receptor agonists that produce intoxication of greater potency and longer duration than marijuana [32,35]. Effects of these substances may be mild, including light sedation and euphoria.

Table 13.2. Selected products containing designer drugs

Products sold as bath salts containing stimulants	Products sold as incense containing synthetic cannabinoids
White Rush	Spice Gold
Cloud Nine	Banana Cream Nuke
Ivory Wave	Black Mamba
Ocean Snow	Blueberry Posh
Charge Plus	Spice Smoke Blend
White Lightning	Genie
Scarface	Yucatan Fire
Hurricane Charlie	Skunk
Red Dove	Sence
White Dove	ChillX
Sextacy	Earth Impact
Zoom	OG potpourri

In more severe cases, hallucinations, severe agitation, tachycardia, hypertension, coma, suicidality, and drug dependence may occur. Because urine drug screening is unreliable, diagnosis depends on a clear history of substance use [32].

Bath salts, sold under names such as White Rush and Cloud Nine, contain active stimulants such as 3,4-methylenedioxy-pyrovalerone (MDPV) or 4-methylmethcathinone (mephedrone). Penders and Gestring (2011) report three similar cases, which presented with paranoid hallucinatory psychosis after ingestion of such products. Patients' clinical presentations featured a drug-induced delirium with inattention, insomnia, and vivid dream-like hallucinations of threatening intruders. They were fearful of others and had incomplete memory of periods of intoxication [36].

The Centers for Disease Control issued a report in May of 2011 chronicling Michigan emergency department (ED) visits for bath salt intoxication between November, 13, 2010, and March 31, 2011 [31]. A total of 35 patients were identified who had ingested, inhaled, or injected bath salts. Among these 35 patients, 17 were hospitalized (9 to the ICU), 15 were discharged from the ED, 2 left against medical advice, and one was dead on arrival. The patient who died received toxicologic studies revealing high levels of MDPV as well as marijuana and other prescription drugs. Patients presented most commonly with agitation (23 patients), tachycardia (22 patients), and delusions/hallucinations (14 patients). Six patients reported suicidality. Seventeen of the patients had urine drug screening obtained; all but one tested positive for other drugs such as marijuana, opiates, benzodiazepines, cocaine, or amphetamines [31].

Functional causes of psychosis

Psychiatric disorders are the most common cause of psychotic symptoms in ED patients. The major disorders include schizophrenia, bipolar mania, schizoaffective disorder, depression with psychotic features, brief psychotic disorder, and delusional disorder. However, patients should be screened for medical (organic) causes of psychosis, especially those patients without known pre-existing psychiatric illness.

Schizophrenia is debilitating and common, affecting approximately 0.4–0.7% of the entire population [37]. It takes hold early in life, is incurable, and contributes to severe psychosocial dysfunction that predisposes to unemployment, homelessness, and suicide [38]. One study showed roughly 10% of people with schizophrenia committed suicide at 40-year follow-up, a suicide rate nearly equal to that of people with bipolar disorder [38].

The symptom constellation in schizophrenia is vast. Delusions; hallucinations; disorganized speech, thoughts, and behavior; catatonia, flattened affect; poverty of speech; and decreased motivation is common. Auditory hallucinations are the hallmark of the disorder, while other causes of psychosis generally predispose to visual hallucinations. Voices often run a streaming commentary on the patient's activities and are usually accusatory, threatening, or claim control of the patient's actions. Sometimes two voices will discuss the patient's behavior among themselves or with the patient. The patient usually locates the voices inside his mind rather than in space around him, and takes them quite seriously, often forming delusions based on what they say. While auditory hallucinations are a core feature of classic schizophrenia, hallucinations of any type can occur [38].

Like schizophrenia, *bipolar disorders* are common and debilitating. Bipolar Disorder I, in which patients endure cycles of mania and depression, has a lifetime prevalence of 1% [39]. Bipolar Disorder II, which is only slightly more prevalent, features episodes of hypomania and depression. In either case, social dysfunction and suicide are common. Among all patients with bipolar disorder, 50% attempt suicide during their lives, and between 11% and 19% successfully kill themselves [40].

A bipolar manic episode may present with features of psychosis, particularly delusions and agitation. Patients experience a persistently elevated, expansive, or irritable mood in which they may experience grandiose delusions, decreased sleep, pressured speech, and flight of ideas. They may be easily distractible, pleasure seeking, or display increased goal-directed activity [41]. In our experience, manic patients are prone to agitation and violence when delusions are challenged.

Other psychiatric disorders presenting as psychosis tend to have features of either schizophrenia or bipolar disorder. Brief psychotic disorder usually occurs after a major life stressor (job loss, death of a loved one). It consists of abrupt-onset psychosis that lasts at least 24 hours and terminates (often without treatment) within 30 days of onset. Patients return to premorbid level of functioning. Schizophreniform disorder is akin to schizophrenia in many ways, but lasts between one and six months only. Patients with schizoaffective disorder meet criteria for schizophrenia and a mood disorder concurrently (major depressive disorder or bipolar disorder), although their psychotic symptoms pre-date the onset of their mood symptoms [42]. Major depressive disorder with psychotic

features is diagnosed in patients with major depressive disorder who have psychotic features, but do not meet criteria for schizophrenia [1]. Patients with delusional disorder have one or more nonbizarre delusions and preserved social function outside of that affected by their delusions. Delusions are plausible, such as being followed, poisoned, infected, loved, or deceived, and last for more than one month [42].

Children with psychosis

Acute psychosis in children and adolescents is an uncommon presenting complaint. The top priorities, as in adults, are to differentiate acute delirium from psychosis and uncover organic etiologies. However, this is more difficult in children, especially younger ones, because patients have limited ability to provide history and physical exam findings are often more subtle.

Psychotic disorders in children, as in adults, can be functional or organic (see Table 13.1). Functional psychotic syndromes include schizophrenia spectrum disorders, and the psychotic forms of mood disorders. Organic psychosis can develop secondary to central nervous system lesions, a consequence of medical illness, trauma, or drug use. The onset of psychosis is an important diagnostic element because acute onset is more commonly associated with a medical cause rather than psychiatric disease. Because psychiatric disorders presenting with psychosis are rare in children under the age of 13, all children presenting with psychosis, including ones with symptoms suggestive of primary psychiatric diagnoses, should undergo a thorough medical evaluation to exclude reversible causes of psychosis.

Organic psychosis in children

Children presenting with psychosis due to a medical condition will almost always have signs and symptoms of delirium such as altered sensorium with waxing and waning deficits in attention and concentration. The differential diagnosis of organic causes of acute psychosis in children is broad (see Table 13.1) and should be tailored to particular features of pediatric medical conditions, especially drug toxicity.

In our experience, substance-induced toxicity (see previous section) is a more common cause of acute delirium in children, and should be considered early in the evaluation. This is because children are more susceptible to the side effects of medications (at therapeutic doses) and adolescents commonly experiment with recreational drugs. A study in 2003 noted that nearly 8% of children 4–17 years of age had been diagnosed with ADHD; more than half of these were taking *stimulant medications*. Hallucinations are a well-known side effect of stimulant medications. Even at therapeutic doses, amphetamine, methyphenidate, atomexitine, and others can cause psychosis and mania, especially in children of 10 years or less. Hallucinations are usually visual or tactile (formication) [43].

Systemic lupus erythematosus (SLE) is an autoimmune multi-system inflammatory condition affecting more than a million Americans. The diagnosis is made before age 21 in 20% [44]. Psychosis is very common in pediatric SLE, affecting 12% [45]. Auditory and visual hallucinations, blunted affect, and paranoid delusions are common features. Other manifestations of the disease are vast, including glomerulonephritis, malar rash, neurologic dysfunction (seizures, cerebrovascular accidents), cardiopulmonary concerns (pericarditis, pleural effusion), and arthritis. Females account for 90% of cases, with black females disproportionately affected. Neuropsychiatric SLE is treated with both antipsychotics and immunosuppressive agents [44].

A few rare *metabolic diseases* can present with acute psychosis in the pediatric age group. Early recognition of psychosis caused by a metabolic disease can lead to early treatment and prevention of permanent neurologic sequelae. These metabolic diseases include: urea cycle defects, acute intermittent porphyria, and Wilson's disease [7].

Wilson's disease, a rare disorder first described in 1912, involves impaired biliary copper excretion leading to multi-organ copper deposition. Major tissues involved include the liver and basal ganglia (among others). Up to 25% of patients present initially with psychiatric symptoms such as depression, mania, and psychosis [46]. More than half of patients are symptomatic before age 15 years, highlighting the importance for consideration of this diagnosis in a young patient with a first-episode of behavioral problems. Other features of the disorder include cirrhosis and jaundice, splenomegaly, thrombocytopenia, bleeding, dysphagia, dsyarthria, limb ataxia, choric movements, and Kayser-Fleischer rings. Laboratory studies and hepatic biopsy confirm the diagnosis. Antipsychotic medicines can be given as needed, but definitive treatment is copper chelation or liver transplantation [47].

Functional psychosis in children

It cannot be overstated that assigning a psychiatric disorder as the primary cause of a child's psychotic episode requires a thorough diagnostic process to exclude medical illness. This is particularly true in children less than 13 years old. While diagnosis of psychiatric illness in children is challenging for emergency physicians, subtle behavioral clues are sometimes helpful. Children who are at a substantial risk for developing a psychiatric illness demonstrate clinical risk factors for subsequent psychosis. These risk factors include: subthreshold psychotic symptoms (those not reported by the patient until questioned), brief psychotic episodes with spontaneous resolution, primary relatives with psychiatric illness, depression, and thought disorganization. Interestingly, cannabis use before age 18 may also be a risk factor for the development of psychiatric illness. Cannabis use is associated with a younger age of schizophrenia onset and increased likelihood of negative symptoms [48]. Early prodromal symptoms of psychiatric disease in children involve mood and anxiety symptoms such as depression, irritability, guilt, mood swings, suicidal ideation, sleep disturbances, and decreased motivation and concentration.

Childhood-onset schizophrenia (COS) is diagnosed before the age of 13. It is a rare (1/40,000 prevalence) and serious form of schizophrenia that persists into adulthood [49]. Whereas auditory hallucinations are the hallmark of schizophrenia at any age, children have increased rates of visual (80% of patients), tactile (60%), and olfactory (30%) hallucinations compared to adults [50]. A family history of schizophrenia should be queried. Because of the rarity of this disorder, a thorough medical screening should be obtained in all children despite the presence of symptoms classically associated with schizophrenia.

Bipolar disorder in childhood and adolescence was once a rare diagnosis, representing only 10% of diagnoses in inpatient psychiatric units in 1996. However, by 2004, bipolar disorder accounted for 34% of diagnoses in children on inpatient psychiatric units. The criteria for diagnosis are the same as those for the adult disorder, but some authors feel aggressive behavior and irritable mood are less common features in children. A manic youngster with delusions of grandeur may indeed reflect bipolar disorder [51].

Identifying risk factors and questioning patient and family regarding prodromal symptoms not only helps the clinician identify children at risk for psychiatric disease but also increases the opportunity to intervene earlier. Studies have demonstrated that early detection of psychotic disorders in children results in greater response to antipsychotics, improved clinical condition with fewer negative psychotic symptoms, decreased suicide risk, improved mood and cognitive scores, and decreased likelihood of re-hospitalization or premature termination of treatment [48].

Geriatric patients with psychosis

The process of separating acute delirium from psychosis in the elderly is similar to that of the younger patient. However, dementia is an additional consideration in the elderly. Dementia (particularly vascular dementia and Alzheimer's disease) predisposes patients to psychosis that may require inpatient psychiatric management. Dementia with psychosis can be difficult to distinguish from delirium because both promote disorientation, unlike pure psychosis. Additionally, episodes of psychosis superimposed on baseline dementia, may be intermittent, mimicking the waxing and waning course that often describes delirium. Patients older than 65 years old are extremely prone to both delirium and dementia. Often these patients present to the emergency department with altered mental status, psychosis, and no information regarding their cognitive baseline, leaving the responsibility to distinguish dementia with psychotic features from delirium solely with the emergency physicians [9].

Dementia is a progressive decline in cognitive function that results in impaired social or occupational functioning. It is most commonly due to Alzheimer's disease, followed by vascular dementia. Parkinsonism, Lewy Body dementia, and frontotemporal dementia are other common types. By age 85, approximately half of all people have dementia [52]. Unless secondary to traumatic brain injury or stroke, dementia is of gradual onset. It features irreversible cognitive impairment with maintained attentiveness and concentration. Unlike delirious patients, those with dementia have normal level of consciousness, organized thinking, and a stable but progressive course [9]. While alteration of perception often signifies delirium, it frequently occurs in late stages of dementia [19].

Delirium affects up to 10% of elderly emergency department patients and, although it is associated with increased rate of mortality, emergency clinicians frequently overlook it [9]. Patients most vulnerable to delirium include the elderly, the demented, and those with medical comorbidities (history of cerebrovascular accident, congestive heart failure, etc.). In such patients, even a minor insult such as administration of a low dose narcotic agent can precipitate delirium [9].

Emergency physicians fail to recognize 57–83% of cases of delirium due to improper screening. Those most commonly overlooked include cases of hypoactive delirium, patients over 80 years of age, visually impaired patients, and those with dementia. Hypoactive delirium mimics lethargy, which may be attributed to the underlying illness and not further investigated as a separate entity. Patients over 80 years or those with known history of dementia may receive improper delirium screening because confusion is simply attributed to dementia. Clinicians may falsely attribute visual hallucinations to baseline visual impairment [9].

Missed delirium in the emergency department portends a six month mortality rate of 31% compared to only 11% among patients in whom delirium was recognized. The Confusion Assessment Model for the Intensive Care Unit (CAM-ICU) provides a sensible screening tool for delirium that takes less than 2 minutes to perform, and can be used easily by emergency physicians [9].

To perform the CAM-ICU, clinicians assess for the following: Is an acute change or fluctuating course in mental status present? If so, is inattention present? If yes again, then is there altered level of consciousness? Positive results for all three assessments indicate the patient is delirious. If the first two items are positive, but the patient's level of consciousness is normal, the clinician next assesses for disorganized thinking, which if present, confirms the patient has delirium [9].

If delirium is present, consider a wide medical differential diagnosis to include neurologic, cardiovascular, pulmonary, renal, and/or hepatic dysfunction. Order appropriate diagnostics and have a low threshold for ICU admission. Management of psychosis is covered in a later section.

Pregnant/postpartum psychosis

Psychosis during pregnancy

Pregnancy does not lead to an increased risk of psychosis, but concerns over fetal safety often lead women to discontinue mood-stabilizing medicines resulting in high rates of relapse of psychotic disorders during pregnancy. In bipolar disorder, medication discontinuation during pregnancy leads to a 2-fold risk of relapse, compared to women who maintain their pharmacotherapy. Relapse may be harder to control requiring higher medication doses than would have been required for maintenance therapy. This is why it is generally recommended to continue psychiatric therapy during pregnancy [53]. Nearly all medications used in the management of acute psychosis are known to pose risk to the fetus. However, agitation and psychosis, if left untreated, may pose a greater risk.

Benzodiazepines such as lorazepam, diazepam, and midazolam, when used in the first trimester, have shown possible association with congenital anomalies such as cleft lip and cleft palate. Expert consensus, however, is that they are not teratogenic. During third trimester, benzodiazepines can promote neonatal sedation, apnea, and floppy infant and withdrawal syndromes. While benzodiazepines carry a class D pregnancy category status, benefits of use in the acutely agitated pregnant patient outweigh potential risks [53].

Antipsychotic agents carry pregnancy class B or C warnings. Anecdotal evidence often cites haloperidol as having the best safety record, but newer atypical agents such as risperidone have not generated concern. Low potency antipsychotics pose a small risk of increased teratogenicity. However, it has been shown that schizophrenia doubles the risk of fetal malformation and demise independent of medication exposure [54]. Antipsychotic treatment is usually recommended during pregnancy especially in severe disease.

Management of the *acutely agitated pregnant patient* is similar to that of a nonpregnant patient. Attempts at verbal de-escalation, followed by physical and chemical restraint use, are necessary. Clinicians should have a low threshold for chemical sedation when agitation puts caregivers, the patient, and her fetus as risk of trauma. While sedative and antipsychotic medications may pose risk to the fetus, a few doses used to control agitation are likely to outweigh risk of fetal trauma. Anecdotal evidence favors the safety of antipsychotics over benzodiazepines in pregnancy. Thus, we recommend the use of a first-generation antipsychotic such as haloperidol or droperidol in the initial treatment of all agitated pregnant patients [55].

Postpartum psychosis

At no other time in a woman's life is she at greater risk for a psychotic episode than during the period following childbirth. Postpartum psychosis (PP) occurs in one to two mothers per 1,000 childbirths, but the rate is 100 times greater for women with previous PP or bipolar disorder [56]. Approximately half of postpartum psychotic episodes represent a first episode of psychosis, while the other half reflect relapse of a previously diagnosed psychiatric illness. Most episodes of psychosis occur within the first 2 weeks after childbirth. Risk factors include personal or family history of postpartum psychosis, history of bipolar disorder, first pregnancy, and recent discontinuation of mood stabilizers like lithium [57]. Suicidal and infanticidal thoughts should be assessed. While the majority of cases are psychiatric in origin, clinicians must consider medical diagnoses and follow the same evaluation process used for all patients presenting with psychosis.

The etiology of PP is unknown but familial susceptibility suggests a genetic link and rapid hormone changes seem to play a triggering role. PP is considered a specific manifestation of bipolar disorder occurring during the postpartum period [56]. Women with bipolar disorder have an increased rate of recurrence in the postpartum period that can manifest as psychosis. However, women with no prior history can present with PP as a first time manifestation of bipolar disorder. Along with bipolar disorder, patients with a history of schizoaffective disorder, schizophrenia, and depression with psychotic features have an increased risk of PP. Among a registry of 120 hospitalized patients with PP, 75% were found to have either bipolar disorder or schizoaffective disorder. Schizophrenia accounted for 12% of this group. The typical manifestations of psychosis (hallucinations, delusions, and thought disorganization) are often combined with symptoms of mania or depression. Patients commonly have insomnia, rapid mood changes, and may become violent or agitated [57].

Psychotic symptoms common among women with PP include command *auditory hallucinations* instructing the mother to harm the infant, and *delusions related to the infant*. A study of 108 women admitted for PP found 53% of mothers had delusions about their baby. The content of these delusions involved thoughts that their baby is evil (52%), or the thought that someone would harm or kill the baby (36%). Many mothers thought the baby was someone else's child. Other delusions included thinking the baby is God, that someone will take the baby away, that the baby was not yet delivered, that the baby is a born-again relative [58].

Infanticide is committed by 4% of all women with PP [56]. Risk factors for infanticide include delusions of the infant being a devil and history of childhood physical or sexual abuse in the mother [58,59]. These mothers often present with *La Belle Indifference*, denial of pregnancy, depersonalization, and dissociative hallucinations [59].

A so-called "late-onset postpartum psychosis" has been described. It generally occurs as a manifestation of psychotic depression in the setting of long-standing postpartum depression. It may occur several months after delivery and commonly features delusions of paranoia and persecution [57].

Management of postpartum psychosis focuses on ruling out medical causes of psychosis. Thoughts of suicide and infanticide thoughts must be queried and risk estimation determined. Agitation is managed as in any other case, with patient-protective sedation. Early psychiatric evaluation and initiation of mood stabilizing medication is recommended.

Management of psychosis in the emergency department

The initial management of a patient with psychosis regardless of the etiology should be the identification and treatment of agitation and violent behavior, because failure to do so can result in risk to staff and patient (Figure 13.1). We believe that untreated agitation also leads to delay in diagnosis, treatment, risk assessment for suicide and homicide, assessment of the patient's ability to care for self, and risk of elopement. Here we discuss the management of agitation, and follow with information on the *medical screening examination*, which allows for ultimate categorization of psychosis (organic or functional) and appropriate disposition.

The first step in the management of the agitated psychotic patient is creating a safe environment. Before administration of chemical or physical restraints, several methods of de-escalation should be attempted. One-to-one observation and verbal calming interventions may be all that is needed to prevent violence. Placing the patient in a quiet room or providing diversionary activities (food, drink, television) may also be helpful. Please see Chapter 21 on de-escalation techniques for further information. If these methods fail, agitated psychotic patients posing a threat to self or others should be chemically and/or physically restrained.

Chemical restraint (i.e., administration of sedative agent(s) to extinguish agitation) should always be considered first because it may prevent the need for physical restraints. This may also decrease the complications of the struggling patient in physical restraints, including hyperthermia, dehydration, rhabdomyolysis, and lactic acidosis [60].

Several medications may be used in the management of agitation and violence (see Figure 13.1 and Table 13.3) [60–63]. The major drug classes to consider are benzodiazepines, typical antipsychotics, and atypical antipsychotics. A brief description of these medication classes and our recommendations follow.

Benzodiazepines such as midazolam and lorazepam are sedative-hypnotic agents that potentiate GABA (γ-aminobutyric acid) transmission in the central nervous system. They promote anxiolysis, sedation, and have anticonvulsant effects. Side effects include respiratory depression, neurologic depression, ataxia, hypotension, and confusion. While serious adverse effects like respiratory depression or hypotension are very uncommon at usual doses, patients with decreased hepatic metabolism or those intoxicated with alcohol or opiates are at increased risk [60]. Whereas lorazepam is the classic benzodiazepine used for agitation, the rapid onset of midazolam makes this drug especially attractive to practitioners seeking rapid tranquilization of violent patients [60].

Antipsychotic medications include older agents like haloperidol and droperidol, as well as atypical agents such as olanzapine. These drugs antagonize dopamine class-2 receptors in the central nervous system and have been used to manage psychosis, vomiting, Tourette syndrome, and singultus. Side effects of these agents are numerous, including QT-interval prolongation, extrapyramidal symptoms, tardive dyskinesia, and neuroleptic malignant syndrome. Among these, emergency clinicians are most likely to encounter extrapyramidal symptoms, which can be treated with diphenhydramine and/or benzotropine.

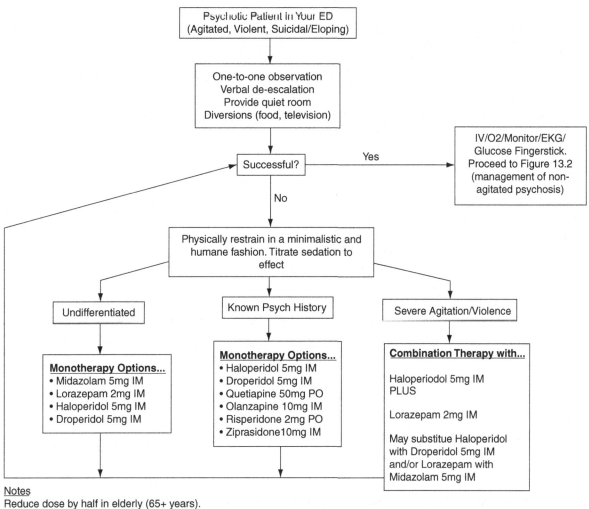

Figure 13.1. Approach to the agitated psychotic patient.

Newer agents such as risperidone and quetiapine can occasionally cause hypotension, tachycardia, and occasionally chest pain. Ziprasidone and olanzapine may worsen dementia and should be avoided in patients with baseline cognitive deficits (Table 13.3) [60,63].

Prolongation of the QT interval and subsequent cardiac arrhythmia are the most feared side effects of antipsychotic agents. While QT prolongation is a class effect and quite rare, only one drug – droperidol – has received a FDA black box warning for this risk [60]. The warning, placed in 2001, states the drug is contraindicated in patients with known long-QT syndrome and additionally states there is risk of fatal QT prolongation in all patients [64]. This warning has substantially decreased use of the drug nationally. Decreased use is likely secondary to fear of litigation born from the blackbox warning more than legitimate risk of fatal arrhythmia. Indeed, a large review of more than 12,000 patients has attested to the safety of

droperidol [65]. The black box warning and subsequent decline in use of droperidol are troubling because the drug's pharmacologic profile makes it arguably the most efficacious medicine for acute agitation [61].

The initial pharmacologic management of acutely psychotic patients can be summarized by the following recommendations (see Figures 13.1 and 13.2). Undifferentiated agitated patients (those with agitation of unknown origin) should receive midazolam, lorazepam, droperidol, or haloperidol as monotherapy. Patients with psychiatric history should receive an antipsychotic as monotherapy (haloperidol, droperidol, quetiapine, olanzapine, risperidone, or ziprasidone). Patients who are severely agitated or violent, posing acute risk to themselves or others require rapid sedation with the administration of haloperidol plus lorazepam as initial therapy. Other options would include either droperidol or midazolam. For cooperative patients with mild agitation, an attempt can be made to give oral medications

Table 13.3. Drugs used in the emergent management of agitation

Drug	Dose[a] and route	Onset	Side effects/notes
Benzodiazepines			Paradoxical excitation is a very rare side effect. All have risk of respiratory neurologic depression; flumazenil is reversal agent
Lorazepam	2–4 mg IM, IV, PO	15–20 min	
Midazolam	1–5 mg IM, IV, PO	0.5–5 min	Hypotension; rapid onset and short duration (1 hr), repeat dosing often needed
Butyrophenone Antipsychotics			All antipsychotics carry risk of QT prolongation, EPS, and NMS, some more than others
Haloperidol	2–10 mg IM, IV, PO	20 min	EPS, QT prolongation, NMS, seizures, bronchospasm
Droperidol	2.5–5 mg IM, IV	3–10 min	Black Box for QT prolongation and risk of torsade de pointes and sudden cardiac death; CI in long-QT syndrome; hypotension, tachycardia, NMS, EPS, bronchospasm; pharmacokinetics are ideal for agitation management
Atypical Antipsychotics			All antipsychotics carry risk of QT prolongation, EPS, and NMS, some more than others
Risperidone	1–4 mg PO	1 hr	Anaphylaxis, hypotension, tachycardia, headache, chest pain, NMS; max 8 mg/24 hr
Ziprasidone	10–20 mg IM, PO	30 min	NMS, QT prolongation, EPS, HTN, hypotension, headache, chest pain; max 40 mg/24 hr
Olanzapine	10 mg IM, SL, PO	15–45 min	EPS, headache, dizziness, chest pain; max 30 mg/24 hr
Quetiapine	25–50 mg PO[b]	1.5 hr	NMS, QT prolongation, hypotension; max 800 mg/24 hr

[a] Reduce dose by half in geriatric patients [1].
[b] Recommend use of immediate release tablets [2].
EPS, extrapyramidal symptoms; NMS, neuroleptic malignant syndrome; CI, contraindicated.

(risperidone, haloperidol, or lorazepam) [61]. For elderly patients, we recommend antipsychotic monotherapy as an initial measure. If benzodiazepines are used, we recommend dose reduction by one half due to concerns for increased sedation and precipitation of delirium.

Physical restraints should be considered a temporary measure in the agitated psychotic patient only after failure of other means. They should be applied in the most minimalistic manner, in a humane manner, and for the least amount of time required to ensure the safety both of the patient and the treatment team. Please see chapter on physical restraints (Chapter 24) for further details regarding their use.

Once agitation is controlled, clinicians should complete a *medical clearance exam* to determine whether the underlying cause of psychosis is organic or functional. The literature is extensive with regard to studies evaluating the most accurate process to differentiate functional from organic causes of psychosis. The common conclusion of these studies recommend focused medical assessment including a thorough *history* with particular attention to new medical complaints, existing medical condition with noncompliance, prior history of psychiatric disease, and substance abuse [61]. This is then followed by a complete *physical exam* looking for signs of underlying or unstable medical conditions with particular attention to

abnormal vital signs, general appearance, cardiopulmonary system, and a focused neurologic exam looking for focal abnormalities that would suggest a CNS lesion [61].

At the completion of a thorough history and physical exam, diagnostic testing is considered. Diagnostic testing as part of the psychiatric medical screening exam has been an area of controversy between psychiatrists and emergency clinicians. Most recommendations suggest diagnostic testing be based on the findings of the history and physical exam rather than mandatory routine testing for all patients with psychosis. Drug screening for patients who are awake and cooperative does not change the initial management but is often requested by psychiatrists because substance abuse frequently coexists or exacerbates psychiatric conditions [61]. Similarly, blood alcohol levels are not useful in a patient who is awake, alert and exhibits decision-making capacity. Alcohol intoxication is diagnosed by clinical examination, not by an increased blood ethanol level. When patients are intoxicated with alcohol, it is recommended that a period of observation be provided, because psychiatric symptoms may improve dramatically as the patient becomes sober [61].

Factors associated with an increased incidence of organic causes of psychosis include: abnormal vital signs, symptoms suggesting illness, physical exam abnormalities, pre-existing or

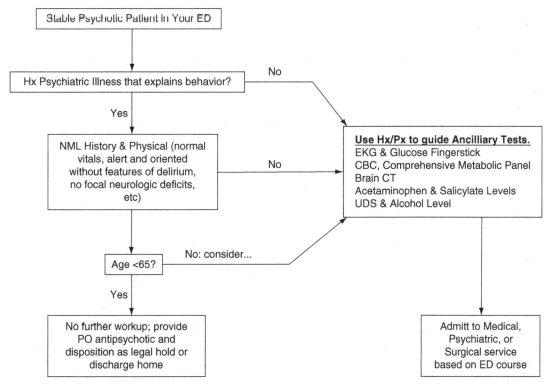

Figure 13.2. Approach to the non-agitated psychotic patient.

new medical complaints, elderly, substance abuse, and patients with no prior history of psychiatric disease. These factors should generate a low threshold for extensive medical evaluation and diagnostic testing before attributing the cause of psychosis to a psychiatric disorder.

Disposition

Not all psychotic patients require automatic hospitalization. It is the evaluating clinician's responsibility to assess the patient for the most reasonable disposition plan. This could include admission to an inpatient psychiatric facility, inpatient medical or surgical service (for management of organic causes of psychosis), or outpatient psychiatric evaluation. The choice is based on the findings of the medical screening exam, risk assessment for harm to self or others, ability to care for self, and the patient's willingness to cooperate with further management goals. Those patients who pose a risk to self or others require involuntary hold until a psychiatrist can perform an emergency psychiatric evaluation and provide treatment for the patient's psychiatric disorder.

Summary

- Psychosis is a disturbance in the perception of reality, often manifested by hallucinations, delusions, and thought disorganization.
- Psychosis can be a presentation of a medical condition (organic) or a psychiatric condition (functional) (see Table 13.1).

- The most common type of hallucination is auditory and frequently associated with a psychiatric disorder. Non-auditory hallucinations, especially visual ones, increase the likelihood of medical illness but are also seen in patients with psychiatric disorders.
- Delirium with psychotic features must be distinguished from psychosis caused by psychiatric disease because the former is almost always due to a reversible medical condition.
- Delirium may present with hallucinations, delusions, and disorganized thought, but additionally have features of alteration in level of consciousness disorientation and abnormalities in vital signs, history, and physical exam.
- Drug exposure and toxicity can cause acute psychosis associated with abnormalities in vital signs, physical exam, as well as specific toxidromes.
- Psychiatric disorders with high rates of psychosis include: Bipolar, schizophrenia, schizoaffective, and depression with psychotic features.
- Symptomatic psychiatric disease is rare in children less than 13 years old. Psychosis in this age group should prompt an extensive search for medical causes.
- Elderly patients with psychosis present a challenge because of high prevalence of both medical problems and underlying dementia making delirium difficult to identify. These patients require a careful evaluation because unrecognized and untreated delirium in this age group portends a 20% absolute increase in mortality.

- Pregnancy does not lead to increased rates of psychosis, but patients with psychiatric disease are more likely to discontinue their mood stabilizers and antipsychotics, increasing the rate of relapse during pregnancy.
- Postpartum psychosis occurs 1–2 weeks after delivery. Risk factors include personal or family history of postpartum psychosis, history of bipolar disorder, first pregnancy, and recent discontinuation of mood stabilizers. Suicide and infanticide risk should be assessed.
- Management of psychotic agitation should be treated early with chemical followed by physical restraints if needed.
- The medical screening exam of patients presenting with psychosis includes a thorough history, complete physical exam, and indicated diagnostic studies based on the findings of the history and physical exam.

References

1. Jibson MD. *Overview of Psychosis.* Waltham, MA: UpToDate; (2010). Available at: http://www.uptodateonline.com (Accessed August 10, 2012).

2. Perala J, Suvisaari J, Saarni S, et al. Lifetime prevalence of psychotic and bipolar I disorders in a general population. *Arch Gen Psychiatry* 2007;**64**:19–28.

3. Nurcombe B, Ebert MH. The psychiatric interview. In: Ebert MH, Loosen PT, Nurcombe B, Leckman JF, (Eds.). *Current Diagnosis & Treatment in Psychiatry,* (2nd Edition, Chapt. 4). New York: McGraw-Hill; 2008.

4. Ropper AH, Samuels MA. Coma and related disorders of consciousness. In: Ropper AH, Samuels MA, (Eds.). *Adams and Victor's Principles of Neurology,* (9th Edition, Chapt. 17). New York: McGraw-Hill; 2009.

5. Patkar A, Mago R, Masand P. Psychotic symptoms in patients with medical disorders. *Curr Psychiatry Rep* 2004;**6**:216–24.

6. Khurana V, Gambhir IS, Kishore D. Evaluation of delirium in the elderly: a hospital-based study. *Geriatr Gerontol Int* 2011;**11**:467–73.

7. Babu K, Boyer E. *Emergency Department Evaluation of Acute Onset Psychosis in Children.* Waltham, MA: UpToDate. Available at: http://www.uptodateonline.com.

8. Ropper AH, Samuels MA. Delirium and other acute confusional states. In: Ropper AH, Samuels MA, (Eds.). *Adams and Victor's Principles of Neurology,* (9th Edition, Chapt. 20). New York: McGraw-Hill; 2009.

9. Han J, Wilson A, Ely E. Delirium in the older emergency department patient: a quiet epidemic. *Emerg Med Clin North Am* 2010;**28**:611–31.

10. Takeuchi A, Ahern TL, Henderson SO. Excited delirium. *West J Emerg Med* 2011;**12**:77–83.

11. Vilke GM, Sloane C, Levine S, et al. Twelve-lead electrocardiogram monitoring of subjects before and after voluntary exposure to the Taser X26. *Am J Emerg Med* 2008;**26**:1–4.

12. Sloane CM, Chan TC, Levine SD, et al. Serum troponin I measurement of subjects exposed to the Taser X-26. *J Emerg Med* 2008;**35**:29–32.

13. Chan TC, Vilke GM, Neuman T. Restraint position and positional asphyxia. *Am J Forensic Med Pathol* 2000;**21**:93.

14. Acioly MA, Carvalho CH, Tatagiba M, et al. The parahippocampal gyrus as a multimodal association area in psychosis. *J Clin Neurosci* 2010;**17**:1603–5.

15. de Araújo Filho GM, da Silva JM, Mazetto L, et al. Psychoses of epilepsy: a study comparing the clinical features of patients with focal versus generalized epilepsies. *Epilepsy Behav* 2011;**20**:655–8.

16. Schlitt M, Lakeman FD, Whitley RJ. Psychosis and herpes simplex encephalitis. *South Med J* 1985;**78**:1347–50.

17. Ropper AH, Samuels MA. Neurologic disorders caused by lesions in specific parts of the cerebrum. In: Ropper AH, Samuels MA, (Eds.). *Adams and Victor's Principles of Neurology,* (9th Edition, Chapt. 22). Waltham, MA: McGraw-Hill; 2009.

18. Loring KE, Tintinalli JE. Central nervous system and spinal infections. In: Tintinalli JE, Stapczynski JS, Cline DM, et al., (Eds.). *Tintinalli's Emergency Medicine: A Comprehensive Study Guide,* (7th Edition, Chapt. 168). New York: McGraw-Hill; 2011.

19. Iglewicz A, Meeks TW, Jeste DV. New wine in old bottle: late-life psychosis. *Psychiatr Clin North Am* 2011;**34**:295–318.

20. Devlin RJ, Henry JA. Major consequences of illicit drug consumption. *Crit Care* 2008;**12**:202.

21. Bishop AG, Tallon JM. Anticholinergic visual hallucinosis from atropine eye drops. *CJEM* 1999;**1**:115–16.

22. Ropper AH, Samuels MA. Disorders of the nervous system caused by drugs, toxins, and other chemical agents. In: Ropper AH, Samuels MA, (Eds.). *Adams and Victor's Principles of Neurology,* (9th Edition, Chapt. 43). New York: McGraw-Hill; 2009.

23. Moore JW, Turner DC, Corlett PR, et al. Ketamine administration in healthy volunteers reproduces aberrant agency experiences associated with schizophrenia. *Cogn Neuropsychiatry* 2011;**6**:1–18.

24. Prybys KM, Hansen KN. Hallucinogens. In: Tintinalli JE, Stapczynski JS, Cline DM, et al., (Eds.). *Tintinalli's Emergency Medicine: A Comprehensive Study Guide,* (7th Edition, Chapt. 182). New York: McGraw-Hill; 2011.

25. Wax Paul M, Young Amy C. Anticholinergics. In: Tintinalli JE, Stapczynski JS, Cline DM, et al., (Eds.). *Tintinalli's Emergency Medicine: A Comprehensive Study Guide,* (7th Edition, Chapt. 196). New York: McGraw-Hill; 2011.

26. DeBellis R, Smith B, Choi S, et al. Management of delirium tremens. *J Intensive Care Med* 2005;**20**:164.

27. Shirley KW, Kothare S, Piatt J, et al. Intrathecal baclofen overdose and withdrawal. *Pediatr Emerg Care* 2006;**22**:258–61.

28. Malhorta T, Rosenzweig I. Baclofen withdrawal causes psychosis in otherwise unclouded consciousness. *J Neuropsychiatry Clin Neurosci* 2009;**21**:476.

29. Dawson KL, Carter ER. A steroid-induced acute psychosis in a child with asthma. *Pediatr Pulmonol* 1998;**26**:362–4.

30. Przeko P, Lee T. Persistent psychosis associated with salvia divinorum use. *Am J Psychiatry* 2009;**166**:832.

31. Centers for Disease Control and Prevention (CDC). Emergency department visits after use of a drug sold as "bath salts" – Michigan, November 13, 2010-March 31, 2011. *MMWR Morb Mortal Wkly Rep* 2011 May 20;**60**:624–7.

32. Hu X, Primack BA, Barnett TE, et al. College students and use of K2: an emerging drug of abuse in young persons. *Subst Abuse Treat Prev Policy* 2011;**6**:16.

33. Zimmermann US, Winkelmann PR, Pilhatsch M, et al. Withdrawal phenomena and dependence syndrome after the consumption of "spice gold". *Dtsch Arztebl Int* 2009;**106**:564–7.

34. NeuroSoup. *List of Synthetic Cannabinoids*. Available at: http://www.neurosoup.com (Accessed September 30, 2011).

35. Rodgman C, Kinzie E, Leimbach E. Bad Mojo: use of the new marijuana substitute leads to more and more ED visits for acute psychosis. *Am J Emerg Med* 2011;**29**:232.

36. Penders TM, Gestring R. Hallucinatory delirium following use of MDPV: "Bath Salts". *Gen Hosp Psychiatry* 2011;**33**:525–6.

37. Saha S, Chant D, Welham J, et al. A systematic review of the prevalence of schizophrenia. *PLoS Med* 2005;**2**:e141.

38. Ropper AH, Samuels MA. The schizophrenias and paranoid states. In: Ropper AH, Samuels MA, (Eds.). *Adams and Victor's Principles of Neurology*, (9th Edition, Chapt. 58). New York: McGraw-Hill; 2009.

39. Merikangas KR, Akiskal HS, Angst J, et al. Lifetime and 12-month prevalence of bipolar spectrum disorder in the National Comorbidity Survey replication. *Arch Gen Psychiatry* 2007;**64**:543–52. Erratum in: *Arch Gen Psychiatry* 2007;**64**:1039.

40. Bellivier F, Yon L, Luquiens A, et al. Suicidal attempts in bipolar disorder: results from an observational study (EMBLEM). *Bipolar Disord* 2011:**13**:377–86.

41. Loosen PT, Shelton RC. Mood disorders. In: Ebert MH, Loosen PT, Nurcombe B, Leckman JF, (Eds.). *Current Diagnosis & Treatment: Psychiatry*, (2nd Edition, Chapt. 18). New York: McGraw Hill; 2008.

42. Shelton RC. Other psychotic disorders. In: Ebert MH, Loosen PT, Nurcombe B, Leckman JF, (Eds.). *Current Diagnosis & Treatment: Psychiatry*, (2nd Edition, Chapt. 17). New York: McGraw-Hill; 2008.

43. Mosholder AD, Gelperin K, Hammad T, et al. Hallucinations and other psychotic symptoms associated with the use of attention-deficit/hyperactivity disorder drugs in children. *Pediatrics* 2009;**123**:611.

44. Muscal E, Nadeem T, Li X, ct al. Evaluation and treatment of acute psychosis in children with Systemic Lupus Erythematosus (SLE): consultation-liaison service experiences at a tertiary-care pediatric institution. *Psychosomatics* 2010;**51**:508–14.

45. Sibbitt WL Jr, Brandt JR, Johnson CR, et al. The incidence and prevalence of neuropsychiatric syndromes in pediatric onset systemic lupus erythematosus. *J Rheumatol* 2002;**29**:1536–42.

46. McDonald LV, Lake CR. Psychosis in an adolescent patient with Wilson's disease: effects of chelation therapy. *Psychosom Med* 1995;**57**:202–4.

47. Ropper AH, Samuels MA. Inherited metabolic diseases of the nervous system. In: Ropper AH, Samuels MA, (Eds.). *Adams and Victor's Principles of Neurology*, (9th Edition, Chapt. 37). New York: McGraw-Hill; 2011.

48. Bhangoo RK, Carter CS. Very early interventions in psychotic disorders. *Psychiatr Clin North Am* 2009;**32**:81–94.

49. Gochman P, Miller R, Rapoport JL. Childhood-onset schizophrenia: the challenge of diagnosis. *Curr Psychiatry Rep* 2011;**13**:321–2.

50. David CN, Greenstein D, Clasen L, et al. Childhood onset schizophrenia: high rate of visual hallucinations. *J Am Acad Child Adolesc Psychiatry* 2011;**50**:681–686.e3.

51. Washburn JJ, West AE, Heil JA. Treatment of pediatric bipolar disorder: a review. *Minerva Psichiatr* 2011;**52**:21–35.

52. Aminoff MJ, Kerchner GA. Nervous system disorders. In: McPhee SJ, Papadakis MA, Rabow MW, (Eds.). *Current Medical Diagnosis & Treatment 2012*, (Chapt. 24). New York: McGraw-Hill; 2011.

53. Lusskin S, Misri S. *Psychosis and Pregnancy*. Waltham, MA: UpToDate. Available at: http://www.uptodateonline.com.

54. Meyer JM. Pharmacotherapy of psychosis and mania. In: Brunton LL, Chabner BA, Knollmann BC, (Eds.). *Goodman & Gilman's The Pharmacological Basis of Therapeutics*, (12th Edition, Chapt. 16). New York: McGraw-Hill; 2011.

55. Ladavac AS, Dubin WR, Ning A, et al. Emergency management of agitation in pregnancy. *Gen Hosp Psychiatry* 2007;**29**:39–41.

56. Spinelli MG. Postpartum psychosis: detection of risk and management. *Am J Psychiatry* 2009;**166**:405–8.

57. Lusskin SI, Misri S. *Postpartum Psychosis: Treatment*. Waltham, MA: UpToDate. Available at: http://www.uptodateonline.com.

58. Chandra PS, Bhargavaraman RP, Raghunandan VN, et al. Delusions related to infant and their association with mother-infant interactions in postpartum psychotic disorders. *Arch Womens Ment Health* 2006;**9**:285–8.

59. Spinelli MG. A systematic investigation of 16 cases of neonaticide. *Am J Psychiatry* 2001;**158**:811–13.

60. Marco CA, Vaughan J. Emergency management of agitation in schizophrenia. *Am J Emerg Med* 2005;**23**:767–76.

61. Lukens TW, Wolf SJ, Edlow JA, et al. American College of Emergency Physicians Clinical Policies Subcommittee (Writing Committee) on Critical Issues in the Diagnosis and Management of the Adult Psychiatric Patient in the Emergency Department. Clinical policy: critical issues in the diagnosis and management of the adult psychiatric patient in the emergency department. *Ann Emerg Med* 2006;**47**:79–99.

62. Kapur R, Fink ES. The violent patient. In: Tintinalli JE, Stapczynski JS, Cline DM, et al., (Eds.). *Tintinalli's Emergency Medicine: A Comprehensive Study Guide*, (7th Edition, Chapt. e293.1). New York: McGraw-Hill; 2011.

63. AccessMedicine. *Drug Monographs*. The McGraw-Hill Companies. Available at: http://www.accessmedicine.com.

64. Kao LW, Kirk MA, Evers SJ, et al. Droperidol, QT prolongation, and sudden death: what is the evidence? *Ann Emerg Med* 2003;**41**:546–58.

65. Shale JH, Shale CM, Mastin WD. A review of the safety and efficacy of droperidol for the rapid sedation of severely agitated and violent patients. *J Clin Psychiatry* 2003;**64**:500–5.

Personality disorders in the acute setting

Dennis Beedle

Introduction

For many healthcare providers, it is the nature of their emotional response to the patient who helps them identify that they are working with a "difficult patient," or potentially a patient with a personality disorder. It is our professional responsibility to work with patients whose personality disorders make it a challenging task to be helpful. Being committed to our professional ethical principles helps to manage the strong emotional responses that are sometimes evoked in caring for patients with personality disorders [1]. A better understanding of the emotional and interpersonal aspect of the process can be helpful to emergency department (ED) staff. The goal in the ED is to help the person with a personality disorder diagnosis address the behavioral or medical problems that resulted in the visit to the ED. Maintaining a therapeutic stance and alliance building are critical in interactions with all patients, but especially those with personality disorders who can engender negative emotional responses and behaviors from ED staff [2].

Prevalence of personality disorders

Personality disorders are fairly frequent psychiatric diagnoses with a recent review suggesting a general population estimate of approximately 6–10% [3]. The recurrent use of the ED is associated with personality disorder diagnoses, which suggests these patients may be commonly encountered in this setting [4]. Personality disorder diagnoses are also associated with an increased prevalence of other medical and psychiatric disorders. A personality disorder diagnosis may be a risk factor for cardiovascular disease and increased mortality [5].

Etiology of personality disorders

The etiologies of personality disorders are actively being investigated. Both genetic vulnerabilities and environmental factors seem to be involved in the development of personality disorders. One recent study estimates the heritable contribution of risk for personality disorders ranges from a low of 20.5% for schizotypal personality to a high of 40.9% for antisocial personality disorder [6]. Epidemiologic research demonstrates a high incidence of severe neglect and abuse in the childhood histories of many patients diagnosed with borderline and antisocial personality disorders [7]. The impact of this early developmental trauma is modulated by protective genetic factors, with some individuals being more resilient to negative outcomes. For example, high expression of the neurotransmitter metabolizing enzyme monoamine oxidase A moderates the effect of childhood maltreatment in the development of later antisocial behaviors [8]. Genetic studies increasingly support the concept of subsyndromal presentation of mental illnesses overlapping with certain personality disorders and styles:

- Obsessive-compulsive personality disorder with obsessive-compulsive disorder [9]
- Schizotypal personality disorder with schizophrenia [10]
- Avoidant personality disorder symptoms with schizophrenia spectrum disorders [11].

Because nature and nurture co-conspire to make us the persons we are, it is not unexpected that the phenotypic presentation of inherited traits can be significantly impacted by current environmental events and childhood experience.

Diagnosis of personality disorders

The ED is a challenging setting for making a diagnosis of a personality disorder. This diagnosis may be inaccurately made when problematic interactions and behaviors are secondary to other mental illnesses: pain, delirium, unrecognized medical issues, intoxicated states, and substance withdrawal. The usefulness of making a personality disorder diagnosis depends on the attitude, knowledge, and skill of the treating ED staff for these often stigmatized disorders. The general diagnostic criteria for personality disorder diagnoses in the current DSM-IV-TR are:

1. Inner experience and behavior that are markedly deviant from the person's cultural background along with two or more of the following:
   · Cognitive distortions of self, other people, and events
   · Abnormalities of affectivity with increased or restricted range, intensity, lability, and inappropriateness of affective responses
   · Interpersonal dysfunction

Behavioral Emergencies for the Emergency Physician, ed. Leslie S. Zun, Lara G. Chepenik, and Mary Nan S. Mallory. Published by Cambridge University Press. © Cambridge University Press 2013.

2. The personality pattern:
   - Is inflexible and pervasive across many personal and social situations
   - Leads to significant distress or impairment in occupation, social, or other important areas of life
   - Is stable and of long duration, with an onset no later than early adulthood
   - Is not a consequence of or better accounted for by another mental disorder
   - Is not the direct effect of a substance or medical condition

In the DSM-IV-TR, the diagnosis of personality disorders is broken down into nine specific personality disorders. These disorders are divided into three clusters. The three personality disorders in cluster A (the odd and eccentric) include:

1. Paranoid
   - Distrust and suspiciousness
   - Others motivations are seen as malevolent
2. Schizoid
   - Detached from social relationships
   - Restricted range of emotional experience
3. Schizotypal
   - Acute discomfort in close relationships
   - Cognitive or perceptual distortions
   - Eccentricities of behavior

The three personality disorders in cluster B (dramatic, emotional, and erratic) include:

1. Borderline
   - Unstable interpersonal relationships
   - Unstable self-image
   - Unstable and intense affects
   - Impulsivity
2. Narcissistic
   - Grandiosity
   - Need for admiration
   - Lack of empathy
3. Antisocial
   - Habitual disregard of others
   - Violation of the rights of others

The three personality disorders in cluster C (anxious and fearful) include:

1. Avoidant
   - Social inhibition
   - Feelings of inadequacy
   - Hypersensitive to negative evaluation
2. Dependent
   - Submissive
   - Clinging
   - A need to be taken care of

3 Obsessive-compulsive
   - Orderliness
   - Perfectionism
   - Control

In addition to the diagnosis of personality disorder NOS may be used under two sets of circumstances:

- The general pattern of personality disorder diagnosis is met
- Traits of several different personality disorders are present
- Criteria for a specific personality disorder are not fully met

The second set of circumstances that a diagnosis of personality disorder NOS may be properly made is:

- General criteria for personality are met
- Category is not present in DSM-IV-TR (This may be used for historical diagnoses such as passive aggressive personality disorder.)

Specific diagnostic criteria exist for each of the nine personality disorder diagnoses in DSM-IV-TR but a more detailed review is beyond the scope of this chapter [12].

The American Psychiatric Association is currently developing the new Diagnostic and Statistical Manual of Mental Disorders 5 (DSM 5), in which the process of personality disorder diagnosis is undergoing a major revision. Although the final version is not complete, it appears certain that the total number of personality disorder diagnoses will be reduced. In addition, a system is being developed to describe areas of difficulty and levels of functioning in personality assessment. The proposed revisions to the DSM V personality disorder section are based on research findings regarding difficulties in the reliability and accuracy of the current system of personality disorder diagnosis. These proposed changes are controversial and the final version of DSM V is anticipated in 2013. The new International Classification of Diseases 11 is also in development and, like DSM V, will be moving toward a dimensional trait model of personality pathology where personality traits are seen as continuous and personality pathology is found at the extremes of normally distributed traits [13,14].

Comorbid addictive illness

The most clinically significant comorbid disorder in patients with personality disorders is alcohol use disorders [15]. Many patients appear to be suffering from personality disorders when either acutely intoxicated or while actively using over a sustained period. Maintaining long-term sobriety is not compatible with the current diagnosis of antisocial personality disorder. In a sample of long-term abstinent alcohol-dependent individuals, 25% retrospectively qualified for a lifetime diagnosis of antisocial personality disorder. None of the abstinent subjects currently met criteria for this diagnosis. It is unclear if this change was related to beneficial effects of sobriety or if subjects met diagnostic criteria for antisocial personality due to the impact of alcohol dependence on their behavior [16].

Patients with personality disorder diagnoses are additionally more likely to have persistent drug use disorders. Antisocial, borderline, and schizotypal personality disorder diagnoses are predictors of continued substance use. In antisocial personality disorder, deceitfulness and lack of remorse are associated with continued use. Identity disturbance and self-damaging impulsivity are associated with continued use in borderline personality disorder. Ideas of reverence and social anxiety are associated with continued use in schizotypal personality disorder [17].

In assessing risk of violence in the ED, younger male patients with personality disorders are at increased risk of multiple episodes of violent behavior in the ED, especially if there is a history of violent behavior, personal victimization, and substance use disorder [18]. Patients with personality disorder diagnosis and substance use disorders are also at increased risk of repeat violence in community settings [19].

Referral to residential treatment programs and inpatient addictions programs are helpful approaches for addiction recovery and many of these programs support 12-step engagement. For many patients with personality disorders and addictive comorbidities, no or very restricted insurance benefits limit availability of these services. Referral to local 12-step meetings is a reasonable approach to the patient with addictive illness and suspect personality disorder diagnosis [20]. It may be useful for the ED to develop relationships with local Alcoholics Anonymous and other 12-step based programs, to facilitate a more effective referral process and to aid in the education of ED staff. Although success rates for 12-step-based programs are controversial, there is evidence that supports better outcomes with this self-help approach and reduced healthcare costs [21].

Comorbid mental illness

Major mental illness is often comorbid with a personality disorder diagnosis. Although all patients with personality disorder appear at increased risk for major depression, patients with borderline, avoidant, and paranoid personality disorders are at particular risk for major depressive disorder [22]. Patients with antisocial personality disorder, conduct disorder, substance use disorder, mood disorder, and non-affective psychosis all have an increased risk of serious suicide attempts compared to healthy controls. Comorbidity among these psychiatric disorders increases the risk of serious suicide attempts. The majority of patients (56.6%) who make serious suicide attempts have two or more of these diagnoses [23]. In a study of 229 completed suicides, personality disorder diagnoses were found in 31% of deaths and were the principal diagnosis in 9% of the cases [24]. Patients with paranoid, schizoid, histrionic, and obsessive-compulsive personality disorders are at increased risk of violent behavior. Comorbidity of these personality disorders with substance use, mood and anxiety disorders is also associated with a further increase of violence [25].

Comorbid medical illness

Antisocial lifestyle is associated with higher rates of death and disability by the age of 48 [26]. It is not clear if the higher rates of medical illness and poorer health outcomes in patients with personality disorders are because of the direct long-term biologic effects of childhood neglect, abuse, and trauma commonly seen in patients with personality disorder diagnoses. Other possible reasons for this finding are less healthy lifestyle choices, delayed help seeking, and poorer compliance with treatment recommendations or a combination of the above factors. Not only are patients with character disorder more likely to have addictions, accidents, mental and physical illnesses, but are more likely to require ED treatment and admission to the hospital than those without character disorder [27]. A patient's compliance with treatment recommendations may be decreased by a personality disorder diagnosis. Suspicion of staff and fear of appearing dependent or vulnerable may be traits that variously interfere with compliance, assessments, and interventions needed for life-threatening conditions. Entitlement and poor frustration tolerance may result in a patient leaving against medical advice when their evaluation is lengthy or delayed.

Interpersonal issues in the personality disordered patient

Interpersonal dysfunction is the *sine qua non* of character disorder diagnosis. The patient with character disorder is often observant and focused on the real behavior and attitude of others. The responsibility for interpersonal conflict is often projected to others with the patient failing to see their own contribution. Most of the patients who cause significant difficulty in the emergency department are patients in the cluster B group. Although patients in the other diagnostic clusters may be somewhat difficult to access and treat, their care is not usually as evocative of intense emotional responses by ED staff. Repeated emergency room visits for contact and reassurance by a patient with dependent personality regarding vague or minor medical issues can be frustration to ED staff. An aging person with a personality disorder may have difficulty being in a dependent relationship with family or caregivers. This difficulty may lead to ED visits when there are unresolved conflicts at home or in long-term care facilities that interfere with compliance with needed medical care.

Personality disordered patients may have difficulty with trust and may be prone to feel shame, which can inhibit their communication of important symptoms. These patients may be reluctant to ask questions that facilitate understanding of and compliance with medical treatment. Patients with antisocial personality disorder may not be truthful in their discussions with staff in the ED due to concerns of legal consequences.

Patients in general are sensitive to the nonverbal communications and facial expressions of healthcare providers. Trying to establish a therapeutic alliance when you are highly upset is not likely to be successful. If a clinical interaction is going badly with a patient with a personality disorder, sending in your replacement can salvage the encounter. You may remain the "bad" caregiver, but the new staff-person may be the good doctor or nurse the patient has been looking for. In such a situation, it is reasonable to acknowledge that there is a conflict and offer the option to work with another person if this is possible. If the patient working with another staff member is not possible, disengaging from the patient for a period of time to regain one's composure is advisable.

A psychodynamic perspective

Strong emotional states, expressed or not, are common in all patients in the ED. Pain and anxiety about the potential seriousness of distressing symptoms and the predictable long wait for the ambulatory ED patient are challenging even for emotionally healthy people. The ED is even more problematic for people with personality disorders, who in general have negative or exaggerated expectations of caregivers, more difficulty regulating emotions, and more sensitivity to any expressed or perceived negativity on the part of the healthcare providers.

Psychodynamic concepts of defense, transference, countertransference, and regression are based on the intense and prolonged interaction with patients in a dependent situation. If generalized to the broader frame of care giving and patient relationships seen in the ED, these observations and ideas can help us understand certain negative emotional interactions seen with patients with personality disorders. Although a detailed review of these concepts goes beyond the scope of this chapter, it may be useful to briefly define them. Defense is the way we cope with our strong emotions. The emotion we are dealing with may be something we are consciously aware of or it may be unconscious. Transference is the process of a patient bringing in old expectations and patterns from relationships in the past into a new relationship. Countertransference is the emotional response of a therapist in a relationship with a patient in which emotional responses are stimulated. Countertransference can be seen as a defect in our own defenses, a response to the defenses of a patient or as our contribution to a co-constructed interpersonal engagement. Regression occurs when strong emotions interfere with healthy adult defenses and a person uses immature or maladaptive defenses.

Projective identification is a form of transference and countertransference reaction first described by the psychoanalyst Melanie Klein [28]. She developed a theory around the splitting of internal states (objects) into good and bad parts. These internal objects are projected outward toward others along with intense affective states. This theory is applied to the clinical experience of a therapist having strong emotional responses to a patient that are out of proportion to the actual overt events occurring in the treatment session. This process may also occur in other everyday relationships. Intense states of fear, anger, and a sense of badness in a person are projected into the therapist who identifies with the affective state of the patient

and struggles defensively with the projected sense of badness and intense affects stirred up in response. This concept of projective identification was further developed by others over time. The adult patient abused as a child can induce hostile feelings in caregivers. The ED staff-person is at risk of becoming the hostile caregiver because of a patient's experience with hostile parents as a child in a dependent or sick state. Occasionally, both patient and therapist are angry or fearful and feel the other person in the room is the cause. Projective identification is not only a challenge for the therapist to control, but can be used to understand the affective state of the patient [29]. These ideas have evolved toward the recognition that the process of transference and countertransference occurs with contributions from both people. Although the underlying mechanism of this process is not well understood, nonverbal communication and recently discovered mirror neurons represent potential biologic underpinnings for this clinical process and experience [30]. One indication of projective identification is that the emotional response is uncharacteristic of the person or disproportional to the apparent provocation. It is common for staff to feel ashamed or guilty about strong emotional reactions toward patients without apparent cause and an understanding of this process can be useful for ED staff.

The approach to a successful interview

An interviewing style that is emotionally sensitive is essential when evaluating patients with personality disorder diagnoses. Initially allowing the patient to talk from their perspective facilitates alliance building before beginning the formal risk assessment. It is best to precede the risk assessment with questions that speak to emotional states including anger or unhappiness that are to be expected from the patient's situation. Paying attention to verbal and nonverbal communication is important. Allowing time for the patient to tell their story, the demonstration of empathy toward the patient's affective state, and normalizing the idea that in such a situation a person might think of harming themselves (ending it all) or hurting another person (doing something) are effective interviewing approaches.

Being homicidal or suicidal are clinical conclusions, not appropriate interview questions. Asking a person if they are feeling suicidal or homicidal may lead to inaccurate assessment of risk. Being suicidal or homicidal is easily confused with being bad, weak, or sick in the patient's mind. Because many patients are aware that being suicidal or homicidal can lead to psychiatric hospitalization, quickly getting to the point can lead to a denial of what may have been disclosed with more appropriately paced questions. Being so angry at another person that you feel like hurting them is part of the human condition that may or may not be associated with mental illness, addiction, or personality disorder diagnosis. A person being unhappy and despondent is also commonly seen, dependent on external circumstances and internal states. The critical clinical assessment in the ED is if action is possible or likely in response to these mood and cognitive states. Patients with personality disorders, addictive, and mental illness diagnoses are more likely to act impulsively at times of intense emotional pain or arousal. Acknowledgment of the normality of dysphoric mood states and anger may allow for a more honest disclosure of the person's symptoms, plans, and potential actions. The patient's sense of being understood and supported in the interview builds trust and enhances free communication. This allows for a better diagnostic assessment and appropriate intervention. A positive interview experience increases the likelihood of the patient agreeing to suggested interventions.

Alliance building with the personality disordered patient

Patients with personality disorders are particularly sensitive to the traditional authority stance of the stereotypic physician. A more collaborative stance with a willingness to hear an initial "no" is important in establishing an alliance. This should be coupled with a willingness to re-approach the patient at a later point, to allow the person to change their decision in a face saving manner.

Managing our countertransference to a patient with a personality disorder and that patient's projections onto us, are important in the process of developing an alliance. In dealing with a patient who has a personality disorder, a more intense emotional response is generally felt by the physician or nurse compared to the response to other patients with similar complaints.

In schizoid and schizotypal personality disorders, there may be a sense of detachment in the emotional response to the patients' needs. A high degree of sympathy may be felt toward a person with a dependent personality disorder. A paranoid patient may induce a sense of fear and distrust in staff. A countertransference problem is particularly likely if there is intense anger toward a patient. Anger most commonly occurs in dealing with cluster B personality disorders. Intense anger in staff may lead to unhelpful and unprofessional behavior toward the patient. Minimally, if not understood and managed, anger may result in a premature closure of the attempt to engage the patient in responsible and informed decisions regarding medical assessment and stabilization.

High volume and emotionally demanding situations are taxing to healthcare providers and may provoke unhelpful responses to character disorder patients. Physicians need to monitor themselves from the perspective of professional behavior and responsibility. Another sign of potential difficulty is seeing a patient as "being bad" even when the issue is clearly medical or psychiatric in nature. The "bad patient" problem is more common with patients who suffer from addiction and who have a personality disorder. The patient who suffers from antisocial personality disorder and engages in illegal behaviors where the rights of others are significantly violated induces emotional responses that can be particularly taxing.

Successful work with a personality disordered patient requires attention to the emotional state of the person, and maintaining a positive attitude, despite one's own natural emotional reactions. Reasonable limits are also appropriate if set in a non-punitive manner. Limit setting needs to be motivated by the desire to be helpful to the patient and to facilitate the evaluation. Evaluation and management of medical issues are often more time consuming when the patient has a personality disorder. This is an additional challenge for busy ED staff.

Management of borderline personality disorder

Borderline personality disorder is a particularly challenging condition for ED staff to assess and manage. Although patients with borderline personality disorder are sometimes thought to only have attempts with low lethality, a significant number of them do kill themselves. The period of greatest risk occurs in the initial phase of follow-up after the identification of the disorder [31]. It is important that there is continuity in the care of the patient with a borderline personality disorder. Mental health providers working with the patient should be contacted by the ED to aid in assessment and to confirm follow-up plans. The patient who is already known to the ED will be easier to complete a risk assessment with because the prior record can be reviewed to aid in the process. It is helpful to assign the assessment and management to a nurse and physician who have worked with the patient in the past.

Patients with more severe character disorders, including borderline personality, benefit by having access to their outpatient provider when in crisis. It is preferred that the patient in crisis first contacts the provider to discuss potential interventions that may include arranging an urgent outpatient appointment or a visit to the ED for further assessment and possible admission. The therapist determines if the patient is reliable enough to go to the ED alone, requires a friend or family member to accompany them or if police assistance is needed. The outpatient provider then communicates the plan to the ED and is available to review the final disposition with the ED staff. It is essential for the ED to communicate with the provider if the patient does not present to the ED as anticipated. In some situations police may need to be contacted to check on the well-being of the patient at home or to bring the patient to the ED for assessment. An outpatient provider may need to set some limits on their availability for phone calls from patients at night. Some visits to the ED for assessment and stabilization are unavoidable in more symptomatic patients who can overwhelm a single therapist. The best strategy is for the ED and outpatient provider to function as a team. Over time the frequency and intensity of crisis visits to the ED is likely to decrease as outpatient treatment progress. The ED becomes a backup for the outpatient provider rather than the center of engagement for the patient. Although such efforts are time consuming, being able to discharge a borderline patient from the ED avoids the potential for further worsening of self-harm and suicidal behavior that may occur after an involuntary admission to a psychiatric unit. The advisability of a hospital admission is increased if the patient does not have an outpatient provider, the provider cannot be contacted, or the patient is new to the ED. If a person with borderline personality disorder is highly traumatized, despondent, hopeless, anxious or in a dissociated state, a brief hospital admission can be life saving. A patient with borderline personality disorder may become acutely self-injurious or suicidal when the decision to hospitalize is communicated to them. One-to-one monitoring to prevent self-injury or escape may be needed in the ED while the patient waits to be admitted. Psychiatric admission should be expedited if possible, because many EDs are not suited for the care of a patient who is actively attempting to self-injure or flee.

Life events' importance in risk assessment

Life events increase suicide risk in patients with personality disorders. Schizotypal, borderline, avoidant, and obsessive-compulsive personality disorders have been shown to have an increase in suicidal attempts in the month of, or month following, a negative life event. The two categories of life events that are predictive relate to intimate relations problems and criminal or legal issues.

Events related to love and marriage included:

- Broken engagement
- Relationship worsening
- Separation from a spouse
- Divorce
- Respondent infidelity
- Spouse infidelity
- Spouse or mate dying
- Ended love affair.

Events related to crime and legal issues included being:

- The victim of a physical assault or attack
- Robbed
- Burglarized
- Accused of a crime
- Arrested
- Sent to jail
- Involved in a court case.

The overall category of love and marriage problems was associated with increased suicide attempts; however, no individual items in this group were significantly associated with increased risk. All events in the category of criminal and legal issues showed significant association with suicide attempts, except being robbed or burglarized. In this study, negative events related to work/school, children/other family matters, money/financial issues, social/recreational issues, and health were not significant predictors of an increase in suicide attempts. Positive events were not associated with an increase in suicide attempts in any of the categories [32].

Another study looking at stressful life events as measured by the Social Readjustment Rating Scale has shown that legal problems and spousal loss are life events that increase the risk of suicide attempts in patients with antisocial personality disorder. Patients with a narcissistic personality disorder diagnosis are at increased risk of suicide at times of specific interpersonal and environmental stress. These life events include domestic, financial, and health problems such as being fired from work, changes in the number of arguments with a spouse, personal injury, illness, and foreclosure of a mortgage or loan. Dependent personality disorder diagnosis is associated with increased risk of attempted suicide with work and sexual problems; these being associated with the loss of interpersonal ties that are emotionally fulfilling. Paranoid and schizotypal personality disorder diagnoses are associated with increased risk in suicidal behavior when there has been a change in social activity such as going to clubs, dancing, movies, and visiting others [33,34].

Risk assessment

The decision to admit or discharge patients with character disorders as either a primary or as a comorbid disorder in the ED in psychiatric crisis is a complicated one. This decision should be based on a careful risk assessment that considers the following issues:

History

- The presence and severity of past suicide attempts or aggressive episodes
- Access to weapons or other means to harm themselves or others
- Identifiable target of aggressive impulses versus a more diffused anger without a specific target or remote unavailable target
- Violence or a suicide attempt immediately following an ED assessment and discharge (short-term unpredictability)
- Noncompliance with prior discharge plans from the ED with escalation of dangerous behaviors.

Symptoms

- Symptom level of comorbid psychiatric illness including depression, mania, and psychosis
- Likelihood of continued binge alcohol and substance abuse in comorbid patients
- Expressed intent to kill themselves or harm others especially if these persist after evaluation and intervention.

Stressors

- Recent negative life events
- Onset of new medical disorders
- Severe conflict with significant others.

Attitude

- The refusal to allow contact with significant others and outside mental health providers who know the patient

- The patient's willingness to stay with supportive friends or family until the crisis has abated contrasted with an insistence to be alone after discharge from the ED
- Willingness to engage in verifiable means of harm reduction
- Premature and vague reassurance by the patient that things will be OK if allowed to go home versus the willingness to engage in a meaningful assessment and aftercare plan
- Statements which indicate coming to the ED was a mistake or attempts to leave abruptly without completing the psychiatric assessment
- "Contracting for safety" is not protective, but the unwillingness to engage in a safety contract is concerning.

Supports

- The availability and attitude of social and family supports
- Current engagement in outpatient treatment
- Availability of outpatient psychiatric providers to help in risk assessment in the ED and follow-up planning post-discharge
- Availability of alternative services such as crisis beds and inpatient or residential level chemical dependency treatment.

Protective factors are noted that reduce the lifetime risk of suicide but are not preventive of immediate risk. Men and women of all races, religions, and ages kill themselves.

Risk assessment in a personality disordered patient is not a process that lends itself to a simple approach. After full assessment, risk is categorized as low, medium, or high. Risk can be assessed along a time dimension as imminent (immediate), short-term (hours and days), intermediate (weeks and months), and long-term (years and lifetime). Certain dynamic risk factors can be seen as warning signs of immediate risk of suicide [35]. Prediction of aggression must consider both static and dynamic risk factors, with a past history of violence being a strong predictor of future violence [36]. Warning signs of suicide and violence include:

- A recent serious suicide attempt that was unreported or only accidentally survived
- A violent episode immediately before coming to the ED
- Severe life stressors
- Severe conflict with family and important others
- Suicidal and/or homicidal ideation with intent and plan present on mental status exam
- Intense rage against an identified person who is characterized as bad
- Intense guilt, shame, or self-loathing
- Preparing for and rehearsing a suicide or homicide
- Severe insomnia
- Severe psychomotor agitation and anxiety
- Verbal and physical threats in the ED.

For risk assessments in which there are no warning signs, the art lies in consideration of the historical (static) and current (dynamic) risks. Specific patterns of vulnerability also may be revealed in the patient's history and may inform treatment and disposition planning. A personality disordered patient with a history of a life-threatening suicide following a romantic breakup is at higher risk of suicide if there is another interpersonal loss. The availability of supports and the patient's attitude toward engagement also should be considered in the acute risk analysis.

One way to conceptualize the risk assessment process is that of a vector analysis. Some factors push a patient out of a central safety zone. Other factors tend to reduce risk, pulling the patient back into a safer configuration. Predicting risk for the personality disorder patient requires a careful history, accurate diagnosis, knowledge of factors associated with risk, determination of the current social situation, and consideration of individual vulnerabilities. The final determination is a clinical judgment that weighs all known factors with an appreciation that important factors may not be known. Countertransference reactions can be useful in risk assessment. If discharging a patient is highly anxiety provoking or associated with the idea that something bad will happen, consultation with a colleague is advised before discharge from the ED.

If it is felt there is a duty to warn a person of threats made against him or her by a patient with a personality disorder, a decision to discharge that patient from the ED should be carefully considered. If the sense of danger to another person rises to this level, it is advisable to offer a voluntary admission to the patient or consider involuntary admission. It may not be possible to involuntary commit a patient with a personality disorder depending on state law. Most states' laws allow for a short period of involuntary admission before the court determination of commitment. This time can be used to clarify diagnosis and to decrease the immediate jeopardy to the other person. Discharge can be delayed from the ED to allow for legal consultation regarding the issues duty to warn and involuntary commitment. A consultation from a psychiatrist regarding the decision to discharge is advisable. When both static and dynamic risk factors are elevated, and adequate interventions to modulate the dynamic risk are not possible, the patient with a personality disorder diagnosis may require involuntary psychiatric admission for the protection of self and others.

Mobilization of social supports

There is limited literature on acute treatment in the ED specific to personality disorders. Psychiatric crisis management involves patient engagement and mobilization of their social supports. This may be useful for a person who is in crisis due to interpersonal loss or conflict. Because heightened rejection sensitivity is seen in certain personality disordered patients, the crisis often can be diminished by having family and friends come to the ED. Patients with dependent but hostile relations with parents or spouse, may benefit from support from more distant family members including siblings, aunts, uncles, and friends. Generally, the patient's self-report of who is supportive can be trusted, although it is important to clarify that the person is not someone who co-abuses substances with the patient. It is a positive sign if the patient allows ED staff to speak to friends or family members. This serves two purposes, first to gain valuable collateral history and second to mobilize supportive people being involved in aftercare.

Attempting to get permission to get collateral history before forming an alliance with a patient with a personality disorder diagnosis can be difficult and problematic. Such collateral history is essential in risk assessment if the patient is not being honest or is minimizing risk factors. The patient may avoid giving permission if such collateral history will not corroborate the patient's own account of their history and recent events. Sometimes shame and embarrassment motivate an unwillingness to allow collateral history and engagement of supports. In such a situation, direct discussion with the patient about the necessity of getting collateral history for risk assessment and allowing significant people to be involved post-discharge may overcome this resistance.

In some personality disorders, such as schizoid and schizotypal, social isolation is frequently present. The situation faced by the ED evaluator is not that the patient opposes engagement, rather that no one may be involved with the person. In these situations, linkage with community resources such as crisis residential services or a crisis team may help address the risk of the patient's social isolation, especially if immediate family cannot be engaged, live in distant locations, or refuse to be involved.

Although contact for collateral history is allowed in an emergency for patients unable to consent such as a catatonic patient, the situation is more difficult when a personality disorder patient explicitly refuses to consent for collateral contact. If a personality disordered patient has overdosed, contact of collaterals against the patient's expressed wish would be permissible to determine what pills were taken if this information was not otherwise available and not knowing placed the patient's life at risk. The general principle is that information can be sought against a patient's will if having the information is essential for the emergency treatment of the patient and there is no other way to assure the patient's safety. The use of written consent for release of information or collateral contact is preferred. The patient's agreement to allow for collateral contact should also be documented in the progress notes. Local ED policy should be followed regarding the need for written consent for collateral history gathering.

Information can or must be disclosed to potential victims and/or local police of a credible threat of violence as part of the Tarasoff "duty to warn" laws that are present in many states [37]. States' laws vary significantly and knowledge of local requirements is essential. Because hospitalization is protective of potential victims, the decision to warn a potential victim can be deferred to the treating psychiatrist if a patient is admitted. These threats should be specifically documented and directly communicated to the treating psychiatrist. Breaking confidentially in an emergency situation can have a negative impact on the alliance with a personality disordered patient. If confidentially is broken, the reasons for doing so should be explained to the patient and documented in the medical record. Being honest about what is being done and why, sends an important message to the character disordered patient. When possible, consultation with a hospital attorney and senior clinical staff should be sought before a breach of confidentiality or after one has occurred. Adamant refusal to identify or allow contact with any source of collateral history may, depending on the overall risk assessment, tip the balance toward hospitalization.

Medication

The benefits of medication are limited in the treatment of character disorders in the ED. A benzodiazepine may be administered to treat high levels of anxiety or to decrease agitation and aggression [38]. After a patient with a personality disorder receives emergency or involuntary medication, an adequate period of observation in the ED is advisable to assure that the acute symptoms remain improved as medication effects decrease. Before such a patient's discharge, the risk assessment should be repeated after the medication effects wear off. For this reason, the use of short-acting benzodiazepines is preferred. The need to use involuntary or emergency medication in the ED increases the advisability of an admission to an inpatient psychiatric unit.

Disposition

It is advisable to give specific discharge instruction to avoid alcohol and substance use for a personality disordered patient in crisis. Even if the person does not meet criteria for a substance use disorder, the disinhibiting effects of intoxication can increase the risk of impulsive action. Specific instruction to avoid contact with a person with whom the patient has a high degree of conflict is also helpful, although it may not be honored. Sometimes suggesting a third party be involved, such as a mutual friend or relative, may decrease the risk of a highly regressive interaction between the patient and the person with whom they are in conflict. This is particularly important if the conflict is because of a separation or threatened separation.

Important alliance building occurs through the manner in which discharge from the ED is managed. As part of the discharge instructions to the patient with a personality disorder, it is important to advise that they return for reassessment if suicidal ideas or aggressive impulses again feel unmanageable. Even when suicidal ideas or anger are long standing, this advice is helpful from a clinical and risk management perspective. Feeling rejected and unwanted, unloved and unlovable are common feelings in those who suffer from severe personality disorders. Being advised to return if things worsen is similar to the advice given to patients with medical illnesses that are difficult to accurately access or whose course is hard to predict. For a person with a personality disorder, such advice may reduce the sense of alienation and rejection they commonly experience. ED staff may be aware that they do not wish to ever see this particular patient again, but this is best understood as a countertransference to the patient's own self-hatred. Understanding and overcoming these emotional challenges adds to professional competency. In addition, one's own self-esteem is justifiably enhanced by doing the right thing for the difficult patient.

Referral and aftercare

The criteria for diagnosis of a personality disorder are often based on interpersonal dysfunction which causes significant stress for a patient. Focus on the stressful interpersonal situation in which patients finds themselves may provide a way to suggest mental health intervention because it is broadly accepted that stress is bad for your health. The primary therapeutic approach to the treatment of personality disorder diagnosis is a psychotherapeutic one [39]. The suggestion of getting some counseling or doing some talking with a therapist about the stress may lead to engagement in outpatient therapy by the person with a personality disorder diagnosis. With the patient's permission, engaging family members or supports in the aftercare plan is helpful. Family therapy may be useful when personality issues impact family functioning or dysfunctional family patterns impact the patient.

Documentation and risk management

Blaming or labeling a patient as bad or wrong in the medical record is not helpful from a risk-management perspective. Writing it down does not prove you are right. Negative emotional responses and attitudes toward the character disordered patient should be controlled, hopefully understood, discussed with a supervisor, but not documented. The urge to document the wrongness or badness of the patients or to prove oneself right in a progress note is certainly a sign of a countertransference reaction. Patients with personality disorders are entitled to review medical records, and documentation that is pejorative may increase the potential for litigation around adverse outcomes. The character disordered patient's initial refusal to consent for evaluation and treatment can be provocative of negative responses from the ED physician. Efforts should be made to calm the anxious or angry patient and on further

alliance building with the distrustful patient. These efforts should be documented if the patient ultimately insists on rejecting important recommendations.

The documentation of the psychiatric assessment should include the standard elements of any psychiatric evaluation. Unless the patient has a well-established diagnosis of personality disorder, it is best to note a differential diagnosis that includes personality disorder as a "rule out." It is useful to document the contact numbers for friends, family, and outpatient psychiatric providers in the ED record for future reference. If there was contact with an outpatient provider for crisis assessment and management, this should be noted in the progress note. If friends and family are involved in the assessment or discharge plan it is important to document this, along with their attitude and apparent reliability. It is also helpful to document any area of sensitivity or vulnerability that was an issue during the evaluation.

Summary and discussion

Patients with severe personality disorders benefit from a coordinated plan with outpatient psychiatric providers. Contact with outpatient providers also helps with risk assessment. An understanding of basic psychodynamic concepts may help staff effectively deal with their emotional responses to the personality disordered patient. Facilitating outpatient psychiatric referral for patients with personality disorder diagnoses is an important goal for the ED.

Emergency departments are becoming increasingly demanding and stressful for staff. The human tendency to regress under stress is universal. Attention to core clinical values can help ED staff manage negative emotional and behavioral responses to patients with character disorders. Professionalism is demonstrated by the capacity to keep the emotional state and needs of the patient with a personality disorder in mind, despite countertransference reactions. Attitudes of ED educators and leadership are critical in improving the approach to stigmatized disorders, including chemical dependency, mental illness, and personality disorder diagnoses.

References

1. Adams J, Murray R, III. The general approach to the difficult patient. *Emerg Med Clin North Am* 1998;**16**:689–700.

2. Spence JM, Bergmans Y, Strike C, et al. Experiences of substance-using suicidal males who present frequently to the emergency department. *CJEM* 2008;**10**:339–46.

3. Samuels J. Personality disorders: epidemiology and public health issues. *Int Rev Psychiatry* 2011;**23**:223–33.

4. Bruffaerts R, Sabbe M, Demyttenaere K. Who visits the psychiatric emergency room for the first time? *Soc Psychiatry Psychiatr Epidemiol* 2006;**41**:580–6.

5. Lee HB, Bienvenu OJ, Cho SJ, et al. Personality disorders and traits as predictors of incident cardiovascular disease: findings from the 23-year follow-up of the Baltimore ECA study. *Psychosomatics* 2010;**51**:289–96.

6. Kendler KS, Aggen SH, Czajkowski N, et al. The structure of genetic and

environmental risk factors for DSM-IV personality disorders: a multivariate twin study. *Arch Gen Psychiatry* 2008;**65**:1438–46.

7. Jonson-Reid M,Presnall N, Drake B, et al. Effects of child maltreatment and inherited liability on antisocial development: an official records study. *J Am Acad Child Adolesc Psychiatry* 2010;**49**:321–32.

8. Caspi A, McClay J, Moffitt TE, et al. Role of genotype in the cycle of violence in

maltreated children. *Science* 2002;**297**:851–4.

9. Fineberg NA, Sharma P, Sivakumaran T, Sahakian B, Chamberlain SR. Does obsessive-compulsive personality disorder belong within the obsessive-compulsive spectrum? *CNS Spectr* 2007;**12**:467–82.

10. Tarbox SI, Pogue-Geile MF. A multivariate perspective on schizotypy and familial association with schizophrenia: a review. *Clin Psychol Rev* 2011;**31**:1169–82.

11. Fogelson DL, Asarnow RA, Sugar CA, et al. Avoidant personality disorder symptoms in first-degree relatives of schizophrenia patients predict performance on neurocognitive measures: the UCLA family study. *Schizophr Res* 2010;**120**:113–20.

12. American Psychiatric Association. *Diagnostic and Statistical Manual of Mental Disorders.* Text Revision (Fourth Edition). Washington, DC: American Psychiatric Association; 2000.

13. Hopwood CJ, Malone JC, Ansell EB, et al. Personality assessment in DSM-5: empirical support for rating severity, style, and traits. *J Pers Disord* 2011;**25**:305–20.

14. Tyrer P, Crawford M, Mulder R, ICD-11 Working Group for the Revision of Classification of Personality Disorders. Reclassifying personality disorders. *Lancet* 2011;**377**:1814–15.

15. Tragesser SL, Trull TJ, Sher KJ, Park A. Drinking motives as mediators in the relation between personality disorder symptoms and alcohol use disorder. *J Pers Disord* 2008;**22**:525–37.

16. Di Sclafani V, Finn P, Fein G. Psychiatric comorbidity in long-term abstinent alcoholic individuals. *Alcohol Clin Exp Res* 2007;**31**:795–3.

17. Fenton MC, Keyes K, Geier T, et al. Psychiatric comorbidity and the persistence of drug use disorders in the United States. *Addiction* 2012;**107**:599–609.

18. Flannery RB Jr, Walker AP. Repetitively assaultive psychiatric patients: fifteen-year analysis of the Assaulted Staff Action Program (ASAP) with implications for emergency services. *Int J Emerg Ment Health* 2008;**10**:1–8.

19. Grann M, Danesh J, Fazel S. The association between psychiatric diagnosis and violent re-offending in adult offenders in the community. *BMC Psychiatry* 2008;**8**:92.

20. Ouimette PC, Gima K, Moos RH, Finney JW. A comparative evaluation of substance abuse treatment IV. The effect of comorbid psychiatric diagnoses on amount of treatment, continuing care, and 1-year outcomes. *Alcohol Clin Exp Res* 1999;**23**:552–7.

21. Humphreys K, Moos RH. Encouraging posttreatment self-help group involvement to reduce demand for continuing care services: two-year clinical and utilization outcomes. *Alcohol Clin Exp Res* 2007;**31**:64–8.

22. Reichborn-Kjennerud T, Czajkowski N, Roysamb E, et al. Major depression and dimensional representations of DSM-IV personality disorders: a population-based twin study. *Psychol Med* 2010;**40**:1475–84.

23. Beautrais AL, Joyce PR, Mulder RT, et al. Prevalence and comorbidity of mental disorders in persons making serious suicide attempts: a case-control study. *Am J Psychiatry* 1996;**153**:1009–14.

24. Henriksson MM, Aro HM, Marttunen MJ, et al. Mental disorders and comorbidity in suicide. *Am J Psychiatry* 1993;**150**:935–40.

25. Pulay AJ, Dawson DA, Hasin DS, et al. Violent behavior and DSM-IV psychiatric disorders: results from the national epidemiologic survey on alcohol and related conditions. *J Clin Psychiatry* 2008;**69**:12–22.

26. Shepherd JP, Shepherd I, Newcombe RG, Farrington D. Impact of antisocial lifestyle on health: chronic disability and death by middle age. *J Public Health (Oxf)* 2009;**31**:506–11.

27. Wagner JA, Pietrzak RH, Petry NM. Psychiatric disorders are associated with hospital care utilization in persons with hypertension: results from the National Epidemiologic Survey on alcohol and related conditions. *Soc Psychiatry Psychiatr Epidemiol* 2008;**43**:878–88.

28. Klein M. Notes on some schizoid mechanisms. *Int J Psychoanal* 1946;**27**:99–110.

29. Racker H. The meanings and uses of countertransference. *Psychoanal Q* 1957;**26**:303–57.

30. Gallese V, Eagle MN, Migone P. Intentional attunement: mirror neurons and the neural underpinnings of interpersonal relations. *J Am Psychoanal Assoc* 2007;**55**:131–76.

31. Pompili M, Girardi P, Ruberto A, Tatarelli R. Suicide in borderline personality disorder: a meta-analysis. *Nord J Psychiatry* 2005;**59**:319–24.

32. Yen S, Pagano ME, Shea MT, et al. Recent life events preceding suicide attempts in a personality disorder sample: findings from the collaborative longitudinal personality disorders study. *J Consult Clin Psychol* 2005;**73**:99–105.

33. Holmes TH, Rahe RH. The Social Readjustment Rating Scale. *J Psychosom Res* 1967;**11**:213–18.

34. Blasco-Fontecilla H, Baca-Garcia E, Duberstein P, et al. An exploratory study of the relationship between diverse life events and specific personality disorders in a sample of suicide attempters. *J Pers Disord* 2010;**24**:773–84.

35. Rudd MD, Berman AL, Joiner TE Jr, et al. Warning signs for suicide: theory, research, and clinical applications. *Suicide Life Threat Behav* 2006;**36**:255–62.

36. Amore M, Menchetti M, Tonti C, et al. Predictors of violent behavior among acute psychiatric patients: clinical study. *Psychiatry Clin Neurosci* 2008;**62**:247–55.

37. Herbert PB, Young KA. Tarasoff at twenty-five. *J Am Acad Psychiatry Law* 2002;**30**:275–81.

38. Allen MH, Currier GW, Carpenter D, et al. The expert consensus guideline series. Treatment of behavioral emergencies 2005. *J Psychiatr Pract* 2005;**11**(Suppl 1):5–108.

39. Matusiewicz AK, Hopwood CJ, Banducci AN, Lejuez CW. The effectiveness of cognitive behavioral therapy for personality disorders. *Psychiatr Clin North Am* 2010;**33**:657–85.

The patient with factitious disorders or malingering in the emergency department

Rachel Lipson Glick

Introduction

In malingering and factitious disorder, the patient pretends to be ill or intentionally causes his or her own symptoms. Physicians, who are trained to trust what patients tell them, have difficulty assessing and treating these patients who lie. This chapter will review the diagnosis, assessment, and management of these, often difficult, patients, providing practical advice to the emergency physician.

Case examples

Malingering

A 22-year-old man comes to the emergency department (ED) complaining of severe pain in his leg. He explains he was in a motorcycle accident a few days before this presentation, and although his leg was not broken it was "bruised and banged up." Nursing staff note that, although he was walking around the waiting room without a limp, when he was aware of being observed he limped and winced in pain when he put weight on this leg. Examination of his leg reveals some bruises and abrasions on his leg that are healing well. When the physician recommends nonsteroidal anti-inflammatory drugs (NSAIDs) for the pain, the patient says he knows he needs Vicodin because that is all that ever works for his pain. A review of his medical records shows he often comes to the ED requesting narcotics and that he has been given small amounts for various injuries in the past. The physician suspects he is exaggerating his pain to get narcotics unnecessarily.

Factitious disorder

A 34-year-old medical assistant is brought to the ED unconscious and is found to have a blood glucose that is dangerously low. She is revived with Dextrose50 and tells the physician that she has diabetes that has never been well controlled. She states that she has had many episodes of both hypo- and hyperglycemia that have led to hospitalizations. She lives in another city and has never been evaluated previously at this hospital. Her mother is at her bedside when the physician comes back to discuss control of her diabetes. Her mother seems surprised,

and says that, as far as she knows, her daughter does not have diabetes. The patient then abruptly starts to dress and asks for paperwork to sign out against medical advice.

Definitions

Somatization is the bodily representation of a psychological need [1]. It is a common way for children to indicate that they need psychological support; such as when a child who is anxious develops a "tummy ache" to avoid going to school. In older children and adults, it is considered a less healthy way to get emotional needs met. When somatization leads to dysfunction, as in the somatoform disorders or in malingering or factitious disorder, it is considered pathologic [1].

Malingering and factitious disorder are both forms of somatization in which the patient is aware of producing or feigning their symptoms [1]. The patient's awareness is what distinguishes these two disorders from the somatoform disorders (see Tables 15.1 and 15.2). In malingering, the patient seeks *secondary gain* by using the symptoms to get something or get out of something, such as avoiding jail time by claiming to be suicidal [2]. In factitious disorder, the motivation is unconscious and leads the patient to desire the sick role but not for any tangible benefit other than taking on this role for psychological purposes. This is referred to as *primary* or *psychological gain*. Primary gain is believed to decrease subconscious stress or anxiety [2].

The idea of malingering and using physical, or psychological, complaints to one's benefit for tangible gains is a relatively easy concept to understand. The desire to take on the sick-role for psychological needs is a more difficult concept to grasp. Regardless, both disorders challenge emergency physicians who see their jobs as taking care of "real" sick patients, not those who do things to themselves, or pretend to have symptoms.

Diagnosis

Malingering

According to *The Diagnostic and Statistical Manual of Mental Disorders, 4th Edition, Text Revision* (DSM-IV-TR), malingering

Behavioral Emergencies for the Emergency Physician, ed. Leslie S. Zun, Lara G. Chepenik, and Mary Nan S. Mallory. Published by Cambridge University Press. © Cambridge University Press 2013.

Table 15.1. Patient awareness in malingering and factitious disorders

Disorder	Mechanism of illness production	Motivation for illness behavior
Somatoform disorders	Unconscious	Unconscious
Factitious disorder	Conscious	Unconscious
Malingering	Conscious	Conscious

Table 15.2. Clinical features in malingering and factious disorder

Malingering	Factitious disorder
Men>woman	Women > men, except in Munchausen's variant
Substance abuse	Employment/training in medical field
Vague, unverifiable history	Vague, unverifiable history
Refuses tests, treatments, AMA	Not bothered by invasive procedures
Antisocial personality disorder	Borderline personality disorder

is given a V-code designation, suggesting it is not in and of itself a diagnosis. Rather, it is an issue that can be the focus of the clinical encounter [3]. It is defined as "the intentional production of false or grossly exaggerated physical or psychological symptoms, motivated by external incentives such as avoiding military duty, avoiding work, obtaining financial compensation, evading criminal prosecution, or obtaining drugs"[4]. The DSM goes on to note that malingering behavior can be adaptive in some instances, e.g., when a prisoner of war feigns illness [4]. The DSM-IV-TR description of malingering lists some situations in which malingering should be suspected. If there is a discrepancy between the patient's level of stress or dysfunction and the objective findings, or if the patient is uncooperative with the assessment [4], the physician might consider malingering. Although to make a final diagnosis, the external incentive that is driving the behavior must be identified and other possible diagnoses ruled-out. The incidence of malingering is unknown. Malingering using psychiatric symptoms appears to be more common in people dealing with the legal system, while physical symptoms are more often associated with financial gain or disability seeking behavior [3].

Factitious disorder

Factitious disorder is diagnosed, according to DSM-IV-TR, when three conditions are met: there is intentional production of, or feigning, of physical or psychological symptoms, the motivation for symptom production is to take on the sick-role, and no external incentives drive the behavior [4]. Proposed changes in the upcoming DSM-V maintain these diagnostic criteria [5]. Case reports of individuals with this disorder demonstrate the lengths to which patients with factitious disorder will go to take on the sick-role [6]. A patient with factitious disorder will do something as seemingly distasteful as injecting feces under her skin to cause cellulitis. Factitious disorder is more common in women than men, and a preponderance of those with the diagnosis have studied or worked in a medical field [7,8].

A sub-category of factitious disorder, Munchausen syndrome, named after the famous 18th century traveling storyteller, Baron von Munchausen, is characterized by patients who travel widely and tell elaborate tales about their illnesses and treatments thus becoming career medical imposters. This term should be reserved for those with the most severe form of factitious disorder [6], but it is often used in the lay press and even in medical settings to describe all patients with factitious disorder rather than just this sub-type. Interestingly, this variant seems more common in men [8].

Some other historical factors suggestive of factitious disorder include multiple hospital admissions, lack of verifiable history, social isolation and few interpersonal connections, early history of serious or chronic illness, multiple scars, failure to respond to typical treatments, and comorbid personality disorder; most often borderline personality disorder [8].

Finally, emergency physicians must be aware of Munchausen syndrome by proxy. In this rare disorder, a parent or guardian causes a factitious illness in a child.

Assessment

Malingering should be suspected in patients who have clear motives for seeking care. Those who are under arrest or facing other unpleasant situations might be using medical complaints to avoid legal or other consequences. Patients who are malingering often have vague, confusing, and unverifiable stories [9]. Their symptoms do not correlate with objective findings. They often refuse testing. They might ask specifically for medications, often controlled medications, and can quickly be labeled "drug-seeking" by nursing staff and physicians. Alternatively, they might demand letters for work, school, attorneys, court, or other entities to verify that they are ill. They often have comorbid antisocial personality disorder and substance use issues [6,8].

The physician should pay careful attention to the patient's affect as well as his or her degree of cooperativeness and guardedness with the examiner. Patients who are malingering may exaggerate their symptoms, or appear to be acting rather than feeling pain or anxiety [10]. It is helpful, if possible, to observe the patient when they do not know they are being observed to see if it still appears that they are in distress [6].

It is also helpful, especially when the patient reports a long history of symptoms, to try to figure out why the patient is in the ED now. What do they need that has led them to seek your help at this particular time? Sometimes just asking this question allows the provider to get to the real reason the patient is presenting now. This opens the way to discuss what they are requesting and explain whether you can or cannot help with it. For example, a patient presents to the ED complaining of pain that started with a car accident 2 years ago. He wears a neck brace and insists that he needs X-rays today. There are no objective findings on exam and X-rays are normal. When the physician questions why he is in the ED now, he explains he needs a doctor to fill out disability forms so he can take them to his new lawyer.

The patient with factitious disorder is rarely even identified as such in the ED setting. Most often they produce findings on exam, falsify lab results, or tell stories that lead to appropriate treatment for the illness they are pretending to have or complications from treatment of that illness [10]. Case reports describe numerous examples of factitious disorder ranging from hypoglycemia caused by use of insulin to sepsis to multiple traumas [11–13].

People with factitious disorder want to be patients. They are more or less compliant in the ED setting, although their histories are often vague and inconsistent. A subtle lack of concern about their sometimes very serious situation and the fact they are not bothered by the prospect of invasive or painful procedures might be a clue to the underlying factitious disorder, but again, this is quite difficult to recognize in the ED. More often, the medical team becomes suspicious of the patient while they are on a medical unit and are not responding to treatment as expected. For example, a young woman with reported diagnosis of Bartter's syndrome is admitted for bradycardia because of low potassium levels. Yet her potassium levels do not increase with supplementation. The team only becomes suspicious of her when the potassium levels remain low. This prompts them to order a furosemide level. The results show that the patient is taking a diuretic to lower her potassium, despite the risk of arrhythmia.

Management

Patients with malingering and factitious disorder can present with almost any symptom or complaint one can imagine. Both malingering and factitious disorder are diagnoses of exclusion. The patient must be evaluated for whatever their physical (or psychological) concern is before a diagnosis of malingering or factitious disorder is made. Patients who have already harmed themselves, such as the patient who has manipulated her skin so that she now has a cellulitis, need medical care regardless of the initial cause.

If either malingering or factitious disorder is suspected, attempts should be made to get collateral information as well as old records, as these can help confirm the diagnosis. Often patients with these disorders will present at off hours when they know less seasoned providers will be on duty [6]. They also may travel from ED to ED, so getting a full history of contacts with the healthcare system can be difficult.

While recognition is the first step in the psychiatric management of malingering and factitious disorder, this is not easy to do when an unknown patient presents to the ED. The ED physician must first focus on ruling out medical illness and treating any true pathology that is found. If deception on the part of the patient is suspected, invasive procedures, extensive evaluations, and admissions to the hospital should be avoided as iatrogenic harm can occur. Second, physicians must be aware of their own reactions toward these patients and remember that these patients are in emotional distress. They simply don't know how to deal with their pain and/or have their needs met in more appropriate ways. Third, appropriate limits should be set. A patient should not be given the medications he or she requests, unless they are needed. For example, the patient who reports severe pain, but does not have objective findings, and is noted to appear to be without pain when he is observed unbeknownst in the waiting area, should not be given opiates.

Psychiatric treatment options for both conditions are limited [8]. Nevertheless, psychiatric consultants may assist in the evaluation and management of these patients, but often their greatest help is not to the patient directly, but rather to the staff who are struggling with their own negative feelings toward the patient.

There is debate in the literature about the wisdom of confronting these patients. Patients who are confronted rarely admit the deception [6]. Patients with both malingering and factitious disorder will often leave the hospital if confronted with medical staff suspicion of their story, as illustrated in the case of factitious disorder described at the beginning of this chapter. A better approach might be to give them a face-saving way out of the situation, but this can be difficult to do.

Documentation should be carefully worded, but should honestly summarize your findings and reasons for your suspicions. Some legal experts suggest describing the patient's manipulative behavior, rather than using the word malingering, as this word can be seen as pejorative. Instead stating, "The patient reported severe pain and inability to walk, but was observed walking with no limp or apparent discomfort in the waiting area, so no opiates were prescribed," is the preferable way to document clinical decision making in the case example above. Table 15.3 summarizes recommendations for the management of malingering and factitious disorders.

Table 15.3. Suggested management of factitious disorder and malingering in the ED

Rule out medical illness
Treat any injuries or conditions produced by the patient
Avoid iatrogenic injuries
Review records/get collateral history if possible
Set limits
Document management and medical decision making
Manage negative feelings toward the patient

Conclusion

Patients with malingering and factitious disorder present unique challenges to the emergency physician. In the busy setting of an emergency service, where some patients face life and death situations, the presentation of a person who is making him or herself sick, or simply pretending to be sick, is extremely frustrating. The physician should try to put aside any negative feelings toward these patients and evaluate them for true medical needs, while setting appropriate limits and carefully documenting objective findings and medical decision making.

References

1. Folks DG, Ford CV, Houcki CA. Somatoform disorders, factitious disorders, and malingering. In: Stoudemire A, (Ed.). *Clinical Psychiatry for Medical Students*, (3rd Edition). Philadelphia: Lippincott-Raven Publishers; 1998.

2. Hollifield MA. Somatization disorder. In: Sadock BJ, Sadock VA, (Eds.). *Kaplan & Sadock's Comprehensive Textbook of Psychiatry*, (8th Edition). Philadelphia: Lippincott Williams & Wilkins; 2005.

3. McDermott BE, Feldman MD. Malingering in the medical setting. *Psychiatr Clin N Am* 2007;**30**:645–62.

4. American Psychiatric Association. *Diagnostic and Statistical Manual of Mental Disorders*, Text Revision (4th Edition). Washington, DC: American Psychiatric Association; 2000.

5. Dimsdale J, Creed F. The proposed diagnosis of somatic symptom disorders in DSM-V to replace somatoform disorders in DSM-IV–a preliminary report. *J Psychosomatic Res* 2009;**66**:473–6.

6. Epstein LA, Stern TA. Factitious disorders and malingering. In: Glick RL, Berlin JS, Fishkind AB, Zeller SL, (Eds.). *Emergency Psychiatry, Principles and Practice*. Philadelphia: Lippincott Williams & Wilkins; 2008.

7. Krahn LE, Li H, O'Connor MK. Patients who strive to be ill: factitious disorder with physical symptoms. *Am J Psychiatry* 2003;**160**:1163–8.

8. Smith FA. Factitious disorders and malingering. In: Stern TA, Rosenbaum JF, Fava M, et al., (Eds.). *Massachusetts General Hospital Comprehensive Clinical Psychiatry*. Philadelphia: Mosby Elsevier; 2008.

9. Schwartz P, Weathers M. The psychotic patient. In: Riba M, Ravindranath D, (Eds.). *Clinical Manual of Emergency Psychiatry*. Washington, DC: American Psychiatric Publishing, Inc; 2010.

10. Simakhodskyay Z, Haddad F, Quintero M, Ravindranath D, Glick RL. Disposition and resource options. In: Riba M, Ravindranath D, (Eds.). *Clinical Manual of Emergency Psychiatry*. Washington, DC: American Psychiatric Publishing, Inc; 2010.

11. Lazarus A, Kozinn WP. Munchausen's syndrome with hematuria and sepsis: an unusual case. *Int J Psychiatry Med* 1991;**21**:113–16.

12. Bretz SW, Richards JR. Munchausen syndrome presenting acutely in the emergency department. *J Emerg Med* 2000;**18**:417–20.

13. Hedges BE, Dimsdale JE, Hoyt DB. Munchausen syndrome presenting as recurrent multiple trauma. *Psychosomatics* 1995;**36**:60–3.

The patient with delirium and dementia in the emergency department

Lorin M. Scher and David C. Hsu

Introduction

Patients with delirium, dementia, and those with both delirium and dementia can be the most challenging patients in the emergency department (ED). Medically and emotionally complex, these patients often require multidisciplinary resources, astute coordination of care, and vigilant observation. ED physicians, psychiatrists, nurses, social workers, primary care physicians, hospitalists, and sometimes geriatricians may comprise the medical team. Family members and caretakers provide necessary perspectives and are recognized and integrated into the evaluation and management process when caring for these patients. Only with teamwork will these patients be cared for optimally.

Dementia most often occur in adults 65 years of age or older. One quarter of all ED visits are for older adults, and of those, one quarter are for cognition-related presentations [1]. Half of all hospital days are for older adults and their care amounts to billions of dollars annually [2]. ED visits for older adults are increasing, and they often present by ambulance with more severe medical illness requiring more tests and longer ED stay [1]. Because studies have shown that ED physicians tend to miss a diagnosis of delirium or other cognitive impairment approximately 75% of the time, the American College of Emergency Physicians and the Society for Academic Emergency Medicine Geriatric Task Force in 2009 have selected "cognitive assessment" as one of the three quality indicators for improvement of geriatric emergency care [3].

Integration of psychiatric emergency services into the ED can help with cognitive assessment and management. Social workers and psychiatrists often are willing to work with ED physicians and nurses directly in a team-care approach. Early consultation with specialists has been shown to decrease future negative outcomes [4].

Approach to the cognitively impaired patient

Delirium and dementia are formally known as "cognitive disorders," with core features of impairment in the cognitive domains. Presentations and associated symptoms are invariably diverse, so an open-minded approach to the cognitively impaired patient is recommended. Recent data suggest that delirium and dementia may reside more on a continuum rather than as two separate disease entities [2]. Patients with either diagnosis have a higher risk of succumbing to the other, and intervention data may support similar treatments based on comparable pathophysiology. For example, depressed mood, as well as psychotic symptoms, can be seen in both. Both disorders seem to have acetylcholine deficiencies. Whereas anticholinergic medications can make both dementia and delirium patients worse, cholinesterase inhibitors can make them better. Generally, patients with delirium tend to improve more quickly than patients with dementia, but newer research describes "persistent delirium," which can last for months [5]. Delirium is more acute, and dementia is more chronic. Patients can also have delirium superimposed on dementia [6], making diagnosis and management more challenging.

Patients with delirium and dementia unfortunately have high mortality rates. It is currently unclear whether the pathophysiology of the mental disorders themselves leads to worse survival rates, but it is clear that patients with these disorders have high comorbid medical conditions. Clinicians who care for patients with terminal illness are familiar with delirium and the associated emotional challenges. Studies have shown that patients with these disorders are severely distressed by them [7]. Medical team members, caretakers, and family members are also severely distressed by these disorders. Caregiving is an independent risk factor for mortality of the caregiver [8]. Common reasons for patients with dementia to present to the hospital are caregiver illness and "nervous exhaustion" by caregivers [9]. Therefore, in this patient population, it is imperative to consider not only quantity of life, but also quality of life, on all fronts, including others in the patient's sphere of influence.

The approach to a cognitively impaired patient in the ED should be as follows [10]:

1. *Differentiate between delirium and dementia.* Many patients will come to the ED with a history that they are "not the same" or they have developed new behaviors. With a history and exam, including attention to the vital signs and the patient's orientation to self and environment, the clinician

Behavioral Emergencies for the Emergency Physician, ed. Leslie S. Zun, Lara G. Chepenik, and Mary Nan S. Mallory. Published by Cambridge University Press. © Cambridge University Press 2013.

should be able to decipher whether the process is acute, chronic, or acute on chronic. A proper assessment will help outline potential management strategies. Consultations may be needed.

2. *Provide supportive measures.* Because some underlying illnesses responsible for acute cognitive changes are life-threatening, immediate assessment and care targeted toward the traditional "A,B,C,D's" of resuscitation may lead to improvements of cognition once baseline ventilation, cardiac function, perfusion, and neurologic function are addressed. As with all ED patients, the evaluation of possible myocardial infarction and stroke must be given top priority. Agitation should be addressed. Communication with families and caretakers, and addressing their emotional needs is important, as often the underlying issues do not, however, immediately resolve.

3. *Search vigilantly for a medical cause.* Delirium is considered a reversible condition. Dementia sub-types can also be reversed, but more commonly, as with Alzheimer's disease, the process is irreversible. In addition to a thorough history and physical exam, medical investigations often include laboratory tests, radiography, and advanced imaging tests like magnetic resonance imaging and computed tomography. Lumbar punctures and electroencephalograms may be indicated.

Delirium

Background

Delirium is considered a medical emergency [11], seen in all age groups, and is common among older patients in the ED. One in ten older ED patients will have delirium [1], and with comparable morbidity and mortality to patients with acute coronary syndromes and sepsis. With reports of emergency physicians missing the diagnosis of delirium up to 75% of the time, this can be conceptualized as a "medical error" [12]. Delirium in the ED has been shown to be an independent predictor of both prolonged hospital stay and six-month mortality. Patients with delirium in the ED had higher mortality rates than those whose delirium was not detected [13]. Although unclear about the care coordination and treatment decisions, approximately 25% of patients with delirium would also be discharged from the ED [14].

Delirium has been written about extensively in general medical and psychiatric literature, especially in the past 20 years. Although it can occur in patients across the lifespan, most studies have focused on older adults, as does this chapter. Most studies of delirium have been conducted in the community or hospital setting. The prevalence of delirium in the general community is 1–2%, but this increases to 14–24% in the hospital setting [11]. At least 20% of older adults will experience complications from delirium during their hospital stay [2]. Postoperative delirium in the elderly can be as high as 53%, and for delirium in the intensive care unit, 87% [11]. Up to 60%

of the elderly in nursing homes will have an episode of delirium, and 83% experience delirium at the end of life [2].

At least one quarter of all patients with delirium will die within 1 year, and 22–76% will die during the hospital admission [2]. Comparable to costs of falls and diabetes, the total cost of delirium when counting ED visits, physician and clinic visits, rehabilitation services, home health care, and institutionalization amounts to more than $100 billion per year [15]. The occurrence rate of in-hospital delirium is a defined marker of quality of care and patient safety by the National Quality Measures Clearinghouse of the Agency for Healthcare Research and Quality [2].

Longitudinal studies of delirium have also revealed chronic negative outcomes. In an observational cohort study of 412 older patients with delirium, one third of them continued to have delirium at 6 months associated with a mortality rate of 39% at 1 year. The study concluded that persistent delirium predicts greater mortality [5]. Over time, delirium also predicted poorer hospital outcomes when measuring length of hospital stay, nursing home placement, and functional decline [16].

Clinical features

The Diagnostic and Statistical Manual of Mental Disorders, 4th Edition, Text Revision (DSM-IV-TR) [17] published by the American Psychiatric Association in 2000 describes "delirium" as a "disturbance of consciousness that is accompanied by a change in cognition ... manifested by a reduced clarity of awareness of the environment." There may be perceptual disturbances, such as hallucinations. Patients often have disturbances of the sleep–wake cycle or may exhibit changes in emotions, which may include fear, anxiety, depression, and euphoria. Motor symptoms vary between hyperactivity or hypoactivity. Hyperactive patients in delirium tend to elicit more hallucinations and agitation.

A prodrome of restlessness, disorientation, or distractibility may precede the full course of delirium, which may last hours to days or weeks to months, often fluctuating throughout the day. The majority of patients with delirium recover fully, but the rates are lower with elderly patients. Finally, delirium is always secondary to an underlying medical condition, so there must be evidence from the history, exam, or laboratory tests that suggests medical illness.

Although having the clinical description of "delirium" may be helpful, diagnosing delirium in the ED may be more challenging due to time constraints. Several published bedside screening instruments can guide the busy clinician in the assessment process. The most popular instruments for efficient screening of patients have been the Mini-Mental State Examination (MMSE), Confusion Assessment Method (CAM), CAM-ICU, Six-Item Screener (SIS), and the Mini-Cog [18,19].

A recent meta-analysis revealed the CAM to be most effective, and the MMSE to be least useful in the diagnosis of delirium [19]. Requiring less than 5 minutes to administer, the CAM assesses (1) acute onset and fluctuating course,

Table 16.1. Popular screening instruments for delirium or dementia

Confusion assessment method (CAM)

1. Acute onset and fluctuating course: Is this new and change from baseline?
2. Inattention: Are they having difficulty focusing?
3. Disorganized thinking: Is the patient rambling or unclear?
4. Altered level of consciousness: alert (normal), vigilant, lethargic, stupor, or coma.

Diagnosis of delirium requires positive or abnormal rating for (1) and (2), plus (3) or (4).

Adapted from Wong CL et al. "Does this patient have delirium? value of bedside instruments." *JAMA* 2010;**304**:779–786 [19].

Six-item screener (SIS)

Ask patient to remember three objects, e.g., GRASS, PAPER, SHOE.

1. What year is this?
2. What month is this?
3. What is the day of the week?
4. Ask for the three objects. "GRASS."
5. "PAPER."
6. "SHOE."

One point each adds up to six points. Two or more errors is high risk for cognitive impairment.

Adapted from Carpenter, CR et al., "The Six-Item Screener and AD8 for the detection of cognitive impairment in geriatric emergency department patients." *Ann Emerg Med* 2011;**57**:653–661 [20].

(2) inattention, (3) disorganized thinking, and (4) altered level of consciousness (Table 16.1). A diagnosis of delirium requires positive or abnormal answers to (1) and (2), plus one of either (3) or (4). The CAM was based on the DSM-III criteria and has a high likelihood ratio of diagnosing delirium if the criteria are used above. A variant of CAM is the CAM-ICU, which can be administered in two minutes and by nursing staff.

The SIS has received attention in the emergency medicine literature [18,20,21]. This cognitive screening test includes six easy-to-remember questions and can be administered in less than 1 minute. ED clinicians found the SIS better suited for the elderly because sometimes these patients had trouble writing or drawing, a requirement of other screening tests. The SIS is purely verbal. The clinician first asks the patient to remember three items, then he or she will ask for orientation of year, month, and day of the week. After the orientation questions, the clinician finally asks for recall of the three objects. Each question is valued at one point. Two or more errors demonstrate cognitive impairment. In three studies, sensitivity for elderly emergency department patients using the SIS was 63–94% with a specificity of 77–86% [18,20,21].

Diagnostic evaluation

Delirium can be due to a wide number of medical and toxicological conditions, so clinicians must be thorough and vigilant in their assessments. Studies have revealed several conditions and risk factors that are most associated with delirium and that should guide the evaluation process: baseline risk factors, precipitating factors, and specific medical conditions.

The five most common baseline risk factors for delirium are dementia, medications, medical illness, age, and male gender. Using a specialized risk calculator, the strongest risk was found in patients with underlying dementia, medical illness, alcohol abuse, and depression [22]. The odds ratio for dementia was 5.2.

Precipitating factors directly precede the onset of delirium, usually within the 24 hours prior, and include the use of physical restraints, malnutrition, three or more newly added medications, insertion of bladder catheter, and iatrogenic events [23]. "Iatrogenic events" were defined as any illnesses or complication due to therapeutic interventions or procedures like a cardiopulmonary complication, hospital-acquired infection, medication-related complication, unintentional injury, new pressure sore, or fecal impaction.

With regard to specific medical conditions, the most common etiologies of delirium were fluid and electrolyte imbalances, infection, drug toxicity, and sensory/environmental issues [24]. Common predictors of delirium were abnormal sodium level, severe illness, chronic cognitive impairment, fever or hypothermia, psychoactive drug use, and azotemia. Associated drugs included narcotics, benzodiazepines, anticholinergic medications, methyldopa, and nonsteroidal anti-inflammatory agents. A 60% rate of delirium occurred in patients with three or more risk factors. For patients with four risk factors, the rate was nearly 100%.

Management

Treatment strategies for managing delirium are divided into nonpharmacologic and pharmacologic interventions and can definitely be implemented in the ED. Prevention of delirium and nonpharmacologic interventions are generally considered first-line approaches to patients with risk factors. A landmark study in delirium, the Yale Delirium Prevention Trial, demonstrated effectiveness in reducing delirium in older hospitalized patients [25]. Researchers followed 852 patients on the general medical service up until their discharge, and delirium was the primary outcome. The intervention, named the Elder Life Program, targeted six main risk factors for delirium. These included cognitive impairment, sleep deprivation, immobility, visual impairment, hearing impairment, and dehydration. The standardized protocols included frequent re-orientation, cognitively stimulating activities, nonpharmacologic sleep agents like warm drinks, relaxation music and back massage, noise reductions and optimization of sleep schedule, early mobilization, visual aids, hearing aids, and early rehydration. Caregivers can be used to help with re-orientation, and they should make frequent eye contact with patients. Physical restraints should be avoided when possible as they tend to prolong delirium and increase the risk of injury.

Pharmacologic agents are used when nonpharmacologic interventions have been unsuccessful, and the patient is at risk for significant harm to themselves or others [2]. Duration of medication treatment should be as short as possible. Risks and benefits of using pharmacologic agents for delirium must be balanced and discussed with caretakers and staff. Antipsychotic medications such as haloperidol, risperidone, olanzapine, and quetiapine have been shown to be efficacious in reducing symptoms of delirium. The mantra of "start low, go slow" is a useful guide when using these medications, especially in elderly patients.

Antipsychotics carry various levels of risk of increased stroke and seizure, prolongation of the QT interval, extrapyramidal symptoms, hyperglycemia, and neuroleptic malignant syndrome. No data exist to suggest one antipsychotic is better than the other, but mindfulness of side-effect profile is warranted [11]. Efficacy of antipsychotic medications has been attributed to the state of dopamine excess in episodes of delirium [26]. Similarly, patients with delirium have been found to have low levels of acetylcholine and GABA. Therefore, limiting the use of anticholinergic medications and benzodiazepines in these patients is indicated, unless there is evidence that delirium was caused by sedative withdrawal, in which case, benzodiazepines would be the treatment of choice.

Disposition

Patients who are found to have delirium in the ED should be admitted to the hospital for evaluation and treatment with few exceptions, such as available skilled nursing care in a patient with a well-understood etiology. Sometimes, upon presentation to the ED, the underlying medical cause is clear, as with sepsis but requires hospitalization. Nonwithstanding, patients should demonstrate stable vital signs and recovery to baseline functioning before discharge. Family members or caretakers should be engaged as early as possible to gain an understanding of the patient's baseline level of functioning to define treatment goals, and to assist with discharge planning.

For some patients with dementia, this may be challenging. Consultation with social workers and psychiatrists may help with the management of patients, and in-patient psychiatrists or consultation-liaison psychiatrists can be helpful. Evidence suggests that referral to psychiatry for diagnosis of delirium led to higher prescription of psychotropic medication, decreased 1-year rehospitalization rate, and decreased discharge to nursing home [4].

Dementia

Background

Dementia is common in elderly ED patients, as are associated medical comorbidity. The prevalence of dementia in the ED in older patients is approximately 20% [14]. They are also more likely to be admitted, however, for a reason other than dementia [27]. Dementia itself is an uncommon reason for admission to the medical hospital, so the ED clinician should be aware of the common ED presentations for patients with concurrent dementia. They generally have more episodes of syncope,

collapse, fractured femur, urinary tract infection, pneumonia, and dehydration, all reasons for potential delirium. Necessary resource usage may be high. One study noted that 26% of patients with dementia, Alzheimer's type, were admitted for behavioral problems, and almost all of the patients received laboratory tests, an electrocardiogram, and chest radiograph. Only approximately 25% of these patients received a cranial computed tomography test [28]. Admissions for social reasons were also more common for patients with dementia.

The clinical course for dementia has been studied extensively. If the age at diagnosis of Alzheimer's disease was in the 60s or early 70s, then families could expect patients to have a median lifespan of 7 to 10 years. When diagnosed in the 90s, lifespan would be shortened to 3 years or less [29]. For patients with advanced dementia, with or without a feeding tube, the median 6-month mortality is 50% [30]. In another study, more than 50% of patients with advanced dementia died by 18 months [31]. The probability of an eating problem was 85.8%. Approximately half of patients would have pneumonia or a febrile episode. Dyspnea and pain were common symptoms. In their last 3 months of life, 40% of patients had a hospitalization, emergency room visit, parenteral therapy, or tube feeding. Patients with dementia stay on average 4 more days in the hospital than patients without dementia, with an additional cost per patient of $4000 [32].

Autopsy studies report the most common cause of death (46%) for patients with dementia to be bronchopneumonia [33], followed by emphysema (36.5%) and pulmonary thromboembolism (17.3%). Evidence of a myocardial infarction (40%) is identified across the age spectrum. Alzheimer's disease (64%) is the most common dementia type, 10.4% with mixed Alzheimer's disease and ischemia or Lewy body disease, 6.4% with diffuse Lewy body disease, and 4.0% with frontotemporal dementia. Cerebral atherosclerosis is seen at autopsy in nearly half the patients with dementia.

Importantly, dementia can be divided into presentations with reversible and irreversible causes. To the extent possible, the ED clinician should investigate the cause of a patient's dementia so that consultation, treatment, and reversal of symptoms may be possible. There is a long list of conditions that can produce dementia syndromes; substance use and depression are among the more common. Metabolic disturbances, neoplastic syndromes, and normal pressure hydrocephalus also have the potential of being reversed (Table 16.2).

The more common irreversible dementias gradually worsen over time. Alzheimer's disease is the most common form of dementia, accounting for 50–80% of cases. Frontotemporal dementia (12–25%), mixed types (10–30%), pure vascular dementia (10–20%), and Lewy body dementia (5–10%) occur with decreasing frequency [34]. Less than 1% of adults will have dementia by the sixth decade, but approximately one third of people over 85 years of age will be diagnosed. Alzheimer's disease is caused by accumulation of the microtubule protein tau, leading to plaques and tangles, as well as neuronal atrophy in the hippocampus [35]. Other dementia subtypes include

Table 16.2. Causes of reversible dementia

1. Structural lesions (primary or secondary brain tumors, subdural hematoma, normal-pressure hydrocephalus)

2. Head trauma

3. Endocrine conditions (hypothyroidism, hypercalcemia, hypoglycemia)

4. Nutritional conditions (deficiency of vitamin B12, thiamine, niacin)

5. Other infectious conditions (HIV, neurosyphilis, *Cryptococcus*)

6. Derangements of renal and hepatic function

7. Neurological conditions (multiple sclerosis)

8. Effects of medications (benzodiazepines, beta-blockers, anticholinergics)

9. Autoimmune diseases (lupus erythematosus, vasculitis, Hashimoto's encephalopathy, neurosarcoidosis)

10. Environmental toxins (heavy metals, organic hydrocarbons)

11. Long-standing substance abuse (alcohol abuse)

12. Psychiatric disorders (depression)

Adapted from the American Psychiatric Association Practice Guideline for the Treatment of Patients With Alzheimer's Disease and Other Dementias, Second Edition (2007) [40].

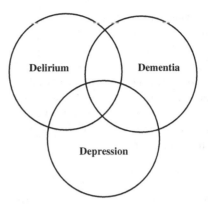

Figure 16.1. The relative overlap of the *three D's* in psychiatry

vascular dementia, dementia with Lewy bodies, frontotemporal dementia, Huntington's disease, Parkinson's disease, Wilson's disease, prion dementias, and dementia after traumatic brain injury [36].

Clinical features

Dementia is a complex neuropsychiatric syndrome, characterized by multiple cognitive deficits and global deterioration of functioning. DSM-IV-TR outlines the diagnostic criteria for dementia of different types, including Alzheimer's dementia and vascular dementia [17]. The cognitive impairments must always include memory impairment, plus one or more of the following: language disturbance (aphasia), impaired motor ability (apraxia), failure to recognize objects (agnosia), or disturbance in planning and organizing (executive functioning). These impairments must also significantly affect social and occupational functioning, as well as demonstrate a major decline from baseline functioning. Vascular dementia has the added criteria of evidence for cerebrovascular disease and is often a contributor to the mixed dementia diagnosis.

Because the course of dementia may progress over several years up to a decade, the ED clinician will see patients with varying degrees of impairment, throughout the natural history of disease. Although unlikely that a patient would present to the ED specifically for an initial evaluation of dementia, recognition of the clinical features of dementia and their associated illnesses and injuries are justifiably in the purview of the emergency physician. Studies show that 29–76% of patients with dementia are not diagnosed by their primary care physician [34], suggesting that the ED team likely has a prominent role in

identifying concurrent cognitive decline when assessing patients for other presenting symptoms. A thorough cognitive assessment will determine the severity of the dementia process, important because more severe dementia may be associated with more medical complication.

Several cognitive screening instruments exist to help the emergency physician assess cognitive abilities, such as the Mini-Mental State Examination (MMSE), Memory Impairment Screen, and Clock drawings [34]. Clinical suspicion and ED screening are important. The MMSE is a reasonable starting point, but follow-up testing is needed for more thorough evaluation. Generally, a score of less than 23 or 24 (with a range from 16 to 26) on the MMSE suggests memory impairment and possible dementia, but the cut-offs range from 16 to 26 [34].

The neuropsychiatric sequelae of dementia can make the diagnosis of a presenting patient more challenging. The relative overlap of the *three D's* in psychiatry, namely dementia, delirium, and depression will, at times, baffle the most experienced clinicians, particularly with time and resource limitations in the emergency department (Figure 16.1). While this chapter focuses on delirium and dementia, interested readers are referred to Chapter 8 on depression for a more comprehensive perspective. Mindfulness and symptom recognition of the *three D's* will frame a differential diagnosis. Performance on bedside screening exams along with direct observation of behavior will allow for additional diagnostic refinements.

Two studies helped to characterize the phenomenology of dementia with regard to associated symptoms. A *JAMA* 2002 study of neuropsychiatric symptoms of dementia revealed that 75% of patients with dementia had neuropsychiatric symptoms in the previous month, with 55% suffering from two or more and 44% with three or more [37]. Patients were noted to have apathy (36%), depression (32%), and agitation/aggression (30%). Since their onset of cognitive impairment, 80% of patients reported having at least one neuropsychiatric symptom, with no difference seen between dementia sub-types. However, the authors noted there was more "aberrant motor behavior" reported in patients specifically with Alzheimer's disease. A recent study in the *American Journal of Psychiatry* reported that psychosis occurred in 41% of patients with Alzheimer's disease, with 36% being delusions and 18% as hallucinations [38].

Dementia with Lewy bodies can be challenging to diagnose, but should be considered before starting an antipsychotic medication [39]. It is characterized by progressive cognitive decline, associated with fluctuations in attention, recurrent visual hallucinations, and parkinsonian motor symptoms. Antipsychotic medication may worsen motor symptoms, and are generally avoided in patients with this type of dementia.

Diagnostic evaluation

The extensive body of literature that exists discussing the risk factors for the development of dementia is beyond the scope of this review and less relevant for emergency physicians. Age, family history of dementia, and vascular risk factors are reasonable cues for the physician when considering laboratory testing or neuroimaging studies. The most important diagnostic dilemma will be differentiating chronic dementia from delirium or reversible dementia. Because dementia is a strong risk factor for delirium and the incidence of delirium is high in these patients, there should be a very low threshold for considering the diagnosis of delirium with new symptoms or behavioral changes.

No substitute exists for a comprehensive history and physical exam. A mental status and neurological exam are warranted. The history taken from the patient and the caretakers will best yield the underlying reasons for and timing of the particular visit. Sometimes, there are additive reasons for the decision to seek care in the ED, and may be as straightforward as the accumulation of various symptoms compounded with caregiver exhaustion. Finally, proceeding through the differential diagnosis of reversible dementia will help guide the ED clinician in potentially discovering etiologies that can be immediately rectified.

Management

Patients with dementia who present to the ED may subsequently require admission to the hospital for various medical or surgical reasons. In addition to careful management of the presenting chief complaint, an important role of the ED team is to gather collateral information about baseline functioning and accurate demographic data, screen for immediate reversible medical diseases, and institute nonpharmacological plans to prevent delirium and agitation. If needed, emergency psychiatric medication, such as low-dose antipsychotics, may stabilize the patient's behavior (Table 16.3), and continuation of patients' previous medications for dementia, such as cholinesterase inhibitors or NMDA antagonists, is reasonable [40]. As always, developing a therapeutic alliance with the family and caregiver is essential.

The U.S. Food and Drug Administration (FDA) has issued public health advisories on antipsychotic medications and their association with increased mortality for patients with dementia [41]. Olanzapine, aripiprazole, risperidone, and quetiapine were associated with a 1.6- to 1.7-fold increase in mortality,

Table 16.3. Antipsychotic treatment for patients with delirium or dementia

Drug	Starting dose
Typical antipsychotic	
Haloperidol	0.5 – 1.0 mg orally twice a day, with as needed doses every 4 hours 0.5 – 1.0 mg intramuscularly
Atypical antipsychotic	
Risperidone	0.5 mg orally twice a day
Olanzapine	2.5 – 5.0 mg orally daily
Quetiapine	25 mg orally twice a day

Adapted from Inouye SK. Delirium in older persons. *N Engl J Med.* 2006;**354**:1157–65 [2].

mostly due to heart-related events and pneumonia. Subsequently, the FDA additionally included conventional or typical antipsychotics, such as haloperidol, in the public health advisory [42]. They noted, "The decision to use antipsychotic medications in the treatment of patients with symptoms of dementia is left to the discretion of the physician. Such use is often called 'off-label' use and falls within the practice of medicine." Caregivers should be advised when feasible.

Special considerations in the ED pertaining to patients with dementia include suicidal ideation, agitation, falls, abuse and neglect, and wandering [40]. Suicidal ideation is common in early dementia, particularly for patients who have insight regarding their likely cognitive decline. Many will develop clinical depression, and the elderly in general, especially elderly men, are at higher risk for suicide. The additional considerations tend to occur in patients at later stages of dementia. Dementia patients are vulnerable adults, requiring vigilance for signs of caretaker abuse or neglect. Adult protective services should be consulted when there is suspicion of elder abuse.

Disposition

Patients with dementia have many comorbid medical conditions that may require hospital admission. Early consultations with Psychiatry, Internal Medicine, Neurology, and Social Work should expedite coordination of care and bring expertise in managing patients with underlying dementia. Specialized Geriatric Medicine, Geriatric Psychiatry, Psychiatry, or Neurology in-patient units may provide expertise beyond a general medical ward. When patients arrive from skilled nursing facilities, early communication regarding expectations for hospitalization can help to solidify future discharge plans without compromising placement.

Conclusion

Clinical presentations involving delirium or dementia are among the most challenging for the emergency physician.

Multi-disciplinary teamwork will enhance assessment, management, and disposition of patients with cognitive impairment. Families and caregivers play an important role. Mindfulness of environmental stressors for patients is important, and non-pharmacological interventions are first-line. Delirium, dementia, and depression tend to overlap, so recognition of associated conditions can help to establish baselines and guide therapy. Several rapid, bedside screening instruments exist to diagnose cognitive impairment in the ED. So as to facilitate appropriate and sometimes time-dependent intervention, emergency physicians should stabilize patients with delirium and recognize the reversible causes of dementia.

References

1. Samaras N, Chevalley T, Samaras D, Gold G. Older patients in the emergency department: a review. *Ann Emerg Med* 2010;**56**:261–9.

2. Inouye SK. Delirium in older persons. *N Engl J Med* 2006;**354**:1157–65.

3. Terrell KM, Hustey FM, Hwang U, et al. Quality indicators for geriatric emergency care. *Acad Emerg Med* 2009;**16**:441–9.

4. Mittal D, Majithia D, Kennedy R, Rhudy J. Differences in characteristics and outcome of delirium as based on referral patterns. *Psychosomatics* 2006;**47**:367–75.

5. Kiely DK, Marcantonio ER, Inouye SK, et al. Persistent delirium predicts greater mortality. *J Am Geriatr Soc* 2009;**57**:55–61.

6. Bellelli G, Frisoni GB, Turco R, et al. Delirium superimposed on dementia predicts 12-month survival in elderly patients discharged from a postacute rehabilitation facility. *J Gerontol A Biol Sci Med Sci* 2007;**62**:1306–9.

7. Breitbart W, Gibson C, Tremblay A. The delirium experience: delirium recall and delirium-related distress in hospitalized patients with cancer, their spouses/caregivers, and their nurses. *Psychosomatics* 2002;**43**:183–94.

8. Schulz R, Beach SR. Caregiving as a risk factor for mortality: the Caregiver Health Effects Study. *JAMA* 1999;**282**:2215–19.

9. Cohen CA, Pushkar D. Lessons learned from a longitudinal study of dementia care. *Am J Geriatr Psychiatry* 1999;**7**:139–46.

10. Smith JSJ. Delirium and dementia. In: Marx JHR, Walls R, (Eds.). *Rosen's Emergency Medicine*, (7th Edition). St. Louis: Mosby; 2009.

11. Fong TG, Tulebaev SR, Inouye SK. Delirium in elderly adults: diagnosis, prevention and treatment. *Nat Rev Neurol* 2009;**5**:210–20.

12. Han JH, Zimmerman EE, Cutler N, et al. Delirium in older emergency department patients: recognition, risk factors, and psychomotor subtypes. *Acad Emerg Med* 2009;**16**:193–200.

13. Kakuma R, du Fort GG, Arsenault L, et al. Delirium in older emergency department patients discharged home: effect on survival. *J Am Geriatr Soc* 2003;**51**:443–50.

14. Hustey FM, Meldon SW, Smith MD, Lex CK. The effect of mental status screening on the care of elderly emergency department patients. *Ann Emerg Med* 2003;**41**:678–84.

15. Leslie DL, Marcantonio ER, Zhang Y, Leo-Summers L, Inouye SK. One-year health care costs associated with delirium in the elderly population. *Arch Intern Med* 2008;**168**:27–32.

16. Inouye SK, Rushing JT, Foreman MD, Palmer RM, Pompei P. Does delirium contribute to poor hospital outcomes? A three-site epidemiologic study. *J Gen Intern Med* 1998;**13**:234–42.

17. American Psychiatric Association. *Diagnostic and Statistical Manual of Mental Disorders DSM-IV-TR* (4th Edition). Arlington, VA: American Psychiatric Publishing, Inc.; 2000.

18. Wilber ST, Lofgren SD, Mager TG, Blanda M, Gerson LW. An evaluation of two screening tools for cognitive impairment in older emergency department patients. *Acad Emerg Med* 2005;**12**:612–16.

19. Wong CL, Holroyd-Leduc J, Simel DL, Straus SE. Does this patient have delirium?: value of bedside instruments. *JAMA* 2010;**304**:779–86.

20. Carpenter CR, DesPain B, Keeling TN, Shah M, Rothenberger M. The Six-Item Screener and AD8 for the detection of cognitive impairment in geriatric emergency department patients. *Ann Emerg Med* 2011;**57**:653–61.

21. Wilber ST, Carpenter CR, Hustey FM. The Six-Item Screener to detect cognitive impairment in older emergency department patients. *Acad Emerg Med* 2008;**15**:613–6.

22. Elie M, Cole MG, Primeau FJ, Bellavance F. Delirium risk factors in elderly hospitalized patients. *J Gen Intern Med* 1998;**13**:204–12.

23. Inouye SK, Charpentier PA. Precipitating factors for delirium in hospitalized elderly persons. Predictive model and interrelationship with baseline vulnerability. *JAMA* 1996;**275**:852–7.

24. Francis J, Martin D, Kapoor WN. A prospective study of delirium in hospitalized elderly. *JAMA* 1990;**263**:1097–101.

25. Inouye SK, Bogardus ST Jr, Charpentier PA, et al. A multicomponent intervention to prevent delirium in hospitalized older patients. *N Engl J Med* 1999;**340**:669–76.

26. Trzepacz PT, Leonard M. Delirium. In: Levenson JL, (Ed.). *The American Psychiatric Publishing Textbook of Psychosomatic Medicine: Psychiatric Care of the Medically Ill*, (2nd Edition). Arlington, VA: American Psychiatric Publishing, Inc; 2011: 71–114.

27. Natalwala A, Potluri R, Uppal H, Heun R. Reasons for hospital admissions in dementia patients in Birmingham, UK, during 2002–2007. *Dement Geriatr Cogn Disord* 2008;**26**:499–505.

28. Nourhashemi F, Andrieu S, Sastres N, et al. Descriptive analysis of emergency hospital admissions of patients with Alzheimer disease. *Alzheimer Dis Assoc Disord* 2001;**15**:21–5.

29. Brookmeyer R, Corrada MM, Curriero FC, Kawas C. Survival following a diagnosis of Alzheimer disease. *Arch Neurol* 2002;**59**:1764–7.

30. Meier DE, Ahronheim JC, Morris J, Baskin-Lyons S, Morrison RS. High short-term mortality in hospitalized patients with advanced dementia: lack of benefit of tube feeding. *Arch Intern Med* 2001;**161**:594–9.

31. Mitchell SL, Teno JM, Kiely DK, et al. The clinical course of advanced dementia. *N Engl J Med* 2009;**361**:1529–38.

32. Lyketsos CG, Sheppard JM, Rabins PV. Dementia in elderly persons in a general hospital. *Am J Psychiatry* 2000;**157**:704–7.

33. Fu C, Chute DJ, Farag ES, et al. Comorbidity in dementia: an autopsy study. *Arch Pathol Lab Med* 2004;**128**:32–8.

34. Holsinger T, Deveau J, Boustani M, Williams JW Jr. Does this patient have dementia? *JAMA* 2007;**297**:2391–404.

35. Blennow K, de Leon MJ, Zetterberg H. Alzheimer's disease. *Lancet* 2006;**368**:387–403.

36. Lobo ASP, Quintanilla MA. Dementia. In: Levenson JL, (Ed.). *The American Psychiatric Publishing Textbook of Psychosomatic Medicine: Psychiatric Care of the Medically Ill*, (2nd Edition). Arlington, VA: American Psychiatric Publishing, Inc; 2011: 115–51.

37. Lyketsos CG, Lopez O, Jones B, et al. Prevalence of neuropsychiatric symptoms in dementia and mild cognitive impairment: results from the cardiovascular health study. *JAMA* 2002;**288**:1475–83.

38. Ropacki SA, Jeste DV. Epidemiology of and risk factors for psychosis of Alzheimer's disease: a review of 55 studies published from 1990 to 2003. *Am J Psychiatry* 2005;**162**:2022–30.

39. National Institute of Neurological Disorders and Stroke. *NINDS Dementia With Lewy Bodies Information Page.* Available at: http://www.ninds.nih.gov/ disorders/dementiawithlewybodies/ dementiawithlewybodies.htm (Accessed December 28, 2011).

40. American Psychiatric Association. Practice guideline for the treatment of patients with Alzheimer's disease and other dementias, second edition. *Am J Psychiatry* 2007;**164**:5–56.

41. U.S. Food and Drug Administration. *Public Health Advisory: Deaths with Antipsychotics in Elderly Patients with Behavioral Disturbances.* Available at: http://www.fda.gov/Drugs/DrugSafety/ PostmarketDrugSafetyInformationfor PatientsandProviders/DrugSafety InformationforHealthcareProfessionals/ PublicHealthAdvisories/ucm053171. htm.

42. U.S. Food and Drug Administration. *FDA Requests Boxed Warnings on Older Class of Antipsychotic Drugs 2008.* Available at: http://www.fda.gov/ NewsEvents/Newsroom/ PressAnnouncements/2008/ucm116912. htm.

The patient with excited delirium in the emergency department

Michael P. Wilson and Gary M. Vilke

Introduction

Excited delirium syndrome (ExDS) is a specific type of extreme agitation. The syndrome itself has been criticized as having been "invented," to classify and ultimately justify deaths that occur in highly agitated individuals during police arrest and restraint. Although the syndrome does not always result in death, ExDS carries a very high mortality compared to other acute behavioral emergencies. Knowledge of ExDS, therefore, is extremely important for both psychiatrists and emergency physicians.

Forensic pathologists and medical examiners have generally applied the term "excited delirium" retrospectively, to describe findings in a subgroup of patients with delirium who died suddenly while in police custody [1]. Patients with ExDS, due to their extreme aggressiveness, have therefore traditionally been encountered by law enforcement and prehospital personnel. As these patients are often transported to an emergency department (ED), they are also cared for by emergency medicine clinicians.

Excited delirium syndrome, also previously called agitated delirium, has defied an easy unifying definition. There are no specific tests or imaging studies that can be used to make the diagnosis, but like other medical syndromes, ExDS is a specific clinical presentation with a host of common features. The more features present, the more likely the diagnosis [2]. ExDS is generally defined as altered mental status due to delirium combined with severe excitement or aggressiveness, in which other medical etiologies have been excluded. This severe agitation often attracts the attention of law enforcement, due to the sometimes bizarre and aggressive public presentations of individuals with ExDS. Although other signs and symptoms are variable, most experts agree that ExDS patients display several of the following [1]:

- Imperviousness to significant pain
- Rapid breathing
- Sweating
- Extreme agitation
- Elevated temperature
- Lack of response to verbal commands by police
- Lack of fatiguing
- Unusual or superhuman strength
- Inappropriate clothing for the environment

Tolerance to pain is an almost-universal feature, displayed by nearly every patient with ExDS. Numerous available Internet videos attest to this particular feature of the syndrome [3,4]. As is suggested in the syndrome's name, these patients also generally have an acute cognitive impairment with a waxing and waning course. Thus, they have a true delirium. This combination of signs and symptoms is particularly lethal, with a rate of sudden death as high as 11% based on limited epidemiologic data [5].

History

ExDS may be related to a phenomenon known as Bell's mania, which was first described in the medical literature in the mid-1800s. In 1849, Dr. Luther Bell, the superintendent of the McLean Asylum of the Insane in Somerville, Massachusetts, described 40 cases of a unique clinical condition which seemed "scarcely suited for the cares of an institution for the insane" [6]. Instead, continued Bell, "His physiognomy and articulation are rather those of fever and delirium." This syndrome had a high mortality rate, with nearly 75% of cases ending in death. Bell's initial report was followed by several subsequent similar reports. A 1934 review by Kraines noted several patients who had a "syndrome of sudden onset, with overactivity, great excitement, sleeplessness, apparent delirium, and distorted ideas; without any clear evidence of a definite toxic infectious factor" [7]. Kraines also noted that a standardized nomenclature for this syndrome did not yet exist, and at that time, was variously referred to in the medical literature as Bell's mania, acute delirious mania, delirium grave, acute delirium, specific febrile delirium, acute psychotic furors, or collapse delirium.

The descriptions of ExDS-like presentations by Bell and Kraines in the late 1800s and early 1900s were noted in the medical literature mainly as case reports until the 1950s, when the introduction of antipsychotics like chlorpromazine became more common in psychiatric facilities for the treatment of agitated patients. As agitated psychotic individuals were more

Behavioral Emergencies for the Emergency Physician, ed. Leslie S. Zun, Lara G. Chepenik, and Mary Nan S. Mallory. Published by Cambridge University Press. © Cambridge University Press 2013.

aggressively treated with pharmacologic therapy, ExDS-like reported deaths essentially disappeared from the medical literature. With effective treatment to interrupt the progressively worsening delirium and excitation, mortality from this condition, which was nearly 75% when first described, fell sharply.

In the 1980s, new reports of an ExDS-like syndrome again appeared in the medical literature, this time in association with cocaine. The first use of the term "excited delirium" was in a 1985 report by Wetli and Fishbain, who described seven cases of an agitated delirium in association with illicit drug use [8]. This report noted that, while all cases were eventually fatal, deaths in these individuals differed from a typical cocaine overdose in two ways. First, these cases had extreme agitation that preceded death, even though postmortem levels of cocaine were more typical of recreational use than overdose. Second, unlike a typical cocaine overdose, none of these seven patients had preterminal seizures. Wetli and Fishbain warned of the potential for sudden death in conjunction with this excited delirium syndrome, and the term is now preferred in the medical literature when describing this syndrome. Despite the many descriptions of ExDS since the time of Bell, some civil rights advocates have claimed that the syndrome was invented by police and lawyers to absolve them of guilt for sudden deaths that occurred while placing and maintaining individuals in police custody. These critics have claimed that ExDS is likely better explained by other diagnoses such as stimulant intoxication or psychosis, and that the custody deaths are caused by police restraint techniques [9,10]. However, in 2004, the National Association of Medical Examiners published a position paper which confirmed the existence of an Excited Delirium syndrome for the first time [11]. In 2009, the American College of Emergency Physicians followed suit by publishing a white paper report on the syndrome [1]. Additionally, several review papers and a textbook have since been written on the topic to improve the understanding of and to provide education about this syndrome, as well as to offer unifying terminology [12–18]. With these publications and the advent of educational resources such as exciteddelirium.org, there is now a greater understanding that ExDS is a medical emergency with potentially lethal consequences [3].

Diagnosis and etiology

Diagnosis of ExDS is often tricky, as many causes and clinical findings of ExDS overlap with other disease states. Stimulant intoxication, hypoglycemia, thyroid storm, seizures, or head injury, for instance, can cause agitation and aggression similar to ExDS [19]. The term ExDS, however, is not intended to include these other conditions, except insofar as they also meet the clinical case definition of ExDS before the identification of an another attribution. Once an alternative medical diagnosis is made for the ExDS-like behavior, the patient is no longer considered to have ExDS.

The exact etiology of ExDS is unknown. Some basic science and epidemiologic investigations have implicated cocaine or other stimulants as well as mental illness [15,16]. Currently, the majority of reported cases of ExDS are associated with stimulant drug use, such as cocaine, methamphetamine, PCP, or LSD, although cases of ExDS still occur in psychiatric patients who are untreated or have abruptly discontinued their medication [1,20–28].

In cases in which illicit stimulants are involved, the presentation is often abrupt and does not involve increased or elevated levels of the drug. Reports demonstrate typical recreational patterns of use. However, postmortem examinations of the brain of chronic cocaine patients have demonstrated a characteristic down-regulation of dopamine transporters in the ventral striatum, which is normally strongly innervated by dopaminergic neurons [29,30]. This allows dopamine to persist in the synapses, and suggests that excessive dopamine transmission, particularly in the striatum, may play a role in the clinical presentation of ExDS.

Regardless of the exact pathophysiologic cause, ExDS is a true medical emergency. All ExDS patients will require emergency medical care for stabilization and treatment. Many current efforts have focused on training prehospital personnel and police to recognize the syndrome. The rest of this chapter, however, will have a slightly different focus, reviewing instead the existing literature on evaluation and treatment considerations.

Initial approach and workup

As noted above, many different conditions can cause a clinical presentation that overlaps with ExDS. Stimulant intoxication, hypoglycemia, thyroid storm, seizures, head injury, serotonin syndrome, heatstroke, pheochromocytoma, and neuroleptic malignant syndrome all have clinical presentations that can be similar to ExDS. Several psychiatric conditions may also have characteristics that overlap with ExDS, including substance intoxication, schizophrenia of the paranoid type, severe mania, and even extreme emotional rage from acute stressful social circumstances. Unlike more subtle clinical presentations, recognizing a severely agitated patient is not difficult. Rather, the main challenge lies in providing their initial management safely. Patients with ExDS should be approached the same way that all patients with agitation are approached: cautiously. Whether in the prehospital environment or in the hospital, providers must keep their own personal safety in mind.

Current expert guidelines on the management of agitated patients recommend verbal de-escalation as the first step, when possible [31,32]. By definition, ExDS patients respond poorly to verbal cues, even police re-direction. Consequently, by the time most of these patients are encountered by medical providers, this initial preferred approach has already failed. Continued verbal communication may still be useful, however, potentially calming both patients and staff during any use of force. Although often ineffective, the patient should be engaged verbally by a single individual, who communicates expectations and give commands in a firm but calming tone. If possible, an effort should be made to reduce environmental stimuli. In the prehospital environment, this may be quite difficult given the inherent chaos in an uncontrolled setting and myriad environmental stimuli from bystanders, family, police dogs, lights, sirens, and additional responding officers. Environmental stimuli can be problematic for physically gaining control of the patient. Although there is little formal scientific evidence on this point, a patient who is experiencing a catecholamine surge from fear is unlikely to respond quickly to pain compliance techniques. Thus, the amount of force needed will correspondingly be greater; use of greater force increases the possibility of injury to both patients and providers.

The ethics of and techniques for proper restraint have been more thoroughly reviewed elsewhere [33]. Related chapters on de-escalation, restraint and seclusion, and rapid treatment for agitated patients in this text merit review. In the pre-hospital setting, the basic principles used by law enforcement to control a patient in ExDS revolve around rapid physical restraint, minimalization of the patient's exertional activity, and safety for all. The use of a taser electronic control device (ECD) is felt by many experts to be preferable to the more traditional physical wrestling for control, because fighting or heavy physical exertion has a more deleterious effect on a patient's acid–base status [34–36]. Additionally, the patient's airway should be carefully protected during any forceful maneuver, and respiratory status carefully monitored both during and after restraint.

Treatment options for ExDS

Once the patient is restrained, rapid medical assessment can begin [37]. Law enforcement officers and prehospital medical providers are not expected to diagnose the cause of an acute behavioral disturbance, because even experienced physicians have difficulty discerning the etiology of a severely agitated state by clinical observation alone. Rather, prehospital personnel should recognize the clinical syndrome of ExDS as an emergency and rapidly initiate therapeutic interventions within their scope of practice. Medical conditions and psychiatric diagnoses are entertained by the emergency physicians and consultants, usually with the help of laboratory and radiographic imaging, before making the final diagnosis of ExDS.

In choosing treatment options, providers should focus on identifying the most likely cause of the agitation [38]. Expert consensus guidelines generally recognize three classes of medications for initial calming of agitated patients: benzodiazepines, first-generation antipsychotics (or FGA), and second-generation antipsychotics (SGA). Some experts include dissociative agents such as ketamine as a 4th class of medication, particularly in severe agitation such as seen in ExDS, although only limited evidence exists for its use. Extremely agitated trauma patients, especially those who have suffered blunt trauma or in whom there is a high suspicion of head injury, should be paralyzed, sedated, and intubated to protect the airway while additional diagnostic workup proceeds. Once

the patient is calmed, other treatment modalities are generally used for supportive care.

The decision of when initially to use each of the classes of antipsychotic medication is not always clear. In general, expert consensus guidelines recommend that providers treat the underlying cause of the agitation if it is known [38]. In most cases, the cause of the agitated delirium will not be known before the need for pharmacological intervention. In these instances, expert consensus guidelines recommend the use of benzodiazepines as a first-line treatment, as most of the cases of ExDS are associated with sympathomimetic illicit drug use [1]. If the patient is known to have a behavioral disorder and the likely ExDS symptomatology is due to medication noncompliance, antipsychotic medications can be used primarily or as adjunctive therapy with benzodiazepines.

Benzodiazepines

Benzodiazepines as a class bind to inhibitory γ-aminobutyric acid (GABA) receptors in the human brain. Drugs in this class include lorazepam, diazepam, and midazolam, which are injectable benzodiazepines widely available to prehospital and hospital personnel. As these medications cause sedation, they are therefore extremely helpful in management of ExDS patients. This is especially true if the source of the agitation is thought to be secondary to stimulant drug use, in which case benzodiazepines are the drug of choice.

Benzodiazapines are most often administered parenterally by intramuscular (IM), intravenous (IV), or intraosseous (IO) routes, although intranasal (IN) formulations also exist for midazolam. Serial doses may be required for sedation, and the doses of benzodiazepines typically are much higher in ExDS patients than those needed for anxious or mildly agitated persons. On the negative side, benzodiazepines may work relatively slowly if given IM (for instance, an onset of 1–5 minutes for midazolam). In addition, potential side effects include over-sedation, respiratory depression, and hypotension. Although the ExDS patient population is typically hyper-stimulated, the clinical course can fluctuate and the potential for sedative side effects exists. Ongoing cardiopulmonary monitoring may be indicated and supportive care is easily managed in the ED setting if needed.

First-generation antipsychotics

Conventional or first-generation antipsychotics (FGAs) are an older class of medications often used for calming. The butyrophenone class, which includes both haloperidol and droperidol, is the most widely used in U.S. emergency departments [19]. These agents likely produce calming by inhibiting dopamine transmission in the brain. In addition, they are structurally similar to GABA, and may interact with GABA receptors at higher doses [39].

Haloperidol and droperidol generally bind tightly to dopamine receptors, with little activity at other receptor subtypes [19]. Each of these medications, however, has important side effects. Both haloperidol and droperidol can lengthen the QT portion of the cardiac cycle, and have been associated with sudden death. Because sudden death is a feature of ExDS and some ExDS deaths have been associated with ventricular dysrhythmias, it is wise to be cautious when administering these medications. In particular, if long QT Syndrome is suspected based either on history or concomitant medications, these medications should be avoided. Of further note, when haloperidol or droperidol are administered, injections are generally given IM for both safety and efficacy in the physically agitated patient. The U.S. Food and Drug Administration (FDA) has issued warnings about sudden death when using both of these medications intravenously. Cardiac arrhythmias can result at higher doses, which may be required in ExDS patients. Lower doses may be effective when given in combination with a benzodiazepine. If given intravenously, cardiac monitoring should be performed, but can be challenging in patients who are sweaty and combative.

A final additional reason for caution with the use of FGAs is hyperthermia. ExDS patients often have elevated temperatures, and there is some theoretical concern that this condition may result from dopamine derangements similar to those with neuroleptic malignant syndrome. If so, dopamine antagonists like the FGAs would be contraindicated. In practice, however, this is rarely seen and seems to be more of a theoretical concern.

Second-generation antipsychotics

Second-generation antipsychotics (SGAs) available in an injectable form include both olanzapine and ziprasidone. Both agents bind more tightly to receptor types other than dopamine, and so have fewer cardiac and movement-related side effects than FGAs. Both ziprasidone and olanzapine are equally as effective as haloperidol alone for calming [40,41]. Unlike FGAs, however, there is limited evidence about the use of SGAs in combination with benzodiazepines. Several retrospective reviews have not noted any significant vital sign abnormalities with the combination of SGAs with benzodiazepines unless the patient is significantly intoxicated with alcohol [42–45]. In these cases, haloperidol or haloperidol with benzodiazepines may be a safer choice [46].

Ketamine

Ketamine is an older medication that is structurally related to PCP. It is a dissociative anesthetic that binds NMDA receptors, and may be given IM or IV. Ketamine rapidly causes a dissociative state with preservation of airway reflexes [47]. Given its rapid onset of action, preservation of airway reflexes, and wide therapeutic range of dosing, ketamine is an attractive agent for use in ExDS. However, there is limited evidence about its use in ExDS, with some theoretical concern for worsening pre-existing hypertension and tachycardia. In addition, ketamine sometimes causes increased oral secretions and is rarely associated with laryngospasm [48]. Despite concern for side effects, several case reports have noted safety with its use in the prehospital setting [49,50].

Initial combination therapy

To increase calming, many clinicians commonly pair benzodiazepines with antipsychotics, especially FGAs. In a 1997 study, Battaglia and colleagues published the largest emergency department investigation of haloperidol and lorazepam [51]. This study compared three different medications: haloperidol alone, lorazepam alone, and haloperidol combined with lorazepam. The researchers noted that side effects from haloperidol were reduced when this medication was combined with a benzodiazepine like lorazepam. Subsequent studies noted a similar reduction in side effects when haloperidol was combined with an anticholinergic such as promethazine, and these studies form part of the current recommendation to always pair haloperidol with an adjunctive medication [19]. The Battaglia study, however, excluded individuals with alcohol intoxication. Thus, it is not known whether this combination would be useful in alcohol-intoxicated patients. There are also no prospective studies specifically comparing treatment options for patients with ExDS. Thus, as with any combination of medications, patients should be monitored carefully for side effects.

At least one case report has described using intramuscular ketamine for initial therapy, followed by benzodiazepines once the patient was calm enough for IV access [49]. Theoretically, these agents have synergistic effects. In addition, benzodiazepines may help prevent emergence phenomena described in some patients after ketamine administration and metabolism.

Other treatment modalities

The goal of calming with any class of medication, whether antipsychotics, benzodiazepines, ketamine, or the combination of these, is to prevent harm to the patient or staff, and to facilitate an examination, assessment, and emergency treatment of the patient [37]. This therapeutic approach should occur with all patients exhibiting signs and symptoms of ExDS, even if the final diagnosis changes after the ensuing workup. As with all ED patients with delirium, the underlying medical explanation is investigated, usually including re-examination, review of medical records, laboratory studies, and neuro-imaging. Hypoglycemia can present as an agitated adrenergic state, and is immediately reversible when recognized with a bedside blood glucose level check. Other identified medical conditions are treated as indicated. When a medical or psychiatric disorder is thought to be the etiology of the delirium and agitation, then the diagnosis of ExDS is no longer applicable. When no correctable etiology is identified, the diagnosis of ExDS is presumed. After effective sedation, appropriate therapeutic measures include intravenous fluids, consideration for sodium bicarbonate, and cooling when appropriate.

Intravenous fluids

Patients with ExDS are commonly hyperthermic. When coupled with agitated and aggressive behavior, patients generally have a large amount of insensible water loss. As such, most have some degree of dehydration. In addition, aggressive behavior and typically violent struggles predispose patients to the development of rhabdomyolysis. Once safely permitted, intravenous fluid administration proceeds unless otherwise contraindicated by underlying medical conditions. If vascular access is needed urgently, interosseous (IO) access is an option. IO access may also be safer, because it is often easier to restrain a limb for this procedure and does not require precise vein cannulation.

Sodium bicarbonate

As with most other treatments, routine use of intravenous sodium bicarbonate has not been evaluated for treatment of metabolic acidosis in ExDS. However, use of this agent makes intuitive sense. Violent struggles cause a lactic acidosis that is associated with electrolyte abnormalities. These electrolyte abnormalities subsequently predispose the patient to the development of ventricular arrhythmias. Urinary alkalization with sodium bicarbonate and intravenous normal saline may be used to help correct an acidosis as well as prevent or minimize renal failure from rhabdomyolysis. Unfortunately, the use of bicarbonate may also predispose the patient to electrolyte abnormalities, particularly hypernatremia and hypokalemia. Clinical evidence is lacking. The risks and benefits must be carefully considered. If a patient goes into cardiac arrest from ExDS, early bicarbonate therapy should be considered.

Cooling

Hyperthermia is present in many patients with ExDS. This hyperthermia can often be assessed clinically with a tactile temperature in lieu of a core temperature measurement if this is not available. Profuse sweating may be evident. Patients who are suffering significant or presumed hyperthermia should be cooled aggressively as soon as is practical. Some experts have noted that significant hyperthermia in the face of ExDS is a predictor of increased mortality, although definitive epidemiologic data is currently lacking [1].

Although often difficult to cool a patient in the prehospital arena, both cooled intravenous fluids and ice packs to the neck, groin, or axillae may be used to initiate the temperature-lowering process. If not already undressed, all ExDS patients should be disrobed. In the emergency department, other techniques such as evaporative cooling with misting across bare skin or using fans, commercial cooling blankets, and ice water immersion are effective. Patients with significant temperature elevations should be cooled by more than one method. When feasible, continuous core temperature measurements are ideal so as not to overshoot normothermia. Although some researchers have likened the dopamine dysfunction in ExDS to neuroleptic malignant syndrome, there has been no work evaluating the use of dantrolene in these patients. Typical management of hyperthermia is therefore more similar to heatstroke or heat-illness protocols.

Conclusions

Although once controversial, ExDS is now accepted as a unique clinical syndrome with a long history, albeit by various names, in the medical literature. Although ExDS is not universally fatal as was originally thought, approximately 1 in 10 patients will nonetheless progress to sudden cardiac death. As of now, the factor(s) responsible for this mortality is not fully understood. Although some associations have been made, the risk factors for sudden death in ExDS have not been identified.

Although much is not known about the pathophysiology of ExDS, most experts agree that early interventions by police, EMS, and emergency department personnel are important and can impact survival in many patients. In a patient with ExDS, timely treatment of patients is needed to save lives from this disease. In the event of a sudden death, careful observations by law enforcement and healthcare providers will assist medical examiners in making accurate determinations of an ExDS attribution.

Once symptoms consistent with ExDS are recognized, providers should attempt de-escalation, provide physical and chemical restraint as quickly and safely as possible, and initiate medical stabilization and evaluation for possible underlying causes of extreme agitation. Difficulty with traditional physical restraint is anticipated due to adrenergic hyperactivity. The use of an electronic control device, such as a taser ECD, may be preferable to prolonged and potentially dangerous efforts to physically subdue a violent patient. Regardless of which restraint technique is used, providers should be mindful of their personal safety. Once the patient is restrained, medical providers should quickly use appropriate medications. When ExDS symptoms are thought to be secondary to stimulant intoxication, benzodiazepines are considered the first-line medication. Cardiopulmonary monitoring is indicated as soon as feasible. Attention to airway maintenance, breathing adequacy, and volume resuscitation, along with rapid treatment of hypoglycemia, hyperthermia, and metabolic acidosis may be life saving.

Increased awareness and education about ExDS will hopefully lead to better and earlier recognition of the syndrome. ExDS is a medical emergency, and cooperative protocols are needed between law enforcement, EMS, and local emergency departments to best manage these patients. Ideal management involves rapid, safe control of patients with a minimum of force by police; aggressive use of medications for calming; IV hydration; cardiac monitoring; transport of patients by EMS; and rapid assessment and treatment in receiving emergency departments. Further research on ExDS is needed to better define these inter-disciplinary protocols, as well as better define ExDS itself. Research identifying the mechanisms and risk factors for sudden death and the best practice approaches will hopefully prevent morbidity and decrease the mortality rate.

References

1. ACEP Excited Delirium Task Force. *White Paper Report on Excited Delirium Syndrome.* 2009. Available at: http://ccpicd.com/Documents/Excited%20Delirium%20Task%20Force.pdf (Accessed June 7, 2011).

2. Hall C, Butler C, Kader A, et al. Police use of force, injuries and death: prospective evaluation of outcomes for all police use of force/restraint including conducted energy weapons in a large Canadian city. *Acad Emerg Med* 2009;**16**:S198–9.

3. Excited Delirium. *Education, Research, and Information.* Available at: http://www.exciteddelirium.org (Accessed January 28, 2012).

4. *Madness.in.the.fast.lane.* Available at: http://www.youtube.com/watch?v=e5oFVHE1-Ko (Accessed January 18, 2012).

5. Stratton SJ, Rogers C, Brickett K, Gruzinski G. Factors associated with sudden death of individuals requiring restraint for excited delirium. *Am J Emerg Med* 2001;**19**:187–91.

6. Bell L. On a form of disease resembling some advanced stages of mania and fever, but so contradistinguished from any ordinarily observed or described combination of symptoms, as to render it probable that it may be an overlooked and hitherto unrecorded malady. *Am J Insanity* 1849;**6**:97–127.

7. Kraines SH. Bell's Mania. *Am J Psychiatry* 1934;**91**:29–40.

8. Wetli CV, Fishbain DA. Cocaine-induced psychosis and sudden death in recreational cocaine users. *J Forensic Sci* 1985;**30**:873–80.

9. Reay DT, Fligner CL, Stilwell AD, et al. Positional asphyxia during law enforcement transport. *Am J Forensic Med Pathol* 1992;**13**:90–7.

10. O'Halloran RL, Lewman LV. Restraint asphyxiation in excited delirium. *Am J Forensic Med Pathol* 1993;**14**:289–95.

11. Stephens BG, Jentzen JM, Karch S, Wetli CV, Mash DC. National Association of Medical Examiners position paper on the certification of cocaine-related deaths. *Am J Forens Med Sci* 2004;**25**:11–13.

12. DiMaio TG, DiMaio VJM. *Excited Delirium Syndrome Cause of Death and Prevention,* (1st Edition). Boca Raton, FL: Taylor & Francis Group; 2006: 1–60.

13. Grant JR, Southall PE, Mealey J, Scott SR, Fowler DR. Excited delirium deaths in custody past and present. *Am J Forensic Med Pathol* 2009;**30**:1–5.

14. Otahbuchi M, Cevik C, Bagdure S, Nugent K. Excited delirium, restraints, and unexpected death: a review of pathogenesis. *Am J Forensic Med Pathol* 2010;**31**:1–6.

15. Takeuchi A, Ahern TL, Henderson SO. Excited delirium. *West J Emerg Med* 2011;**12**:77–83.

16. Vilke GM, DeBard ML, Chan TC, et al. Excited Delirium Syndrome (ExDS): defining based on a review of the literature. *J Emerg Med* 2011 [Epub ahead of print].

17. Vilke GM, Payne-James J, Karsch SB. Excited Delirium Syndrome (ExDS): redefining an old diagnosis. *J Forens Legal Med* 2012;**19**:7–11.

18. Vilke GM, Bozeman WP, Dawes DM, DeMers G, Wilson MP. Excited delirium syndrome (ExDS): treatment options and considerations. *J Forensic Leg Med* 2012;**19**:117–21.

19. Vilke GM, Wilson MP. Agitation: what every emergency physician should know. *Emerg Med Rep* 2009;**30**:1–8.

20. Escobedo LG, Ruttenber AJ, Agocs MM, Anda RF, Wetli CV. Emerging patterns of cocaine use and the epidemic of cocaine overdose deaths in Dade County, Florida. *Arch Pathol Lab Med* 1991;**115**:900–5.

21. Ruttenber AJ, Sweeney PA, Mendlein JM, Wetli CV. Preliminary findings of an epidemiologic study of cocaine-related deaths, Dade County, Florida, 1978–85. *NIDA Res Monogr* 1991;**110**:95–112.

22. Mirchandani HG, Rorke LB, Sekula-Perlman A, Hood IC. Cocaine-induced agitated delirium, forceful struggle, and minor head injury: a further definition of sudden death during restraint. *Am J Forensic Med Pathol* 1994;**15**:95–9.

23. Wetli CV. Mash D, Karsch SB. Cocaine-associated agitated delirium and the neuroleptic malignant syndrome. *Am J Emerg Med* 1996;**14**:425–8.

24. Hick JL, Smith SW, Lynch MT. Metabolic acidosis in restraint-associated cardiac arrest: a case series. *Acad Emerg Med* 1999;**6**:239–43.

25. Ruttenber AJ, McAnally HB, Wetli CV. Cocaine-associated rhabdomyolysis and excited delirium: different stages of the same syndrome. *Am J Forensic Med Pathol* 1999;**20**:120–7.

26. Allam S, Noble JS. Cocaine-excited delirium and severe acidosis. *Anesthesia* 2001;**56**:385–6.

27. Gruszecki AC, McGwin G, Robinson A, Davis GG. Unexplained sudden death and the likelihood of drug abuse. *J Forensic Sci* 2005;**50**:1–4.

28. Bunai Y, Akaza K, Jiang WX, Nagai A. Fatal hyperthermia associated with excited delirium during an arrest. *Leg Med (Tokyo)* 2008;**10**:306–9.

29. Mash DC, Duque L, Pablo J, et al. Brain biomarkers for identifying excited delirium as a cause of sudden death. *Forensic Sci Int* 2009;**190**:e13–19.

30. Mash DC. Biochemical brain markers in excited delirium deaths. In: Kroll MW, Ho JD, (Eds.). *TASER Conducted Electrical Weapons: Physiology, Pathology, and Law.* New York, NY: Springer; 2009: 365–77.

31. Richmond JS, Berlin JS, Fishkind A, et al. Verbal de-escalation of the agitated patient: consensus statement of the American Association for Emergency Psychiatry Project BETA De-escalation Workgroup. *West J Emerg Med* 2012;**13**:17–25.

32. Wilson MP, Zeller SL. Introduction: reconsidering psychiatry in the emergency department. *J Emerg Med* [Epub ahead of print].

33. Wilson MP, Sloane C. Chemical restraints, physical restraints, and other demonstrations of force. In: Jesus J, (Ed.). *Ethical Problems in the Emergency Department.* New York: Wiley-Blackwell; [In press].

34. Ho JD, Dawes DM, Nelson RS, et al. Acidosis and catecholamine evaluation following simulated law enforcement "Use of force" encounters. *Acad Emerg Med* 2010;**12**:E60–6.

35. Ho JD, Dawes DM, Cole JB, et al. Lactate and pH evaluation in exhausted humans with prolonged TASER® X26 exposure or continued exertion. *Forensic Sci Int* 2009;**190**:80–6.

36. Ho JD, Dawes DM, Bultman LL, et al. Prolonged TASER® use on exhausted humans does not worsen markers of acidosis. *Am J Emerg Med* 2009;**27**:413–18.

37. Nordstrom K, Zun LS, Wilson MP, et al. Medical evaluation and triage of the agitated patient: consensus statement of the American Association for Emergency Psychiatry Project BETA Medical Evaluation Workgroup. *West J Emerg Med* 2012;**13**:3–10.

38. Wilson MP, Pepper D, Currier GW, Holloman GH, Feifel D. The psychopharmacology of agitation: consensus statement of the American Association for Emergency Psychiatry Project BETA Psychopharmacology Workgroup. *West J Emerg Med* 2012;**13**:26–34.

39. Richards JR, Schneir AB. Droperidol in the emergency department: is it safe? *J Emerg Med* 2001;**24**:441–7.

40. Zeller SL, Rhoades R. Systematic reviews of assessment measures and pharmacologic treatments for agitation. *Clin Ther* 2010;**32**:403–25.

41. Citrome L. Comparison of intramuscular ziprasidone, olanzapine, or aripiprazole for agitation: a quantitative review of efficacy and safety. *J Clin Psychiatry* 2007;**68**:1876–85.

42. Wilson MP, MacDonald K, Vilke GM, Ronquillo L, Feifel D. *Use of Intramuscular Ziprasidone by ED Clinicians and its Effect on Vital Signs.* National Behavioral Emergencies Conference, December 1–2, 2011; Las Vegas, Nevada.

43. Wilson MP, MacDonald KS, Vilke GM, Feifel D. A comparison of the safety of olanzapine and haloperidol in combination with benzodiazepines in emergency department patients with acute agitation. *J Emerg Med* 2011 [Epub ahead of print].

44. Wilson MP, MacDonald KS, Vilke GM, Feifel D. Potential complications of combining intramuscular olanzapine with benzodiazepines in agitated emergency department patients. *J Emerg Med* 2010 [Epub ahead of print].

45. Macdonald K, Wilson MP, Minassian A, et al. A retrospective analysis of intramuscular haloperidol and intramuscular olanzapine in the treatment of agitation in drug- and alcohol-using patients. *Gen Hosp Psychiatry* 2010;**32**:443–5.

46. Zeller SL, Wilson MP. Acute treatment of agitation in schizophrenia. *Drug Discov Today Ther Strateg* 2011;**8**:25–9.

47. Green SM, Roback MG, Kennedy RM, et al. Clinical practice guideline for emergency department ketamine dissociative sedation: 2011 Update. *Ann Emerg Med* 2010;**57**:449–61.

48. Burnett AM, Watters BJ, Barringer KW, et al. Laryngospasm and hypoxia after intramuscular administration of ketamine to a patient in excited delirium. *Prehosp Emerg Care* 2012;**16**:412–14.

49. Roberts JR, Geeting GK. Intramuscular ketamine for the rapid tranquilization of the uncontrollable, violent, and dangerous adult patient. *J Trauma* 2001;**51**:1008–10.

50. Hick JL, Ho JD. Ketamine chemical restraint to facilitate rescue of a combative "jumper". *Prehosp Emerg Care* 2005;**9**:85–9.

51. Battaglia J, Moss S, Rush J, et al. Haloperidol, lorazepam, or both for psychotic agitation? A multicenter, prospective, double-blind, emergency department study. *Am J Emerg Med* 1997;**15**:335–40.

Medical illness in psychiatric patients in the emergency department

Victor G. Stiebel and Barbara Nightengale

Comorbidity incidence/prevalence

Comorbidity is a noun that describes the simultaneous presence of two chronic diseases or conditions in a patient. It is a given that medical illness is common in psychiatric patients and that psychiatric pathology is common in medical conditions. A summary of the Collaborative Psychiatric Epidemiology Surveys, 2001–2003 [1] noted that 25% of the adult population of the United States suffered from any mental disorder. Those diagnosed with any medical condition constitute 58%. In the area of overlap, 68% of adults with mental disorders have some medical condition and 29% of those with medical conditions have a mental disorder.

The number of physical symptoms reported during a primary care office visit has been shown to strongly correlate with the likelihood of a psychiatric disorder, ranging from 2% to almost 60% [2]. Lipowski [3] was one of the first to identify that between 30 and 60% of medical inpatients will suffer from some psychiatric condition. Within the emergency department, psychiatric patients make up one of the major diagnostic categories [4]. A survey looking for occult psychiatric diagnoses using the PRIME-MD found 42% of a consecutive sample of general emergency department patients received a psychiatric diagnosis [5]. Unfortunately, this diagnosis is frequently missed by the emergency department (ED) physician for a variety of reasons including time constraints, lack of training and overall resources, and overall acuity level of other patients [6].

Into this confused picture steps the busy ED physician, with variable training and experience in psychiatry. As we will see, psycho-social stressors may play a role at least as important as pure medical or psychiatric issues, but social services are limited in most emergency departments, and even more limited in which of the limited community services can be used. Trying to ensure that both medical and psychiatric parts of the clinical picture come into focus equally and at the same time is clearly of great importance.

Emergency physicians are experts at evaluation based on complex thought processes including pattern recognition, laboratory testing, and heuristic strategies to rule out the worst-case scenario. However, these methods, inherently imperfect, allow bias to enter our thought processes. In the setting of a patient with both medical and psychiatric diagnoses, this can have catastrophic results. Medical diagnoses and psychiatric conditions do not occur in a vacuum, are often interrelated, and one will frequently impact adversely on the other. Additionally, psychosocial factors can add an exponential degree of complexity to a clinical situation. An open mind and avoidance of early diagnostic closure are vital.

Limited medical access

Mental health follow-up is becoming a medical crisis even in urban areas. Over the past 20 years, there has been a remarkable shift in the delivery of health care from the inpatient to the outpatient setting. This has had profound effects on mental health as it transformed from long-term care to relatively brief crisis-oriented inpatient stabilization with community-centered outpatient care. This care is often heavily dependent on dwindling public funds. For a variety of social reasons, these patients may enter a cycle of downward social drift resulting in loss of social support, financial hardship, and isolation. Loss of pre-existing insurance coverage quickly follows, leading to the loss of primary care as well. A 1990 study from New York City found that 27% of the uninsured used the emergency department for primary care services [7]. In 2007, a national survey noted 12% of emergency department visits involved mental illness or substance abuse [8]. Access to medical care is further limited by lack of transportation, inadequate or unsupervised housing, and frequent moves between service areas. If patients do see a medical provider, it is often at the mental health center, and the encounter focus will usually be on medications, not primary care or preventive health monitoring. The end result of this process is medical care being provided on an ad hoc and often emergency basis. This is germane in the emergency department where time limits care to specific presenting complaints and discharge planning is frequently limited. A typical discharge will simply direct the patient to follow-up with mental health. Rhodes et al. [9] found that among simulated patients with insurance, follow-up appointment rates were 22% but for those without insurance, it was only 12%. The typical default referral is to the local community mental health center. Resources are

Behavioral Emergencies for the Emergency Physician, ed. Leslie S. Zun, Lara G. Chepenik, and Mary Nan S. Mallory. Published by Cambridge University Press. © Cambridge University Press 2013.

limited; for example, one such local facility has 1.5 full time equivalent psychiatrists for over 2000 chronically mentally ill patients. Often patients lack the resources to get to the follow-up appointment, even if they are motivated to do so. The three classic pillars of ensuring medical follow-up, giving an appointment time, providing the means to get to it and giving the name of a provider who will be expecting the referral are therefore frequently not realistic from the emergency setting.

Medication noncompliance

Medication noncompliance is a well-known problem in the medically ill in general. Patients often suffer from side effects and the number of pills to be taken in any given day can be daunting. Understanding of medication regimens is frequently limited. Even the most motivated patient will find the task of keeping track of a handful of pills challenging. The mentally ill patient with medical comorbidities must often take additional medications. Psychiatric symptoms also affect compliance. A patient with paranoid delusions may begin to incorporate their medications into their delusional system and refuse to take them. A patient with manic-depression may describe medications as mind dulling or numbing and discontinue them. Depressed patients may simply not have the energy to take their medicine. Further complicating the clinical situation is that patients frequently self-medicate with alcohol, medications (obtained both legally and otherwise), and illicit substances. Demented patients may simply forget to take their pills, take them all at once, or use them incorrectly. Almost all patients can be confused by trade names versus generics. Patients learn to identify their pills by shape or color, details which can change depending on the pharmacy or manufacturer.

For various reasons, physicians may overlook cost concerns when prescribing. Marketing may contribute to trade name prescribing, even when less-expensive generic alternatives are available. There are, however, practical issues driving prescribing practices, such as once daily or depot dosing versus several times per day regimens with many generics. Enteric-coated pills are better tolerated than their uncoated, often cheaper, alternatives. The difference per month between generic haloperidol and a name brand second-generation antipsychotic can be hundreds of dollars each month. Finally, in any given city, two different insurance plans may have different preferred formularies. Even patients with a traditional Medicare plan who are prescribed "covered" medications can find themselves facing huge pharmacy bills when they enter the co-pay "donut-hole" of Medicare Part D. The end result is that a clinician may not realize there is a problem until a patient's condition starts to deteriorate and questions are asked.

Duality of approach

The initial evaluation of the medically ill patient with an unexplained symptom in a medical setting tends to focus on medical diagnoses. Conversely, the initial evaluation of a mentally ill patient with unexplained symptoms in a mental health setting will tend to focus on psychopathology. When this same medical patient is seen in a psychiatric clinic, or visa versa, there can be a tendency to early diagnostic closure, eliminating potential alternative diagnoses, again with potentially catastrophic results. This artificial dichotomy of "either medical or psychiatric" can result in an evaluation that will be heavily influenced by which part of the clinical picture is being brought into focus first.

The basic problem is that patients and clinical conditions do not exist independently. We noted earlier that between 30% and 80% of medical patients seen in a primary care setting will actually have a psychosocial diagnosis [3]. It is also known that patients with psychiatric diagnoses have an overall morbidity and mortality rate significantly higher than that of matched controls [10,11]. We have already mentioned the high prevalence of occult and diagnosed psychiatric conditions in the emergency department. The SADHEART [12] studies looked at antidepressant use following myocardial infarction. They found that mortality doubled over 6.7 years compared with controls in patients who had not been treated with antidepressants regardless of whether the patient had depression or not. A review in JAMA notes that depression was associated with a significantly increased risk of stroke [13]. Trying to impose a rigid boundary between medical and psychiatric conditions is diagnostically limiting, and could result in clinical errors.

A dualistic approach would conceptualize comorbid medical and psychiatric conditions as a diagnostic continuum that must be approached from multiple views with a very high degree of suspicion and a holistic approach to the patient. "Primary" disorders typically refer to classical psychiatric disorders such as mania and schizophrenia. "Secondary" usually refer to conditions due to other medical conditions, drugs/alcohol, or medications. Evaluation of pre-existing and comorbid psychiatric conditions and their treatments, which can have a profound impact on the patient's medical evaluation, differential diagnosis, and treatment plan should quickly follow stabilization of the emergency condition. During the next tier of investigation, one can begin to evaluate potential comorbidities in developing the differential diagnosis and management plan. In almost all cases, a new psychiatric diagnosis is one of exclusion in the emergency setting.

With this approach in mind, cause-and-effect consideration must be given to a patient with worsening physical symptoms being the result of deterioration in their underlying psychiatric condition. One example would be the anxious or somatic patient presenting with pain in some body part. Another might be a chronic schizophrenic who presents with a fever and a low blood count. However, these same clinical scenarios could represent a case of angina, sepsis, or neuroleptic malignant syndrome. Because patients may not know the specifics of their condition, and medication lists may be unavailable or incorrect, we are reminded of the need to collaborate with mental health providers, just as we would with a primary care physician.

Risk factor assessment

Assessing risk factors for medical illness in patients with psychiatric disorders is essential but often overlooked. There is increased use of harmful substances, exposure to unhealthy environments, side effects from medications used to treat psychiatric disorders, and a lack of resources which all contribute to higher risk of medical comorbidities. Also, despite the fact that patients who present to physicians with primary concerns of mental illness frequently are known to have higher risk for cardiovascular disease and other medical problems, there are many barriers to screening for them and modifying the associated unhealthy habits that contribute to medical illness.

Substance use in mental illness is prevalent. According to the National Comorbidity Survey, approximately 50% of the U.S. population with any mental disorder also has a substance use disorder at some point in their lifetime. More than half of patients with severe mental illness such as bipolar disorder and schizophrenia are dually diagnosed with substance use disorder. In patients with mental disorders, 15% have a substance use disorder within the 12 months before their diagnosis of mental disorder, which contrasts with 8% of the general population having a substance use disorder within the past year. Of the 15% comorbid substance use disorder and mental disorder cases, less than half of the cases received any treatment for the substance use disorder within those 12 months [14]. Many theories exist as to why comorbid mental illness and substance use is so prevalent. They include substance-induced psychiatric disorders, psychiatric disorders causing substance use, the common factor model which attributes substance use and mental illness to underlying variables that increase the risk for development of both disorders, and bidirectional models that suggest that psychiatric disorders can induce substance use disorder that then exacerbates the initial psychiatric condition.

Tobacco use is one of the most common substances of dependence in patients with a psychiatric disorder. In the past, there was a strong social and behavioral drive that encouraged smoking. Cigarettes were used as a reward for desired behaviors, an opportunity to leave a locked unit, and an opportunity to bond with other residents or staff. Although smoking is now banned in most healthcare settings, current smoking rates are upward of 41% in patients with a past-month mental illness as compared to 22% in patients without mental illness [15]. Tobacco use plays a role in both causing medical comorbidities as well as altering the effects of medications. Nicotine can lead to cardiovascular disease by causing increased myocardial work through transient blood pressure elevation and coronary artery vasoconstriction, hypercoagulable state, dyslipidemia, and endothelial dysfunction. Also, nicotine withdrawal can be severe and persist for up to a month. Nicotine binds to nicotinic acetylcholine receptors and has a mild stimulatory effect, which results in withdrawal symptoms of irritability, restlessness, poor concentration, dysphoric or anxious mood, and insomnia. Lastly, nicotine can decrease levels of some psychotropic medications by inducing cytochrome P450 metabolism by means of the hepatic enzyme CYP1A2. This can be relevant if a relapse of symptoms is observed in a patient who was a stable inpatient while not smoking and then began smoking again once discharged to outpatient.

Screening for abuse and dependence of common substances such as alcohol, cocaine, sedatives, and opioids is essential to recognize intoxication and prevent complicated withdrawal, to assess for risk of medical comorbidities, and to provide preventive care. Alcohol is a CNS depressant that modulates neurotransmission by enhancing GABA receptor-mediated inhibition and reduces glutamate NMDA receptor-mediated excitation. With consistent, heavy alcohol use, there is up-regulation of glutamate receptors that leads to increased neuro-excitation upon alcohol withdrawal. Common alcohol withdrawal syndromes generally begin within 24 hours of the last drink and can last several days and range from minor symptoms such as anxiety, nausea, anorexia, insomnia, and headache to alcoholic hallucinosis, which is a transient state of auditory, visual, or tactile hallucinations with intact sensorium and normal autonomic function. Delirium tremens is a medical emergency that requires intensive care unit (ICU) admission and is characterized by disorientation, agitation, hallucinations, autonomic instability such as increased heart rate, blood pressure, diaphoresis, or fever. It occurs most frequently between 2 to 3 days after the last drink and is more likely to occur in patients with a history of delirium tremens or withdrawal seizures or with a current severe medical illness. It is associated with a 5–15% mortality rate. Withdrawal seizures are usually tonic–clonic and occur in the first 1 to 2 days after cessation of alcohol. Patients with alcohol use disorders are at risk for many more chronic medical problems, with some of the most severe complications including Wernicke's encephalopathy, Korsakoff's dementia, cirrhosis and its associated complications, cardiomyopathy, pancytopenia.

While those with a psychiatric disorder compared to those without have significantly increased odds ratios of using tobacco and alcohol, the highest comorbidity of mental illness and addictive disorder is illicit substance use. According to the NIMH Epidemiologic Catchment Area Program, more than half of those that abuse drugs have a psychiatric comorbidity with an odds ratio of 4.5 [16]. There are many significant possible adverse effects of illicit substances, thus discussion will be limited to some of the most severe. Benzodiazepine use can lead to physiologic dependence with moderate to high dosage for greater than 2 weeks, with the exception being alprazolam which can have significant withdrawal after only a short period of use. Due to a similar mechanism of action on $GABA_A$ receptors, benzodiazepine withdrawal is similar to alcohol withdrawal. Seizures can occur within days of last use depending on the half-life of the benzodiazepine. Barbiturate withdrawal carries higher risk of seizure, however, use is less prevalent than benzodiazepines. Overdose of benzodiazepines, like alcohol, can result in respiratory and CNS depression. With opioids, aside from risk of CNS and respiratory depression, the majority of medical complications arise from intravenous use. Co-occurrence of HIV and hepatitis B and C in intravenous drug users is very high with one in five individuals having HIV and more than half having hepatitis C. Other risks of intravenous drug use include development of abscesses or endocarditis, due to both dirty needles and impurities in the drug, which can subsequently lead to emboli resulting in end-organ damage. With higher doses of cocaine and other stimulants, cardiovascular complications can occur. Stimulants increase monoamine activity through dopamine, norepinephrine, and serotonin. This sympathetic stimulation can cause coronary vasospasm that most often leads to transient chest pain but sometimes results in acute myocardial infarction. Arrhythmias, hypertension, and stroke can also be a consequence of stimulant-induced vasospasm. Hallucinogen medical complications most often arise from accidental or self-inflicted injury from psychotic behavior, but PCP has also been associated with rhabdomyolysis and acute kidney injury. Lastly, the negative impacts of cannabis are primarily secondary to the smoke inhalation, which can result in various pulmonary complications.

While the substances that patients use may cause medical comorbidities, there is also risk of iatrogenic medical problems from medications used to treat psychiatric illness. The prevalence of obesity, metabolic syndrome diabetes, and cardiopulmonary disease in the mentally ill population are estimated to be double that of the general population [17]. Monitoring for metabolic syndrome in patients with antipsychotic use is extremely important. Metabolic syndrome is defined by the 2001 National Cholesterol Education Program / Adult Treatment Panel [ATP] III guidelines as having three of the following five criteria: waist circumference greater than 40 inches in men and greater than 35 inches in women, triglycerides greater than or equal to 150 mg/dL, HDL cholesterol less than 40 mg/dL in men and less than 50 mg/dL in women, blood pressure greater than or equal to 130/85 mmHg, fasting blood glucose greater than or equal to 100 mg/dL. Note that patients on drug treatment for any of the last four criteria count as having met that criteria. Side effects of antipsychotics, particularly the second-generation antipsychotics, increase risk for metabolic syndrome. Clozapine, olanzapine, and quetiapine are associated with the most risk for development of metabolic disorder features [18]. Screening includes taking an annual personal and family history of cardiovascular diseases, risk factors, and equivalents, including hypertension, dyslipidemia, diabetes, tobacco use, coronary artery disease, aortic aneurysm, and cerebrovascular disease. Body mass index should be calculated monthly, and waist circumference should be measured every 3 months. Blood pressure readings can quickly be taken at every visit, but at a minimum should be recorded every 3 months. Lastly, obtaining fasting lipid panel and either fasting blood sugar or HbA1C at 3 months and then yearly after initiating an antipsychotic helps screen for development of hyperlipidemia or diabetes.

Additional psychosocial factors play a role in the poor overall health of psychiatric patients. Psychologically, it is difficult to be motivated for exercise or even basic physical activity when much of the day is spent dealing with the ongoing challenge of overwhelming depression and despair or paranoid delusions. Socially supports and fitness program infra-structure are often lacking, unavailable, or too expensive. Supervised residences do not always promote healthy meals and dietary monitoring programs are lacking. The mentally ill homeless patient may have significant nutritional deficiencies. Efforts at promotion of healthy lifestyles have been only marginally successful.

Finally, a multitude of other environmental and clinical factors lead to increased medical complications in patients with psychiatric illness. Living situations may be suboptimal due to financial constraints as well as by impaired hygiene and regard for self-care as a result of severe mental illness. Access to medical care is often limited due to poor organizational skills or insufficient income for transportation. Inpatient psychiatric hospitalization focuses on stabilization of mental illness, and often screening opportunities are missed. Also, the stigma of mental illness can lead to clinicians focusing on the psychiatric condition rather than addressing other medical problems. This is compounded by the fact that dysfunction of thought processes may result in mentally ill patients giving poor histories when medically ill, having poor follow-up, or being reluctant to embrace interventions. In addition, follow-up for mental health concerns may trump medical concerns, so the patient may be frequently seen by a psychiatrist and rarely seen by other health professionals.

Polypharmacy is a growing national problem, not just in the comorbid medical–psychiatric patient, and is noted especially in select patient populations like nursing homes, a growing referral source for many emergency departments. One study found that patients in this cohort presenting to the emergency department took an average of four medications per day (range 1–17) but adverse drug events accounted for 11% of all emergency visits [19]. Howard et al.'s [20] sample found a median of 24 prescriptions had been filled in the previous year. Psychotropic medications specifically may carry a significant side-effect burden. First-generation antipsychotics (haloperidol and others) have been associated with cardiac arrhythmias, extra pyramidal side effects, and neuroleptic malignant syndrome. Second-generation agents (olanzepine, risperdol and others) have a tendency toward weight gain resulting in metabolic syndrome and have been associated with stroke. Traditional tricyclic antidepressants (amitriptyline and others) are highly anticholinergic and often sedating, while serotonin specific reuptake inhibitors (fluoxetine, sertraline, others) can cause agitation, gastrointestinal distress, and possibly effect platelet function. Benzodiazepines carry a risk for addiction and dependence as well as sedation. Anticonvulsants used as mood stabilizers (valproic acid) can cause weight gain, hair loss, and toxic blood levels. Even the "safe" serotonin specific receptor inhibitors (fluoxetine, sertraline, others) can be sedating or activating, sometimes are associated with gastrointestinal distress, and can paradoxically cause worsening anxiety or agitation. Many of the newer medications, while being targeted to specific neurotransmitters, also have very specific cytochrome P450 metabolic pathways, leading to inadvertent toxicity. The foregoing should not be seen as an indictment of psychopharmacology, but rather a reminder of the importance of obtaining a full history, reviewing medication lists, and maintaining an open mind with regard to differential diagnosis.

Clinical syndrome: agitation

The psychiatric differential diagnosis of agitation includes manic states, schizophrenia, psychotic disorders, intoxications, and confusional states. These patients present with agitation or threatening behaviors, hallucinations or delusions and impaired reality testing. A good history and clinical assessment will often help to determine if the person is suffering from a psychiatric diagnosis, a medical diagnosis such as delirium or pain, or some psychosocial stressor not medically related. While florid mania is relatively uncommon, delirium can be present as much as 89% in an ICU setting [21]. Two studies looked specifically at the prevalence in the emergency department and both found that delirium was present in 10% of the populations but that overall detection rates were only 23% [22,23].

Historical information is vital to determine etiology. Auditory hallucinations are most common in psychiatric disorders such as schizophrenia. Tactile hallucinations are classically associated with drug abuse or seizure disorders. Visual hallucinations are particularly common in delirious states. Medications and over-the-counter remedies need to be reviewed, particularly for anything newly added or changed. Polypharmacy as noted above is pervasive, widespread, and especially affects the elderly. The more medications a patient takes results in an exponential increase in the potential for adverse effects or drug–drug interactions. Medics can often provide vital additional information. Physical examination may reveal hypoxia, hypertensive emergencies, hypoperfused states, or sepsis. Evidence of poisoning or intoxication can sometimes be observed. Medical evaluation will often include screening for drugs of abuse, thyroid functions, leukocytosis, and chemistries. Treatment must focus on the underlying cause, however, agitation does carry a significant risk of mortality and emergency treatment should not be delayed.

Clinical syndrome: depression

In contrast to the agitated and/or psychotic patient, depressed patients tend to be quiet, withdrawn, and can easily be forgotten in the back areas of a busy emergency department. Kessler and colleagues [24] found that depression has a lifetime prevalence of 16%. Estimates of depression in the ED are as high as 30% [25]. Virtually all medical conditions are associated with some depressive complaints, with diabetes, heart and lung disease, and arthritis being most common. Not all these patients are suffering from a major depressive disorder. Patients are often being faced with catastrophic life changes, including physical appearance, pain, isolation, financial uncertainty, and changed relationships. Being sad can be a normal and expectable consequence of medical illness in these situations. A follow-up report from the SADHART 9 series noted that mortality doubled over 6.7 years in patients not treated with antidepressant medication.

Obtaining solid historical information from the patient and any other sources is vital. Laboratory testing to include electro-cardiogram (ECG), chemistries, thyroid function, pregnancy, and urine may help clarify an underlying diagnosis. Drug and alcohol testing should be considered. Physical examination may be particularly informative, especially in patients who have not been previously diagnosed with depression. Many medications have depression as a frequent side effect. Weakness and fatigue can be a sign of myocardial infarction, hypothyroid states, or fibromyalgia, as well as a symptom of depression. Fluid and electrolyte disorders can profoundly affect a person's mood and general demeanor. Neuropsychiatric conditions including Parkinson's disease, stroke, and dementia will sometimes present with a depressed demeanor.

One of the difficulties in making a diagnosis of depression in the medically ill is that there is an exceptional amount of symptom overlap, the duality that recurs during this discussion. Schwab et al. [26] in 1966 suggested that psychological symptoms of depression are often experienced by medically ill patients even though they may not be suffering from the clinical entity we call depression. The DSM-IV-TR criteria for major depression include duration of at least 2 weeks and include complaints of poor appetite, insomnia, loss of interest, and/or energy and feelings of worthlessness, among others [27]. A patient, boarded in the emergency department for 18 hours, not eating, sleep deprived, and scared will likely positively endorse symptoms about energy, appetite, worry, and fear. This will only be magnified after time in an ICU setting.

Several alternative methods have been suggested as being more useful to screen for depression in the medically ill patient. Endicott [28] working with the previous edition of DSM found that substituting four criteria increased diagnostic accuracy. These were a fearful or depressed appearance, not being able to be cheered up, social withdrawal, or general pessimism. A patient who could not be cheered up, did not smile, or did not respond to good news was believed to be a good marker of a severe depression in cancer patients [29]. These papers simply re-emphasize the importance of obtaining as much history from as many sources as possible.

Although it is vital to keep the possibility of anxiety or panic in the differential diagnosis, a psychiatric diagnosis is unlikely to cause acute morbidity or mortality. Any patient with a reasonable clinical presentation of chest pain should be fully evaluated. Gastrointestinal emergencies need to be considered in a patient with acute abdominal pain. New or unexplained neurological symptoms will likely warrant a complete evaluation. In many of these cases admission is going to be the most prudent course of action. However, two caveats should be mentioned. If, based on solid clinical judgment, a somatic cause of the patient's symptoms is felt to be less likely, then an evaluation may be more focused. The other is that in the emergency setting, the clinician may have access to information that the admitting team may not have. Therefore documentation and a complete transfer of information is vital.

Clinical syndrome: chronic obstructive lung disease

Chronic obstructive lung disease, COPD, as an end result of smoking, is a frequent finding in psychiatric patients. COPD can also be a primary cause of anxiety and depression. Major depression and anxiety may be as high as 44% in patients with COPD [30]. Common treatments for asthma and COPD include steroids and beta-agonists, both of which can worsen depression and anxiety. Mortality is also significantly higher in these comorbidly ill patients [31]. The essential feature of generalized anxiety disorder is "excessive worry," but trouble concentrating, fatigue, and trouble sleeping are symptoms common to depression as well. In the emergency setting, making a determination of "excessive worry" is problematic, and establishing that depressive symptoms are not related to the medical illness is challenging. These patients do in fact suffer from fatigue that comes from the physical effort of breathing, the fear of suffocation and have difficulty with sleep due to positioning, CPAP (continuous positive airway pressure) machines, and medications. Social factors such as not being able to leave the house, loneliness, concern over self-image, and being dependent on oxygen will contribute to the overall disease picture. Treatment for these patients should focus first on optimizing their respiratory status. Medications such as benzodiazepines can be very useful for the emergent control of anxiety, although their long-term use can pose challenges due to sedation and tolerance. The use of low-dose antipsychotic medication has a place in the treatment armentarium, but their potential side-effect profile should be considered in the risk–benefit analysis. COPD patients suffering from anxiety spectrum disorders may benefit from psychological interventions such as cognitive behavior therapy, group support, and relaxation training.

Clinical syndrome: cardiovascular disease

Cardiovascular disease remains one of the leading causes of death and overall morbidity in the United States. It was long felt that there was a strong relationship between depression and heart disease. Stress, "Type A" personality types, and unhealthy lifestyle choices were among the factors cited. As noted above, it is also known that once a patient became depressed, other issues such as obesity, smoking, and sedentary lifestyles become increasing factors. Depression has consistently been found in almost 20% of patients with cardiovascular disease [32]. Frasure-Smith et al. [33] in 1993 first confirmed that depression increased mortality following acute myocardial infarction by a factor of three. A 2003 study found that heart patients coincidentally treated with selective serotonin reuptake inhibitors (SSRIs) had fewer deaths or recurrent MI [34]. Fleet et al. [35] found, however, that 25% of their sample of chest pain patients actually had an undiagnosed panic disorder. The SADHEART studies noted earlier provide further justification for the prudent clinician maintaining an open mind toward the duality of comorbid illnesses.

The evaluation of these patients should begin with a thorough medical evaluation. A standard cardiac evaluation including ECG and iso-enzymes is an important starting point. In fact, at the minimum, an overnight admission to a monitored bed is generally going to be required. While carefully ruling out organic pathology, it may not be unreasonable to consult with Psychiatry early in the course of admission. Aggressive treatment of anxiety and despondency, even if only with short-acting benzodiazepines, could bring significant relief to this population. If a patient in this cohort became a frequent visitor to the emergency department, obtaining cardiac catheterization may ultimately be the best option to clarify their medical status.

Clinical syndrome: gastrointestinal disorders

Since before the time of Freud, there has been a known relationship between the gastrointestinal (GI) system and psychiatric disorders. Peptic ulcer disease, inflammatory bowel, including ulcerative colitis and Crohn's disease, were the classically described illnesses. Psychiatric comorbidity included anxiety, depression, and somatization. Often this balance tended toward psychiatric or so-called "functional" illnesses. As our understanding broadened, we learned that this was not always correct, as when bacteria or anti-inflammatory drugs were found to be associated with peptic ulcer disease. Still, it is estimated that as many as 20% of peptic ulcer disease patients and up to 30% of those suffering from inflammatory bowel disease will be diagnosed with depression [36].

Perhaps the biggest mental health factor associated with these disorders is overall quality of life. Guthrie and colleagues [37] demonstrated that physical function, role limitation, pain, and overall health perception were significantly worse in this comorbid cohort. However, this is a complex association. A patient suffering from depression could have worsened bowel symptoms but the patient with severe bowel disease is likely to depressed. Many of the medications used to treat either symptom cluster can have side effects on the other. Social stress can become profound. It becomes increasingly more difficult for patients to leave home, go to work, or meet friends. A vicious cycle ensures.

A detailed history can sometimes tease apart the two clinical presentations. It is vital to note time of symptoms onset. Depression is marked by depressed mood, decreased interest, poor concentration and feelings of worthlessness, to name a few. The Rome criteria for irritable bowel disease focus on pain, features of the bowel symptoms, and time course aimed to eliminate some of the diagnostic uncertainty inherent in this disease. Clearly there can be an overlap of symptom clusters. These patients can be referred early to mental health with subsequent untreated physical suffering. More often, the diagnosis and treatment focus on the physical, with mental anguish being treated symptomatically, if at all. This then becomes a dilemma for the busy emergency department with a frequent visitor refusing to consider the possibility of a comorbid situation. Sometimes, great progress will be made with a patient by simply listening and letting them know you are trying to understand their situation.

Definitive pharmacologic interventions will rarely be started in the emergency department. A focus on the acute presentation is probably the best starting point, and short-acting benzodiazepines are certainly reasonable to consider. Pain needs to be addressed. Traditional tricyclic antidepressants have been shown to be effective over placebo [38]. The benefit of these medications is likely due to a combination of anticholinergic properties as well as some analgesic effect. Duloxetine, a serotonin and norepinephrine reuptake inhibitor was marketed with a specific indication as an analgesic, although most of the SSRIs likely share some of this benefit. It is important to identify whether these medications are being started for their antidepressant or analgesic properties. In conjunction with the primary care provider, an emergency physician may have a window of opportunity, when a patient is in crisis, to initiate this type of medication.

Clinical syndrome: pain

Pain is another area of comorbidity with substantial overlap of symptom clusters. These patients will often be labeled as having somatization disorder. This is a very difficult term with multiple meanings ranging from any patient with physical complaints to a DSM-IV-TR diagnosis of a psychiatric patient with multiple somatic complaints. The label can be descriptive or pejorative. As always, a good history is vital and diagnostic accuracy very important. Pain is an extremely common presenting complaint in the emergency department and chronic pain can effect up to 35% [39]. A survey for the World Health Organization found that almost 70% of patients suffering from depression reported pain as an initial symptom [40].

Pain, however, can cause a range of psychosocial distress short of major depression. These patients are inwardly focused and acutely aware of every bodily sensation resulting in objectively minor complaints presenting as an impending catastrophe. This can quickly lead to isolation due to fears of leaving the home, overuse of medications, frequent calls to the doctor or visits to the ED, and burnout of friends and caregivers. Self-reported depression, feelings of worthlessness, and anhedonia (a pervasive inability to experience pleasure) are more likely to reflect a primary psychiatric disorder. A patient in severe pain may report feelings of being better off dead as a way to end the suffering, but not really interested in taking their own life. Anxiety complaints can be directly related to the pain, or fear of the pain, even if not currently present. Anger at the doctor's inability to find a resolution to their condition can quickly lead to an impasse limiting proper evaluation and effective treatment.

Until proven otherwise, a complaint of pain should be taken at face value and the measurement of pain is one of several "5th vital signs" that is tracked by The Joint Commission (TJC). In an ideal setting, pain management would be tailored to the specific causes of the pain, whether that is neuropathic, central, or psychiatric. However, the emergency department is rarely ideal. Physicians still tend to undermedicate pain with inadequate dosing and/or improper frequency. Many reasons are given for this including overcrowding, fears of causing addiction, overmedication causing complications, and poor understanding of basic pharmacokinetics. In addition, psychiatric medications are often unfamiliar, comorbid psychopathology is frightening and fears of making the mental health patient worse can be added obstacles. Opioids are probably the "gold standard" of pain control with the added benefit of being effective anxiolytics and rarely contraindicated due to drug–drug interactions. Combination therapy with a nonsteroidal anti-inflammatory agent can have additive benefits. Psychiatric patients are often taking adjunctive medications such as tricyclic antidepressants, anticonvulsants, and benzodiazepines that can be adjusted to serve dual therapeutic purpose. In the acute setting, overtreatment and possible sedation is probably a better result than undertreatment and needless suffering.

Conclusion

Bias is an inherent part of the human psyche but is not inherently detrimental to patient care. Not being aware of bias, however, can be catastrophic. Medical and psychiatric illnesses often represent an overlapping and complex spectrum of symptoms and diagnoses. Both emergency physicians and psychiatrists must avoid early diagnostic closure and look at the whole patient. A duality of approach will almost always result in improved overall care.

References

1. Alegria M, Jackson JS, Kessler RC, Takeuchi D. *Collaborative Psychiatric Epidemiology Surveys, 2001–2003.* Ann Arbor, MI: Institute for Social Research, Survey Research Center; 2007.

2. Kroenke K, Spitzer RL, Janet BW, Williams DSW. Physical symptoms in primary care: predictors of psychiatric disorders and functional impairment. *Arch Fam Med* 1994;**3**:774–9.

3. Lipowski ZL. The interface of psychiatry and medicine: towards integrated health care. *Can J Psychiatry* 1987;**32**:743–8.

4. Curran GM, Sullivan G, Williams K, et al. Emergency department use of persons with comorbid psychiatric and substance abuse disorders. *Ann Emerg Med* 2003;**41**:659–67.

5. Schriger DL, Gibbons PS, Langone CA, et al. Enabling the diagnosis of occult psychiatric illness in the emergency department: a randomized, controlled trial of the computerized, self-administered PRIME-MD. *Ann Emerg Med* 2001;**37**:132–40.

6. Santucci KA, Sather J, Baker MD. Emergency medicine training programs' educational requirements in the management of psychiatric emergencies: current perspective. *Pediatr Emerg Care* 2003;**19**:154–6.

7. Billings J, Parikh N, Mijanovich T. Emergency department use in New York City: a substitute for primary care? *Issue Brief (Commonw Fund)* 2000;**433**:1–5.

8. *Mental Illness Accounts for Large Portion of ED.* Psychiatric News, August 20, 2010.

9. Rhodes KV, Vieth TL, Kushner H, et al. Referral without access: for psychiatric services, wait for the beep. *Ann Emerg Med* 2009;**54**:272–8.

10. Felker B, Yazel JJ, Short D. Mortality and medical comorbidity among psychiatric patients: a review. *Psychiatr Serv* 1996;**47**:1356–63.

11. Mykletun A, Bjerkeset O, Overland S, et al. Levels of anxiety and depression as predictors of mortality: the HUNT Study. *Br J Psychiatry* 2009;**195**:118–25.

12. Glassman AH, Bigger T, Gaffney M. Psychiatric characteristics associated with long-term mortality among 361 patients having an acute coronary syndrome and major depression. *Arch Gen Psychiatry* 2009;**66**:1022–9.

13. Pan A, Sun Q, Okereke O, et al. Depression and risk of stroke morbidity and mortality: a meta-analysis and systematic review. *JAMA* 2011;**306**:1241–9.

14. Kessler RC. The epidemiology of co-occurring addictive and mental disorders: implications for prevention and service utilization. *Am J Orthopsychiatry* 1996;**66**:17–31.

15. Lasser K, Boyd JW, Woolhandler S, et al. Smoking and mental illness-a population-based prevalence study. *JAMA* 2000;**284**:2606–10.

16. Darre A, Regier MD, Farmer ME, et al. Comorbidity of mental disorders with alcohol and other drug abuse results from the Epidemiologic Catchment Area (ECA) Study. *JAMA* 1990;**264**:2511–18.

17. Scott D, Happell B. The high prevalence of poor physical health and unhealthy lifestyle behaviours in individuals with severe mental illness. *Issues Ment Health Nurs* 2011;**32**:589–97.

18. Newcomer JW, Haupt DW. The metabolic effects of antipsychotic medications. *Can J Psychiatry* 2006;**51**:480.

19. Corinne MH, Dankoff J, Colacone A, et al. Polypharmacy, adverse drug-related events, and potential adverse drug interactions in elderly patients presenting to an emergency department. *Ann Emer Med* 2001;**38**:666–71.

20. Howard M, Dolovich L, Kaczorowski L, et al. Prescribing of potentially inappropriate medications to elderly people. *Fam Pract* 2004;**21**:244–7.

21. McNicoll L, Pisani MA, Zhang Y, et al. Delirium in the intensive care unit. *J Am Geriatr Soc* 2003;**51**:591–8.

22. Hustey FM, Meldon SW. The prevalence and documentation of impaired mental status in elderly emergency department patients. *Ann Emerg Med* 2002;**39**:248–53.

23. Elie M, Rousseau F. Prevalence and detection of delirium in elderly emergency department patients. *Can Med Assoc J* 2000;**163**:977–81.

24. Kessler RC, Berglund P, Demler O, et al. The epidemiology of major depressive disorder: results from the National Comorbidity survey replication. *JAMA* 2003;**289**:3095–105.

25. Claassen CA, Larkin GL. Occult suicidality in an emergency department population. *Br J Psychiatry* 2005;**186**:352–3.

26. Schwab JJ, Clemmons RS, Bialow M, et al. The affective symptomatology of depression in medical inpatients. *Psychosomatics* 1966;**7**:214–17.

27. American Psychiatric Association. *Diagnostic and Statistical Manual of Mental Disorders*, (4th Edition) Text Revision. Arlington, VA: American Psychiatric Association; 2000.

28. Endicott J. Measurement of depression in patients with cancer. *Cancer* 1984;**53**:2243–8.

29. Akechi T, Ietsugu T, Sukigara M, et al. Symptom indicator of severity of depression in cancer patients: a comparison of the DSM-IV criteria with alternative diagnostic criteria. *Hosp Psychiatry* 2009;**31**:225–32.

30. Ng TP, Niti M, Tan WC, et al. Depressive symptoms and chronic obstructive pulmonary disease: effect on mortality, hospital readmission, symptom burden, functional status, and quality of life. *Arch Intern Med* 2007;**167**:6–7.

31. Abrams TE, Sarrazin MV, VanderWeg MW. Acute exacerbations of chronic obstructive pulmonary disease and the effect of existing psychiatric comorbidity on subsequent mortality. *Psychosomatics* 2011;**52**:441–9.

32. Shapiro PA, Lidogoster L, Glassman AH. Depression and heart disease. *Psychiatr Ann* 1997;**27**:347–52.

33. Frasure-Smith N, Lespérance F, Talajic M. Depression following myocardial infarction. Impact on 6-month survival. *JAMA* 1993;**270**:1819–25.

34. Berkman LF, Blumenthal J, Burg M, et al. Enhancing Recovery in Coronary Heart Disease (ENRICHD). *JAMA* 2003;**289**:3106–16.

35. Fleet RP, Dupuis G, Marchand A, et al. Panic disorder in emergency department chest pain patients: prevalence, comorbidity, suicidal ideation, and physician recognition. *Am J Med* 1996;**101**:371–80.

36. Craig TKJ. In: Brown GW, (Ed.). *Abdominal Pain, in Life Events and Illness.* New York: Guilford; 1989: 233–59.

37. Guthrie E, Jackson J, Shaffer J, et al. Psychological disorder and severity of inflammatory bowel disease predict health-related quality of life in ulcerative colitis and Crohn's disease. *Am J Gastroenterol* 2002;**97**:1994–9.

38. Jackson JL, OMalley PG, Tomkins G, et al. Treatment of functional GI disorders with antidepressant medications. *Am J Med* 2000;**108**:65–72.

39. Hanley O, Miner J, Rockswold E, Biros M. The relationship between chronic illness, chronic pain and socioeconomic factors in the ED. *Am J Emerg Med* 2011;**29**:266–93.

40. Simon GE, VonKorff M, Piccinelli M, et al. An international study of the relation between somatic symptoms and depression. *N Engl J Med* 1999;**341**:1329–35.

Chapter 19

Acute care of eating disorders

Suzanne Dooley-Hash

Introduction

Eating disorders (EDs) are unique among mental illnesses in that they are frequently associated with both psychiatric comorbidities and medical complications that can be severe, and at times, even fatal. Eating disorders, in fact, have the highest mortality rates of any mental illness with a standardized mortality rate that is 6–12 times higher than age-matched controls [1]. Approximately two thirds of the deaths seen in ED patients are due to either suicide or cardiac causes, both of which are likely to initially present to an emergency department or other acute care setting. Given that the majority of ED patients do not readily self-disclose their illness to healthcare providers, it is imperative that all physicians and other providers be able to recognize the signs and symptoms of the common eating disorders and maintain a high index of suspicion for the potentially life-threatening associated medical complications. The purpose of this chapter is to (1) give a brief overview of the eating disorders, (2) discuss recognition of eating disorders and commonly associated medical complications and their management in the acute setting, and (3) provide suggestions for definitive, long-term treatment referral.

Impact of eating disorders

Despite their relatively low prevalence in the general population, eating disorders are among the most prevalent psychiatric problems in adolescents and young adults, and are third only to obesity and asthma as the most common chronic illnesses in these age groups [2]. In fact, some experts estimate that as many as 14% of adolescents have some form of clinically significant eating disorder [2,3] and rates as high as 7–21% of EDs have been found in screening studies in both the general population and primary care settings [4–6]. Patients with EDs have also been found to have overall increased usage of all healthcare services including emergency departments [7,8]. At least one study has shown that the average number of emergency department visits was increased in ED patients who eventually died from their illness, when compared to controls [9]. This finding raises concerns that the ED patients who present to the emergency department for care may also have an increased severity of disease and, therefore, be at an increased risk of mortality.

In addition to having increased rates of overall healthcare usage patients are also at significantly increased risk of death when compared to their peers. Anorexia nervosa has an estimated lifetime mortality rate of 10% making it the deadliest mental illness [1,10–12]. It is notable that as many as half of ED-related deaths are attributable to suicide [13,14]. The standardized mortality rate (SMR) for suicide in a patient with anorexia nervosa (AN) is 32.4. This means that a patient with AN is more than 32 times more likely to die by suicide than a healthy person of the same demographics. This figure is even more striking when compared to an SMR for suicide of 27.8 for major depressive disorder, 18.2 for alcohol abuse, and 8.0 for schizophrenia [1]. Fewer data are available for eating disorders other than AN, but a recent study showed similar overall mortality rates for all EDs [15]. Other studies have shown that between 13–31% of all bulimia nervosa (BN) patients will attempt suicide at least once during the course of their illness [16]. In addition, there is evidence that shows weight and low self-esteem associated with poor body image affects quality of life, leading to an increased risk of suicide in patients with binge eating disorder (BED) and/or morbid obesity, including those who undergo bariatric surgery [14].

In addition to an increased risk of suicide, ED patients also have high rates of other psychiatric comorbidity. Compared to the general population they have an increased incidence of mood and anxiety disorders, obsessive-compulsive disorder, and substance abuse, all of which can contribute to increased usage of the healthcare system. The emergency department and other acute care settings represent important points of entry into the healthcare system for many people and may be the only available access for some ED patients. An emergency department visit may also represent an ideal "teachable moment" during which a patient is more receptive to information concerning their disorder. The same visit may be the only opportunity for any healthcare provider to recognize the ED and intervene on behalf of the patient. It is, therefore, very important that all physicians and other healthcare providers be aware

Behavioral Emergencies for the Emergency Physician, ed. Leslie S. Zun, Lara G. Chepenik, and Mary Nan S. Mallory. Published by Cambridge University Press. © Cambridge University Press 2013.

of the signs and symptoms that are consistent with eating disorders, and be prepared to treat them appropriately.

Prevalence and types of eating disorders

Although AN is the first diagnosis that many think of in relation to eating disorders, it is actually the least common diagnosis. Traditional estimates for a lifetime prevalence of AN are consistently around 0.5%-1% based on strict diagnostic criteria as defined in the Diagnostic and Statistical Manual of Mental Disorders, 4th Edition (DSM-IV). Recent studies, however, suggest this may have increased over the past few decades to be as high as 0.9%-2.2% [17]. AN is characterized by a refusal to maintain body weight at or above a minimally normal weight for age and height (< 85% of that expected), an intense fear of gaining weight or becoming fat, and an undue influence of body weight or shape on self-evaluation. Patients with AN also often deny the seriousness of their illness despite very low body weights [18]. AN can be either of a purely restrictive type or a binge/purge type. Current DSM-IV criteria also include amenorrhea as a diagnostic criteria for AN, but this has recently been under debate and will likely be removed in the upcoming DSM-V due to its inapplicability in many patients (all males and premenarchal females or those on oral contraceptives) and lack of diagnostic utility [19]. Multiple other changes in the diagnostic criteria for all eating disorders are anticipated in the upcoming DSM-V, which is scheduled for release in May 2013.

Bulimia nervosa (BN) also involves self-evaluation that is unduly influenced by body shape and weight. BN is, however, characterized by recurrent episodes of binge eating that are accompanied by a sense of lack of control over eating during the episode as well as recurrent inappropriate compensatory behavior, or purging, to prevent weight gain. Compensatory methods of purging include self-induced vomiting, misuse of laxatives, diuretics, enemas or other medications, fasting, and/or excessive exercise [18]. These behaviors occur, on average, at least twice a week for 3 months. By definition, patients with BN do not meet weight criteria for AN (< 85% of expected) and their weight is often normal or above normal. Lifetime prevalence estimates for BN are usually around 1–3%, and have been as high as 4.6% in some studies [17,20].

The final diagnostic category for eating disorders is currently the one most commonly used. Eating disorder not otherwise specified (EDNOS) encompasses any clinically significant eating disorder (one that causes distress and/or impairment) that does not meet full criteria for either AN or BN [21]. Recent prevalence studies estimate a current prevalence for EDNOS of approximately 4% [22], while other studies have suggested that as many as 5.3–10.6% of the general population will suffer from some form of EDNOS during their lifetime [23,24]. Binge eating disorder (BED), which is the most common form of EDNOS, is defined by recurrent episodes of binge eating without any compensatory behaviors. BED has been included as a provisional diagnosis for DSM-V and is significant due to its frequent association with obesity [19,25]. BED is unique among EDs in that approximately 40% of cases occur in males. It has a total lifetime prevalence of 5.5% or approximately 3.5% in women and 2.0% in men [25].

Although EDs can occur in anyone, they most often have their onset during adolescence and young adulthood and are thought to be much more common in females than males. Traditional estimates place a 10:1 female to male ratio for most EDs. Some recent studies, however, have seen much higher rates in males, and it has been suggested that this gender gap is closing [26]. Minorities now also have rates of EDs equivalent to those of Caucasian populations [27]. Other individuals at high risk for the development of an ED are athletes, especially those involved in sports that emphasize weight or extreme fitness such as ballet, gymnastics, running, wrestling, and body-building. Adolescent females with Type I diabetes mellitus and post-bariatric surgery patients are other high-risk groups [28,29].

Medical complications of eating disorders

There are a multitude of medical complications associated with EDs (see Table 19.1). These complications can be either directly related to the effects of starvation and/or to the frequency and type of purging behaviors used, and range in severity from very mild to potentially life-threatening. Many of these complications will be covered in the following sections. It is important to note that patients with EDs are often quite reluctant to disclose their illness to healthcare providers and may present to the emergency department with vague non-specific complaints rather than complaints directly attributable to their ED. Identification and proper management of these patients requires the healthcare provider to maintain a high index of

Table 19.1. Signs and symptoms of eating disorders

General	Hematologic
– Marked weight loss, gain, or fluctuations in weight	– Pancytopenia
– Failure to gain/grow as expected in child or adolescent	– Decreased erythrocyte sedimentation rate
– Cold intolerance	Endocrine
– Weakness	– Poor glycemic control in diabetics/DKA
– Fatigue	– Amenorrhea or irregular menses
– Dizziness/syncope	– Loss of libido
– Oral/facial	– Decreased bone density/osteoporosis/fractures
– Oral trauma	– Infertility
– Dental erosion/caries	– Thyroid abnormalities – euthyroid sick syndrome
– Parotid gland enlargement	– Hypercortisolemia
– Perimyolysis	– Neurogenic diabetes insipidus
– Cheilosis	– Arrested growth

Table 19.1. (cont.)

– Sore throat	– Hypoglycemia
Cardiovascular	Metabolic
– Bradycardia	– Hypokalemia
– Hypotension	– Hyponatremia
– Mitral valve prolapse	– Hypophosphatemia (refeeding)
– Sudden cardiac death	– Dehydration
– Chest pain	– Nephropathy
– Palpitations	– Metabolic acidosis
– Arrhythmias	– Pseudo-Bartter's syndrome
– Cardiomyopathy (emetine)	– Hypothermia
– Peripheral edema	Neurologic
– Orthostasis	– Seizures
Pulmonary	– Decreased concentration
– Dyspnea	– Memory loss
– Aspiration	– Insomnia
– Spontaneous pneumothorax	– Peripheral neuropathy
– COPD	– Cerebral atrophy
– Respiratory failure	Psychiatric
Gastrointestinal	– Depression
– Abdominal pain	– Anxiety
– Gastroparesis	– Self-harm
– Prolonged gastric transit/delayed gastric emptying	– Suicide
– GERD	– Irritability/mood changes
– Hematemesis/Mallory-Weiss tear	Dermatalogic
– Hemorrhoids and rectal prolapsed	– Lanugo hair
– Constipation	– Alopecia
– Hepatitis	– Yellowish skin discoloration (carotenoderma)
– Pancreatitis (refeeding)	– Brittle nails
– Acute gastric dilatation/rupture	– Dry skin
– Esophageal rupture	– Pruritis
– SMA syndrome	– Callus/scar on dorsum of hand (Russell's sign)
	– Poor wound healing
	– Acrocyanosis

a Life-threatening complications are in darker shading.

suspicion for these illnesses and to readily recognize signs and symptoms consistent with ED pathology. Common presenting complaints include headache, mood changes, sore throat, dizziness/syncope, palpitations, fatigue/generalized weakness, sports-related or overuse injuries, and gastrointestinal (GI) complaints such as indigestion, abdominal pain, bloating, constipation, and hematemesis, but many others are possible.

Cardiovascular complications

Cardiovascular complications are common in ED patients and may appear early in the illness. Patients may present with complaints of chest pain, palpitations, lightheadedness/syncope or they may have asymptomatic electrocardiogram (ECG) changes. Any of these complaints should prompt a thorough evaluation which includes a complete blood count (CBC), basic metabolic panel (BMP), magnesium and phosphorus levels, and an ECG. Arrhythmias, particularly sinus bradycardia, and ECG changes are the most frequent abnormalities seen [30]. Sinus bradycardia (HR < 60) in AN is an adaptive physiologic response to starvation and is thought to be mediated by increased vagal tone to cardiac muscle [31]. The degree of bradycardia correlates significantly with the severity of the illness as measured by BMI [32]. It is important to note that almost all significantly undernourished patients will be bradycardic [32]. A "normal" heart rate (70–90 bpm) in an AN patient who has a baseline rate of 50 bpm is a cause for concern and should trigger further evaluation for the etiology of this relative tachycardia [33]. Other ECG changes include low voltage tracings, right axis deviation, nonspecific ST-T segment changes, U waves, conduction disturbances, and prolonged QTc interval [30]. The cause of prolonged QTc in these patients is not always clear, but may be related to electrolyte abnormalities. Due to its association with malignant arrhythmias and death, this finding should always prompt admission to a monitored bed and further evaluation for underlying etiology [30]. Some investigators have proposed that it is actually increased QTc dispersion (interlead variation of QTc), which can also be seen in these patients, rather than the prolonged QTc that leads to an increased risk of ventricular arrhythmia and sudden cardiac death, but studies have had inconsistent findings to date [32,34]. Electrolyte abnormalities such as hypokalemia or hypocalcemia also contribute to the development of arrhythmias and ECG changes and should be treated aggressively with supplementation when discovered.

Hypotension is also frequently seen in ED patients and is likely multifactorial in nature. In addition to volume depletion due to fluid restriction and/or purging, structural changes to the heart contribute to a significant decrease in BP in many of these patients. Cardiac muscle atrophy results in decreased left ventricular wall muscle mass, diminished force of myocardial contraction, and decreased cardiac output all of which contribute to hypotension. Autonomic dysfunction can also lead to decreased blood pressure response to exercise, and decreased heart rate variability, as well as decreased peripheral vascular tone with resultant orthostasis. These changes are generally reversible with adequate nutrition and weight restoration [35]. A word of caution regarding treatment of these patients in the acute setting – avoid aggressive IV fluid resuscitation in the ED patient who is hypotensive but otherwise hemodynamically stable. It is important to recognize that a BP of 78/50 may be baseline for a young woman with a significantly low body mass index and that rather than improving BP, rapid infusion of fluids may quickly lead to volume overload and resultant congestive heart failure in a patient whose heart has been weakened by starvation [17]. Slow continuous infusions of 50–75 cc/hour are generally recommended in the tachycardic and/or hypotensive ED patient who is alert, mentating appropriately and otherwise at baseline [33].

In addition to cardiomyopathy related to starvation, some ED patients may develop a potentially fatal cardiomyopathy that results from the use of Syrup of Ipecac to induce vomiting. The active ingredients in Ipecac are potent alkaloids, cephalin, and emetine. Emetine is directly toxic to both cardiac and skeletal muscle. With repeated use over a relatively short period of time (a few months) emetine accumulates in muscle tissue. A cumulative dose as low as 1250 mg (~40 doses at 32 mg emetine/dose) can lead to irreversible damage to the myocardium with resultant arrhythmias, valvular insufficiency, cardiomegaly, decreased ejection fraction, and congestive heart failure (CHF). These patients may present in the acute care setting with shortness of breath, decreased exercise tolerance, pulmonary edema, increased jugular venous distension, and other signs of heart failure. Treatment of these patients is the same as for other causes of cardiomyopathy (diuresis, preload reduction, etc.) as there are no specific antidotes or other treatments for an emetine-induced cardiomyopathy [33,36].

Other cardiac complications that are seen in ED patients are of unclear clinical significance. Mitral valve prolapse (MVP) has an increased incidence in ED patients. It has been reported in as many as 20% of those with AN and is thought to be related to the relatively large size of the mitral valve in relation to the atrophied left ventricular wall that results from starvation. MVP is associated with an increased risk for arrhythmias, but is otherwise generally a benign condition. Pericardial effusion is also frequently seen in AN patients, but is usually small and does not cause significant compromise. Both of these findings resolve with weight restoration [30].

Pulmonary complications

Although less common than some other ED-related problems, pulmonary complications are seen and can be life threatening. Self-induced vomiting can lead to aspiration pneumonitis, pneumothorax, pneumomediastinum, and subcutaneous emphysema [17]. Spontaneous pneumothorax has been seen in AN patients who may also develop early COPD possibly related to decreased surfactant levels [33]. In addition, weakened respiratory muscles can lead to the development of respiratory insufficiency with hypoxia and hypercarbia. As for any patient presenting to the emergency department with complaints of dyspnea, decreased exercise tolerance, cough, and/or chest pain, appropriate laboratory studies (complete blood count, basic metabolic panel, blood cultures if febrile), a chest X-ray, and possibly an ECG should be obtained. Supplemental oxygen should be provided as needed. Intubation should be considered in any patient in significant respiratory distress, but only after a careful evaluation for unilateral decreased breath sounds consistent with pneumothorax to avoid development of tension physiology that may be associated with positive pressure ventilation of a patient with a pneumothorax. Tube thoracostomy may be required if a significant pneumothorax is present. Arterial blood gases may help to determine the level of respiratory insufficiency and need for respiratory support.

Gastrointestinal complications

Gastrointestinal (GI) complaints such as abdominal pain, bloating, and constipation are among the most common symptoms for which ED patients seek medical care. These symptoms may reflect relatively mild disease, or may indicate a life-threatening condition. Indigestion or heartburn may be caused by repeated exposure of the esophagus to gastric acids from recurrent vomiting which can lead to gastroesophageal reflux (GERD), esophagitis, and esophageal spasm. Hematemesis can result from small lacerations of the esophageal mucosa, known as Mallory-Weiss tears, or may indicate more serious pathology such as esophageal rupture due to forceful vomiting (Boerhaave's syndrome) [37]. The complaint of increased chest pain with yawning is concerning for Boerhaave's. Any concern for this syndrome should prompt a thorough evaluation for esophageal rupture that includes a chest X-ray, direct visualization of the esophagus (endoscopy), and/or computed tomography scan of the chest. Mediastinitis with sepsis can develop rapidly in these patients and carries a high mortality rate [38].

Prolonged starvation, chronic vomiting, and chronic laxative abuse can all lead to significant slowing of the entire GI tract. Gastroparesis, or delayed gastric emptying, may be due to prolonged starvation and/or recurrent vomiting [33,39]. It results in nausea and vomiting, as well as abdominal bloating and discomfort which are increased with food intake. Treatment is mostly supportive using IV fluids, antiemetics, and promotility agents such as metoclopramide. Abdominal X-rays, which will be normal or show nonspecific changes in gastroparesis, may be necessary to differentiate this condition from others such as small bowel obstruction (SBO), which can manifest with similar symptoms. Acute gastric dilatation can also present with abdominal pain, distension, and vomiting. Although relatively rare, gastric dilatation has been reported in ED patients both as the result of massive bingeing and during the process of refeeding, and can lead to fatal gastric rupture [39]. Constipation is also related to slowed GI (colonic) motility and may develop as a consequence of chronic laxative abuse, electrolyte abnormalities, hypovolemia, and starvation. Long-term use of stimulant laxatives may directly damage colonic nerves and result in cathartic colon syndrome or a complete lack of colonic motility [39].

Less common GI complications reported in ED patients include acute hepatitis secondary to fatty infiltration, fulminant hepatic failure, pancreatitis, and superior mesenteric artery (SMA) syndrome [30,33,40]. Biliary colic and/or cholecystitis can also be seen, even in very malnourished ED patients who have had rapid weight loss or repeated cycles of gaining and losing weight. In addition to a basic metabolic panel, liver function tests and pancreatic enzyme levels should also be assessed in ED patients who present with significant complaints of epigastric or right upper quadrant abdominal pain with or without vomiting. SMA syndrome refers to a functional obstruction of a portion of the duodenum due to its compression between the aorta, vertebral column and the SMA and will manifest with symptoms similar to a SBO. Acute treatment is short-term bowel rest, IV fluids, and gastric decompression. The syndrome is caused by loss of the fat pad that normally surrounds the SMA and, although it will resolve with weight gain, some patients may require temporary placement of feeding tube distal to the point of obstruction [33].

Metabolic and electrolyte abnormalities

There are many electrolyte disturbances commonly associated with eating disorders. These are more common in patients who purge and are largely related to the most frequently used method of purging which can include self-induced vomiting, laxative and/or diuretic abuse. Restriction of fluid intake and starvation can also result in significant abnormalities. Electrolyte abnormalities affect nearly every organ system, and their consequences can be potentially life threatening. It is important to note, however, that many ED patients, particularly those with restrictive anorexia, will have normal laboratory studies despite severe malnourishment. Therefore, the lack of electrolyte abnormalities does not necessarily exclude severe malnourishment or other ED complications.

Hypokalemia is the most frequent electrolyte abnormality seen in ED patients. Decreased potassium can be seen in any ED patient, but seriously decreased levels (< 2.5 mEq/L) are almost exclusively related to purging behaviors such as vomiting or laxative/diuretic abuse. In fact, in the absence of other possible causes of vomiting such as viral illness, the unexpected finding of significant hypokalemia in an otherwise healthy appearing adolescent or young woman is very specific for BN and should prompt further investigation for possible purging behavior. Mild hypokalemia (3.0–3.5 mEq/L) is often asymptomatic and can be treated with oral potassium supplementation over 1–2 days. It is important to remember that serum potassium levels measure only extracellular potassium and may not accurately reflect the total body depletion. A general rule of thumb is that each 0.5–1.0 mEq/L deficit in serum potassium will require 100–200 mEq/L of oral potassium supplementation to normalize [33]. More significant hypokalemia, however, predisposes patients to the development of potentially fatal cardiac arrhythmias [17]. Any patient with a potassium of < 2.5 mEq/L should be admitted to the hospital for IV potassium supplementation and continued cardiac monitoring. In the presence of a significant hypochloremic metabolic alkalosis, ongoing renal losses of potassium will prevent adequate potassium repletion until the alkalosis is resolved. This is secondary to ongoing secretion of aldosterone that is triggered by dehydration. This will cause ongoing renal potassium losses until the dehydration and alkalosis are

corrected. In such cases, patients with less severe hypokalemia (2.5–3.0 mEq/L) should be admitted for treatment as well. Judicious use of IV fluids containing sodium chloride (50–75 cc/hr for 1–2 L) will correct the underlying dehydration and allow for adequate potassium replacement. Rapid IV fluid administration can lead to peripheral edema without resulting in intravascular volume repletion and should be avoided [33,41].

Hyponatremia may be due to dehydration or can be related to excess water intake, or "water-loading," in a patient who has a decreased ability to clear free water due to low renal solute load. Use of diuretics and selective serotonin reuptake inhibitors may exacerbate hyponatremia in these patients [17]. Serum sodium levels below 120 mEq/L can result in seizures and death. Treatment of hyponatremia in ED patients depends on its cause and is similar to that caused by other conditions. Administration of normal saline (NS) should be carefully monitored with a goal of increasing the serum sodium by 4–6 mEq/L in first 1–2 hours and no more than 8–10 mEq/L in the first 24 hours. Rapid increases in serum sodium should be avoided due to the risk of central pontine myelinolysis and the use of hypertonic (3%) saline should be reserved for symptomatic patients.

Other electrolyte abnormalities such as hypochloremia and hypocalcemia, as well as micronutrient deficiencies, can also be seen in ED patients. Low magnesium levels are often found concomitantly with hypokalemia and can be associated with muscle cramping, weakness, paresthesias, and arrhythmias. Oral magnesium supplementation is usually sufficient except in severe cases [37]. Hypophosphatemia associated with refeeding is potentially fatal and will be discussed later in the chapter.

Metabolic alkalosis is the most common acid–base disturbance seen in patients who purge, and a serum bicarbonate of >38 is highly suggestive of self-induced vomiting [33]. Severe diarrhea secondary to laxative abuse may result in a non-ion gap metabolic acidosis acutely, but with chronic use most patients develop a mild metabolic alkalosis and severe hypokalemia. Renal dysfunction in ED patients may also contribute to acid–base disturbances. Most renal abnormalities are pre-renal in nature secondary to purging or decreased fluid intake; however, chronic AN patients are also at risk for intrinsic renal disease and renal failure [37].

Patients with very low body weight may also be hypothermic. This is a reflection of the reduced basal metabolic rate that results from chronic starvation and usually indicates severe malnutrition.

Endocrine complications

Long-term complications of EDs include infertility, amenorrhea or irregular menses, osteoporosis, arrested growth, hypercortisolemia, and thyroid abnormalities and are beyond the scope of this chapter. Acute endocrine abnormalities such as significant hypo- or hyperglycemia in ED patients, however, can be life-threatening. Hypoglycemia is usually mild, but when severe has resulted in the death of patients with AN [42,43]. In addition, adolescent and young adult females with Type I diabetes mellitus (DM) have a well-documented increased risk for eating disorders. The incidence of DM-related EDs has been increasing over the past decade and has recently led to the use of the term "diabulimia" to describe the unique ED behaviors of some patients with DM. This term refers to the intentional manipulation of insulin to result in weight loss. The result is poor glucose control. These patients are at high risk for recurrent diabetic ketoacidosis (DKA) in the short term, and have much higher incidence of many of the long-term complications of diabetes [43]. These patients are also at risk of suicide by insulin overdose. Treatment of DKA in these patients is similar to that of other patients, and includes IV fluids, electrolyte replacement, and insulin [43]. The physician, however, should be cognizant of the fact that severely malnourished patients are at risk for cardiomyopathy related to decreased cardiac muscle mass. They, therefore, have increased potential for fluid overload and resultant pulmonary edema with aggressive fluid resuscitation, and should be monitored very closely for the development of related symptoms [33].

Neurologic complications

Brain imaging has shown significant cerebral atrophy and ventricular enlargement in very malnourished ED patients. This atrophy may manifest as complaints of cognitive impairment such as decreased concentration and memory loss [44]. Peripheral neuropathies are also seen in AN patients and may be related to vitamin B and/or other micronutrient deficiencies [30]. These changes are generally reversible with weight restoration, but some patients may experience permanent cognitive deficits. Seizures have also been reported in ED patients and may be related to medications (e.g., buproprion) and/or hypoglycemia.

Other complications

Although not acutely life-threatening, some of the classic signs and symptoms of EDs are quite helpful in recognizing patients with an occult ED. Parents may bring their child or adolescent in for concerns of weight loss or failure to grow. Older patients might complain of generalized fatigue or weakness, cold intolerance, or dizziness – none of which are diagnostic in and of themselves, but when taken in consideration with other findings, should heighten suspicion for an eating disorder.

Other commonly described findings include the development of lanugo hair (fine hair growth in places where hair doesn't normally grow); alopecia; carotenoderma (skin discoloration due to high levels of carotene); brittle nails; dry, itchy skin; poor wound healing; and acrocyanosis. Russell's sign (callus or scar on dorsum of hand that has been used repeatedly to induce vomiting) is considered a classic sign of BN, but in fact is seen very infrequently in patients. Absence of this sign does not necessarily mean the absence of self-induced vomiting, as many seasoned bulimics can force vomiting by voluntary abdominal muscle contraction. Oral trauma, dental erosion, perimyolysis (increased erosion on lingular surface of maxillary teeth), cheilosis (cracking and erythema at the corners of the mouth), and parotid gland enlargement can also be seen [17,33].

Significant hematologic abnormalities are not commonly seen in ED patients. Mild iron deficiency anemia may be present but is often masked by volume contraction such that the patient's complete blood count appears normal. Starvation is one of the few causes of decreased sedimentation rate, but this is a very nonspecific finding. Pancytopenia can be seen in severe AN cases due to bone marrow hypoplasia, but is generally rapidly reversible with adequate nutrition [17].

Guide to the eating disorder patient's medicine cabinet

Many of the complications seen in ED patients may be related to the use or abuse of several medications. As discussed above, abuses of laxatives and diuretics is common in ED patients and can lead to dehydration, metabolic and electrolyte abnormalities, renal failure, and other problems.

Other medications frequently used for appetite suppression in ED patients are stimulants. The use of prescription stimulants for the treatment of attention-deficit/hyperactivity disorder has increased dramatically over the past two decades. Their increased availability on many high school and college campuses has undoubtedly contributed to their increased misuse and abuse over the same time period [45]. Signs and symptoms suggestive of inappropriate stimulant use include tachycardia, mydriasis, sweating, and agitation. Abuse of other substances, including alcohol, is also increased in ED patients. Some studies find that as many as 41% of patients with EDs will also be affected by a substance use disorder at some point in their illness [46].

It is also important to remember that many ED patients have psychiatric comorbidities and may be on any number of psychotropic medications which are frequently used in suicide attempts/overdose [30]. Signs and symptoms related to these medications depend on the particular drug involved, but many cause arrhythmias (tricyclic antidepressants), QTc prolongation (antipsychotics), seizures (buproprion), hypotension, respiratory suppression, altered mental status (benzodiazepines), and even death. A full toxicological evaluation including ECG and basic laboratory studies as well as salicylate, acetaminophen, and ethanol levels is warranted in any patient suspected of overdose. Treatment is mostly supportive with airway protection as needed, IV fluids and cardiac monitoring being critical.

Complications of recovery

In addition to the multiple complications directly associated with eating disorder behaviors, there are a few other problems that arise in ED patients once they begin refeeding and/or cease purging. While the most severely malnourished patients are usually initially treated and stabilized in an inpatient setting, there is an increased emphasis on family-based outpatient treatments of many ED patients, some of whom are at increased risk for complications during the initial recovery period. These complications include relatively benign conditions such as sialadenosis. Sialadenosis is caused by chronic hypertrophy of the parotid glands due to chronic vomiting and overproduction of saliva. It usually appears 3–4 days after the cessation of vomiting and may cause patients to present for evaluation due to painless or mildly painful bilateral swelling of the parotid glands. This is a benign, self-limiting condition, and reassurance is the only treatment necessary [33].

Other problems that can arise in the recovery period, however, are much more serious and can lead to fatal complications. Purging and/or diuretic use can lead to chronic dehydration which stimulates renal aldosterone production. During the first 2–3 weeks after these patients stop purging, they are at risk for developing severe edema along with worsening metabolic alkalosis and electrolyte abnormalities, most notably hypokalemia and hypomagnesemia. This condition is known as Pseudo-Bartter's syndrome and is due to the chronic hyperaldosteronism related to dehydration and purging [33,41]. The key to treating these patients is volume repletion with slow IV fluid replacement (50–75 cc/hr. of NS) along with potassium and magnesium supplementation. Rapid boluses of large volumes of IV fluid should be avoided, and some patients may initially benefit from low-dose spironolactone which will block excess aldosterone production and stop ongoing renal potassium losses [33].

Refeeding syndrome is another very serious condition that can develop in the ED patient's initial recovery period [17,30,33]. This syndrome was first described during World War II when it was noted that many of the newly released concentration camp victims died shortly after being rescued and given food by well-meaning soldiers. It was later discovered hypophosphatemia primarily contributed to refeeding syndrome. Prolonged starvation causes many fluid and electrolyte shifts. The body maintains homeostasis by shifting intracellular electrolytes to the extracellular space such that measured serum levels may appear relatively normal despite severe total body depletion. In the early stages of refeeding, release of insulin leads to an increased cellular uptake of phosphorus and other electrolytes. Serum levels can rapidly drop to dangerous levels if refeeding occurs too quickly or without adequate monitoring and replacement of electrolytes. While it is true that the most severely malnourished patients are likely to be hospitalized during the early stages of refeeding and, therefore, unlikely to present to an emergency department for care, significant hypophosphatemia can also develop in patients who are much closer to or even at a normal weight. A patient with only a slightly low weight is still at significant increased risk if they have had little or no nutritional intake for >5 days, a history of alcohol abuse and/or the use of medications including insulin, chemotherapy, antacids, or diuretics [33]. This means that a patient who appears normal or only slightly underweight and is undergoing outpatient treatment for an eating disorder (or who is attempting to recover on their own) may indeed present to the emergency department with signs and symptoms of refeeding syndrome. These symptoms are largely related to hypophosphatemia and include neurologic (confusion, seizures, coma), cardiac (arrhythmias, heart failure), hematologic (hemolysis), and muscular (weakness, rhabdomyolysis, diaphragm weakness leading to respiratory failure) complications [30,33]. Refeeding syndrome can be prevented by careful monitoring during the early refeeding process. For the emergency physician it is important to note that, even in a hypotensive patient with symptoms of refeeding syndrome, IV fluids should be used very cautiously. Rapid administration of IV fluids can lead to volume overload, pulmonary edema, and worsening heart failure. Emergency department treatment of patients with suspected refeeding syndrome includes slow administration of IV fluids (50–70 cc/hour of NS), aggressive replacement of electrolytes and hospital admission to a monitored, or possibly intensive care, bed.

Management of eating disorder patients in the acute care setting

It is imperative that all healthcare providers maintain a supportive, nonjudgmental stance toward the patient. With all minors (less than 18 years old) and, whenever possible, with adult patients, involve family members and the patient's significant other. It is also imperative that the EM physician recognizes and treats all potentially life-threatening abnormalities. In general, management of acute symptoms in ED patients is quite similar to treatment of those same symptoms in any other patient. There are a few caveats to this, however. It is important to remember that a severely malnourished patient with AN will likely be hypotensive (SBP < 90 mmHg) and bradycardic (HR < 60). This is true in both adults and younger patients. A "normal" heart rate in a severely underweight patient is actually a cause for concern and a thorough search for the etiology of this relative tachycardia should be undertaken. Look for sources of fever, dehydration, and signs of decompensation such as altered mental status.

Equally important to consider is the judicious use of IV fluids in the ED patient. As with every patient, use fluids as needed to stabilize vital signs, but avoid "flooding" the patient with excess fluids. Many of these patients will have significant heart muscle atrophy and excess fluids can quickly lead to volume overload, pulmonary edema, and heart failure. In addition, edema caused by rapid administration of IV fluids can be very counterproductive in these patients who are so attuned to their body size and shape and may result in worsening of restriction, diuretic use, etc., to compensate for the excess fluids.

Electrolyte replacement is also very important in these patients. Significant abnormalities in electrolytes can also be a clue to ED behaviors in an otherwise asymptomatic patient who denies any ED symptoms. Hypokalemia is very common in BN patients and in AN patients who purge. Any young, otherwise healthy patient who presents with significantly low potassium (< 3.0 mEq/L) and/or elevated bicarbonate (>35 mEq/L) should be suspected of purging. Also keep in mind that psychiatric comorbidities are common in these patients and they should all be screened for suicidal ideation.

Disposition

In addition to generally accepted indications for hospital admission for any patient, there are specific indications for admission of an eating disordered patient. Table 19.2 contains guidelines from the Society for Adolescent Health [47] concerning these indications. The American Psychiatric Association has published similar guidelines for use in adult patients, with the main difference being a weight recommendation which is ≤85% of ideal body weight (IBW) for an adult (IBW=100 lbs for a person 5 ft. tall + 5 pounds for every inch over 5 ft.)

The majority of patients with EDs recover fully; however, prognosis is much improved by early diagnosis and effective early treatment. The risk of developing a chronic, treatment-resistant ED increases with every year that the patient goes un- or inadequately treated [2,48]. Successful, definitive treatment is most often quite lengthy (3–5 years) and will obviously not be accomplished in the acute care setting. It is imperative, however, that any healthcare provider in an acute care setting, such as the emergency department, who has identified a patient who likely suffers from an ED, refer this patient for appropriate specialty care. For patients who do not require hospitalization, it is very important to ensure adequate follow-up care with the patient's primary care provider (PCP) and/or ED specialist. ED-related resources should also be given directly to the patient and family members. Ideally, the EM provider who has concerns for an occult ED in a patient will relate these concerns to the PCP whenever possible. It is also helpful to know the local resources available in your area. If you are unsure, or there are not any, there are several online sources of information on eating disorder treatment specialists throughout the country. These include the Academy for Eating Disorders (http://www.aedweb.org), the National Eating Disorders Association (http://www.neda.com), and ED Referral (http://www.EDReferral.com), among others.

Screening

Patients with severe AN are often easier to identify due to their obvious emaciation, but less severe cases are often overlooked by healthcare providers and other professionals. Patients with BN or EDNOS, on the other hand, are normal to overweight and may have no obvious abnormalities at first glance. Also, time constraints in the ED or other acute care facility limit the utility of widespread screening for EDs. All healthcare providers must, therefore, maintain a high index of suspicion for these potentially fatal illnesses. Targeted screening of individuals at high risk for EDs, especially in the presence of potentially ED-related complaints can lead to early identification and treatment and vastly improved outcome for these patients. Although there are many screening tools for EDs available, the majority of them are too lengthy or difficult to administer in the emergency department. The SCOFF questionnaire (Table 19.3), however, is a brief screening tool that is easy to remember and administer and that has been shown to have good sensitivity and specificity for identification of patients with EDs in several different patient care settings [49]. Assessment of associated psychiatric comorbidities such as substance use, depression, and/or suicidal ideation is strongly recommended in these patients as well.

Conclusions

Eating disorders are serious mental illnesses that have multiple psychiatric and medical comorbidities and high rates of mortality. Effective interventions do exist and most patients recover fully with good treatment. ED and other healthcare visits represent an opportunity for early recognition and intervention in patients who are often otherwise reluctant to disclose their illness secondary to denial and/or embarrassment.

Table 19.2. Society for Adolescent Health guidelines for hospitalization of an eating disorder patient [47]

Severe malnutrition (weight ≤ 75% average body weight for age, sex, and height)
Dehydration
Electrolyte disturbances (hypokalemia, hyponatremia, hypophosphatemia)
Cardiac dysrhythmia
Physiologic instability – Severe bradycardia (heart rate < 50 awake, < 45 sleeping) – Hypotension (BP <N 80/50 mmHg) – Hypothermia (body temperature < 96°F or 35.6°C) – Orthostatic changes in pulse (>20 beats per minute) or blood pressure (>10 mmHg)
Arrested growth and development
Failure of outpatient treatment
Acute food refusal
Uncontrollable bingeing and purging
Acute medical complications of malnutrition (e.g., syncope, seizures, cardiac failure, pancreatitis, etc.)
Acute psychiatric emergencies (e.g., suicidal ideation, acute psychosis)
Comorbid diagnosis that interferes with the treatment of the eating disorder (e.g., severe depression, OCD, severe family dysfunction)

Table 19.3. The SCOFF questionnaire [49]

1.	Do you make yourself Sick because you feel uncomfortably full?
2.	Do you worry you have lost Control over how much you eat?
3.	Have you recently lost Over 14 pounds[a] in a 3-month period?
4.	Do you believe yourself to be Fat when others say you are too thin?
5.	Would you say that Food dominates your life?

[a] Changed from one stone in original version of SCOFF from the United Kingdom [1]. 1 stone = 14 pounds.

It is important that all providers be aware of the signs and symptoms of eating disorders and maintain a high index of suspicion for these illnesses especially in high-risk populations. If you suspect an eating disorder in one of your patients – say something! A visit to the emergency department is a frightening experience for many ED patients. It may also represent an excellent "teachable moment" and opportunity to provide life-saving intervention and referral.

References

1. Harris E, Barraclough B. Excess mortality of mental disorder. *Br J Psychiatry* 1998;**173**:11–53.

2. Chamay-Weber C, Narring F, Michaud P. Partial eating disorders among adolescents: a review. *J Adolesc Health* 2005;**37**:417–27.

3. Fairburn C, Cooper Z, Doll H, Norman P, O'Connor M. The natural course of bulimia nervosa and binge eating disorder in young women. *Arch Gen Psychiatry* 2000;**57**:659–65.

4. Hautala L, Junnila J, Alin J, et al. Uncovering hidden eating disorders using the SCOFF questionnaire: cross-sectional survey of adolescents and comparison with nurse assessments. *Int J Nurs Stud* 2009;**46**:1439–47.

5. Johnston O, Fornai G, Cabrini S, Kendrick T. Feasibility and acceptability of screening for eating disorders in primary care. *Fam Pract* 2007;**24**:511–17.

6. Mond J, Myers T, Crosby R, et al. Screening for eating disorders in primary care: EDE-Q versus SCOFF. *Behav Res Ther* 2008;**46**:612–22.

7. Ogg E, Millar H, Pusztai E, Thom A. General practice consultation patterns preceding diagnosis of eating disorders. *Int J Eat Disord* 1997;**22**:89–93.

8. Striegel-Moore R, Dohm F, Kraemer H, et al. Health services use in women with a history of bulimia nervosa or binge eating disorder. *Int J Eat Disord* 2005;**37**:11–18.

9. Crow S, Praus B, Thuras P. Mortality from eating disorders – a 5- to 10-year record linkage study. *Int J Eat Disord* 1999;**26**:97–101.

10. Birmingham C, Su J, Hlynsky J, Goldner E, Gao M. The mortality rate from anorexia nervosa. *Int J Eat Disord* 2005;**38**:143–6.

11. Fichter M, Quadflieg N, Hedlund S. Twelve-year course and outcome predictors of anorexia nervosa. *Int J Eat Disord* 2006;**39**:87–100.

12. Hoek H. Incidence, prevalence and mortality of anorexia nervosa and other eating disorders. *Curr Opin Psychiatry* 2006;**19**:389–94.

13. Keel P, Dorer D, Eddy K, et al. Predictors of mortality in eating disorders. *Arch Gen Psychiatry* 2003;**60**:179–83.

14. Pompili M, Girardi P, Tatarelli G, Ruberto A, Tatarelli R. Suicide and attempted suicide in eating disorders, obesity and weight-image concern. *Eat Behav* 2006;**7**:384–94.

15. Crow S, Peterson C, Swanson S, et al. Increased mortality in bulimia nervosa and other eating disorders. *Am J Psychiatry* 2009;**AiA**:1–5.

16. Franko D, Keel P, Dorer D, et al. What predicts suicide attempts in women with eating disorders? *Psychol Med* 2004;**34**:843–53.

17. Agras W, editor. *The Oxford Handbook of Eating Disorders*, (1st Edition). New York, NY: Oxford University Press; 2010.

18. American Psychiatric Association *Diagnostic and Statistical Manual of Mental Disorders*, (4th Edition). Waltham, MA: American Psychiatric Association; 1994.

19. Striegel-Moore R, Wonderlich S, Walsh B, Mitchell J, (Eds.). *Developing an Evidence-Based Classification of Eating Disorders*. Scientific Findings for DSM-V, (1st Edition). Arlington, VA: American Psychiatric Association; 2011.

20. Keel P, Heatherton T, Dorer D, Joiner T, Zalta A. Point prevalence of bulimia nervosa in 1982, 1992, and 2002. *Psychol Med* 2006;**36**:119–27.

21. American Psychiatric Association *Diagnostic and Statistical Manual of Mental Disorders*: DSM-IV-TR, (4th Edition). Waltham, MA: American Psychiatric Association; 2000.

22. Crowther J, Armey M, Luce K, Dalton G, Leahey T. The point prevalence of bulimic disorders from 1990 to 2004. *Int J Eat Disord* 2008;**41**:491–7.

23. Favaro A, Ferrara S, Santanastaso P. The spectrum of eating disorders in young women: a prevalence study in a general population sample. *Psychosom Med* 2003;**65**:701–8.

24. Wade T, Bergin J, Tiggermann M, Bulik C, Fairburn C. Prevalence and long-term course of lifetime eating disorders in an adult Australian twin cohort. *Aust N Z J Psychiatry* 2006;**40**:121–8.

25. Hudson JI, Hiripi E, Pope H G Jr, Kessler R C. The prevalence and correlates of eating disorders in the National Comorbidity Survey Replication. *Biol Psychiatry* 2007;**61**:348–58.

26. Domine' F, Berchtold A, Akre' C, Michaud P, Suris J. Disordered eating behaviors: what about boys? *J Adolesc Health* 2009;**44**:111–17.

27. Shaw H, Ramirez L, Trost A, Randall P, Stice E. Body image and eating disturbances across ethnic groups: more similarities than differences. *Psychol Addict Behav* 2004;**18**:12–18.

28. Young-Hyman D, Davis C. Disordered eating behavior in individuals with diabetes: importance of context, evaluation and classification. *Diabetes Care* 2010;**33**:683–9.

29. Segal A, Kinoshita Kussunoki D, Larino M. Post-surgical refusal to eat: anorexia nervosa, bulimia nervosa or a new eating disorder? A case series. *Obes Surg* 2004;**14**:353–60.

30. Katzman D. Medical complications in adolescents with anorexia nervosa: a review of the literature. *Int J Eat Disord* 2005;**37**(Suppl):S52–9.

31. Nudel D, Gootman N, Nussbaum M, Shenker I. Altered exercise performance and abnormal sympathetic responses to exercise in patients with anorexia nervosa. *J Pediatr* 1984;**105**:34–7.

32. Panagiotopoulos C, McCrindle B, Hick K, Katzman D. Electrocardiographic findings in patients with eating disorders. *Pediatrics* 2000;**105**:1100–5.

33. Mehler P, Anderson A. *Eating Disorders: a Guide to Medical Care and Complications*, (2nd Edition). Baltimore, MD: The Johns Hopkins University Press; 2010.

34. Swenne I, Larsson P. Heart risk associated with weight loss in anorexia

nervosa and eating disorders: risk factors for QTc prolongation and dispersion. *Acta Paediatr* 1999;**88**:304–9.

35. Mont L, Castro J, Herreros B, et al. Reversibility of cardiac abnormalities in adolescents with anorexia nervosa after weight recovery. *J Am Acad Child Adolesc Psychiatry* 2003;**42**:808–13.

36. Silber T. Ipecac syrup abuse, morbidity, and mortality: isn't it time to repeal its over-the-counter status? *J Adolesc Health* 2005;**37**:256–60.

37. Pomeroy C, Mitchell J. *Medical complications of anorexia nervosa and bulimia nervosa.* In: Fairburn CG, Brownell UD (Eds), *Eating Disorders and Obesity: A Comprehensive Handbook,* (2nd Edition). New York: Guilford Press; 2002: 278–85.

38. Chen K, Chen J, Kuo S, et al. Descending necrotizing mediastinitis: a 10-year surgical experience in a single institution. *J Thor Cardiov Surg* 2008;**136**:191–8.

39. Zipfel S, Sammet I, Rapps N, et al. Gastrointestinal disturbances in eating disorders: clinical and neurobiological causes. *Auton Neurosci* 2006;**129**:99–106.

40. Mitchell J, Crow S. Medical complications of anorexia nervosa and bulimia nervosa. *Curr Opin Psychiatry* 2006;**19**:438–43.

41. Mitchell J, Pomeroy C, Seppala M. Pseudo-Bartter's Syndrome, diuretic abuse and eating disorders. *Int J Eat Disord* 1988;**7**:225–37.

42. Mattingly D, Bhanji S. Hypoglycaemia and anorexia nervosa. *J R Soc Med* 1995;**88**:191–5.

43. Goebel-Fabbri A. Disturbed eating behaviors and eating disorders in type 1 diabetes: clinical significance and treatment recommendations. *Curr Diab Rep* 2009;**9**:133–9.

44. Lask B, Gordon I, Christie D, et al. Functional neuroimaging in early onset anorexia nervosa. *Int J Eat Disord* 2005;**37**:S49.

45. Bogle K, Smith B. Illicit methylphenidate use: a review of prevalence, availability, pharmacology, and consequences. *Curr Drug Abuse Rev* 2009;**2**:157–76.

46. Piran N, Robinson S. Associations between disordered eating behaviors and licit and illicit substance use and abuse in a university sample. *Addict Behav* 2006;**31**:1761–75.

47. Golden N, Katzman D, Kreipe R, et al. Eating disorders in adolescents: position paper of the society for adolescent medicine. *J Adolesc Health* 2003;**33**:496–503.

48. Steinhausen H. The outcome of anorexia nervosa in the 20th century. *Am J Psychiatry* 2002;**159**:1284–93.

49. Hill L, Reid F, Morgan J, Lacey J. SCOFF, the development of an eating disorder screening questionnaire. *Int J Eat Disord* 2010;**43**:344–51.

Chapter 20

Management of the emergency department patient with co-occurring substance abuse disorder

David S. Howes and Alicia N. Sanders

Introduction

Serious mental illness (SMI) with concomitant substance use disorder (SUD) has been referred to in the following terms: dual diagnosis, comorbidity, or, as we will be using in this chapter, co-occurring disorder (COD). According to the Co-occurring Center for Excellence, a COD is defined as a person who "has one or more substance-related disorder[s] as well as one or more mental disorders." The Co-occurring Center for Excellence was created in 2003 by the Substance Abuse and Mental Health Services Administration (SAMHSA) to be the leading national resource for the topic of COD [1].

In this chapter, we will describe the epidemiology of COD, discuss its assessment and suggest the use of simplified diagnostic criteria to confirm substance use disorder in a patient with known or suspected serious mental illness (SMI), assess and treat the patient with known or suspected SMI for a concurrent drug intoxication, and discuss disposition of the COD patient who is no longer acutely intoxicated, withdrawing or suffering from an acute medical condition. We will review the relevant literature that specifically addresses the acute ED evaluation and management of such patients in support of our recommendations.

Epidemiology

Increasingly appreciated over the last several decades, SMI and SUD co-occur at high rates. A frequently quoted large study by Kessler et al. [2] reviewed the epidemiology of co-occurring addictive and mental disorders with regard to implications for prevention and service usage. They found that up to 66% of non-institutionalized adults living with a lifetime addictive disorder also had at least one co-occurring mental disorder; conversely, 51% of people living with one or more lifetime mental illnesses had at least one co-occurring addictive disorder [2].

Of note, in studying the prevalence of COD, most investigations use patients with an SMI as the base population to examine the rates of co-occurring substance use. Few reports address the risk of patients with lifetime SUD developing an SMI. Also, much of the SMI literature focuses primarily on those suffering from schizophrenia, mood disorders, and/or

anxiety disorders. A classic older report found that 47% of schizophrenics had at least one SUD in their lifetime, 32% of those with mood disorder had at least one SUD, and up to 15% of patients with anxiety disorders had a co-occurring SUD. In this large 1990 study, the most frequently associated co-occurring substance of dependence or abuse was alcohol, especially in schizophrenia and mood disorders such as dysthymia and bipolar, followed by cannabis and cocaine [3].

More recent data from Drake and Mueser show that alcohol abuse by schizophrenic patients remains prevalent and in the range of previous reports [4], although there has been an increase in cocaine use in this population [5]. However, a report by Clarke et al. reveals a dramatic doubling in the rate of SUD in patients with mood disorders, rising to greater than 60% over the last two decades [6].

Epidemiologic studies of COD show varying rates in specific populations. Study of geographic residence has shown that rural residents with SMI have higher rates of SUD than their urban counterparts [7]. Mericle et al. [8] reported that rates of COD varied significantly by race/ethnicity with 8.2% of whites, 5.8% of Latinos, 5.4% of blacks, and 2.1% of Asians meeting criteria for lifetime COD. Whites were more likely than persons in each of the other groups to have lifetime COD. In all groups, the majority of patients with COD reported that symptoms of SMI preceded SUD. Only rates of unemployment and history of psychiatric hospitalization among individuals with COD were found to vary significantly by racial/ethnic group [8]. Overall, it has been found that among all populations, those with CODs experience more poor health episodes and poorer lifetime health outcome, are more likely to be non-domiciled, and have higher rates of unemployment than patients with either SMI or SUD alone [9].

Assessment in the emergency department setting

The differences between the management of a patient in the outpatient setting and the emergency department (ED) are evident in a passage from the Treatment Improvement Protocol (TIP) for "Substance Abuse Treatment for Persons with Co-Occurring Disorders" (2005) promulgated by the Center for Substance

---

Behavioral Emergencies for the Emergency Physician, ed. Leslie S. Zun, Lara G. Chepenik, and Mary Nan S. Mallory. Published by Cambridge University Press. © Cambridge University Press 2013.

Abuse Treatment: "Many may think of the typical person with COD as having a severe mental disorder combined with a severe substance use disorder, such as schizophrenia combined with alcohol dependence. However, counselors working in addiction agencies are more likely to see persons with severe addiction combined with mild- to moderate-severity mental disorders; an example would be a person with alcohol dependence combined with a depressive disorder or an anxiety disorder. Efforts to provide treatment that will meet the unique needs of people with COD have gained momentum over the past two decades in both substance abuse treatment and mental health services settings" [10].

In the ED setting, patients with potential or known COD typically present with acute behavioral disturbance. The primary issue is to discern whether the presentation is primarily due to the underlying mental disorder or acute drug intoxication. Less frequently, a withdrawal syndrome or acute medical illness should be considered. We know that the majority of patients with COD have SMI symptoms before emergence of symptoms of SUD [8]; therefore, the clinician might first attempt to elicit a history of mental illness. The vast majority of ED patients with a history of SMI will have evidence of such a diagnosis in previous ED visits or will admit to same. Thus, the first issue to be resolved is whether or not the patient is now presenting with an acute drug intoxication complicating the assessment of the underlying mental disorder [10,11]. This is a two-stage process; if the patient is able to cooperate, they should be screened for a history of substance abuse, and then assessed for an acute drug intoxication syndrome. We offer a novel ED screening examination for SUD that consists of seven questions that is brief, straightforward, easily (and quickly) administered and interpreted. The Drug Abuse Screening Test Modified for ED (DAST-ED) is adapted for specific use in the ED and is based on two well-known drug abuse screening tests that have been well studied and validated for use in the outpatient setting (Table 20.1) [12,13].

Once the ED physician has established that the patient has a history of SMI and, more likely than not, has SUD, then a tentative diagnosis of COD is likely – at this point, *an acute intoxication should be ruled out:*

- Attention to the vital signs (VS) is paramount. If the blood pressure (BP) and pulse (P) are high, a sympathomimetic intoxication, e.g., cocaine, methamphetamine, MDMA, or phencyclidine may be present. If the BP, respiratory rate (RR), and/or oxygen saturation are low, then opioid, barbiturate, or benzodiazepine intoxication should be suspected.
- Fever, if present, mandates a careful search for an infectious or environmental cause.
- Check the pupils – they are dilated in sympathomimetic intoxications and constricted in acute opioid use.
- Ask the patient – the history of acute intoxicant use as reported by the patient has been assessed in both the outpatient and ED settings and has been found to be both highly sensitive and specific as compared to results of a clinical assessment for the presence of a toxidrome and formal drug testing [11,14,15].
- Ask the family and friends for corroborating evidence.
- Assess the patient's orientation to person, place, and time. Disorientation favors an acute delirium due to intoxication or medical illness rather than primary acute mental illness.
- The ED patient presenting with isolated acute phase mental illness should have a steady gait, be awake and alert, and is usually able to cooperate with a history and physical examination.
- *The most important management strategy in the initial evaluation of the ED patient with acute behavioral disturbance is to evaluate for the presence of an acute intoxication or other medical condition and stabilize the patient* (Table 20.2).

Table 20.1. Drug Abuse Screening Test Modified for ED (DAST-ED).
"Drug" includes prescription, over-the-counter (OTC), herbal therapies, and illicit drugs.
- Three or more positive = high likelihood of substance abuse problem
- 1–2 positive = possible substance use disorder
- 0 positive = substance use disorder unlikely (or noncompliance, sociopathy)

1.	Do you ever feel bad or guilty about your drug use?
2.	Have you neglected your family, friends, or missed work because of your use of a drug?
3.	Does your spouse, parents or other family members ever complain about your involvement with any drug?
4.	Have you gone to anyone for help for a drug problem?
5.	Have you ever been arrested or brought to the ED for unusual behavior while under the influence of a drug?
6.	Have you ever experienced withdrawal symptoms (felt sick) when you stopped taking any drug?
7.	Have you ever gone to the ED or been hospitalized for a medical problem related to drug use?

This table adapted from two versions of the Drug Abuse Screening Test (DAST) and questions have been modified to specifically address the ED population. The original DAST developed in 1982 consisted of 28 questions [12]. The more recent DAST was modified in 1989 to include 20 questions (http://counsellingresource.com/lib/quizzes/drug-testing/drug-abuse/) and both have been validated for inpatient and outpatient use [13].

Table 20.2. Clinical features and ED treatment of drug intoxication syndromes

Drug class	Clinical features	ED treatment (Rx): All receive supportive care (IVF +/- cardiac monitor) + specific Rx below
Alcohol	VS okay (although can be tachycardic), pupils constricted or midrange, can be very obtunded or belligerent, slurred speech, unsteady gait, + sniff for ETOH	Low–moderate dose antipsychotic, e.g., haloperidol or ziprasidone, useful for agitation (minimize benzodiazepine use); restrain, prn,
Cocaine	BP and P high, pupils dilated, amped up, impulsive, aggressive, agitated	Benzodiazepine drug of choice
Cannabis	VS OK, pupils midrange, slowed speech, lethargic, unsteady gait, disoriented, repeating phrases, food stigmata, +sniff for cannabis odor	Low dose antipsychotic if reassurance does not reduce paranoid reaction
Methamphetamine	BP and P high, pupils dilated, amped up, impulsive, aggressive, agitated, belligerent, can be scary	Benzodiazepine drug of choice
Opioids	RR and O_2 saturation low, pupils constricted, slurred speech, lethargic	Supplemental O_2; naloxone
MDMA	BP and P high, pupils dilated, awake and mellow, oral issues and "connected to everyone"	Reassurance, bite block?
Benzodiazepines	VS OK, pupils midrange, but comatose or headed that way	*Avoid reversal agent, e.g., flumazenil*; O_2, respiratory support as indicated
Barbiturates	BP, RR, and temp low, pupils midrange, comatose	O_2, respiratory support as indicated
Ketamine	BP and P high, eyes bobbing, catatonic	Restrain as indicated; low–moderate dose benzodiazepine for agitation
PCP	BP and P high, pupils dilated, amped up, repeating phrases, aggressive, agitated, belligerent, strong and scary	Restrain as indicated; moderate- high dose benzodiazepine for agitation
LSD/psilocybin/ mescaline	BP and P high, pupils dilated, "lights on but no one home," groovy	Restrain as indicated; late Beatles – Ravi Shankar music in background?

VS, vital signs; BP, blood pressure; P, pulse rate; RR, respiratory rate; O_2, oxygen.

A common-sense approach to the ED patient with acute behavioral disturbance primarily involves a brief clinical assessment as noted above and will serve as an effective initial screening tool. Keep in mind that drug-induced intoxications, drug withdrawal syndromes, metabolic disturbance, and infectious conditions can induce mental status changes that may mimic acute mental illness, and this is an important management strategy in the initial approach to the behaviorally disturbed patient. If an acute intoxication, withdrawal state or other medical condition is found, the patient must be stabilized and observed until sobriety is attained and/or the acute medical condition has resolved in a manner that allows an appropriate psychiatric interview and assessment.

The *assessment of the acute phase of SMI* is straightforward and should include the following:

- Psychiatric history
  - What's the diagnosis and how long is the SMI history?
  - Outpatient treatment history – last visit?
  - Last psychiatric hospitalization? How many in last year?
- Medications? Taking them? If not, when stopped?
- Are they working or going to school? (important to know level of functioning)
- Living situation?
- Family/friends in the picture?
- Current substance abuse?

- Current prescribed medications, over-the-counter medications, and herbal treatments?
- Is the patient at imminent risk of harm to self or others for psychiatric reasons?
- Can they take care of themselves?
- Does the patient have a safe place to stay if discharged?

Treatment of the ED patient

Treatment of the ED patient with acute behavioral disturbance initially focuses on stabilization of the patient, addressing and promptly correcting abnormal VS, treating specific target symptoms and vital sign abnormalities based on the presence of a suspected drug intoxication(s), and additional supportive care with observation until such time as the patient is no longer exhibiting signs of intoxication, withdrawal, or mental status changes due to an acute medical condition.

Keeping in mind the recommendations for treatment of specific drug intoxications offered in Table 20.2 (Clinical features and ED treatment of drug intoxication syndromes), the following general guidelines in the treatment of the patient with acute behavioral disturbance can be helpful:

- Anxiety and low grade agitation should be treated with reassurance and small doses of a benzodiazepine, e.g., lorazepam, 1 mg, po, IM, or IV. Please wait 20–30 minutes before re-dosing.

- Psychosis should be addressed with antipsychotics, e.g., start with haloperidol, 5 mg po, IM, or IV or ziprasidone, 25 mg po or 10 mg IM or IV.
- Severe agitation and psychosis should be treated with:
  - Restraints – protect the patient and the staff.
  - A combination of an antipsychotic and benzodiazepine, e.g., haloperidol 5–10 mg and lorazepam 1–2 mg IM or IV. Please wait 20–30 minutes before re-dosing.

Disposition from the ED setting

Once the patient is sober, unrestrained, alert, stable on their feet, and cooperative, they may be assessed for underlying acute SMI as discussed above. The patient who now denies or has never had suicidal or homicidal ideation or intent during the ED visit, can care for themselves, and has a safe place to return may be discharged with referrals to outpatient treatment [16–18]. If the patient does not meet these criteria, further evaluation by a psychiatric healthcare professional and consideration for admission to an inpatient mental health facility is indicated. This is especially important in the adolescent population when suicidal ideation is present [19,20], the older male patient, or the patient who has few resources to assure medication compliance and adherence to an appropriate follow-up regimen [16].

Treatment in the outpatient setting

Treatment strategies for COD have evolved over the past two decades. In the past, many clinicians were trained to treat either SMI or SUD. Recent approaches to the treatment of the COD patient focuses on integrated care as studies have shown that COD patients have higher rates of relapse and poorer treatment outcomes than those with only SMI or SUD [21]. These patients are also more frequently hospitalized and have longer hospital stays [22].

Treatment targeted to an SUD may also effectively treat the patient's comorbid SMI. For example, in patients who suffer from schizophrenia, olanzapine appears more effective than first- or second-generation antipsychotics in reducing SUD cravings, specifically for cocaine [5,23]. For depression, the most studied associated SUD has been alcohol. A small study has shown that combined treatment with naltrexone and sertraline resulted in a higher rate of 14-week abstinence than treatment with either drug alone [24]. For bipolar disorder and concomitant alcohol use, recent recommendations support a combination of the mood stabilizers lithium carbonate and valproic acid [25].

Psychosocial treatments shown to be effective include motivational interviewing, cognitive behavioral therapy, and social skills training. Although the trends in such interventions are popular and may be helpful in selected patients, research fails to support their superiority over routine care [26].

Summary

Patients with co-occurring disorders (COD), defined as serious mental illness (SMI) and concomitant substance use disorders (SUD) are common ED patients. We have stressed the importance of careful assessment of both the SMI and SUD components of the COD patient who presents to the ED with acute behavioral disturbance. Development of a management plan should emphasize stabilization of the patient, address and promptly correct abnormal VS, treat specific target symptoms based on specific drug intoxication syndromes, and provide supportive care and observation until such time as the patient no longer exhibits signs of intoxication, withdrawal, or mental status abnormalities attributable to an acute medical condition. When the patient is sober, cooperative and can engage the examiner sufficiently to complete a brief evaluation of the underlying mental illness issues, a determination of safe disposition from the ED can then follow [27].

References

1. U.S. Department of Health and Human Services. *About Co-occurring*. Substance Abuse and Mental Health Services Administration Newsletter. U.S. Department of Health and Human Services. Available at: http://www.samhsa.gov/co-occurring/ (Accessed December 22, 2011).

2. Kessler RC, Nelson CB, McGonagle KA, et al. The epidemiology of co-occurring addictive and mental disorders: implications for prevention and service utilization. *Am J Addict* 1996;**66**:17–31.

3. Regier DA, Farmer ME, Rae DS, et al. Comorbidity of mental disorders with alcohol and other drug abuse. Results

from the Epidemiologic Catchment Area (ECA) Study. *JAMA* 1990;**264**:2511–18.

4. Drake RE, Mueser KT. *Co-Occurring Alcohol Use Disorder and Schizophrenia*. National Institute on Alcohol Abuse and Alcoholism, National Institutes of Health, November 2002. Available at: http://pubs.niaaa.nih.gov/publications/arh26-2/99-102.htm

5. Sayers SL, Campbell EC, Kondrich J, et al. Cocaine abuse in schizophrenic patients treated with olanzapine versus haloperidol. *J Nerv Ment Dis* 2005;**193**:379–86.

6. Clark RE, Samnaliev M, McGovern MP. Treatment for co-occurring mental and

substance use disorders in five state Medicaid programs. *Psychiat Serv* 2007;**58**:942–8.

7. Simmons LA, Havens JR. Comorbid substance and mental disorders among rural Americans: results from the national comorbid survey. *J Affect Disord* 2007;**99**:265–71.

8. Mericle AA, Ta Park VM, Holck P, Arria AM. Prevalence, patterns, and correlates of co-occurring substance use and mental disorders in the United States: variations by race/ethnicity. *Compr Psychiatry* 2011 [Epub ahead of print].

9. Roberts A. Psychiatric comorbidity in white and African-American illicit substance abusers: evidence for

differential etiology. *Clin Psychol Rev* 2011;**20**:667–77.

10. Center for Substance Abuse Treatment. *Substance Abuse Treatment for Persons With Co-Occurring Disorders.* Treatment Improvement Protocol (TIP) Series 42. DHHS Publication No. (SMA) 05-3922. Rockville, MD: Substance Abuse and Mental Health Services Administration; 2005. Available at: http://www.ncbi.nlm.nih.gov/books/NBK25700/.

11. Lee MO, Vivier PM, Diercks DB. Is the self-report of recent cocaine or methamphetamine use reliable in illicit stimulant drug users who present to the Emergency Department with chest pain? *J Emerg Med* 2009;**37**:237–41.

12. Skinner HA. The drug abuse screening test. *Addict Behav* 1982;**7**:363–71.

13. Gavin DR, Ross HE, Skinner HA. Diagnostic validity of the Drug Abuse Screening Test in the assessment of DSM-III drug disorders. *Br J Addict* 1989;**84**:301–7.

14. Kellerman A, Fihn SD, LoGerfo JP, Copass MK. Impact of drug screening in suspected overdose. *Ann Emerg Med* 1987;**16**:1206–16.

15. Perrone J, De Roos F, Jayaraman S, Hollander JE. Drug screening versus history in detection of substance use in ED psychiatric patients. *Am J Emerg Med* 2001;**19**:49–51.

16. Owens PL, Mutter R, Stocks C. *Mental Health and Substance Abuse-related Emergency Department Visits, 2007.* AHRQ Statistical Brief #92, July 2010. Available at: http://www.hcup-us.ahrq.gov/reports/statbriefs/sb92.pdf.

17. Caton CL, Hasin DS, Shrout PE, et al. Stability of early-phase primary psychotic disorders with concurrent substance use and substance-induced psychosis. *Br J Psychiatry* 2007;**190**:105–11.

18. Ries RK, Yuodelis-Flores C, Comtois KA, Roy-Byrne PP, Russo JE. Substance-induced suicidal admissions to an acute psychiatric service: characteristics and outcomes. *J Subst Abuse Treat* 2008;**34**:72–9.

19. King CA, O'Mara RM, Hayward CN, Cunningham RM. Adolescent suicide risk screening in the emergency department. *Acad Emerg Med* 2009;**16**:234–41.

20. Esposito-Smythers C, Spirito A, Kahler CW, Hunt J, Monti P. Treatment of co-occurring substance abuse and suicidality among adolescents: a randomized trial. *J Consult Clin Psychol* 2011;**79**:728–39.

21. Pages KP, Russon JE, Wingerson DK, et al. Predictors and outcome of discharge against medical advice from the psychiatric units of a general hospital. *Psychiat Serv* 1998;**49**:1187–92.

22. Ding K, Yang J, Cheng G, et al. Hospitalizations and hospital charges for co-occurring substance use and mental disorders. *J Subst Abuse Treat* 2011;**40**:366–75.

23. Smelson DA, Ziedonis D, Williams J, et al. The efficacy of olanzapine for decreasing cue-elicited craving in individuals with schizophrenia and cocaine dependence: a preliminary report. *J Clin Psychopharmacol* 2006;**26**:9–12.

24. Pettinati HM, Oslin DW, Kampman KM, et al. A double-blind, placebo-controlled trial combining sertraline and naltrexone for treating co-occurring depression and alcohol dependence. *Am J Psychiatry* 2010;**167**:668–75.

25. Salloum IM, Cornelius JR, Daley DC, et al. Efficacy of valproate maintenance in patients with bipolar disorder and alcoholism: a double-blind placebo-controlled study. *Arch Gen Psychiatry* 2005;**62**:37–45.

26. Cleary M, Hunt G, Matheson S, Siegfried N, Walter G. Psychosocial interventions for people with both severe mental illness and substance misuse. *Cochrane Database Syst Rev* 2008;**1**:CD001088.

27. Agency for Healthcare Research and Quality. *Detoxification and Substance Abuse Treatment: Co-occurring Medical and Psychiatric Conditions.* National Guideline Clearinghouse. Agency for Healthcare Research and Quality. December 2011. Available at: http://www.ngc.gov/content.aspx?id=9119.

Chapter

21

Use of verbal de-escalation techniques in the emergency department

Janet S. Richmond

Introduction

In a busy emergency department (ED), agitation requires immediate attention and intervention. When one thinks about agitation, one usually thinks of the wildly out of control patient who requires immediate restraint and/or medication. However, agitation should be considered to be on a continuum: the patient who begins to become upset may be able to calm down and cooperate with staff without medication but with skilled interviewing techniques, while the patient who is brought in acutely psychotic or handcuffed by the police, may not be able to cooperate through a verbal exchange [1,3].

This chapter will address methods of verbal de-escalation for the patient who is agitated, but still in control, or who can regain control without the need for restraints or medication, but who, without some verbal intervention, could escalate into full-blown agitation and behavioral dyscontrol. This chapter addresses effective verbal de-escalation techniques which are easy to learn and quick to implement. Verbal de-escalation takes no more than five or ten minutes. These recommendations are in part based on the author's clinical experience and a consensus panel of emergency psychiatry clinicians [1].

The patient is stressed and the clinician may be as well. The patient may be unwilling or unable to provide much history, and may give conflicting information. Additionally, other patients and the physician, often pressed for time, can be pulled, with the patient into irrational thinking [1,2]. De-escalation is a team effort, and any member of the staff can do whatever he can to help. Generally, the first person to approach the patient should be the one to engage the patient. Other ED staff – nursing staff, security often have years of experience and special interest in the management of agitated patients, and are skillful at de-fusing tense situations. It is best if only one person talks to the patient to avoid excessive stimulation for the patient. Thus, as in a cardiac code, one staff-person (preferably someone skilled and comfortable with de-escalation and/or who knows the patient) should be in charge of the de-escalation and talk to the patient. If that person is not comfortable, then another staff member should take over.

Agitation: definition

Agitation can be defined as a hyperaroused state in which the individual exhibits excessive, repeated, purposeless motor or verbal behavior. Examples of such behavior is pacing, fidgeting, clenching fists or teeth, a prolonged stare, picking at clothing or skin, threatening to or actually throwing objects, or responding to internal stimuli, usually auditory or visual hallucinations. Such patients often look around the room trying to "track" or locate the source of the voices. Agitation should be considered to be on a continuum ranging from anxiety to outright violence.

Types of agitation

The following diagnostic categories are those in which agitation may be the presenting symptom or become a prominent feature (Tables 21.1, 21.2, and 21.3).

Signs of escalating agitation

Increased pacing, irritability, impatience, frustration, verbal outbursts, slamming or banging objects, an exaggerated startle response, and increased sweating or hyperventilation are all signs of escalating agitation. Labile affect and paranoia can also lead to increased agitation. Defiant, demanding, or threatening behaviors are also signs of escalation [2,3].

The clinician needs to monitor any changes in behavior or affect minute-by-minute and respond quickly to avoid further escalation. Furthermore, the clinician must pay careful attention to his own minute-by-minute reactions and feelings, which are diagnostic indicators of the patient's emotional state [2,4]. The BARS is a standardized instrument that can also be used to measure a patient's level of agitation. A score of four indicates the presence of increasing agitation [5].

Goals of treatment of the agitated patient

Symptom reduction and management is what emergency physicians do best, and this applies to agitation as well. Agitation like

Behavioral Emergencies for the Emergency Physician, ed. Leslie S. Zun, Lara G. Chepenik, and Mary Nan S. Mallory. Published by Cambridge University Press. © Cambridge University Press 2013.

Table 21.1. Conditions that may cause agitation

1. COGNITIVE IMPAIRMENTS
   Deliriuim
   Drug/EtOH Intoxication /withdrawal
   Dementia
   Mental Retardation/Developmentally delayed
   Traumatic brain injury (TBI)

2. PERCEPTUAL DISTURBANCES
   Paranoia
   Psychosis including mania

3. MOOD DISORDERS
   Anxiety
   Depression with agitation

4. TRAUMATIC EVENTS
   Acute trauma
   PTSD

5. PAIN
   Acute pain

6. DRUG REACTIONS
   Akathisia

7. METABOLIC
   hyper/hypoglycemia,
   hyperthyroidism-myxedema

8. NEUROLOGIC
   Acute head trauma
   partial complex seizure disorder/temporal lobe epilepsy

9. OTHER
   Hypoxia
   Personality disorders
   Medication-seeking/substance abusers

Adapted from Zun L: Optimizing ED Neurological Emergency Patient Care FERNE (Foundation for Education and Research in Neurological Emergencies, UIC University of Illinois at Chicago) / MEMC V 2009. Accessed 8/14/11 [3].

Table 21.2. Summary of approaches to the agitated patient

Determine level of agitation of the patient
Elicit patient's "request"
Show willingness to listen
Be genuine, flexible, honest
Recognize your own reactions
Provide empathic responses
Observe for rapidly fluctuating emotional changes
Assure back-up and your own safe exit

any other acute symptom must be addressed directly and swiftly, even when the etiology is not readily apparent. Because a patient cannot be treated until he is cooperative, the goal of any encounter with an agitated patient is to help him become cooperative, stay in control and prevent further escalation.

Why verbal de-escalation?

Medication and restraint have been traditionally considered standard treatment for agitation. However, it is time consuming

Table 21.3. Summary of interviewing techniques

Be empathic
Be honest and flexible
Talk to the patient from the doorway if this is safer than sitting in room with patient
Appeal to the patient's rational side
Agree with the patient as much as you can
Leave the exam room when necessary
Take a break
Summarize
Bargain
Offer choices
Set limits
State consequences of behavior

in that it requires many staff-persons and planning. Moreover, it puts the patient in a submissive position. Nonphysical interventions such as negotiation and discussion are a means of role modeling for the patient using methods of resolving conflicts without violence. When restraints are used, what is reinforced is that physical force is the only method of conflict resolution, which the agitated patient already believes to be true. It also reinforces that it is others, not he, who ultimately have the ability to contain his behavior [1]. Restraint and seclusion are no longer considered treatment but coercive techniques to be avoided unless there is imminent danger without any alternative [6]. Furthermore, these procedures can be dehumanizing, humiliating [7], traumatizing, (see Chapter 32), and in some cases can actually lead to further escalation of agitation [1,6,8–12].

In its policy, the Massachusetts Department of Mental Health states that alternatives to seclusion and restraint use a "strength-based, patient-driven approach" that "enhance(es) self-esteem," provides "modeling, mentoring, supervision... foster(s) a healing environment for patients and a supportive environment for staff" [6]. Staff morale is enhanced because "managing a behavioral emergency competently can be very rewarding" [2].

Beck et al. [13] found that the use of restraints correlated with an increased rate of inpatient admissions.

While the effectiveness of verbal de-escalation is mentioned in the literature, very little has been written about the actual techniques in how to do this, with few exceptions [1,2,14,15]. One emergency medicine textbook does discuss the need for establishing rapport and recommends sound principles: be fully engaged with the patient, be polite, do not argue with the patient or family, and attempt to negotiate whenever there is a conflict [16].

There is indirect evidence from pharmacologic [17] and other studies of agitation [18] that verbal techniques can be successful in a large minority of patients. In a recent study

[17], patients were excluded from a clinical trial of droperidol if they were successfully managed with verbal de-escalation. However, specific verbal de-escalation techniques were not identified.

Safety: the environment

If the clinician or other staff do not feel safe, then no treatment can occur. Thus, the environment and the type and quantity of staff are important. Because existing emergency departments have different physical layouts, each facility must deal with their particular space limitations. It is generally recommended, however, that a quiet area away from the more active ED with accessibility to emergency restraints and medication is ideal. Also, physical proximity of the psychiatric area to the main ED is desirable for medical issues and any extra staff that might be needed.

Movable furniture allows for flexible and equal access to exits for both patient and staff. Also, the ability to quickly take furniture out of the area can expedite the creation of a safe environment. Objects which can be thrown or otherwise used as weapons (such as pens, books, etc.) should be removed as well. Some emergency departments prefer stationary furniture, so that the patient cannot use the objects as weapons, but this may create a false sense of security. TV monitors can also be helpful so that patients can be monitored from the nursing station. It is also advised that agitated patients, who may have come with items which can be used as weapons (medications, shoelaces, pens, matches as well as overt weapons such as knives and guns) require close observation and depending on the policy of each ED, most likely will benefit from a clothing search. Some facilities call this a "health and safety" search, done by either nursing personnel or security.

Staffing

When working with an agitated patient, staff must always be prepared for the worst-case scenario, which generally involves physical restraint of the patient. Thus, working with an agitated patient is a team effort and there must be an adequate number of people to fill each role on the team. Placing a patient in restraints should ideally involve six people – one for each limb, one for the head and one to apply restraints, but at least four should be present – one person per limb. A "show of force" in an emergency department requires less staff than in other situations, such as a contained inpatient setting, A show of force not exceeding six people is considered best, and these people should be the team members assigned the specific roles noted above. It is best if these roles are assigned at the beginning of a shift with backup available if a team member is unavailable when needed [1]. Larger numbers of staff (as may be needed on an inpatient unit) are inappropriate for the ED, because many strangers can increase the patient's sense of fear and loss of control. However, this does not rule out calling for backup from stronger staff members, security officers, or police, if the situation cannot be handled by hospital personnel.

General approaches to the agitated patient

The best treatment for agitation is to prevent it, or prevent it from escalating. To that end, the following recommendations are discussed for the emergency physician who does not readily have a psychiatric clinician available to him.

The goals of verbal de-escalation are to contain the patient's emotional turmoil, define the problem(s) [2] and elicit what Lazare et al. [19] have described as a "request." These goals also help build a therapeutic alliance. These goals help build rapport.

Establishing rapport: working together on a problem

Establishing rapport is the basis of every doctor–patient relationship, and this is critical with the agitated patient. The patient needs to know that the physician will work with him to resolve his dilemma. There is evidence that the better the relationship, the less likelihood of further escalation of agitation or violence [20].

In building this relationship, caution should be given to presuming a working relationship prematurely, or dwelling too long on establishing one when it is already assumed by the patient [2]. For example, by virtue of the physician's role as a helper and healer, there may be an a-priori alliance. Just walking in with a white coat, stethoscope, and a caring attitude establishes enough for many patients. However, this too is not always the case. Past unpleasant or even traumatic experiences with medical staff or with an ED can generalize to all physicians and all hospitals. Past traumatic events such as difficult past medical treatments or procedures may make the patient more wary of the physician (e.g., the child who fears "a shot" or a patient who has undergone grueling chemotherapy can be "triggered" by being once again in a hospital, which he associates with pain and suffering). (See Chapter 32.)

Finally, some patients perceive the very need to seek help as being humiliating and shameful, causing them anxiety that can escalate to agitation. Lazare suggests that physicians, too, mainly because of their training, can be exquisitely sensitive to humiliation [7]. Power struggles can ensue when both patient and doctor feel disempowered and (fear being) humiliated.

The clinician's demeanor

Body language, speech, and attitude

Physical posture is important. The clinician must demonstrate by body language that he will not harm the patient, that he wants to listen, and wants everyone to be safe. Normal, friendly eye contact should be used, but excessive eye contact, especially staring, can be interpreted as an aggressive act. If the patient is pacing, one recommendation is to walk with the patient, but at a slower pace [15] as is stooping so as to make oneself appear smaller is also a consideration [1,15,21,22].

Both the patient and clinician should have equal access to the exit; neither should feel "trapped." The clinician should not crowd the patient and should stand or sit at least an arm's length from the patient. If a patient tells you to get out of the room, do so [1,21].

Direct eye contact may be too threatening to the patient. Hands should be visible and not clenched. Concealed hands, either behind one's back or in one's pockets, can raise the patient's suspicion that the clinician may have a concealed weapon [1,15,21,22]. Closed body language, such as arm folding or turning away can communicate lack of interest. The message, verbal and otherwise, is that "I want to help, I'm here to listen. Let's talk about this."

For an escalating patient, offering food, water, a blanket or allowing the patient to make a telephone call might well decrease the degree of agitation.

Slow, repetitive, soft speech is best with the escalating patient to help him regain control [1,21,22]. This is referred to as the "broken record" technique [23], which is surprisingly very effective because it eventually forces the patient to stop his activity and pay attention to the clinician's attempts to contain the situation [1].

Agitated patients can be provocative, and may challenge the authority, competence, or credentials of the clinician. Some patients, to deflect their own sense of vulnerability, are exquisitely sensitive in detecting the clinician's vulnerability and focusing on it. In these instances, the clinician should understand his own vulnerabilities, tendencies to retaliate, argue, or otherwise become defensive [2,24]. Such behaviors on the part of the clinician only serve to worsen the situation and create iatrogenic escalation.

If the physician can remind himself that the patient's behavior is not willful, but part of his psychophathology, that can help diminish some of the frustration [1].

For example, the delirious, psychotic, intoxicated, or intellectually disabled patient is impaired in their ability to cooperate. Others with dysfunctional personality traits are demonstrating ingrained, automatic behavior developed during childhood either due to psychological trauma or other problem with early infant–parent attachment. These are the only strategies these patients know that will get their needs met and are automatic because they are so ingrained. Patients do not come to the ED purposely to frustrate or get into arguments with the physician, but it may seem that way in a busy ED with a boisterous and agitated patient.

Finally, flexibility, spontaneity, and authenticity (being "real" and nondefensive) are very useful character traits for working with the agitated patient.

Eliciting the patient's "request"

Patients come to EDs with wants and needs, not always verbalized [19,25]. As stated earlier, eliciting the patient's "request" is a major part of establishing rapport. Lazare et al. [19] identify many "requests" that patients have, even if not verbalized. Examples include succorance, the wish to vent to an empathic listener, a request for medication, some administrative intervention, such as a letter to an employer or intervening with a difficult spouse or parent. Whether or not the request can be granted, all patients need to be asked what their request is. The aggressive patient is no exception. Thus, a statement like, "I really need to know what you expected when you came here" is as essential, as is the caveat "Even if I can't provide it; I would like to know, so we can work on it" [1]. If an agitated patient comes to the ED demanding medication, it may be best to give him the desired medication if appropriate, even if the way it was requested was not. Given the need for quick symptom reduction, honoring the patient's request may be very useful, as the patient knows best what works for him. By not addressing the request, the patient may feel dismissed, misunderstood, and unheard. At least a discussion about the medication should ensue.

Sometimes the answer to the request is "not yet." Consider the following interchange:

PATIENT: "I want to get the f____ out of here!"
STAFF: "Great. That's my job, to start the process of your getting out. The bottom line is that people will need to see that it's safe for you to go. Maybe I can help with that" [1].

Cultural, ethnic, age, and gender issues

Attention to the patient's gender, age, ethnic, and cultural background is not to be overlooked [2,14]. For example, direct eye contact and handshaking in some cultures is unacceptable. Some cultures require a same-sexed physician to examine the patient. However, if this is not possible, the patient needs to know. "I regret that I cannot do as you ask. I understand that it would be more comfortable/acceptable for you to be examined by a female physician, but I am the only physician covering the emergency room this evening. I will certainly ask (a female staff-person) to be in the room when I perform my examination." If the patient's cultural needs are unfamiliar to the physician, asking the patient to educate him can also build an alliance. These techniques empower him through teaching the physician something about which he is an expert. Another consideration is whether the patient needs or wants an interpreter. Interpreters ideally should not be family, but part of the professional interpreters.

Communication techniques

Sympathy

If the physician can sympathize with the patient and his situation, the patient will sense this. For example, one can readily sympathize with someone who is frightened or who has waited a long time to be seen.

Empathy and honesty are the hallmarks of dealing with an agitated patient. Some measured self-disclosure may be helpful: "I can't concentrate on your needs if I'm worried about my own safety" or, asking the patient quite upfront: "do I need to worry about my safety in here?" Sometimes saying, "I'm not feeling comfortable in here, are you having the same feeling?" A general rule is that this type of self-disclosure can have a salutary effect on the patient, without violating boundaries or undermining the physician's role [1,2]. These are advanced interviewing techniques which take practice and require the physician to be self-aware and confident enough to disclose his vulnerability. Such a technique requires the examiner to monitor and recognize minute-by-minute responses by the patient (and his own internal feeling state) and modify them quickly. These techniques are extremely useful and worth practicing because they demonstrate to the patient that the physician is human, can talk about feeling vulnerable, and be strong at the same time. It demonstrates the "realness" and "genuine" character of the physician and models for the patient that talking about feelings is a valid alternative to violence and that the physician cares about safety, including his own [2]. This teaches the patient that it is OK to take care of oneself.

Capture the patient's attention

The patient is absorbed with his own feelings and thoughts. Distraction can be a helpful strategy.

Appeal to the patient's rational side [2], which puts the patient in equal role to the physician in attempting to keep the peace. For example, statements such as, "You know, there are some very ill and distressed people here who need things to be quiet." This technique can also distract the patient from his own agitation.

Talking to the patient from the doorway is an option if the physician feels unsafe to enter the exam room, even when the patient attempts to seduce the clinician – "Oh, it's OK, doc, I'd never hit you. . . .do you think I'm gonna hurt you? I wouldn't hurt a doctor/woman," etc. Another strategy is to have police or other staff on standby: "Oh, doc, did you call them because of me? That's not necessary." The clinician may respond: "I want to make sure that things stay calm" or "I take safety very seriously. They're here for everyone in this ED."

Leaving the exam room [1,21,22] is clearly the thing to do if the patient tells you to get out. If the physician becomes anxious while in the exam room, an option is to leave the room quickly and call for help.

Taking a break [1,2] is a technique used by this author. Remembering that the exam cannot continue if the physician is too frightened of or angry with the patient, he must recognize signs of either emotion bubbling to the surface and prevent his own escalation. Thus, if things are "getting too hot in here" or the patient is starting to get under the physician's skin, suggesting a break is helpful. "OK, let's take a break for a few minutes. . .things seem to be getting too hot in here. . .. Let's both calm down and I'll be back in 10 minutes." It is essential to be back as stated in 10 minutes. Sometimes this process has to be repeated several times until the patient and doctor can have a reasonable conversation.

The message to the patient, however, stated or implied is, "I want to treat you with dignity and respect; you need to afford me the same."

Summarization can help slow down things and ensure that the physician is really trying to understand the patient: "So let me see if I have this straight. . ." The patient then can add or correct to his story.

Bargaining [1,22] is another technique: "I'll let you have a glass of juice, but then I need you to allow the nurse to draw some blood."

Offer choices

For example, stating "You can take the medication by mouth or we can give you an injection ("shot"). Which would you prefer?" gives the patient some control over the general decision, which is not in his control. Or, "Signing in to the hospital voluntarily is preferable to being forced. It says that you're willing to cooperate with the staff, and this may help get you out of the hospital faster, although I can't guarantee that." [1,22].

Set limits

The goal of limit setting is to distract the patient from his own agitation and to put the attention on telling his story [1,22]. Less-experienced clinicians may be at greater risk of being assaulted because they may be more hesitant to set limits and, therefore, more likely to allow threatening behavior to escalate [2,26].

Give instructions

Clear statements such as "You need to demonstrate that you can stay in control so that I can be of help to you" or "I want you to put down the chair," [27] or stating that violence will not be tolerated can be useful [1,22]. The patient may be startled into attentiveness by the physician's directness.

Confrontation is a technique that can quickly lead to further escalation, and needs to be used very judiciously. However, properly timed confrontation can be very useful. An example might be an observational confrontation: "You appear to want to pick a fight. I don't understand why you to want to do this?"

State consequences to the behavior [1,22]. The consequences of disruptive behavior must be stated in a matter of fact manner, giving the patient the facts without humiliating him or coming across as punitive. For example, state clearly and calmly to the patient, "We need the blood drawn; you can either do this willingly or we will have to restrain you to do this." Caution is that such statements should NOT be said until ample staff and equipment is available to act on the consequence should the patient escalate.

Agree with the patient as much as you can

If the patient states that he is being followed by aliens, get more of the story: "Tell me about that; how long has that been going on? Has this happened before? What have you done (recently and in the past) to stop this? How does this make you feel?"

159

If the patient challenges you, "You don't believe me, do you?" the response could be "I have never personally had that experience, but I can agree that I wouldn't like that either." [1, 21].

If the impatient patient challenges the physician because he believes he has waited too long to be seen ("How would you feel if you had to wait this long?"), the physician can agree that "Waiting is difficult" or if true, "Yes, I don't like to wait either," and if it has indeed been a long wait, by all means apologize for the wait, explain why you were late ("There were several critical things I had to attend to before I was able to be free to see you"), be humble and gracious ("I regret that you had to wait so long and I want to thank you for doing so"), and make the wait worthwhile ("but now that I'm free, you have my complete attention" and mean it). These recommendations follow along the principles of the correct method of giving an apology, according to Lazare [28]: (1) identify the offense, (2) give an explanation for the wrong-doing – not an excuse, but an explanation (keeping the explanation as simple and general as possible so as to retain confidentiality), (3) be humble and genuine, and (4) make restitution.

Avoiding interview mistakes

Avoiding the following behaviors can prevent the risk of iatrogenic escalation:

Arguing with the patient is never effective, professional or recommended. If the physician finds himself becoming annoyed with the patient, either excuse yourself or have a discussion about this if the patient appears able to listen: "When you do/say that, I feel annoyed. If I am annoyed, I can't be attentive to your needs" [1,2,15,16,21,22].

Being judgmental or stating something in a judgmental way is another route to argument, and should be avoided.

Empathic failures

An example of an empathic failure is assuming you know how the patient feels. For example, "You must feel scared" might provoke the following response: "No! I'm furious! I'm going to get those...!" Another example of an empathic failure would be to not address the patient's request once it is elicited. As noted earlier, if not addressed, the patient may feel dismissed, misunderstood, and unheard.

Trying to dissuade a fixed belief or delusion

If a patient states that he is being followed by aliens, the physician may gently challenge this belief to determine how fixed the belief is [1,2,21,22]. However, it is of no use to suggest that it is impossible. Similarly, if the patient believes that all doctors are "quacks," it is useless to attempt to dissuade him of this belief. A better approach is to get a history as to how the patient came to that belief. Attempts to persuade the patient that you are not a quack will result in increased arguments from the patient and can lead to an impasse. A more useful response might be, "You don't know me; perhaps you can give me a try. I,

too, may prove to be like all the other doctors, but you haven't given me a chance." Such statements can catch the patient's attention because the physician is not challenging the patient's assumptions (which the patient expects), and gives him an alternative and a chance to save face.

Being punitive or threatening

Consequences of a patient's behavior cannot be said with anger or over-emotion.

Provoking the patient

If the physician becomes angry and gets into an argument with the patient, all objectivity has obviously been lost [1]. People can disagree, but conflict between doctor and patient is rarely resolved through aggression. A neutral third party may help, asking another physician to take over the case, and apologizing to the patient once you regain composure all can be useful. Apology [28] if done well is another indicator of the physician's ability to self-reflect, admit his errors, and role model proper behavior for the patient.

Some patients who appear to be drug seeking can provoke the physician into provocative statements. Try not to get seduced into this – the patient *is* attempting to wear down the physician into giving him what the physician deems inappropriate. Again, the physician can be firm, hold his ground, but still be empathic, calmly stating, "I understand that you believe this medication is the only thing that helps you. I do not agree/believe this to be the case....You have refused alternative treatments I have proposed...I'm sorry this is all I can do for you." Some patients will need to be escorted off the grounds. Using this technique, however, the physician is being sympathetic, addressing the patient's request, and politely disagreeing or not giving what the patient wants. It is this author's experience that when such a statement is said politely but firmly in a matter of fact manner, patients generally do not return to wreak further havoc, become violent, or threatening.

Humiliating the patient

According to Lazare and Levy [29], humiliation is an aggressive act where a person has threatened another person's integrity and very self. In some cases, humiliation itself can be traumatic. Therefore, do not challenge the patient, insult him, or do anything else that can be perceived as humiliating. These behaviors, as well as any form of coercion, can destroy this relationship and must be avoided.

Traumatizing or re-traumatizing the patient

As stated earlier, some patients have had bad experiences with medical providers or either have been abused by authority figures. If a patient is acting in an agitated manner, simply asking, "Did anyone ever hurt you before?" may be useful in getting that history.

Inadvertently accepting the patient's projections

Consider the following situation. The patient is provocative, and projects his anger onto the physician, waiting for the physician to make a "slip," and "prove" to the patient that the physician is indeed punitive. The physician can indeed accept the projection, unconsciously "slip" into irrational thinking and behave in a manner that proves to the patient that he is correct. The patient feels vindicated while the physician may feel as though he is someone else usually because he is feeling the patient's anger – the patient's sadistic parent, or a victim himself.

Special presentations

The *anxious patient* can become increasingly agitated and can even become violent if anxious enough. Reassurance and frequent checks by staff are helpful if there is a long wait to be seen. Anxious patients often cannot contain their anxiety and when that happens, they can become irritable and even hostile or aggressive.

The *delirious patient* is disoriented, usually paranoid, and may be experiencing hallucinations, including visual and tactile. Reassurance, cold compresses, blankets, food, and water may help the agitated patient calm down, and repeated, low-toned reminders as to where the patient is, why they are in the ED, and the physician and other staff's roles are key. A family member or other familiar person may be able to reassure the patient. If the patient cannot calm down with these techniques, offering medication to calm them may be necessary, but also may be wanted by the patient. Careful explanations and repetitive orientation are verbal techniques which appear to apply best to the delirious patient. Because the level of arousal waxes and wanes, it may be difficult to contain the patient and medication may be the best alternative.

If possible, one staff-person assigned to the patient to repeatedly explain, orient, and speak calmly to the patient may spare increased agitation.

The *demented patient* may erupt quickly into agitation. Similar principles apply to the demented patient: ideally one staff-person or family member calming the patient, as well as careful watching for signs of increased agitation.

The *paranoid patient* is defensive, secretive, irritable, and quick to react in a hostile manner to a perceived threat [2]. He may crouch in a corner, appear frightened, and be scanning the environment. If staff moves in too quickly, the patient, who is misinterpreting cues may be frightened enough to attack out of self-protection. With paranoid patients, stating what one is doing at every move is essential. "I'm going to sit down here," with the underlying message, "I don't want to startle you." However, the paranoid patient is also frightened of intimacy, and may perceive overly empathic statements as threatening [2].

Overly empathic statements served to disengage the guarded or paranoid patient who is uncomfortable with intimacy. By acknowledging the patient's difficulty with trust, the interviewer can, at times, elicit some capacity to participate in the evaluation [2,30].

The *traumatized patient* fears being re-traumatized or humiliated, and may become defensive quite quickly. He may appear frightened, even paranoid, and defend himself through anger and other distancing behaviors.

It is essential for the clinician not to accept the patient's projection, lest the physician begin to feel like he is the patient's tormentor. Acknowledging the intensity of the patient's emotions, and provide reassurance as best as possible can decrease anxiety.

The *disorganized/psychotic patient*. The psychotic patient's thinking can become quite loose and tangential. When interviewing acutely psychotic patients, the clinician should assess symptoms without attempting to use logic or to convince the patient that his or her perceptions are wrong [1,2,30].

Addressing physical pain

Patients in acute pain can become quite agitated, and management of the pain will alleviate agitation. Patients with chronic pain are often irritable because they do not understand that the nature of their pain is that it does not disappear, that it waxes and wanes, and that other treatments other than pain medications often help to decrease the attendant anxiety/agitation which can contribute to increased pain.

Approaching the patient about psychiatric medication

Offering medication can help the patient feel cared for. Like food or water, giving medication can be soothing. Ask the patient "what has worked for you in the past?"

However, if the patient is resistant, it is best to use incremental techniques [1,22]. After offering, if the patient refuses, an authoritative, educational role is best: "It is important for you to calm down, and medication can do that."

If the patient still refuses, again, an authoritative (not authoritarian) technique can be implemented: "It is my opinion that medication is necessary" and then give a choice: would you prefer (drug X or drug Y, and explain some of the benefits and side effects if the patient is unfamiliar with them); would you prefer the medication orally or by injection?

Finally, stating "This is an emergency, and I have ordered and I am going to give (name of the medication)." In these situations, it is clearly best to prepare for such statements, having both oral and injectable forms of the medication available, and an ample number of staff to implement the plan, should physical restraint become necessary [1].

Conclusion

Agitation is a common presentation in the emergency department. This chapter has addressed techniques of verbal de-escalation that the emergency physician can quickly learn and implement as an alternative to seclusion and restraint. Ultimately, verbal de-escalation improves staff morale and patient adherence, because it uses a non-coercive, patient-centered approach. Verbal de-escalation takes no more than five to ten minutes and enhances the doctor–patient relationship, while seclusion and restraint require more staff and takes more time to implement. The offering of medication can be considered part of verbal de-escalation, and methods of introducing the subject of taking medication can be done in increments as outlined in this chapter.

References

1. Richmond JS, Berlin JS, Fishkind AB, et al. Verbal de-escalation of the agitated patient: consensus statement of the American Association for Emergency Psychiatry Project BETA De-escalation Workgroup. *West J Emerg Med* 2012;**13**:17–25.

2. Kleespies PM. Evaluating behavioral emergencies: the clinical interview. In: Kleespies PM, (Ed.). *Behavioral Emergencies: An Evidence-based Resource for Evaluating and Managing Risk of Suicide, Violence, and Victimization.* Washington, DC: American Psychological Association; 2009: 33–55.

3. Zun L. *Optimizing ED Neurological Emergency Patient Care* 2009. Available at: http://www.ferne.onrg/Lectures/memc_2009/pdf/ferne_memc_2009_zun_agitated.pdf. (Accessed December 9, 2011).

4. Hillard J. *Handbook of Emergency Psychiatry.* Washington, DC: American Psychiatric Association; 1990.

5. Swift RH, Harrigan EP, Cappelleri JC, Kramer D, Chandler LP. Validation of the behavioural activity rating scale (BARS): a novel measure of activity in agitated patients. *J Psychiatr Res* 2002;**36**:87–95.

6. Childs E. *Commonwealth of Massachusetts Department of Mental Health Seclusion and Restraint Philosophy Statement.* Department of Mental Health, Commonwealth of Massachusetts 2004. Available at: http://www.nasmhpd.org/general_files/publications/ntac_pubs/SR%20Project%20Huang/Huang%20I.1%20MA%20RS%20PhilosophyStatement%20-FINAL-%203.26.04.doc (Accessed August 14, 2011).

7. Lazare A. Shame and humiliation in the medical encounter. *Arch Intern Med* 1987;**147**:1653–8.

8. Richmond JS, Hughes DH, Milner K, editor. *Clinical Management of Violent Patients in the Emergency Room.* Workshop. Institute on Psychiatric Services; 1997; Washington, DC: American Psychiatry Association.

9. Metzner JL, Lion J, Reid WH, et al. Resource document on the use of restraint and seclusion in correctional mental health care. *J Am Acad Psychiatry Law* 2007;**35**:417–25.

10. Patel Y, Garmel GM. Management of intoxicated/violent patients. In: Mattu A, Goyal DG, (Eds.). *Emergency Medicine: Avoiding the Pitfalls and Improving the Outcomes.* Malden, MA: Blackwell Publishing; 2007; 99–108.

11. Vorvick L. *Agitation: Overview.* 2008. Available at: http://www.umm.edu/ency/article/003212trt.htm (Accessed August 26, 2011).

12. Ferris M. *Protecting Hospitalized Elders from Falling: A Recent History of Fall Prevention.* Topics in Advanced Practice Nursing eJournal [Internet]. Available at: http://www.medscape.com/viewarticle/585961_2 (Accessed August 26, 2011).

13. Beck JC, White K, Gage B. Emergency psychiatric assessment of violence. *Am J Psychiatry* 1991;**148**:1562–5.

14. Shea SC. *Psychiatric Interviewing: The Art of Understanding,* (2nd Edition). Philadelphia: WB Saunders; 1998.

15. Novitsky MA Jr, Dubin WR. Non-pharmacological management of violence in psychiatric emergencies. *Prim Psychiatry* 2009;**16**:49–53.

16. Eisendrath S, Lichtmacher JE. Common psychiatric disorders: post-traumatic stress disorder. In: McPhee SJ, Papadakis M, (Eds.). *Current Medical Diagnosis and Treatment,* (49th Edition). New York: McGraw Hill; 2010: 938–9.

17. Isbister GK, Page CB, Stokes B, Bryant JL, Downes MA. Randomized controlled trial of intramuscular droperidol versus midazolam for violence and acute behavioral disturbance: the DORM study. *Ann Emerg Med* 2010;**56**:392–401.

18. Downey LV, Zun LS, Gonzales SJ. Frequency of alternative to restraints and seclusion and uses of agitation reduction techniques in the emergency department. *Gen Hosp Psychiatry* 2007;**29**:470–4.

19. Lazare A, Eisenthal S, Wasserman L. The customer approach to patienthood. *Arch Gen Psychiatry* 1975;**32**:553–8.

20. Beauford JE, McNiel DE, Binder RL. Utility of the initial therapeutic alliance in evaluating psychiatric patients' risk of violence. *Am J Psychiatry* 1997;**154**:1272–6.

21. Fiskind A. Calming agitation with words not drugs. *Curr Psychiatry* 2002;**1**:32–40.

22. Fishkind A. Agitation II: de-escalation of the aggressive patient and avoiding coercion. In: Glick RL, Berlin JS, Fishkind A, Zeller S, (Eds.). *Emergency Psychiatry: Principles and Practice.* Philadelphia: Wolters Kluwer Health/Lippincott Williams & Wilkins; 2008: 125–36.

23. Smith MJ. *When I Say No, I Feel Guilty: How to Cope – Using the Skills of Systematic Assertive Therapy.* New York: Dial Press; 1975.

24. Pope K, Tabachnick B. Therapists' anger, hate, fear, and sexual feelings: National survey of therapist responses, client characteristics, critical events, formal complaints, and training. *Prof Psychol Res Pr* 1993;**24**:142–52.

25. Allen MH, Sheets J, Miccio B, et al. What do consumers say they want and need during a psychiatric emergency? *J Pract Psychiatry* 2003;**9**:29–58.

26. Guy J, Brady JL. The stress of violent behavior for the clinician. In: Kleespies PM, (Ed.). *Emergencies in Mental Health Practice Evaluation and Management.* New York: Guilford Press; 1998: 398–417.

27. Malavade KMM. A general approach to the emergency psychiatry patient.

In: Riba M, Ravindranath D, (Eds.). *Clinical Manual of Emergency psychiatry*. Washington, DC: American Psychiatric Association; 2010: 2–11.

28. Lazare A. *On Apology*. New York: Oxford University Press; 2004.

29. Lazare A Levy RS. Apologizing for humiliations in medical practice. *Chest* 2011;**139**:746–51.

30. Jesse S, Anderson G. Emergency services. In: Levy S, Ninan P, (Eds.). *Schizophrenia: Treatment of Acute Psychotic Episodes*. Washington, DC: American Psychiatric Press; 1990: 27–43.

Chapter 22

Use of agitation treatment in the emergency department

Marc L. Martel, Amanda E. Horn, and William R. Dubin

Introduction

The management of acute agitation is a complex medical issue. Emergency physicians are frequently required to care for unknown patients with acute undifferentiated agitation. The emergency physician must not only ensure the safety of the patient, but must consider the safety of ancillary caregivers as well as other patients and visitors. In these circumstances, the etiology of the patient's agitation must be rapidly determined, and although commonly associated with psychiatric disorders such as bipolar disorder, schizophrenia, and alcohol and illicit substance abuse, several life-threatening medical causes need to be considered in the differential diagnosis. Treating the patient's agitation allows both further examination and assessment, and limits agitation-related physiologic and psychological stress.

Agitation is defined by one or more of the following; motor restlessness, heightened responsiveness to stimuli, irritability, inappropriate and/or purposeless verbal or motor activity, decrease sleep and fluctuation of symptoms over time. Aggressive and violent behaviors are clearly linked to agitation, but predicting when aggression will occur is challenging [1]. Additionally, defining the level of a patient's agitation can be difficult. Several scales exist for research and inpatient assessment, but validation in the ED has had little research to assist clinicians in a meaningful manner [2].

Agitation is known to be associated with several other psychiatric and medical causes. In addition to schizophrenia and bipolar disorder, major depression, generalized anxiety disorder, panic disorder, and personality disorder are common etiologies. Several forms of dementia have been linked to agitation, including Parkinson's and Alzheimer's diseases.

Alcohol and illicit substances, particularly cocaine, PCP, and amphetamine intoxication and alcohol and benzodiazepine withdrawal are associated with acute agitation. The degree of agitation resulting from stimulants can be variable. Considered a life-threatening condition, excited delirium is an extreme on the spectrum. Excited delirium is characterized by confusion, anxiety, disorientation, psychomotor agitation, violent behavior, and hyperthermia. This severe form of agitation is believed to cause significant metabolic acidosis and is closely linked to sudden, unexpected death [3]. This syndrome highlights the importance of early and aggressive treatment of agitation by frontline practitioners. It also highlights the need for emergency physicians to have a clear algorithm for management of these patients.

Agitation, regardless of the etiology, is a behavioral emergency. It requires immediate intervention to treat the patient's symptoms, prevent injury, and facilitate medical and/or psychiatric evaluation.

Medications
Antipsychotics

Both typical (first-generation) and atypical (second-generation) antipsychotics are frequently used in the management of agitation. The specific mechanism of action is not known, but these drugs have varying effects on dopamine, serotonin, and other neurotransmitter function [4].

Typical antipsychotics are generally classified into low-, medium-, and high-potency classes. The reference to "potency" is related to dosing of the drugs rather than efficacy. Low-potency antipsychotics are generally more sedating and often cause orthostatic hypotension, dizziness, and anticholinergic symptoms. High-potency antipsychotics are considered less sedating but are more often associated with extrapyramidal side effects. These effects most commonly manifest as tremors, rigidity, acute dystonia, and akathisia. Medium-potency antipsychotics have mixed effects between high- and low-potency medications.

The atypical antipsychotics represent a newer generation of drugs developed primarily to treat schizophrenia and bipolar disorders. These medications tend to more selectively block central dopaminergic receptors or inhibit serotonin reuptake.

It is believed that atypical antipsychotic agents have less sedation, fewer extrapyramidal effects, a lower incidence of tardive dyskinesia, and less effect on QT prolongation.

It is important to note that both types of antipsychotic medications have been associated with significant adverse events. As a result, the U.S. Food and Drug Administration (FDA) has placed several warnings, including the more serious "black box" warnings, on both classes of drugs. The two that apply to acute management of agitation are outlined below; further details on

Behavioral Emergencies for the Emergency Physician, ed. Leslie S. Zun, Lara G. Chepenik, and Mary Nan S. Mallory. Published by Cambridge University Press. © Cambridge University Press 2013.

Table 22.1. Common typical antipsychotics used in the treatment of acute agitation

Name	Potency	Duration (half-life in hours)	U.S. FDA black box warnings
Butyrophenones			
Haloperidol	High	21–24	QT Prolongation, Torsades de pointes, Increased risk of death in elderly
Droperidol	High	2.2	QT Prolongation, Torsades de pointes, Increased risk of death in elderly
Phenothiazines			
Chlorpromazine	Low	23–37	Increased risk of death in elderly
Thioridazine	Intermediate	24	QT Prolongation, Increased risk of death in elderly
Perphenazine	Intermediate	9–12	Increased risk of death in elderly
Trifluoperazine	High	18	Increased risk of death in elderly
Fluphenzaine	High	14.7–15.3	Increased risk of death in elderly
Thioxanthenes			
Loxapine	Intermediate	3–4 (oral), 12 (IM)	Increased risk of death in elderly
Thiothixene	High	34	Increased risk of death in elderly

Table 22.2. Common atypical antipsychotics used in the treatment of acute agitation

Name	Duration (half-life in hours)	U.S. FDA black box warnings
Aripipazole	75	Increased risk of death in elderly, Increased risk of suicide in children
Olanzapine	21–54	Increased risk of death in elderly
Risperidone	20 (oral); 3–6 days (IM)	Increased risk of death in elderly
Quetiapine	6	Increased risk of death in elderly, Increased risk of suicide in children
Ziprasidone	7	Increased risk of death in elderly

the specific medications are listed in Tables 22.1 and 22.2. There is some dispute about the rationale for the black box warning.

The FDA has warned "that both conventional and atypical antipsychotics are associated with an increased risk of mortality in elderly patients treated for dementia-related psychosis" [5]. A meta-analysis conducted by the FDA in 2005 found a 1.6 to 1.7 times increase in the risk of death in patients treated with atypical antipsychotics versus placebo when used for dementia-related behavioral disorders. In 2008, this black box warning was added to the typical antipsychotics. A review of two observational epidemiological studies found that these drugs also increase the risk of death in elderly patients with dementia-related psychosis [5].

Several of the typical antipsychotics have been associated with QT prolongation and torsades de pointes. Although the QTc interval does not directly correlate with an individual patient's risk of developing a malignant cardiac arrhythmia, QT prolongation raises the concern of abnormal cardiac conduction. The FDA recommends reserving these medications for patients who fail alternate treatment and encourage the evaluation of the QTc interval before administration [6]. At a minimum, if electrocardiographic data is available before administration, the QTc

interval should be assessed and considered. Cardiac monitoring may not be possible before initiating control of a patient's agitated state. If this is the case, the danger the patient poses to himself and the healthcare team is more likely to be the acute medical risk. If aggressive behavior is exhibited, the potential risk of medication-induced QT prolongation or cardiac arrhythmias bows to the real risk of violence. In this situation, emergency physicians are expertly trained to handle any cardiac or respiratory situation that may arise.

Other acute adverse effects of antipsychotic use in the treatment of acute agitation include the following.

Anticholinergic effects

These effects are frequent and can be relatively variable. Sedation is common, but is desirable clinically in the management of acute agitation. Other anticholinergic effects include dry mouth, blurred vision, constipation, urinary retention, and adynamic ileus. Dysarthria, mydriasis, and delirium can be seen as a result of the central effects of these medications.

Anticholinergic-related cardiovascular effects are often clinically evident. Most common with thorazine, orthostatic hypotension and tachycardia may be compounded by the medications' adrenergic effects. Hypotension is typically responsive to intravenous fluids.

Movement disorders

Acute antipsychotic-induced movement disorders include akathisia and acute dystonia. Both are likely caused by alterations in the dopaminergic pathways of the basal ganglia, specifically the D2 receptors of the nigrostriatum [7]. These reactions are unfortunately common, with one study reporting more than 60% of chronic use associated with at least one form of antipsychotic-induced movement disorder [8].

Akathisia is an uncomfortable sense of motor restlessness manifested by an intense desire to move, usually the legs. It can also be manifested with an inner sense of restlessness, a feeling of being tense or "wired," or a feeling of "going to explode." These feelings can occur in the absence of motor symptoms. This side effect can occur with acute or chronic use, and is worsened if misdiagnosed and inappropriately treated as progressive agitation. Anticholingergics, including benztropine (1–2 mg IM or po) or diphenhydramine (25–50 mg IM/IV/po) and benzodiazepines (lorazepam 1–2 mg IM/IV) are generally effective in acute reversal. Patients may benefit from ongoing treatment after discharge to prevent reoccurrence [9].

Acute dystonia is typically an idiosyncratic reaction to antipsychotic medications. Dystonic reactions are characterized by intermittent spasmodic or sustained involuntary contractions of the face, neck, trunk, or extremities. More serious forms of dystonia manifest clinically as oculogyric crisis and laryngospasm. Anticholinergics including benztropine (1–2 mg IM or po) or diphenhydramine (25–50 mg IM/IV/po) are indicated, and can be combined if symptoms are resistant to either independently. Benzodiazepines can be added if necessary. Patients should be continued on the reversal agent(s) for 3–5 days to prevent recurrence.

Neuroleptic malignant syndrome

Neuroleptic malignant syndrome (NMS) is a rare, idiosyncratic reaction to the antipsychotics. The high-potency agents are more frequently associated with the syndrome, but both typicals and atypicals have been implicated. NMS is life-threatening disorder characterized by fever, muscular rigidity, autonomic instability, and altered mental status. Mortality has been reported as high as 20% and is related to respiratory failure, cardiovascular collapse, acute renal failure, arrhythmia, and/or disseminated intravascular coagulation. Management is predominantly supportive, and includes discontinuation of antipsychotics, hydration, temperature regulation (cooling), and possibly dantrolene or bromocriptine to reduce rigidity.

Benzodiazepines

Benzodiazepines are commonly used in the acute management of agitation. They may be administered independently, but are more frequently combined with an antipsychotic for agitation control. There are several approved medications available for use in the United States. Several of the available agents are outlined in Table 22.3.

The main distinguishing features between the benzodiazepines are route of administration and duration of action. In the management of acute agitation, the shorter-acting, parenteral medications are preferred. Both midazolam and lorazepam are used extensively in the United States.

Benzodiazepines, particularly the oral formulations, have a wide therapeutic window. Aside from the intended sedation that can be excessive, adverse effects include respiratory suppression, hypoventilation, apnea, hypotension, amnesia, dizziness, and ataxia. Midazolam carries a black box warning issued

Table 22.3. Common benzodiazepines available for use in the treatment of acute agitation

Name	Route of administration	Duration (half-life in hours)
Alprazolam	Oral	9–20
Chlordiazepoxide	Parenteral and Oral	24–48
Clonazepam	Oral	30–40
Clorazepate	Oral	48
Diazepam	Parenteral, Oral and Rectal	35
Lorazepam	Parenteral and Oral	10–20
Midazolam	Parenteral and Oral	1.8–6.4
Oxazepam	Oral	4–15
Triazolam	Oral	1.5–5.

by the FDA related to the risk of respiratory suppression. The recommendations encourage the use of midazolam solely in settings where continuous respiratory and cardiac monitoring, airway management equipment, resuscitative drugs, and providers skilled in airway management are available.

Ketamine

Ketamine is a dissociative anesthetic with clinical indications for anesthesia induction and anesthesia maintenance. The rapid sedative effects are particularly useful in the ED management of acute agitation and ketamine is already commonly used in the ED for procedural sedation [10–13]. In addition to rapid sedation, ketamine's short duration of action, parenteral administration, and in particular the preservation of protective airway reflexes, are attractive properties in the management of patients with acute agitation. Intramuscularly, sedation occurs within 3–4 minutes lasting for up to 30 minutes. The sedative effects of ketamine are profound and in conjunction with its onset of action, agitation control can occur quickly, allowing for rapid stabilization in potentially dangerous situations. After achieving initial sedation, intravenous access can be obtained and additional ED evaluation and subsequent titrated sedation can be performed. Reports of use have been limited to several small cohorts [14,15], although nationally, emergency medical services appear to be adding ketamine to their formularies for use in excited delirium cases [16].

Routes of administration

As outlined above, several treatment modalities exist for the management of acute agitation. Many of the medications are available in both oral and parenteral formulations. A systematic review of published articles on pharmacologic treatments for agitation by Zeller and Rhoades in 2010 suggested that oral, intramuscular, and intravenous administration modalities may all be effective, but noted that the onset of action varied according to the route of administration [17]. The American College of Emergency Physicians (ACEP) recommends oral medications in "agitated but cooperative patients" [18]. This guideline highlights the dilemma clinicians face when managing patients with acute agitation. Although the truly "ideal" medications for acute agitation would have a rapid onset, be short acting and be painlessly administered (needleless), the inherent nature of the patient's presentation frequently precludes oral administration [17]. Similarly, the intravenous route of administration is also dependent on patient compliance to establish intravenous access. As a result, intramuscular injection is typically required.

Several other issues merit clinical consideration when selecting a medication and its route of administration. Liquid and rapid dissolving preparations limit the effects of "cheeking," or not swallowing meds. Parenteral medications, whether intramuscular or intravenous, require the use of a needle and may place providers at an increased risk of blood-borne pathogen exposure through needle-stick injuries. The physician–patient relationship may be improved if injections can be avoided and patient preference is considered when possible [19].

Use of a proprietary, inhaled delivery system may provide an additional alternative to parenteral administration of sedatives in the future. A recent trial of inhaled loxapine showed significant agitation reduction in consenting patients who were able to follow study protocol [20]. This method does, however, require patient cooperation similar to oral formulations.

Special populations

Elderly

For frail elderly patients, patients with renal impairment, or elderly patients who appear to be medically compromised, smaller doses of a single agent is preferable. The medications should be used cautiously and judiciously. The issue of QTc prolongation with antipsychotic medication in the elderly has received much attention recently. This risk can be minimized by staying within dosing guidelines and adhering to recommendations regarding QTc interval checks [21]. These recommendations suggest that a baseline QTc interval is obtained. A patient should not be considered a candidate for intravenous haloperidol if the QTc interval is 450 milliseconds or greater in a male or 470 milliseconds or greater in a female (21). Additionally, any patient whose QTc interval is prolonged beyond 25% of baseline during treatment should have haloperidol discontinued [21].

The following medications are recommended [21]:

- Haloperidol IV 0.25 mg to 0.5 mg every 6 hours
- Haloperidol concentrate or tablets 0.5 mg to 1 mg every 6 hours
- Risperidone 0.25 mg to 0.5 mg solution, dissolving tablet or pill every 6 hours
- Lorazepam 1 mg IM or solution.

Pregnant

There are no outcome studies for treating the agitated pregnant patient [22]. The fetal risk of using several doses of psychotropic medication to treat agitated pregnant women remains unknown. In the absence of safety data, clinicians should use the minimal amount of medication necessary to reduce agitation and aggression in these patients. All efforts should be made to avoid physical restraints, especially in the second or third trimesters, as restraints may pose significant risks to the pregnant patient [22].

Children and adolescents

There are also no data on the treatment of adolescents and children who are severely agitated. Because children and adolescents are more vulnerable to side effects from antipsychotic medication, lorazepam is a preferable alternative. Dosing is 0.5–2 mg orally or IM every hour as needed to achieve sedation. Some authors have also recommended antihistamines such as diphenhydramine or hydroxyzine for children and adolescents with less severe symptoms [23].

Physical restraints

Clinicians at the front-line of managing patients with acute agitation must be aware of U.S. federal regulations related to restraint use. The use of both chemical and physical restraints must be closely monitored and recorded, respecting these guidelines. Chemical restraints, defined as a drug or medication "used as a restriction to manage the patient's freedom of movement and is not a standard treatment or dosage for the patient's condition," fall under the same regulatory guidelines as physical restraints [24].

According to The Joint Commission Standards, restraints (or seclusion) can only be used when clinically justified or when warranted by patient behavior. In practice, restraints may only be used in accordance with institutional policies *and* to protect the immediate physical safety of the patient and others, in the least restrictive manner possible, and must be discontinued as early as possible regardless of the order expiration. Restraints cannot be used to coerce, discipline, or retaliate against the patient, and cannot be used under "as needed" (prn) or standing orders. Within 1 hour, all patients must undergo a formal, face-to-face evaluation by a licensed practitioner if a sedative is ordered for "violent or self-destructive behavior." Monitoring must occur by a specifically trained staff member in accordance with institutional guidelines.

Both chemical and physical restraints will need to be used to safely care for selected agitated patients. An appropriate understanding of the guidelines is required. It is crucial to only use these techniques when appropriate and as part of a cohesive treatment plan for an individual patient. Consultation with legal counsel concerning federal (and any state) regulations is advisable for any practitioner who commonly cares for patients who require agitation control.

QTc prolongation present or concerns for possible cardiac arrhythmias?		
	Yes	**No**
History of dementia? **Yes**	• Lorazepam 2mg IM/IV • Ketamine 4mg/kg IM or 1-2mg/kg IV	
History of dementia? **No**	• Lorazepam 2mg IM/IV • Ketamine 4mg/kg IM or 1-2mg/kg IV • Olanzapine 10mg IM	• Lorazepam 2mg IM/IV • Droperidol 2.5mg IM/IV • Haloperidol 5mg IM/IV • Olanzapine 10mg IM • Ziprasidone 20mg IM

Figure 22.1. Pharmacologic selection I for the management of acute agitation.

Additional recommendations

The real-world management of patients with acute agitation is exceedingly complex. As outlined, a variety of options for medical therapy exist and physical restraints may be necessary. Several research-based protocols that use single drug as well as multi-drug therapies are available and can be easily implemented. A simple algorithm incorporating both clinical features and drug specific warnings is suggested in Figure 22.1.

Length of stay

Safe medical and/or acute psychiatric evaluation is required after management of acute agitation, but ultimately, safe transfer to definitive care is frequently necessary. A significant issue in the management of acute agitation is the time after sedation is administered until the patient may be transferred to definitive care either for psychiatric consultation or admission. The duration of action and depth of sedation must be sufficient to safely allow evaluation and transport, but not excessively long or deep to delay these components of care.

As implied by the delay in onset of action for the oral formulations, lengths of stay may be affected by route of administration as well as medication choice and patient response. Although comparing agents based on half-lives may suggest superiority with respect to throughput times in the ED, no clinical trials to date have specifically addressed this issue. Short-acting agents may encourage more rapid recovery or atypical antipsychotics may provide less sedation. Further study is required.

References

1. Lindenmayer JP. The pathophysiology of agitation. *J Clin Psychiatry* 2000;**61** (Suppl 14):5–10.

2. Zun LS, Downey LS. Level of agitation of psychiatric patients presenting to an emergency department. *J Clin Psychiatry* 2008;**10**:108–13.

3. Wetli CV, Mash D, Karch SB. Cocaine associated agitated delirium and the neuroleptic malignant syndrome. *Am J Emerg Med* 1996;**92**:110–3.

4. Laruelle M, Frankle WG, Narendran R, Kegeles LS, Abi-Dargham A. Mechanism of action of antipsychotic drugs: from dopamine D(2) receptor antagonism to glutamate NMDA facilitation. *Clin Ther* 2005;**27**(Suppl 1): S16–24.

5. U.S. Food and Drug Administration. Available at: http://www.fda.gov/drugs/drugsafety/postmarketdrugsafety informationforpatientsandproviders/ucm124830.htm (Accessed September 28, 2011).

6. U.S. Food and Drug Administration. Available at: http://www.fda.gov/Safety/MedWatch/SafetyInformation/Safety AlertsforHumanMedicalProducts/ucm173778.htm (Accessed September 28, 2011).

7. Marsden CD, Jenner P. The pathophysiology of extrapyramidal side-effects of neuroleptic drugs. *Psychol Med* 1980;**10**:55–72.

8. Janno S, Holi M, Tuisku K, Wahlbeck K. Prevalence of neuroleptic-induced movement disorders in chronic schizophrenia inpatients. *Am J Psychiatry* 2004;**161**:160–3.

9. Vinson DR. Diphenhydramine in the treatment of akathisia induced by prochlorperazine. *J Emerg Med* 2004;**26**:265–73.

10. Green SM, Rothrock SG, Lynch EL, et al. Intramuscular ketamine for pediatric sedation in the emergency department: safety profile in 1,022 cases. *Ann Emerg Med* 1998;**31**:688–97.

11. Green SM, Roback MG, Kennedy RM, Krauss B. Clinical practice guideline for emergency department ketamine dissociative sedation: 2011

update. *Ann Emerg Med* 2011;**57**:449–61.

12. Miner JM, Gray RO, Bahar J, Patel R, McGill JW. Randomized clinical trial of propofol versus ketamine for procedural sedation in the emergency department. *Acad Emerg Med* 2010;**17**:604–11.

13. Sener S, Eken C, Schuyltz CH, Serinken M, Ozsarac M. Ketamine with and without midazolam for emergency department sedation in adults: a randomized controlled trial. *Ann Emerg Med* 2011;**57**:109–14.

14. Le Cong M, Gynther B, Hunter E, Schuller P. Ketamine sedation for patients with acute agitation and psychiatric illness requiring aeromedical retrieval. *Emerg Med J* 2012;**29**:335–7.

15. Melamed E, Oron Y, Ben-Avraham R, Blumenfeld A, Lin G. The combative multitrauma patient: a protocol for prehospital management. *Eur J Emerg Med* 2007;**14**:265–8.

16. SoRelle R. ExDS protocol puts clout in EMS hands. *Emergency Medicine News.* September 2, 2010.

17. Zeller SL, Rhoades RW. Systematic reviews of assessment measures and pharmcologic treatment for agitation. *Clin Ther* 2010;**32**:403–25.

18. Lukens TW, Wold SJ, Edlow JA, et al. Clinical policy: critical issues in the diagnosis and management of the adult psychiatric patient in the emergency department. *Ann Emerg Med* 2006;**47**:79–99.

19. Allen MH, Carpenter D, Sheets JL, Miccio S, Ross R. What do consumers say they want and need during a psychiatric emergency? *J Psychiatr Pract* 2003;**9**:39–58.

20. Lesem MD, Tran-Johnson TK, Riesenberg RA, et al. Rapid acute treatment of agitation in individuals with schizophrenia: multicentre, randomised, placebo-controlled study of inhaled loxapine. *B J Psychiatry* 2011;**198**:51–8.

21. Liptzin B, Jacobson SA. *Kaplan and Sadock's. Comprehensive Textbook of Psychiatry*, (9th Edition, Volume 2). Philadelphia: Wolters Kluwer/ Lippincott Williams & Wilkins; 2009: 4066–73.

22. Ladavac AS, Dubin WR, Ning A, et al. Emergency management of agitation in pregnancy. *Gen Hosp Psychiatry* 2007;**29**:39–41.

23. Heyneman E. The aggressive child. *Child Adolesc Psychiatr Clin N Am* 2003;**12**:667–77.

24. *Department of Health and Human Services Centers for Medicare and Medicaid Services.* Available at: www.cms.hhs.gov/ CFCsAndCoPs/downloads/ finalpatientrightsrule.pdf (Accessed September 30, 2011).

Chapter 23

Management of aggressive and violent behavior in the emergency department

Amanda E. Horn and William R. Dubin

Introduction

Violence within healthcare settings is a well-described phenomenon. However, the exact incidence of violent acts within hospitals, acute care facilities, and medical offices is unknown. This is due in part to the fact that violent acts or threats against healthcare workers do not require mandatory reporting to hospital administration or law enforcement agencies. While it is impossible to know the exact prevalence of assaultive behavior inflicted on healthcare workers, the Bureau of Labor Statistics publishes yearly data on workplace assaults which lead to days off from work. Between 2003 and 2007, roughly 10,000 nonfatal workplace assaults occurred annually in healthcare facilities, which accounts for almost 60% of the nation's total reported workplace assaults. Three quarters of these assaults were by patients or residents of healthcare facilities such as nursing homes [1].

The emergency department (ED) is one of the most dangerous places to work in a hospital. A recent survey of emergency departments in the United States found that nearly 25% of ED staff "sometimes, rarely, or never" felt safe. Of all ED staff surveyed, nurses felt the least safe [2]. Another study of emergency medicine residents and attending physicians reported that more than three quarters of those surveyed experienced at least one violent act at work in the preceding year [3]. While community and academic emergency departments are prone to violence from patients or visitors, there was a higher likelihood of workplace violence in EDs with higher volumes (>60,000 patient visits/year) [3]. Yet, less than half of survey respondents worked in EDs that screened for weapons or had metal detectors, despite the frequency of threats or violent gestures experienced by physicians [3].

There are multiple reasons for the high risk of violence that occurs in emergency departments. These include the fact that patients in the ED are a largely unscreened population, have a high proportion of substance abuse and psychiatric illness, may possess weapons, and many times are brought in under police custody [3–5]. In addition, patient and visitor frustration with wait times, a lack of understanding of the triage system, overcrowding, and uncomfortable surroundings contributes to the tension in an already inherently stressful and chaotic setting [6–8]. A lack of

staff education regarding threat recognition and management may also contribute to ED violence. Studies have found that few EDs provide formal training in techniques to deal with aggressive or combative individuals [2,3]. Yet, such training may be one of the most important steps that an institution can take to ensure clinician and staff safety [9–11]. With the risk of violence being so high in the emergency department, it's essential for ED physicians and staff to have an understanding of the progression of violence and the appropriate de-escalation techniques to defuse potentially violent situations. Insuring the safety of patients, clinicians, and staff is essential to the functioning of an ED.

Medical illness as a cause of violence

Violence can be a manifestation of an underlying medical illness. The incidence of patients presenting with psychiatric illness who have a medical etiology for their symptoms varies from 15% to 90% [12]. Medical examinations of psychiatric patients in the ED are often limited in scope. However, even in violent patients, ED physicians must maintain a high index of suspicion for underlying medical problems and thus may need to initiate laboratory or other studies. Clinical history, signs, and symptoms that are suggestive of a medical etiology include [13]:

- Patients older than 40 or younger than 12 years of age with no previous psychiatric history
- Acute onset (hours to weeks)
- Fluctuating course
- Impaired attention or intermittent somnolence during interview
- Visual or olfactory hallucinations
- Abnormal vital signs
- Disorientation
- Known medical illness or neurological symptoms
- Memory impairment
- Medication that may cause agitation or psychotic symptoms
- Alcohol or drug use.

Shah et al. (2010) describe an effective screening tool to rule out serious medical illness in patients presenting to the ED for psychiatric complaints [14]. This includes vital sign

---

Behavioral Emergencies for the Emergency Physician, ed. Leslie S. Zun, Lara G. Chepenik, and Mary Nan S. Mallory. Published by Cambridge University Press. © Cambridge University Press 2013.

Table 23.1. Medical screening of patients with primary psychiatric complaints

Stable vital signs (T <100.5, HR 50–119, RR <25, DBP < 120, Pox > 94%)
No prior psychiatric history OR age <30
Oriented times four OR Folstein >23
No evidence of acute medical problem
No visual hallucinations present

measurement (temperature < 100.5, heart rate 50–119, respiratory rate <25, diastolic blood pressure < 120, pulse oximetry > 94%); lack of the presence of visual hallucinations; a history of psychiatric problems or age less than 30; orientation to person, place, time and situation, or Folstein score >23 on the Mini-Mental Status Exam [15]; and no evidence of an acute medical problem. These criteria are listed in Table 23.1. A retrospective review of 500 consecutive patients presenting to an academic medical center with primarily psychiatric complaints demonstrated that if these criteria were met, the patient did not need further medical evaluation beyond a history and physical examination [14].

Signs of impending violence

Anticipating the potential for aggression increases ED safety. There are several risk factors for violent behavior that have been extensively documented in the psychiatric literature [4,16–18]. The most reliable predictor for violence is a past history of violent behavior. Other predictors include a history of childhood abuse, borderline or antisocial personality disorder, substance abuse, and patients who are young, male, and of a lower socioeconomic status. In the ED setting, patient histories may not be available initially. However, electronic medical records (EMRs) may play a role to alert ED clinicians of patients who have been violent during past visits. This has been demonstrated to be effective in the ambulatory setting in the past [19]. Drummond, Sparr, and Gordon [19] described a program that reduced the number of violent incidents in the Portland Veterans Administration Medial Center by over 91%. This was done by identifying patients at risk for violence and entering a flag in the patient's computerized database within the medical center. The flag alerted staff to the patient's potential for violence and security immediately sat with the patient throughout the visit. Just as many EMR systems can import medication allergies from past visits into current visits, there may be a role to "flag" potentially violent patients.

Violent outbursts rarely occur without warning. There is often a behavioral prodrome which should be recognized by the healthcare provider. During this prodromal period, patients begin to display increasing levels of anxiety and tension. Frequently this is manifested by a fixed, staring facial expression, clenched fists or jaws, or a rigid, tense posture. Loud, threatening, and insistent speech or escalating verbal profanity and abuse are warning signs of further escalation. The culmination of the escalation toward violence is motor hyperactivity. The patient becomes increasingly restless and begins to pace [4,12]. *This motor activity is a red flag for impending violence and should be evaluated and managed immediately.* It is at this time that appropriate clinician intervention may prevent overtly aggressive acts.

Clinically significant agitation may be defined as abnormal and excessive verbal or physical aggression, purposeless motor behaviors, heightened arousal, and significant disruption of patient's functioning. Behaviors that have been considered most typical of clinically significant agitation that can lead to violence include the following [20]:

- Explosive and/or unpredictable anger
- Intimidating behavior, restlessness, pacing, or excessive movement
- Physical and/or verbal self-abusiveness
- Demeaning or hostile verbal behavior
- Uncooperative or demanding behavior or resistance to care
- Impulsive or impatient behavior
- Low tolerance for pain or frustration.

De-escalation

Multiple options exist for de-escalation of a potentially violent patient as well as management of a patient who has become acutely violent. It is important that the treating physician and the other ED support staff (nurses, medical technicians, and security guards) have protocols in place for managing aggressive patients to minimize harm to both patient and caregivers. Techniques for de-escalation should occur in a step-wise pattern beginning with verbal techniques, followed by the offering of a pharmacologic intervention, a show of force, and finally physical restraint. At times, it may be necessary to use physical restraints until parenteral medications have had their desired effect. While it is important to protect both patient and staff, the clinicians should attempt to preserve patient autonomy even when he/she presents with agitation and aggression.

Nonpharmacologic interpersonal intervention strategies

If possible, patients should be placed in a quiet room away from the rest of the ED population. The area should be free of sharp objects, or equipment that can be thrown or used as a weapon. Visitors or family who escalate a patient's agitation should be asked to wait in another area of the ED. Intervention using talk-down strategies during this period of escalation will frequently avert violent behavior. In an escalating situation, the clinician must be sure that the patient can hear and respond. A patient who is under the influence of alcohol or drugs is not a good candidate for talk-down techniques.

The clinician should speak to the patient in a calm, non-confrontational manner. It is important to avoid an overtly angry or hostile tone. Violence in patients is often a reaction to feelings of helplessness, tension, and frustration [16,21]. Therefore, the clinician should convey concern for the patient's well-being while also firmly conveying that aggressive or disruptive behavior will not be tolerated [9]. For example, the clinician may say, "I understand that you came to the emergency department because you're in pain, and I'm happy to try to help you with this, but it's hard to help you when you raise your voice or threaten people here because it's making the staff and other patients uncomfortable." The patient should be told the consequences of continued aggressive behavior, for example, "If you're not able to calm down and talk to me, then I will need to give you medication so that you don't harm yourself or anyone else". By treating the patient with empathy and respect, more invasive techniques for de-escalation may be avoided.

Emotionally distraught patients require an active response from a clinician. Active eye contact and body language that signal attentiveness and connectedness to the patient will reduce the probability that the patient will need to explode or assault to get his/her point across [22]. It is important to be honest and precise when responding to patients. In all situations, the clinician should keep a proper physical distance from the patient [22]. Assaultive patients have a larger body buffer zone and a rule of thumb is to keep two quick steps or at least an arm's distance from the patient. A personal space can be visualized as an oval zone extending 4 to 6 feet all around [23].

In the very early stages of agitation and aggression, ED staff may consider offering the patient food or drink to show concern for the patient's well-being. The offer of food or drink symbolizes caring, concern, and nurturing and will often significantly attenuate a patient's agitation. By using a soft assertive voice and short sentences the clinician can rapidly determine if the patient is paying attention. Volume, tone, and rate of speech should be lower than the patient's; although, if too low, the patient may perceive it as a threat. The clinician should talk-down a patient by agreeing with him and not arguing. It is important not to respond to the content of the patient's speech. The patient should be overdosed with agreement. An escalating patient should be approached from the front or side as an approach from behind is extremely threatening and the clinician should never turn his/her back to the agitated or threatening patient [23]. Ideally, this intervention should take place in a secure room in which the clinician has safe and rapid egress should aggression worsen. The door to the room should swing outward so that the patient cannot block escape or barricade himself inside the room. The clinician should stay closer to the door to allow for prompt exit.

The main strategy for de-escalating a potentially violent patient is to directly address their anger or hostility. Often the patient who is overwhelmed with angry feelings intimidates the clinician who responds with logical and rational explanations. This type of response only inflames the patient. Rather than address the content of the patient's statements the clinician should address the anger and hostility. For instance, a patient becomes verbally abusive because they believe that they had to wait too long to be seen by the ED physician. Instead of trying to

explain all of the complicating factors in the ED that caused the long wait the clinician might say, "I can see how angry this makes you. I would feel the same way if I had to wait. I am sorry." Another example is the agitation of a family waiting to speak with the physician who is caring for their critically ill family member. It would be appropriate for the nursing staff or ED physician to say to the family, "I know how upsetting this is to you. I can try and answer some of your questions now but I will have to go back in a few minutes to see how your family member is doing." Even with limited time this brief response demonstrates empathy for the patient and their family.

Pharmacologic interventions

The goal of pharmacologic intervention is to calm the patient without sedation so that he/she can participate in the evaluation and treatment. Target symptoms include agitation, anxiety, motor hyperactivity, and restlessness. Disorganized thoughts, hallucinations, and delusions do not remit with several doses of antipsychotic medication and require longer-term treatment. The use of oral liquid or dissolving tablets is the least threatening and coercive pharmacologic intervention. These interventions have an onset of action which is comparable to injectable medications [24]. Even very agitated patients will often agree to take oral medication.

The most frequently used medication strategies consist of benzodiazepines, second-generation antipsychotic medications alone or in combination with a benzodiazepine, and haloperidol (Haldol) alone or in combination with a benzodiazepine [25–27]. The most commonly used benzodiazepine is lorazepam (Ativan). A very common practice is to combine haloperidol 5 mg IM or PO with lorazepam 2 mg IM or PO. This has been demonstrated to be safe and effective [28]. Droperidol (Inapsine) use has significantly diminished because of a black box warning about the potential for QT prolongation and torsades de pointes. If droperidol is used, a pretreatment electrocardiogram and cardiac monitoring are recommended [29]. Midazolam (Versed) is a short-acting benzodiazepine which may cause significant hypotension when administered IV but has little cardiopulmonary effect when given IM [29]. Recommended treatment options are summarized in Table 23.2 [25,26].

While all of these medications are effective there is a significant difference in cost; haloperidol and lorazepam are much less expensive than other agents. Whether there is a difference in adverse side effects in using these medications for one or two doses to treat acute agitation has never been systematically studied.

The most common side effects with antipsychotic medications are dystonic reactions. Dystonia typically manifests as sustained contractions of the extraocular muscles (oculogyric crisis), or muscles of the head and neck (torticollis). Laryngospasm can occur if muscles of the larynx are affected, which can be potentially life threatening. A dystonic reaction can effectively be treated with benztropine (Cogentin) 2 mg IM

Table 23.2. Medication recommendations for violent patients

Oral medication dose	Dosing interval	Precautions
Haloperidol (Haldol) 5–10 mg concentrate	Every hour up to 20 mg/24 hours	
Risperidone (Risperdal) 2 mg, orally disintegrating or liquid	Every one to two hours up to 6 mg /24 hours	
Olanzapine (Zyprexa) 5–10 mg, orally disintegrating	Every one to two hours up to 20 mg /24 hours	Benzodiazepines should not be used in combination with olanzapine because of the risk of cardiorespiratory depression.
Aripiprazole (Abilify) 5–10 mg	Every 2 hours up to 30 mg/24 hours	
Lorazepam (Ativan) 2 mg solution	Every one to two hours up to 12 mg/24 hours	
Intramuscular Medication-Dose	Dosing Interval	Precautions
Haloperidol (Haldol) 5 mg IM or IV	Every one to two hours up to 20 mg/24 hours	
Ziprasidone (Geodon) 20 mg IM	Every 4 hours up to 40 mg/ 24 hours	Do not use with increased corrected QT interval
Aripiprazole (Abilify) 9.75 mg IM	Every two hours up to 30 mg/24 hours	
Olanzapine (Zyprexa) 5–10 mg IM	Every one to two hours up to 20 mg /day.	Benzodiazepines should not be used in combination with olanzapine because of the risk of cardiorespiratory depression.
Lorazepam (Ativan) 2 mg IM	Every one to two hours up to 12 mg/day.	

every 15 to 30 minutes or diphenhydramine (Benadryl) 50 mg IM or IV every 15 to 30 minutes. Usually the dystonic reaction will resolve with one or two doses. The most common side effects with benzodiazepines are sedation and ataxia.

A show of force

A show of force is the last opportunity to manage a patient without using restraints. A show of force involves the use of adequate numbers of security staff and/or ED staff to visually demonstrate to a patient that he/she will not be allowed to lose control and injure others or themselves. This should be done in

a nonconfrontational manner. The physician or ED staff will feel more confident and can make one more effort to explain to the patient the assessment and treatment that is necessary to help them. There should always be enough staff and/or security available to place the patient in restraints if the show of force does not work. A show of force cannot be haphazard. There should be a designated leader and the ED should have a well thought out protocol that all staff and security personnel are aware of and understand how to implement. Such a protocol has to be a joint effort between ED staff and security staff. Clinical staff should always be present as they are the most knowledgeable about the patient's medical/psychiatric condition.

Physical restraints

When verbal and pharmacological interventions fail to reduce a patient's agitation, physical restraints may be used to prevent imminent harm to the patient or staff or to prevent serious disruption of the treatment setting or significant damage to property [13]. Once the decision is made to restrain a patient, the restraint process should be implemented immediately and without negotiation but with rigorous attention to the patient's safety. Restraints rather than seclusion (i.e., separation of the patient from the rest of the therapeutic environment) may be preferable or necessary in the patient with an unstable medical condition including infection, cardiac illness, body temperature instability, or metabolic illness [30]. Patients with delirium or dementia may experience a worsening of symptoms secondary to the sensory isolation induced by seclusion. Patients prone to serious and uncontrollable self-abuse and self-mutilation are also at risk in seclusion [30].

A sufficient number of staff should be used to restrain a patient. Five staff is a minimum with one staff member for each limb and one for the head to prevent the patient from biting and to make sure that the patient's airway is not compromised [30]. Once a decision to restrain is made the immediate clinical area should be cleared. The patient should be given a few and clear behavioral options without undue verbal threat or provocation [30]. The team should position itself around the patient in such a manner as to allow for rapid access to the patient's extremities. At a predetermined signal, the team should commence with physical restraints, with each staff member seizing and controlling the movement of each limb at its joint [30].

Patients should be placed with a slight elevation of the head to prevent aspiration or in a prone position on their side if there is a significant risk of aspiration [5]. It is important to note that patients should never be placed in the "hog-tie" prone position, in which the person is lying on their abdomen with hands behind their back and legs secured to restrained hands, as this has been linked to positional asphyxia. In addition, all efforts should be made to avoid physical restraints in pregnant women while in their second and third trimesters, as this can pose significant risks [31]. Patients can be medicated as outlined in Table 23.2. Even in restraints patients may take oral medications. While a patient is in restraints, continuous monitoring of the patient should occur to prevent injury (15 minute checks of extremities to ensure adequate circulation, adequate hydration, and exercise limbs when appropriate). All clinical efforts should focus on removing the patient from restraints as quickly as is clinically possible. A patient may be released from restraints when he/she is under control and no longer poses a threat to self or others. Patients can be gradually released from restraints and observed before completely removing the restraints. One arm can be released, followed by the contralateral leg, and then the final two restraints can be released. A patient should never be left with only one limb restrained as patients can hit staff if they begin to escalate again. They can also fall off of the gurney pulling it on top of them if they are confused and restless after being medicated. Tardiff and Lion (2008) comprehensively review the restraint procedure [30].

In all restraint episodes, documentation should clearly outline the behavior requiring restraint, the interventions that were made to reduce the patient's agitation before restraints, and all efforts to remove the patient from restraints. All clinicians and emergency department staff should review and thoroughly understand the restraint guidelines, polices, and procedures of their institution and of the Joint Commission and Center for Medicare Services, whose standards are proscriptive and specific.

Weapons screening

The risk of weapons being brought into the ED is considerable [32,33]. The use of metal detectors to increase the safety of the ED has been controversial. Among concerns are that metal detectors suggest a sense of danger, and that metal detectors project a bad image to the community [5,34]. However, studies have demonstrated that metal detectors have actually enhanced patients' sense of safety and that patients felt protected by the presence of a metal detector [34,35]. In a discussion of the subject in the monograph *Emergency Department Violence: Prevention and Management* [5], it is recommended that metal detectors be in secure, isolated areas away from the waiting rooms to minimize the possibility of a confrontation that could involve innocent bystanders. The use of metal detectors requires a thoughtful plan that involves the following issues [36]:

- Access control
- Traffic flow
- Security hardware
- Staff/personnel buy-in and training
- Development of policy and procedures
- Legal counsel and support.

Thompson and Kramer exhaustively review these issues and also offer a sample policy and procedure to address Emergency Department screening [36].

Weapons screening/metal detectors need not only involve a fixed device at the entrance of the ED. Hand-held wand devices can also be used at the bedside to detect hidden weapons. This is particularly helpful for those patients who arrive at the ED by means of ambulance and those who are ill enough as to require immediate medical attention. One study which assessed retrospectively the effect of a new ED security system on weapon confiscation showed that just over 40% of those weapons appropriated were in those patients who had arrived by ambulance [37].

The most important aspect of weapons screening in the ED is that it be performed uniformly, for all patients and visitors. Although there are certain types of patients who are more likely to become violent while in the ED, less is known about which people carry weapons into the emergency department. Indeed, at one large urban, level 1 Trauma center, weapons were confiscated from people of all ages – from the elderly to the young, and in both females and males [36].

Managing the armed patient

If a patient appears in a treatment setting with a weapon, as few people as possible should be exposed to the risk of injury [18]. Staff should retreat to a secure location if possible and keep clear of the subject. Otherwise, attempts should be made to position doors, stretchers, or heavy objects between the subject and the staff and bystanders. Police should be notified; once law enforcement arrives, medical staff should not interfere and let the security officers and/or police handle the incident [5].

If the clinician is confronted face to face with an armed patient, he/she should be calm and not become counteraggressive or threatening. Counterthreats or physical aggression by the clinician are more likely to result in the patient firing the weapon or result in serious injury. The clinician should encourage the patient to talk during the initial phases of the confrontation and repeat the patient's concerns. The firearm is almost invariably an expression of feelings of inadequacy and fear. If a short time passes without the patient actually firing the gun, the likelihood of its eventual use is diminished. Initially, however, the clinician should comply with whatever demand the patient may make and take special care to avoid further upsetting the patient. There should be no attempt to take the weapon from the patient. A suggestion should be made to have the patient put the weapon down gently. However, the clinician should not reach for the gun or tell the patient to drop the gun because it might discharge [18].

If a hostage situation occurs in the ED, the actual control of the incident is best left to experienced authorities. The ED can best be prepared for a hostage crisis by developing well-defined procedures for securing the area, for alerting the appropriate law enforcement agencies, and by designating clear lines of authority. These procedures may be developed in collaboration with law enforcement officials who are trained and experienced in dealing with hostage incidents. Resistance and heroics by unarmed and inexperienced civilians are extremely risky [5].

Violence and legal issues in the ED

A comprehensive discussion of legal issues related to violence is beyond the scope of this chapter. One issue that the ED physician should always be cognizant of is liability related to restraints [38]. The key to reducing liability in restraint episodes is documentation [38]. Even though legal support exists for the use of restraints physicians are still at risk for legal action from patients [38]. Sixteen percent of EDs in teaching hospitals reported at least one legal action made against the ED staff over a 5-year period [39]. Six percent of these cases were for failing to restrain a patient, while another 5% were for injuries that occurred in the restraint process [39]. The ED should always review restraint protocols with hospital administration and the hospital legal department and establish an ongoing training and education program for all ED staff on restraint procedures and policy.

References

1. Bureau of Labor Statistics. *Assault by Person(s), Health Care and Social Assistance, Private Industry, 2003–2007.* Available at: http://www.bls.gov/opub/cwc/sh20100825ar01p1.htm (Accessed June 15, 2011).

2. Kansagra SM, Rao SR, Sullivan AF, et al. A survey of workplace violence across 65 U.S. emergency departments. *Acad Emerg Med* 2008;**15**:1268–74.

3. Behnam M, Tillotson RD, Davis SM, Hobbs GR. Violence in the emergency department: a national survey of emergency medicine residents and attending physicians. *J Emerg Med* 2011;**40**:565–79.

4. Dubin WR, Ning A. Violence toward mental health professionals. In: Simon RI, Tardiff K, (Eds.). *Textbook of Violence Assessment and Management.* Washington, DC: American Psychiatric Publishing, Inc; 2008: 461–81.

5. American College of Emergency Physicians. *Emergency Department Violence: Prevention and Management.* Dallas, TX: American College of Emergency Physicians; 1988.

6. Osbahr AJ, chair. *Violence in the Emergency Department.* Report of the Council on Science and Public Health (I-10) 2010.

7. Gates D, Boss CS, McQueen L. Violence against emergency department workers. *J Emerg Med* 2006;**31**:331–7.

8. Taylor JL, Rew L. A systematic review of the literature: workplace violence in the emergency department. *J Clin Nurs* 2010;**20**:1072–85.

9. Kelen GD, Catlett CL. Violence in the health care setting. *JAMA* 2010;**304**:2530–1.

10. Petit JR. Management of the acutely violent patient. *Psychiatr Clin N Am* 2005;**28**:701–11.

11. Goldberg SB, Lion JR. Violence in the emergency department. In: Lion JR, Dubin WH, Futrell D, (Eds.). *Workplace Security: Effective Policies and Practices in Health Care.* Chicago: Hospital Association Press; 1996: 265–76.

12. Zun LS. Evidence-based evaluation of psychiatric patients. *J Emerg Med* 2004;**28**:35–9.

13. Baron DA, Dubin WR, Ning A. Other psychiatric emergencies. In: Sadock BJ, Sadock VA, Ruiz P, (Eds.). *Kaplan and Sadock's Comprehensive Textbook of Psychiatry*, (9th Edition, Volume 2). Philadelphia: Wolters Kluwer/Lippincott Williams & Wilkins; 2009: 2732–45.

14. Shah SJ, Fiorito M, McNamara RM. A screening tool to medically clear psychiatric patients in the emergency department. *J Emerg Med* 2010 [Epub ahead of print].

15. Folstein MF, Folstein SE, McHugh PR. "Mini-Mental State" A practical method for grading the cognitive state of patients for the clinician. *J Psychiatr Res* 1975;**12**:189–98.

16. Novitsky MA, Julius RJ, Dubin WR. Non-pharmacologic management of violence in psychiatric emergencies. *Prim Psychiatry* 2009;**16**:49–53.

17. Rocca P, Villari V, Bogetto F. Managing the aggressive and violent patient in the psychiatric emergency. *Prog Neuropsychopharmacol Biol Psychiatr* 2006;**30**:586–91.

18. Tardiff K. Clinician safety. In: Tardiff K, (Ed.). *Assessment and Management of Violent Patients*, (2nd Edition). Washington, DC: American Psychiatric Press, Inc; 1996.

19. Drummond DJ, Sparr LF, Gordon GH. Hospital violence reduction among high-risk patients. *JAMA* 1989;**261**:2531–4.

20. Allen MH, Currier GW, Carpenter D, et al. The expert consensus guideline series: treatment of behavioral emergencies. *J Psychiatr Pract* 2005;**11** (Suppl 1):1–108.

21. Dubin WR. Management and treatment of violent patients. In: Flach F, (Ed.). *Directions in Psychiatry*, (Volume 17). New York, NY: The Hatherleigh Company; 1997.

22. Eichelman BS. Strategies for clinician safety. In: Eichelman BS, Hartwig AC, (Eds.). *Patient Violence and the Clinician.* Washington, DC: American Psychiatric Press; 1995: 139.

23. Berg AZ, Bell CC, Tupin J. Clinician safety: assessing and managing violent patients. *New Dir Ment Health Serv* 2000;**86**:9–29.

24. Currier GW, Medori R. Orally versus intramuscularly administered antipsychotic drugs in psychiatric emergencies. *J Psychiatr Pract* 2006;**12**:30–40.

25. Jibson MD. Psychopharmacology in the emergency room. *J Clin Psychiatry* 2007;**68**:796–7.

26. Battaglia J. Pharmacological management of acute agitation. *Drugs* 2005;**65**:1207–22.

27. Currier GW, Simpson GM. Risperidone liquid concentrate and oral lorazepam versus intramuscular haloperidol and intramuscular lorazepam for treatment of psychotic agitation. *J Clin Psychiatry* 2001;**62**:153–7.

28. Battaglia J, Moss S, Rush J, et al. Haloperidol, lorazepam, or both for psychotic agitation? A multicenter, prospective, double-blind, emergency department study. *Am J Emerg Med* 1997;**15**:335–40.

29. Coburn VA, Mycyk MB. Physical and chemical restraints. *Emerg Med Clin N Am* 2009;**27**:655–67.

30. Tardiff K, Lion JR. Seclusion and restraint. In: Simon RI, Tardiff K, Eds.). *Textbook of Violence Assessment and Management.* Washington, DC: American Psychiatric Publishing, Inc; 2008: 339–56.

31. Ladavac AS, Dubin WR, Ning A, Stuckeman P. Emergency management of agitation in pregnancy. *Gen Hosp Psychiatry* 2007;**29**:39–41.

32. Irvin CB, Habas RC. Weapon changes over time after initiation of a comprehensive weapon surveillance system. *Am J Emerg Med* 1999;**17**:323–4.

33. Ordog GJ, Wasserberger J, Ordog C, Ackroyd G, Atluri S. Violence and general security in the emergency department. *Acad Emerg Med* 1995;**2**:151–4.

34. McNamara R, Yu DK, Kelly JJ. Public perception of safety and metal detectors in an urban emergency department. *Am J Emerg Med* 1997;**15**:40–2.

35. Mattox EA, Wright SW, Bracikowski AC. Metal detectors in the pediatric emergency department: patron attitudes and national prevalence. *Pediatr Emerg Care* 2000;**16**:163–5.

36. Thompson BM, Kramer TL. Weapons screening policies and practices. In: Lion JR, Dubin WR, Futrell DE, (Eds.). *Creating a Secure Workplace: Effective Polices and Practices in Health Care.* Chicago: American Hospital Publishing, Inc; 1998: 209–34.

37. Rankins RC, Hendey GW. Effect of a security system on violent incidents and hidden weapons in the emergency department. *Ann Emerg Med* 1999;**33**:676–9.

38. Blanchard JC, Curtis KM. Violence in the emergency department. *Emerg Med Clin North Am* 1999;**17**:717–30.

39. Lavoie FW, Carter GL, Danzl DF, Berg RL. Emergency department violence in United States teaching hospitals. *Ann Emerg Med* 1988;**17**:1227–48.

Chapter 24

Restraint and seclusion techniques in the emergency department

John Kahler and Anita Hart

Introduction

Given the prevalence of violence in our society, it is not surprising that emergency departments (EDs) and hospitals are forced to manage it in a clinical environment. Although no area of health care is immune, certain arenas have been shown to be more prone to violence such as emergency departments, waiting rooms, psychiatry wards, and geriatric units [1]. EDs are highly susceptible to violence due to a variety of factors: high stress environment, long waiting and treatment times, overcrowding, confusion, fragmented communication, staff shortages, and financial issues to name a few [1]. Various reports on the incidence of healthcare providers being victims of violence have been reported as high as 50% [2]. Several predictors of violent behavior in the ED have been cited and include: male gender, substance abuse, victims of violence, and psychiatric illness [3].

Restraints

Definition

A physical restraint is defined as any manual method, physical or mechanical device, material, or equipment that immobilizes or reduces the ability of a patient to move his or her arms, legs, body, or head freely [4]. Casts, slings, or collars that have a therapeutic benefit are not considered to be a restraint if the patient has agreed to the therapeutic intervention. Positioning a patient for a surgery is generally not considered a restraint, as the positioning is considered part of the informed consent for the procedure.

A drug or medication is considered a chemical restraint when it is used to manage the patient's behavior or restrict the patient's freedom of movement and is not a standard treatment or dosage for the patient's condition [4]. Giving a schizophrenic patient who has been off their antipsychotics a dose of haloperidol for symptom control or treating an alcoholic with an active withdrawal syndrome with a benzodiazepene is treating their underlying illness. Administering so much drug that the patient is unable to meaningfully participate in their own care is considered a restraint.

The use of restraints is considered a violation of Patient Rights and as such is regulated by the Center for Medicare and Medicaid Services. The use of restraints is *always* a last resort.

Indications

Restraint may be imposed to ensure the immediate physical safety of the patient, a staff member, or others and must be discontinued at the earliest possible time. There are clinical situations where the judicious use of restraints is warranted but their use is never to be considered to be part of routine practice. Before initiating restraint use, the active consideration of alternatives is an expectation for all clinicians.

Restraints are used in the healthcare setting primarily in two general situations: (1) violent and/or self-destructive situations when the patient has demonstrated or poses an imminent danger to themself or another, and (2) disruption of therapy or nonviolent, non–self-destructive situations. Well-meaning medical personnel may underappreciate the risk of restraints in patient care compared to their perceived benefit. One such example is incorrectly assuming that a patient who is a fall risk meets the definition of imminent danger. Restraints are associated with increased risk of falls and other injury [5,6].

If a patient is harmful to self or another and cannot be managed using de-escalation techniques, restraints may be appropriate. If the restraint is needed to prevent disruption of therapy, such as life-sustaining lines and tubes, and alternatives are not a viable option, then this too would be an appropriate indication for restraints. If a healthcare advocate or proxy decision maker is available, obtaining informed consent is essential [7].

Chemical restraints are defined as the use of medications to control a patient's behavior and restrict their freedom of movement. It is an effective form of management with the combative or agitated patient in the emergency department and is used for the safety of the patient, healthcare providers and to facilitate diagnostics or treatment. Healthcare providers in the emergency setting are burdened with the task of patient's safety and outcomes regardless of the situation, without advanced notice, and often with superimposed urgency. It is for these reasons that proper assessment and diagnosis must occur as

Behavioral Emergencies for the Emergency Physician, ed. Leslie S. Zun, Lara G. Chepenik, and Mary Nan S. Mallory. Published by Cambridge University Press. © Cambridge University Press 2013.

soon as possible. Patients, due to several different reasons, often can't cooperate with the healthcare assessment. Strategies must be used to overcome these barriers. These strategies may involve verbal de-escalation and body language but in some cases only physical or chemical restraints will achieve safe, therapeutic outcomes.

Chemical restraint can take the form of light sedation of the agitated patient in physical restraints to rapid tranquilization of the combative patient. The decision to use chemical restraints is an important one which can significantly improve a physician's ability to manage a patient safely. Caution is taken to prevent further harm, as adverse outcomes, including death, have occurred due to improper use of both physical and chemical restraints. Rapid tranquilization involves the aggressive administration of a medication (such as ketamine, haloperidol, or lorazepam) to quickly control a patient whose behavior is out of control, demonstrating violence, or physically combative. An example might be the confused, combative patient brought into the resuscitation area of the ED without any history. It becomes urgent to determine the underlying etiology which can be traumatic, toxicologic, psychiatric, infectious, or neurologic. Applying rapid tranquilization allows the providers to safely examine, obtain intravenous access, send blood for testing, and provide necessary monitoring until a better understanding of the severity is known and further diagnostics are enabled. The case example in Figure 24.1 illustrates how important diagnostics can be performed and life-saving interventions can be provided for an uncontrolled patient when rapid tranquilization is used.

Table 24.1. Indications for chemical restraint

To calm behavior and facilitate assessment in a combative patient with unknown diagnosis
To enhance patient comfort and safety when physically restrained
To provide safety and treatment for an agitated patient with psychosis

Table 24.2. Most commonly used medications for chemical restraint

Drug	Dosage	Route	Onset of action
Lorazepam	1–2 mg	IV, IM, PO	5–20 min IV, IM
Haloperidol	2–5 mg	IV, IM	20–30 min IV, IM
Ketamine	1–2 mg/kg	IV, IM	30 sec IM, 3–4 min IM

Light sedation, on the other hand, is used to calm the agitated patient in restraints. In many instances patients tolerate physical restraints and do not require sedation. However, when a patient remains assaultive (spitting, biting) or shows increased agitation due to the restraints, light sedation may be indicated for patient safety. This creates an environment safe for the patient and the healthcare providers. Once a patient is sedated, they cannot protect themselves or seek help when needed. The use of chemical restraints is not to be taken lightly, putting a greater responsibility on the provider to ensure the safety of the patient, with close, frequent monitoring, and reassessments. Deaths have occurred when monitoring was not performed for the restrained patient. Restraint should not be used as a form of convenience or punishment. There are several different clinical scenarios in which it is effectively used (Table 24.1).

Chemical restraints are an effective and safe tool in caring for patients when used wisely. As with conscious sedation, the provider must be thoroughly familiar with any drug used, specifically the indications, contraindications, dosage, side effects, and drug interactions. The intent of this chapter is to provide an overview of the pharmacology, indications, side effects, and dosages of the three most commonly used medications (Table 24.2) for chemical sedation. The reader is referred to reference texts for a more in-depth discussion. Some of the more common drugs used in these situations are lorazepam, haloperidol, and ketamine. Others exist but are beyond the scope of this chapter.

Lorazepam (Ativan) is a benzodiazepine with sedative hypnotic actions. It is one of the more commonly used drugs for sedation, seizures, anxiolysis, and chemical restraint in the ED. When used properly it provides safe and effective therapy in most patient populations. A safety advantage of the benzodiazepine class is that they have relatively few drug interactions. The main risk is excessive sedation or respiratory depression and it can be unpredictable in the setting of additional sedatives or opiates. In certain patient populations it should be avoided or used with caution such as intoxicated patients, the elderly, those with sleep apnea, and pulmonary impairment. Lorazepam may be administered PO, IV, or IM, which enhances its clinical utility. The initial dose is generally 1–2 mg by means of either route and it should be dose adjusted for the patient's age and comorbidities.

Haloperidol (Haldol) is an antipsychotic that has been around for a long time. It produces safe and effective sedation in the

A 24-year-old male is brought in by EMS with unknown history. He is altered and combative and medics are unable to obtain vital signs. In the trauma bay it is not possible to examine him because he is confused, uncooperative, and combative. Ketamine 1.5mg/kg is administered IM and he becomes calm. A full physical exam is performed, an IV placed, he is placed on cardiac and pulse oximetry monitors and vital signs are obtained. His temperature is noted to be 104° F. Rocephin is administered within minutes. Later in his ED stay, he is found to have bacterial meningitis by lumbar puncture.

Figure 24.1. Case scenario using effective sedation for emergent medical assessment.

combative patient. It is often used in combination with loraze-pam to rapidly control the agitated patient. The initial dose is usually 2–5 mg IV or IM but the starting dose in the elderly can be as low as 0.5 mg for a total dose of 2 mg daily. Side effects are uncommon but can include tremors, constipation, confusion, urinary retention, postural hypotension, tardive dyskinesia, and torsades de pointes in patients with prolonged QT interval. Haloperidol is contraindicated in Parkinson's patients or those with Parkinsonian features such as Lewy body dementia. It should be used with caution in patients with prolonged QT interval, electrolyte abnormalities, cardiovascular disease, seizure history, hepatic impairment, and elderly and demented patients (especially females). There are a variety of drug interactions that should be reviewed before usage.

Ketamine is a short-acting anesthetic that produces a dissociative state and has analgesic properties. It induces a sedative state in which the patient appears awake but is unconscious. It has some unique characteristics that make it useful in certain patient populations. Being a centrally acting stimulant of the sympathetic nervous system, it can increase blood pressure and cardiac output. This can be useful when trying to avoid hypotension, e.g., the combative trauma patient. On the other hand, it is less desirable in older populations who may be hypertensive and/or have coronary and cerebrovascular disease. One unique adverse effect is an emergence reaction. These may include a range of psychologic manifestations varying from pleasant hallucinations to unpleasant delirium. Emergence reactions occur in up to 12% of cases and usually last for a few hours. They are generally benign without residual effects. Small doses of benzodiazepines or barbiturates can prevent and/or treat these phenomena.

Contraindications to the use of ketamine include hypertension, stroke, head trauma, intracranial mass, or hemorrhage. Caution is recommended in alcoholic patients, those with elevated intraocular pressures, coronary disease, or if thyrotoxicosis is suspected.

Drugs may be used alone or effectively in combination. The combination of haloperidol and lorazepam results in more rapid tranquilization with less extrapyramidal system symptoms [8]. Appropriate monitoring must be provided to any patient sedated or chemically restrained in the ED. This involves frequent physical assessments by nursing such as mental status, vital signs, pulse oximetry, IV access, and in if needed cardiac monitoring. The care provider should perform frequent neurologic and hemodynamic assessments to ensure no physical deterioration of the patient.

Physical restraint application requires training and the demonstrated competency of involved staff. Incorrect application of restraints can lead to injury of the patient and others. All staff must have an understanding of triggers for the use of restraints and appropriate nonphysical intervention skills. An individual assessment needs be performed to select the least restrictive method, safely apply the restraint, and then subsequently assess the physical and psychological state of the patient to determine when discontinuation is indicated. In addition, the staff is required to have cardiopulmonary

resuscitation and first aid certification [4]. To maintain the integrity of the patient and provider relationship, the supervising provider should not participate in the application of restraint.

Physical restraints can take many forms, from tucking someone's blanket so tightly over them that they cannot move their limbs freely to a locked limb restraint on each extremity. The freedom to move one's head and limbs defines the restraint. If a patient cannot put the bedrail down on their own to exit the bed and both bedrails are left in the upright position, it is considered a restraint. One bedrail up and one bedrail down, which provides a safe exit from the bed, is not considered a restraint. Padded bedrails for seizure precautions or both rails up for transportation are considered a safety precaution.

Alternatives to restraint use

Alternatives to both chemical and physical restraints should always be explored before their initiation. In addition to the medical causes for behavior change one should also consider other causes of the behavior change such as pain, discomfort, fear, loneliness, and address these as well. There are a variety of disguises and distractions which can alleviate the need for restraints. For example, covering a line or tube with extra gauze and a long-sleeved shirt may successfully keep an elderly patient with dementia from pulling out an IV. Selective use of abdominal binders may keep surgical drains from being tugged at by a delirious patient [14]. Providing companionship and redirection by inviting families to stay with their loved ones can also be successful (Table 24.3).

Table 24.3. Causes and alternative management of agitation

Causes	Interventions/alternatives
Medical	**Medical**
Infection, Electrolyte imbalance, Dehydration, Renal failure, Encephalopathy, Drug overdose or withdrawal, Sensory deprivation, Sleep-wake disruption	Identify and treat underlying condition, Provide access to sensory aids, Perform frequent observation, Provide adequate pain management, Promote sleep hygiene
Physical	**Physical**
Hunger, Thirst, Fatigue Elimination needs Fever Pain Environmental irritant	Provide calm environment, Proactively toilet Remove offending agent (iv, catheter, tube) if not needed. Use abdominal binders, skin sleeves, iv shields, other methods to disguise as necessary, Adapt environment as needed Activity/ambulation as tolerated
Emotional	**Emotional**
Anger, Sadness, Fearfulness, Loneliness Boredom, Anxiety, Panic	Encourage family visiting, Provide familiar items, Give choices

Documentation

To maintain regulatory compliance, a licensed independent practitioner (e.g., NP, PA, MD, DO) must sign an order authorizing the use of restraints within an hour of the restraint's initiation. Nursing may initiate the restraint without an order when there is imminent danger but cannot maintain the restraint without an order from a licensed independent practitioner. In addition to the order itself, the practitioner must document all alternatives attempted or why they would be considered ineffective in that specific case. Nursing performs periodic re-assessments and must discontinue restraints as soon as the behavior necessitating the restraint episode has resolved.

Complications

Physical restraint has been associated with an increased risk of falls, psychological distress, deconditioning, serious injury (asphyxiation, aspiration, rhabdomyolysis, cardiac events), increased hospital length of stay, and death [5,6,13]. The risks involved must be weighed with serious deliberation. The use of restraints came to national attention in 1998 when the Hartford Courant revealed 142 patients had died in restraints or in seclusion in the previous decade. Now, any death or serious injury while in restraints is considered a Quality Never Event and is reportable.

Policy

Each hospital is required to maintain a policy regarding the use of restraints within their institution. Centers for Medicare and Medicaid Services (CMS) standards provide definitions and delineates guidelines for restraint usage and documentation.

Seclusion

Seclusion is another form of behavior control used in emergency departments and hospitals and is simply defined as the confinement of a patient in a closed space for a specific amount of time. There are a variety of clinical scenarios in which seclusion may be used with the most common reason being violence [9]. Seclusion is of limited utility in the ED due to the need for access to the patient for ongoing medical assessment and treatment. It is contraindicated in certain patient populations (Table 24.4). Although seclusion rates do vary across the country, it is not commonly used in the United States [10]. One of the greatest obstacles to using seclusion in the ED are physical plant issues or lack of clinically appropriate space for placing a patient in seclusion [9].

Seclusion of patients involves risk and therefore is heavily regulated by external agencies. The law supports the use of seclusion in the clinical setting to protect patients from themselves and others when violence seems imminent. Convenience for the healthcare providers is not considered a legitimate reason to seclude a patient and must be avoided [11].

In order for seclusion to be used safely and legally several things must be in place. First, an appropriate room must be

Table 24.4. Seclusion contraindications

Unstable patients requiring close monitoring
Suicidal patients
Self-mutilating patients
Self-abusive patients
Intoxicated patients and those with toxic ingestions

Table 24.5. Seclusion room requirements

Enough space for one patient and six staff members
Impact resistant walls with sound barrier
Direct observation (nonbreakable window and/or video)
Ceilings of at least 3 meters
No mobile furniture or other projectiles
Heavy duty door (steel) that opens outward to prevent the patient from barricading inside
Nonbreakable mirror to view any blind spots in the room
Light fixtures that are ceiling mounted, flush, and non-breakable
Heavy-duty mattress resistant to tearing
Tamperproof smoke and fire detectors
Intercom and alarm system
Soft paint color on walls

available that is designed specifically for seclusion [12]. It must be free of obstacles that a patient could use to injure self, others, or property. For example, furniture should be non-mobile and there should be no objects in the room that can be thrown. Patients must be observed through a nonbreakable window or video monitoring. A more complete list of room considerations is noted in Table 24.5. Very few emergency departments have dedicated space for this type of activity. Policies regarding its usage (indications, monitoring, documentation) must be in place and adequately trained staff must be employed.

A healthcare provider initiating an order for seclusion must weigh the risk/benefits. To do this effectively, knowledge of complications and contraindications is critical. Risks of seclusion include but are not limited to, unrecognized patient deterioration, patient self-injury, neglect, and undue mental stress. Contraindications to the usage of seclusion include the need for close monitoring of an unstable patient, patients who are suicidal, self-abusive, self-mutilating, or have reported or are suspected of an overdosage or ingestion.

Documentation

Documentation for any patient placed in seclusion must include a comprehensive patient assessment, judgment of patient capacity, indication for seclusion, appropriate monitoring, and reassessment. Protocols and hospital policies, in line with CMS and other federal guidelines, must be in place. Staff must be educated. Of note, CMS requires reporting of any death that occurs to a patient while in seclusion or restraints [16].

Summary

Healthcare professionals, and in particular those in EDs, must routinely assess and treat confused, combative, and sometimes violent patients with underlying, but undifferentiated medical, surgical, toxicological, and psychiatric symptoms. When verbal de-escalation and other less restrictive means of managing these behavioral symptoms fail, the judicious and knowledgeable application of physical restraints, administration of chemical restraint, and rarely seclusion, can facilitate emergent assessment and treatment of the patient and provide safety for all parties.

References

1. Coburn VA, Mycyk MB. Physical and chemical restraints. *Emerg Med Clin North Am* 2009;**27**:655–67.

2. Mahoney BS. The extent, nature, and response to victimization of emergency nurses in Pennsylvania. *J Emerg Nurs* 1991;**17**:282–91.

3. Citrome L, Volavka J. Violent patients in the emergency setting. *Psychiatric Clin North Am* 1999;**22**:789–801.

4. Medicare and Medicaid Programs. *Hospitals Conditions of Participation: Patients' Rights (42 CFR Part 482)*. Published in the Federal Register on December 8, 2006 (Volume 71, Number 236; pages 71,378–428).

5. Evans D, Wood J, Lambert L. Patient injury and physical restraint devices: a systematic review. *J Adv Nurs* 2003;**41**:274–82.

6. Mohr WK, Petti TA, Mohr BD. Adverse effects associated with physical restraint. *Can J Psychiatry* 2003;**48**:330–7.

7. Annas GJ. The last resort – the use of physical restraints in medical emergencies. *N Engl J Med* 1999;**341**:1408–12.

8. Battaglia J, Moss S, Rush J, et al. Haloperidol, lorazepam, or both for psychotic agitation? A multicenter, prospective, double-blind, emergency department study. *Am J Emerg Med* 1997;**15**:335–40.

9. Zun LS, Downey L. The use of seclusion in emergency medicine. *Gen Hosp Psychiatry* 2005;**27**:365–71.

10. Betemps EJ, Somoza E, Buncher CR. Hospital characteristics, diagnosis, and staff reasons associated with use of seclusion and restraint. *Hosp Community Psychiatry* 1993;**44**:367–71.

11. Wexler DB. Seclusion and restraint: lessons from law, psychiatry, and psychology. *Int J Law Psychiatry* 1982;**5**:285–94.

12. Royal College of Psychiatrists. *Not Just Bricks and Mortar*. Council report CR62, Jan 1998. London: Royal College of Psychiatrists.

13. Miles SH, Irvine P. Deaths caused by physical restraints. *Gerontologist* 1992;**32**:762–6.

14. Colorado Foundation for Medical Care. *Restraint Reduction*. Available at: www.cms.gov/CFCsAndCoPs/downloads/restraintreduction.pdf

Use of psychiatric medications in the emergency department

Alvin Wang and Gerald Carroll

Introduction

Psychiatric medications are encountered daily in the emergency department, and a familiarity with their pharmacodynamics and pharmacokinetics is essential to our practice. In this chapter, we will review the most common psychiatric medications used in the emergency setting and discuss the larger group of psychiatric medications we encounter daily on our patients' medication lists.

Antidepressants

The most commonly prescribed psychiatric medications are the antidepressants, subdivided into four classes:

- Tricyclic antidepressants (TCAs)
- Heterocyclic antidepressants
- Selective serotonin reuptake inhibitors (SSRIs)
- Monoamine oxidase inhibitors (MAOIs).

These medications have revolutionized our ability to treat depression and have become safer as each class has been invented [1]. These medications have become so common on everyday medication lists of patients of all ages that they are easily overlooked or ignored. As a group, they can be responsible for a wide range of side effects, and in some cases can be fatal in overdose. Antidepressants generally have a large volume of distribution and thus cannot be removed by dialysis.

Tricyclic antidepressants (TCAs) have been in use for more than 50 years and are related in structure to phenothiazines. These medications have broad effects and are used for depression, movement disorders, sleep regulation, migraine headache prophylaxis, and neuropathic pain. Their primary mechanism of action is by means of norepinephrine and serotonin uptake inhibition. They are incompletely absorbed, undergo extensive first-pass metabolism, are fat soluble, and have a large volume of distribution. Several TCAs have active metabolites that prolong their duration of action. For example, amitriptyline is metabolized to nortriptyline. There are variations in side-effect profiles among the TCAs, with some agents displaying more than others. The primary drawbacks of the TCAs are their myriad side effects and lethality in overdose.

Side effects of tricyclic antidepressants are myriad [2]:

- Antimuscarinic actions (dry mouth, blurred vision, constipation, confusion, urinary retention)
- Sympathomimetic actions (tremor, insomnia, palpitations)
- Cardiovascular effects (hypotension, arrhythmias)
- Metabolic-endocrine effects (weight gain, sexual dysfunction, loss of libido)
- Neurologic effects (sedation, seizures)
- Psychiatric effects (worsening of psychosis).

Tricyclic antidepressants are extremely effective for mood disorders and revolutionized the treatment of depression over 40 years ago. However, because of the side-effect profiles and low LD50, their use has been generally supplanted by newer agents. In current practice, they are more likely to be used for chronic neuropathic pain and refractory depression. Nevertheless, TCAs are an important group of medications that every emergency physician should feel comfortable assessing as part of a medication list, in a patient with new side effects, and crucially in overdose.

Signs and symptoms of TCA overdose often present as amplification of the side effects listed above, however, initial symptoms can be minimal and progress to life-threatening central nervous system (CNS) and cardiovascular symptoms within hours. Acute TCA ingestions of 10–20 mg/kg (approximately 5 times the normal therapeutic dose of 2–4 mg/kg/day) can cause significant symptoms [3]. Although serum assays exist to measure TCA level, these data may not always be readily available in all hospital systems. Electrocardiogram (ECG) analysis is an immediately available and relatively sensitive bedside test which can help identify and risk-stratify patients at risk for development of significant symptoms. The most common ECG finding in TCA overdose is sinus tachycardia. Two studies have demonstrated that a limb QRS interval greater than 100 ms or a terminal R wave in lead aVR greater than 3 mm are relatively sensitive indicators of toxicity and can be used to predict an increased incidence of adverse events. In addition, in these studies, no patient with a QRS duration less than 100 ms went on to developed seizure or ventricular dysrhythmia [4–6].

Behavioral Emergencies for the Emergency Physician, ed. Leslie S. Zun, Lara G. Chepenik, and Mary Nan S. Mallory. Published by Cambridge University Press. © Cambridge University Press 2013.

Treatment for TCA toxicity focuses on management of seizures and treatment of life-threatening dysrhythmias. Seizures should be treated with benzodiazepines. Refractory seizures can be treated with barbiturates and/or propofol. Patients with prolonged status epilepticus refractory to all the above treatments may benefit from neuromuscular blockade, intubation, and sedation, however, continuous electroencephalogram (EEG) monitoring should be initiated as well. Conflicting data exists regarding the safety and effectiveness of phenytoin in patients with TCA toxicity. One animal study demonstrated that phenytoin was ineffective in terminating seizures induced by imipramine [7]. Some data suggest that cardiotoxic effects of phenytoin are additive while others suggest that phenytoin may occasionally be effective in terminating ventricular dysrhythmias [8].

Cardiovascular toxicity, namely wide complex dysrhythmias and conduction delays are generally treated by means of alkalinization with sodium bicarbonate which has been shown to be the most efficacious therapy in several systematic reviews [9]. Dosing strategies vary, but in general, 1–2 mEq/kg boluses can be given until the QRS narrows and blood pressure normalizes. After these boluses, a sodium bicarbonate drip can be used to maintain serum pH at approximately 7.50. Hypertonic saline can also be administered to provide additional sodium to help counteract the sodium-channel blocking effect of TCAs. Although no studies have proven the efficacy of lidocaine for ventricular dysrhythmias, it has been used successfully in the past. [8] Class IA and IC antiarrhythmics are contraindicated because they can increase sodium-channel inhibition and further prolong the QT interval. Tricyclic antidepressants generally have a large volume of distribution and thus cannot be removed by dialysis, but this same property may allow the use of intravenous lipid emulsion for the treatment of overdose. A case report documents the successful use of intravenous lipid emulsion in patients with refractory dysrhythmias from TCA overdose [10]. Overall, data on the efficacy of lipid emulsion remains mixed [11].

Heterocyclic antidepressants are a more heterogeneous grouping of medications. The medications from this class in everyday use include trazodone, mirtazipine, bupropion, and venlafaxine. Like their tricyclic precursors, the heterocyclics undergo significant first-pass metabolism and some have active metabolites. Trazedone, bupropion, and venlafaxine have short half-lives, and are often dosed twice daily or supplied in extended-release forms. They have variable effects on norepinephrine and serotonin uptake and on selective subsets of these receptors. Some of these effects are dose dependent. At lower dosage, venlafaxine shows serotonin reuptake inhibitor effects but at higher doses it provides more norepinephrine uptake inhibition, and when tolerated, is more activating. Importantly bupropion and venlafaxine can lower the seizure threshold. Trazedone has mild antidepressant effects, but is useful for its sleep-inducing hypnotic properties and is often used with more activating antidepressants.

Side effects are agent-dependent in this class.

- Venlafaxine: anxiety, hypertension, nausea, sweating, sexual disturbances
- Bupropion: dry mouth, dizziness, seizures, tremor
- Mirtazapine: increased appetite, dizziness, weight gain.

The heterocyclic antidepressants are generally safe in overdose. Some of the older agents in this class, such as amoxapine and maprotiline, can cause neurologic and cardiac toxicity. Both agents are rarely encountered today, but may prompt toxicology consultation. Venlafaxine, bupropion, and mirtazipine are generally safe and well tolerated. In overdose, supportive care is generally sufficient.

Selective serotonin reuptake inhibitors (SSRIs) as their name implies are more selective, improving tolerability and safety profile. Compared to TCAs, SSRIs exhibit less antimuscarinic and antihistaminic side effect, improving medication tolerance. Many SSRIs are on the market. Fluoxetine was the first followed by sertraline, paroxetine, fluvoxamine, citalopram, ecitalopram, and now there are total of 12 SSRIs on the market. They have fairly similar side-effect profiles, tolerability, and efficacy, although some patients respond better to one than another. There are a wide range of studies comparing the SSRIs to tricyclics and to each other often with conflicting results. A systematic review from 2009 evaluated 117 randomized control trials and found clear benefits and differences between various SSRIs. Two agents: ecitalopram and sertraline appear to be superior in efficacy and acceptability [12].

The main pharmacological differences among the SSRIs are in half-life and their variable CYP P450 inhibition. Fluoxetine's pharmacokinetics are notable for an active metabolite, norfluoxetine, with a half-life of 7–9 days. This property can be advantageous for some patients as weekly dosing may be effective. Side effects of SSRIs, while generally mild when compared with the TCAs, can be significant enough to lead to medication noncompliance [13]:

- Decreased libido
- Gastrointestinal symptoms
- Insomnia
- Sexual dysfunction.

Generally SSRIs are safe and cause deleterious effects rarely, unless in very large dosage. With overdose, treatment is generally supportive. Clinicians should be familiar with the toxidrome of serotonin syndrome which may manifest during overdose.

Serotonin syndrome is caused by excessive stimulation of 5-HT2 receptors. It can occur when SSRIs are administered in combination with other SSRIs, MAOIs (monoamine oxidase inhibitors), or atypical antipsychotics, or even with SSRI monotherapy. Symptoms may be mild, including insomnia, tachycardia, and restlessness, or major presenting as altered mental status, myoclonus, hyperthermia, and even coma. In contrast to neuroleptic malignant syndrome (NMS), onset of symptoms with serotonin syndrome occurs more rapidly, generally within 24 hours, after initiation of the medication or a change in dose.

The diagnosis of serotonin syndrome is made clinically because serum levels do not correlate with clinical findings. In 2003, the Hunter criteria were shown to be more sensitive and specific than the previously used Sternbach's criteria [14].

Diagnostic Hunter criteria for serotonin syndrome include the presence of serotonergic agent and *one* of the following criteria or sets of criteria:

- Spontaneous clonus
- Inducible clonus *and* agitation *or* diaphoresis
- Oculor clonus *and* agitation *or* diaphoresis
- Tremor *and* hyper-reflexia
- Hypertonia *and* hyperpyrexia (>38 C) *and* ocular clonus *or* inducible clonus.

Treatment of serotonin syndrome includes the discontinuation of inciting agent(s), sedation, and treatment of autonomic instability. Hyperthermia can be treated with direct and indirect cooling. Antipyretics are not useful. Tachycardia can be treated with short-acting agents-beta-blockers, or direct venodilators. Refractory agitation and autonomic instability can be treated with cyproheptadine, an H1 receptor blocker [15]. Bromocriptine and dantrolene are not recommended [16].

Monoamine oxidase inhibitors (MAOIs) block monoamine oxidase, the enzyme responsible for deaminating serotonin, norepinephrine, and dopamine. Their use was first discovered in 1951 when iproniazid, an analog of isoniazid, was found to be ineffective in the treatment of tuberculosis, but was incidentally noted to elevate the mood of patients receiving it [17]. Monoamine oxidase generally consists of two isomers; MAO-A which is found in the brain and intestine, and MAO-B which is found in the brain and in platelets. MAO-A inhibition is thought to be responsible for most of the antidepressant activity of MAOIs, but is also responsible for the infamous tyramine reaction associated with MAOI therapy. Side effects of MAOIs can be significant and include dizziness in more than 50% of patients, hypotension, headache, dry mouth, and gastrointestinal upset. In addition, there are significant drug interactions associated with MAOIs. Their use is contraindicated with any other medication which inhibits reuptake of serotonin, norepinephrine, and/or dopamine, contains precursors to any of these neurotransmitters, or acts as a sympathomimetic. Administration of any one of these agents to a patient who is taking an MAOI can result in serotonin syndrome or a hyper-adrenergic crisis.

There are four U.S. Food and Drug Administration (FDA) approved MAOIs for the treatment of major depression in the United States; isocarboxazid, phenelzine, tranylcypromine, and selegiline. The last bears additional FDA approval for the treatment of Parkinson's disease and was recently made available in a transdermal formulation (EmSam patch), which may reduce the adverse effects of MAOI by means of bypass of the gastrointestional tract [18,19]. The fifth MAOI, rasagiline, is a selective MAO-B inhibitor with FDA approval for the treatment of Parkinson's disease only. Because of these significant

drug–drug interactions and need for careful dietary restriction, use of MAOIs for the treatment of depression is generally reserved for severe cases that are refractory to all other interventions [20].

MAOI overdose can produce a biphasic response, classically resulting initially with central nervous system (CNS) stimulation and followed by coma and cardiovascular collapse [21]. A significant delay between ingestion and onset of clinical symptoms can occur. Hyperthermia can be treated with direct cooling and indirect cooling measures. Antipyretics are unlikely to be helpful. Hypertension can be treated with short-acting alpha-blocking agents such as phentolamine. Nonselective beta-blockers may be contraindicated due to the theoretical phenomenon of unopposed alpha-receptor stimulation with accelerated hypertension. Hypotension is treated with direct sympathomimetics such as norephinephrine and epinephrine. Dopamine is generally ineffective due to inhibition of norepinephrine synthesis but synergism may also cause profound hypertension. Management of MAOI toxicity and interactions can be complex. Toxicologist consultation is generally recommended.

Symptoms of acute withdrawal from MAOI therapy may include seizures, agitation, and psychosis. Treatment is supportive and may require restarting the discontinued medication.

Antipsychotics

Psychosis and schizophrenia are still poorly understood at biological and genetic levels, although great strides have been taken in pharmacotherapy of these diseases. Despite multiple theories concerning various receptor involvement, genetic predispositions, and environmental factors, no unifying evidence- based theory has emerged. In many ways, understanding of this disease or diseases is still in its infancy. However, neuroleptic medications have been around for some time and are far better understood. Antipsychotics, despite numerous side effects, have revolutionized the treatment of schizophrenia, allowing patients who once had to be hospitalized to live fairly normal lives.

Antipsychotics can be organized biochemically into four classes, but in practice they are grouped by therapeutic effect and side-effect profiles into two classes: typical and atypical. This system offers a rational framework for learning about and working with the various neuroleptic medications.

Typical antipsychotics affect a myriad of receptors in varying degrees. These include dopamine-2 receptors in the cortical striatal areas and serotonin 5-HT2a, alpha 1, histaminic, and muscarinic receptors. The efficacy and side-effect profile of each agent is due to its variable effects on involved receptors. Typical antipsychotics are lipophilic, giving them a large volume of distribution and a concomitantly long half-life. They are metabolized primarily by CYP-2D6, and significant sedation can be seen in "slow metabolizers" by means of this pathway.

Older or "typical" antipsychotics cause a wide range of side effects:

- Akathesia
- Bradykinesia
- Extrapyramidal (parkinsonian) symptoms of rigidity
- Tardive dyskinesia
- Tremor.

Additionally the typical antipsychotics can cause hyperprolactinemia and QT prolongation. The class is associated with neuroleptic malignant syndrome; rarely seen, but with significant morbidity and mortality. Indications include acute psychosis, long-term management of schizophrenia, bipolar disorder with psychotic features, postpartum psychosis, and delirium. Various typical antipsychotics are supplied in oral, intravenous, and depot formulations.

Typical antipsychotics encompass three of the four classes of neuroleptics: phenothiazines, butyrophenones, and the thioxanthines. In clinical practice, those classes offer little insight into the strength, efficacy, or side-effect profile. A more intuitive method of classification involves categorizing these medications as either high or low potency. High potency typical antipsychotics are the most commonly prescribed and in general use include haloperidol and droperidol. These medications offer little sedation and are less anticholinergic, but are more commonly associated with weight gain and extrapyramidal symptoms.

Haloperidol is the prototypical high potency typical antipsychotic medication, and is the most widely prescribed. Orally it undergoes extensive first-pass metabolism of up to 60%, with a half-life approaching 20 hours. It is widely used for acute agitation at a dose of 2–10 mg intramuscularly, with peak effect after 20 minutes. It is also available in a decanoate formulation that clears in 21 days. Depot therapy mitigates noncompliance in the chronic outpatients, preventing acute decompensations often associated with emergency hospitalization.

Droperidol is only for parenteral use and has a faster onset of action than haloperidol with a half-life of approximately 2 hours. In addition to the management of acute psychosis, it was commonly used by anesthesiologists and emergency physicians for nausea until it received a black box warning from the FDA for QT prolongation. Clinically significant sequelae such as sudden cardiac death have not been seen in smaller studies and case studies [22,23]. Haloperidol is now more commonly used for acute psychosis and/or agitation despite its slower onset of action.

Low potency typical antipsychotics are less commonly encountered. Chlorpromazine is used mostly in children and is associated with weight gain. Thioridazine also has a black box warning for its frequency of QT prolongation and is rarely used.

Atypical antipsychotics have less dopamine D2 blockade and a higher serotonin 5-HT2 blockade to D2 ratio compared to typical antipsychotics, postulated to be responsible for the decrease frequency of extrapyramidal symptoms as compared with the typical antipsychotics. One exception discussed later is aripiprazole (Abilify), which is a partial dopamine agonist.

Some atypical antipsychotics also bind to the D2 receptor differently. Clozapine and quetiapine bind D2 loosely and turn over in minutes while typicals bind for hours which may also influence their lower incidence of extrapyramidal symptoms.

The atypical antipsychotics, while generally well tolerated, do have their own side-effect concerns. The clinically relevant side effects vary between agents in frequency and intensity:

- Diabetes
- Extrapyramidal symptoms – (much lower than "typicals")
- Increased mortality in elderly dementia patients
- Hyperlipidemia
- Hyperprolactinemia
- Neuroleptic
- Malignant syndrome
- Tardive dyskinesia
- Weight gain.

Supplied in various formulations including for oral and parenteral administration, atypical antipsychotics are a heterogeneous class and require discussion of their individual properties.

Risperidone (Risperdal) – is often referred to as the most typical of the atypical antipsychotics. It has a rapid absorption and half-life of approximately 20 hours. In addition to D2 and 5-HT2 antagonism it has a small amount of muscarinic blockade, lacking anticholinergic affects. The specific side-effect profile includes mild sedation, moderate weight gain, and a small increase in pituitary adenomas. Among the atypical antipsychotics, risperidone is more commonly associated with extrapyramidal side effects, particularly at higher doses. Its generic availability has contributed to its widespread use. Some data support its use and equivalence to Haldol in severe agitation and psychosis. Risperdone is supplied as an oral tablet, or liquid, rapidly dissolving wafers, and as a depot solution for intramuscular injection.

Olanzipine (Zyprexa) is associated with serious metabolic side effects. It is gradually absorbed with a half-life of approximately 30 hours, and like most atypical antipsychotics, can be dosed once daily. In addition to D2 and 5-HT2 antagonism, olanzipine is a potent anticholinergic and antihistamine. It has 160 times the histamine effect of diphenhydramine [24]. Its side-effect profile is notable for weight gain, hyperlipidemia, hyperglycemia, sedation, dry mouth, and postural hypotension. Hyperlipidemia and hyperglycemia are most pronounced in adolescents taking olanzipine. There are case reports of oversedation when mixed with benzodiazepines [25,26].

Ziprasidone (Geodon) is slowly absorbed with half-life of approximately 7 hours. When administered orally, it must be taken with food to ensure adequate and predictable absorption. It has low histaminic and no muscarinic effects, but has been shown to cause QT prolongation and should not be combined with other medications that also prolong the QT interval. While other atypical antipsychotics are useful for acute agitation, ziprasidone carries an FDA approval for acute agitation and, after haloperidol, is the most commonly used antipsychotic for this indication [27]. Ziprasidone carries a black box warning about use in elderly patients with dementia with data showing an increased mortality in this population.

Quetiapine (Seroquel) is rapidly absorbed with a 6–7 hour half-life. It is generally unsuitable for acute psychosis due to its lack of intramuscular formulation, and the manufacturer's recommended five day dose escalation to avoid over-sedation. However, there are data supporting titration as fast as 2 days [28]. In addition to D2 and 5-HT2 effects, it also antagonizes histaminic, cholinergic, and alpha-1 adrenergic receptors. Its side-effect profile includes mild sedation, orthostatic blood pressure changes, dry mouth, mild weight gain, and akathesia. It has not been shown to affect prolactin levels. Unlike the other atypical antipsychotics, Seroquel may cause respiratory depression in overdose [29].

Aripiprazole (Abilify) has a unique mechanism of action, but in practice it has efficacy comparable to the other atypical antipsychotics. It is a partial agonist rather than direct antagonist at dopamine D2 receptors and serotonin 5-HT2 receptors and is absorbed slowly with a half-life of 75 hours. Aripiprazole has a more benign side-effect profile than other atypical antipsychotics with comparatively, fewer metabolic effects and sedation vs. olanzapine, and less dystonias, cholesterol elevation, and QT prolongation than risperdone [30]. Nevertheless aripiprazole has significant side effects including: insomnia, tremor, and constipation.

Clozapine (Clozaril) is uniquely efficacious among the atypical antipsychotics in treating the positive symptoms of schizophrenia. Unfortunately, it remains a therapy of last resort due to the significant risk of compromised immune function. Agranulocytosis is seen in 1–2% of patients taking this medication, generally occurring within weeks to months of treatment initiation As a result, clozapine requires regular laboratory monitoring, and a pharmacy database to help ensure that adversely affected patients are not accidentally restarted on the medication.

Newer atypical antipsychotics include paliperidone, iloperidone, asenapine, and lurasidone. Paliperidone, an active metabolite of risperidone, is noteworthy for not requiring dose adjustments in patients with mild hepatic impairment. With little available clinical data, the advantages and disadvantages they may hold over the more established atypical antipsychotics have yet to be demonstrated.

Mood stabilizers

Several medications are considered mood stabilizers, also referred to as antimania medications. They include lithium, carbamazapine, valproic acid, and some atypical antipsychotics. In the limited studies comparing efficacy, the available evidence does not demonstrate superiority between agents [31]. Some patients are effectively treated with monotherapy, but many will require a second agent, generally an antipsychotic [32].

Lithium is the most widely studied and prescribed antimania medication. Lithium is a small, monovalent cation, absorbed over 6–8 hours. Excreted largely unchanged in the urine, it undergoes no appreciable metabolism. Despite extensive use and experience treating and maintaining bipolar patients with lithium, the mechanism of action remains unproven [33]. Lithium is similar to sodium in its ability to generate action potentials. Theories include effects on ion transport and electrolyte levels, changes in neurotransmitter release, and a wide range of second messenger effects, and will hopefully become clearer as genetic and biochemical research progresses.

Generally well-tolerated by patients, lithium does have significant side effects and toxicity:

- Neurotoxicity: tremor is most common; ataxia, dysarthria, aphasia, confusion
- Thyroid: decreased thyroid function, generally subclinical, rarely causes mild thyroid swelling; recommend interval TSH monitoring
- Renal: nephrogenic diabetes insipidous, decreased glomerular filtration rate, and rarely nephrotic syndrome
- Cardiac: sinus node depression; contraindicated in patients with sick sinus syndrome
- Pregnancy: increased glomerular clearance in pregnancy requires increased dose; conversely, decreased after delivery to avoid postpartum toxicity; excreted in breast milk.

The common complication of chronic lithium therapy is nephrogenic diabetes insipidus. In acute overdose, neurologic and renal manifestations predominate. Mild overdose can be treated with IV hydration and monitoring. Severe overdoses may require hemodialysis.

Carbamazepine is an anticonvulsant medication that has demonstrated efficacy in treatment of bipolar disorder and has indications for bipolar disorder, epilepsy, and trigeminal neuralgia. It is a tricyclic compound similar in structure to imipramine and other first-generation antidepressants with several pharmacodynamic effects including sodium-channel blockade, decreased synaptic transmission, possible GABA (γ-aminobutyric acid) potentiation, and inhibition of norepinephrine release and uptake. None of these mechanisms clearly explains its role as a mood stabilizer. Carbamazepine's half-life is initially approximately 36 hours, but metabolism induction rapidly decreases this to approximately 20 hours, requiring a dose adjustment in the first few weeks.

Carbamazepine has several side effects and is variably tolerated by patients:

- Neurologic: ataxia, and diplopia are common; drowsiness.
- Gastrointestinal: common.
- Hematologic: rarely, idiosyncratic blood dyscrasias: aplastic anemia, agranulocytosis; more common in the elderly, and seen in the first four weeks of therapy.

Carbamazepine overdose can be severe, potentially lethal, with toxicity similar to other tricyclic compounds.

Valproic acid (VPA) has shown efficacy in the treatment of mania and is widely used for bipolar disorder. Data support its superiority in subsets of patients with rapid cycling or with frequent episodes of mania [7]. It is also widely used as a second agent in patients who have only a partial response to lithium. VPA was initially discovered to have anticonvulsant properties while being used as a solvent for other potential anticonvulsant compounds. Therapeutic both as an acid and its salt, valproate, it is completely ionized into its active form at body pH regardless of formulation. With an 80% bioavailability, VPA concentration peaks at two hours and is confined to the extracellular space. Valproate has a half-life of 9–18 hours, and, at higher levels, its clearance is dose dependent. The mechanisms of action in reducing mania and providing mood stabilization are unclear. Valproate has been shown to blockade NMDA receptors, possibly increase GABA, and may increase potassium conduction across cell membranes and at lower doses hyperpolarize cell membranes.

Side effects are few:

- Neurologic: tremor at high doses
- Hepatotoxicity: rare idiosyncratic reaction that seems more common in children less the two years of age; can be fatal; liver function testing recommended in the first months of treatment
- Teratogenicity: rare reports of increased spina bifida, cardiovascular, orofacial, and digital abnormalities in children of pregnant women taking valproate.

Pharmacotherapy for the agitated patient

Chemical restraint of the agitated patient is perhaps the most common reason psychiatric medications are used in the emergency department. With a fair amount of contradictory data on efficacy and safety, many emergency physicians have strong opinions about the agents they favor. The most common medications used for chemical restraint are haloperidol, droperidol, ziprasidone, olanzipine, lorazepam, and midazolam [34]. Local agitation treatment protocols may be developed based on physician experience, patient age, comorbidities, and in collaboration with emergency psychiatrists.

Traditionally, physicians have prescribed a combination of typical antipsychotics and benzodiazepines for acute agitation in the emergency department. However, these interventions are not without risk. Both theoretical and real concerns about QT prolongation, over-sedation, and extrapyramidal side effects may be encountered. The significant clinical experience physicians have with these regimens balanced against the questionable efficacy but possible improved safety profile of the newer agents, suggests room for variability in agent selection, particularly when underlying conditions and current medication lists are known.

QT prolongation is associated with typical and some atypical antipsychotics and poses a theoretical chance of inducing cardiac arrhythmias, specifically the lethal polymorphic ventricular tachycardia known as "torsades de pointes". Before the black box warning about QT prolongation was issued in 2001, droperidol was widely used for its faster onset of action when compared with haloperidol. Despite continued contention over the degree and clinical relevance of QT prolongation with droperidol, it has disappeared from many hospital pharmacies, and is now used infrequently by many emergency physicians [35–38]. Despite years of emergency department use and a dearth of reported adverse outcomes, QT prolongation continues to be a concern when choosing haloperidol and ziprasidone. In recent years efficacy data on intramuscular use olanzapine and aripiprazole has become available [39–41]. The small amount of literature has only proved efficacy rather than superiority to other agents [42,43]. There are data to suggest that olanzapine and to a greater extent aripiprazole cause less QT prolongation than other agents [23,44,45].

Oversedation is another concern with pharmacologic restraints. Benzodiazepines are known sedatives, and the various typical and atypical antipsychotics have variable sedating properties. Lorazepam and midazolam are the most commonly used benzodiazepines in acute agitation management, with the major difference shorter duration of action with midazolam. In susceptible patients or at larger doses, respiratory depression and apnea can be seen. Typical antipsychotics are minimally sedating so most practitioners focus on the amount of benzodiazepines when titrating level of sedation. Atypical antipsychotics, however, are more variable in their sedative properties. Whereas ziprasidone has a similar sedation profile to the two typical antipsychotics, olanzipine has been found to be very sedating and should be used with caution when combined with a benzodiazepine.

The atypical antipsychotics are increasingly being used for acute agitation. Ziprasidone and olanzipine both have intramuscular formulations but have limited data supporting their use for acute agitation. Both are associated with lower incidence of extrapyramidal symptoms. Ziprasidone can prolong the QT interval similar to the typical antipsychotics, while olanzapine has been shown to have little or no effect on the QT interval. As mentioned, over-sedation and respiratory depression are a concern when these agents are combined with benzodiazepines. The lack of QT prolongation, extrapyramidal symptoms, and rapid onset of action of this class make them promising agents. Lastly, there are limited data that intramuscular aripiprazole may also be safe and efficacious when treating the agitated patient. More definitive studies will hopefully help stratify the risks of and guide patient selection in the use of the atypical antipsychotics. Current data are limited to non-inferiority trials sponsored by the pharmaceutical industry, clearly showing efficacy without clear superiority. As cost merits consideration, currently ziprasidone, aripiprazole, and olanzipine are far more expensive than the generics, haloperidol and droperidol.

In summary, although data exist to support efficacy of all the agents listed above, there is no clearly superior agent. The typicals antipsychotics have the benefits of experience and cost, while the atypicals antipsychotics have better side-effect profiles, but are more expensive, and have less data and provider experience associated with them. If, and how, to combine benzodiazepines with newer antipsychotics remains more art than science.

References

1. Williams JW Jr. A systematic review of newer pharmacotherapies for depression in adults: evidence report summary. *Ann Intern Med* 2000;**132**:743–56.

2. Katzung B, Potter W. Antidepressant agents. In: Katzung B (Eds.), *Basic and Clinical Pharmacology*, (Chapt. 30), New York: McGraw-Hill; 2001: 486–94.

3. Liebelt EL. Cyclic antidepressants. In: Goldfrank LR, Nelson LS, Hoffman RS, et al. (Eds.), *Goldfrank's Toxicologic Emergencies*, (9th Edition, Chapt. 73), New York: McGraw-Hill; 2011.

4. Caravati EM, Bossart PJ. Demographic and electrocardiographic factors associated with severe tricyclic antidepressant toxicity. *J Toxicol Clin Toxicol* 1991;**29**:31–43.

5. Boehnert M, Lovejoy FH. Value of the QRS duration versus the serum drug level in predicting seizures and ventricular arrhythmias after an acute overdose of tricyclic antidepressants. *N Engl J Med* 1985;**313**:474–9.

6. Liebelt EL, Francis PD, Woolf AD. ECG lead aVR versus QRS interval in predicting seizures and arrhythmias in acute tricyclic antidepressant toxicity. *Ann Emerg Med* 1995;**26**:195–201.

7. Beaubien AR, Carpenter DC, Mathieu LF, MacConaill M, Hrdina PD. Antagonism of imipramine poisoning by anticonvulsants in the rat. *Toxicol Appl Pharmacol* 1976;**38**:1–6.

8. Foianini A, Joseph Wiegand T, Benowitz N. What is the role of lidocaine or phenytoin in tricyclic antidepressant-induced cardiotoxicity? *Clin Toxicol (Phila)* 2010;**48**:325–30.

9. Blackman K, Brown SF, Wilkes GJ. Plasma alkalinization for tricyclic antidepressant toxicity: a systematic review. *Emerg Med* 2001;**13**:204–10.

10. Carr D, Boone A, Hoffman RS, Martin K, Ahluwalia N. Successful resuscitation of a doxepin overdose using intravenous fat emulsion. *Clin Toxicol* 2009;**47**:702–65.

11. Jamaty C, Bailey B, Larocque A, et al. Lipid emulsions in the treatment of acute poisoning: a systematic review of human and animal studies. *Clin Toxicol* 2010;**48**:1–27.

12. Cipriani A. Comparative efficacy and acceptability of 12 new-generation antidepressants: a multiple-treatments meta-analysis. *Lancet* 2009;**373**:746–58.

13. Gartlehner G. Comparative benefits and harms of second-generation antidepressants: background paper for the American College of Physicians. *Ann Intern Med* 2008;**149**:734–50.

14. Dunkley EJ, Isbister GK, Sibbritt D, et al. The Hunter Serotonin Toxicity Criteria: simple and accurate diagnostic decision rules for serotonin toxicity. *QJM* 2003;**96**:635–42.

15. Graudins A, Stearman A, Chan B. Treatment of the serotonin syndrome with cyproheptadine. *J Emerg Med* 1998;**16**:615–19.

16. Boyer EW, Shannon M. The serotonin syndrome. *N Engl J Med* 2005;**352**:1112–20.

17. Crane GE. The psychiatric effects of iproniazid. *Am J Psychiatry* 1956;**112**:494–501.

18. Krishnan KR. Revisiting monoamine oxidase inhibitors. *J Clin Psychiatry* 2007;**68**:35–41.

19. Amsterdam JD. A double-blind, placebo-controlled trial of the safety and efficacy of selegiline transfermal system without dietary restrictions in patients with major depressive disorder. *J Clin Psychiatry* 2003;**64**:208–14.

20. American Psychiatric Association. *Treatment of Patients with Major Depressive Disorder {revised 2010 Nov}* in American Psychiatric Association Practice Guidelines. Available at: http://psychiatryonline.org/guidelines.aspx (Accessed November 26, 2011).

21. Linden CH, Rumack BH, Strehlke C. Monoamine oxidase inhibitor overdose. *Ann Emerg Med* 1984;**13**:1137–44.

22. Martel M, Miner JR, Lashkowitz S, et al. QT Prolongation and cardiac arrhythmias associated with droperidol use in critical emergency department patients. *Acad Emerg Med* 2003;**10**:510–11.

23. Albert KK, Chua SE. Effects on prolongation of Bazett's corrected QT interval of seven second-generation antipsychotics in the treatment of schizophrenia: a meta-analysis. *J Psychopharmacol* 2011:**25**;646–66.

24. Currier GW. Atypical antipsychotic medications in the psychiatric emergency service. *J Clin Psychiatry* 2000;**61**(Suppl 14):21–6.

25. Berg JE, Slatsve K, Bjorland S, Sever C. An unexpected reaction to treatment with benzodiazepines and olanzapine in a woman with a manic condition. *Clin Neuropsychol* 2009;**6**:35–8.

26. Wilson MP, Macdonald K, Vilke GM, Feifel D. Potential complications of combining intramusculoar olanzapine with benzodiazepines in emergency department patients. 2010 [Epub ahead of print].

27. Brook S, Lucey JV, Gunn KP. Intramuscular ziprasidone compared with intramuscular haloperidol in the treatment of acute psychosis. Ziprasidone I.M. Study Group. *J Clin Psychiatry* 2000;**61**:933–41.

28. Smith MA. Rapid dose escalation with quetiapine: a pilot study. *J Clin Psychopharmacol* 2005;**25**:331–5.

29. Ngo A. Acute quetiapine overdose in adults: a 5-year retrospective case series. *Ann Emerg Med* 2008;**52**:541–7.

30. Komossa K, Rummel-Kluge C, Schmid F, et al. Aripiprazole versus other atypical antipsychotics for schizophrenia. *Cochrane Database Syst Rev* 2009;**47**:606.

31. Smith LA, Cornelius V, Warnock A, et al. Pharmacological interventions for acute bipolar mania: a systematic review of randomized placebo-controlled trials. *Bipolar Disord* 2007;**9**:551–60.

32. Hirschfeld RMA. Practice guideline for the treatment of patients with bipolar disorder (revision). *Am J Psychiatry* 2003;**1**:64–110.

33. Swann AC, Bowden CL, Morris D, et al. Depression during mania. Treatment response to lithium and divalproex. *Arch Gen Psychiatry* 1997;**54**:37–42.

34. Battaglia J, Moss S, Rush J, et al. Haloperidol, lorazepam, or both for psychotic agitation? A multicenter, prospective, double-blind, emergency department study. *Am J Emerg Med* 1997;**15**:335–40.

35. Kao LW, Kirk MA, Evers SJ, Rosenfeld SH. Droperidol, QT prolongation, and sudden death: what is the evidence? *Ann Emerg Med* 2003;**41**:546–58.

36. White PF. Droperidol: a cost-effective antiemetic for over thirty years. *Anesth Analg* **95**:789–90.

37. Lischke V. Droperidol causes a dose-dependent prolongation of the QT interval. *Anesth Analg* 1994;**79**:983–6.

38. Habib AS. Food and Drug Administration black box warning on the perioperative use of droperidol: a review of the cases. *Anesth Analg* 2003;**96**:1377–9.

39. Meehan K, Zhang F, David S, et al. A double-blind, randomized comparison of the efficacy and safety of intramuscular injections of olanzapine, lorazepam, or placebo in treating acutely agitated patients diagnosed with bipolar mania. *J Clin Psychopharmacol* 2001;**21**:389–97.

40. Jones B, Taylor CC, Meehan K. The efficacy of a rapid-acting intramuscular formulation of olanzapine for positive symptoms. *J Clin Psychiatry* 2001;**62** (Suppl 2):22–4.

41. Andrezina R, Josiassen RC, Marcus RN, et al. Intramuscular aripiprazole for the treatment of acute agitation in patients with schizophrenia or schizoaffective disorder: a double-blind, placebo-controlled comparison with intramuscular haloperidol. *Psychopharmacology (Berl)* 2006;**188**:281–92.

42. Tran-Johnson TK, Efficacy and safety of intramuscular aripiprazole in patients with acute agitation: a randomized, double-blind, placebo-controlled trial. *J Clin Psychiatry* 2007;**68**:111–19.

43. Wright P. Double-blind, placebo-controlled comparison of intramuscular olanzapine and intramuscular haloperidol in the treatment of acute agitation in schizophrenia. *Am J Psychiatry* 2001;**158**:1149–51.

44. Czella J. Analysis of the QTc interval during olanzapine treatment of patients with schizophrenia related psychosis. *J Clin Psychiatry* 2001;**62**:191–8.

45. Glassman AH. Antipsychotic drugs: prolonged QTc interval, torsades de pointes, and sudden death. *Am J Psychiatry* 2001;**158**:1774–82.

Chapter 26

The patient with neuroleptic malignant syndrome in the emergency department

Omeed Saghafi and Jeffrey Sankoff

Introduction

The neuroleptic malignant syndrome (NMS) (*Syndrome Neuroleptique Malin*) was first described in 1960 by French psychiatrists as a tetrad of muscular rigidity, fever, autonomic dysfunction, and altered consciousness [1]. Although NMS was originally believed to be an idiosyncratic reaction to neuroleptics, it is now recognized as an uncommon, but life-threatening, reaction to dopamine blockade that can occur with the use of antipsychotics, non-antipsychotic dopamine antagonists, and withdrawal from dopamine agonists. Supportive care is the primary treatment for NMS. Dantrolene and bromocriptine are possible adjuncts to therapy; however, their use remains controversial.

Epidemiology

Initial estimates of the prevalence of NMS during the 1980s were 2.44%; however, more recent data from 2004 suggest a prevalence of 0.01–0.02% in patients prescribed psychotropic medications [2]. The reasons for the declining prevalence are unclear. The increased use of atypical antipsychotics in place of antipsychotics more commonly associated with NMS is partially responsible for the declining prevalence. Alternatively, NMS may be precluded by clinicians who have become more attuned to recognizing and treating the early signs of drug reactions [3]. Despite the decreasing incidence of NMS, nearly 2,000 cases of NMS are diagnosed annually in the United States. NMS is associated with an expected mortality rate of approximately 10% and healthcare costs of $70 million a year in the United States [4].

Multiple risk factors for NMS have been investigated. While initial case reports implied that males were more likely than females to develop NMS [5,6], more recent research suggests that sex and age are in fact not correlated with the development of the disease [7,8]. Agitation, pre-existing catatonia, dehydration, and the use of restraints have been linked to the development of NMS [6,9]. In addition, most reported cases of NMS occur in the setting of physical exhaustion and dehydration. A prior episode of NMS is noted in 15–20% of cases [10].

In addition to patient susceptibility, drug characteristics may also increase the risk of NMS. High-potency conventional antipsychotics are associated with a greater risk than are atypical antipsychotics (Table 26.1) [6,11,12]. Patients with NMS due to conventional antipsychotics are also more likely to have concurrent extrapyramidal side effects (EPS) and a higher mortality rate than patients with NMS due to atypical antipsychotics. In fact, there have only been three cases of reported deaths from NMS due to atypical antipsychotics [11]. An increased risk of NMS is also seen with higher total doses, more rapid titration, and parenteral administration of antipsychotics (95% of cases reported before 1985 followed a rapid increase in dose of antipsychotic administered) [13].

Lithium, a commonly used mood stabilizer with an unclear mechanism of action, is believed to partially affect dopamine activity. Although there have been case reports suggesting that this drug is associated with the development of NMS, case control studies have not supported this association [14,15].

Pathophysiology

There is currently no proven pathophysiologic explanation for the development of NMS. The most widely accepted hypothesis is that NMS is caused by decreased activity of D_2 dopamine receptors. Dopamine blockade manifests itself clinically as altered mental status, muscular rigidity, and autonomic instability.

The evidence for the hypothesis that dopamine blockade is central to NMS is mostly circumstantial, but is related to the fact that NMS is precipitated by antipsychotics that block dopamine receptors. Furthermore, NMS has also been described after the use of non-antipsychotic dopamine antagonists such as metoclopramide, prochlorperazine, and amoxapine or with the withdrawal of dopamine agonists offering more support to a role for the dopamine receptor in the development of NMS. The finding of decreased concentrations of the dopamine metabolite homovanillic acid in the cerebrospinal fluid of patients with NMS lends further credence to this hypothesis [16].

The clinical manifestations of NMS can also be explained by this dopamine receptor theory. The blockade of dopamine

Behavioral Emergencies for the Emergency Physician, ed. Leslie S. Zun, Lara G. Chepenik, and Mary Nan S. Mallory. Published by Cambridge University Press. © Cambridge University Press 2013.

receptors in the basal ganglia, especially within the nigrostriatal pathway, results in muscular rigidity and resultant rhabdomyolysis similar to that seen in NMS. Dopamine receptors in the hypothalamus are integral to the regulation of body temperature and their blockade results in hyperthermia and autonomic instability. Again, this is consistent with the clinical picture of NMS.

Table 26.1. Examples of high- versus low-potency typical antipsychotics and atypical antipsychotics

High-potency typical antipsychotics	Atypical antipsychotics
Fluphenazine (0.80,[a] 15[b])	Clozapine (0.01,[c] 21[d])
Thioridazine (2.30, 5)	Risperidone (0.05, 23)
Haloperidol (4, 28)	Ziprasidone (0.09, 19)
Low-potency typical antipsychotics	Olanzapine (0.36, 5)
Chlorpromazine (19, 8)	Aripiprazole (1, 0)
Loxapine (17)	Quetiapine (1.84, 5)

[a] Ki value for D_2 dopamine receptor affinity in nM, where Ki is the dissociation constant or equivalently the concentration of medication in molar units (M) at which half of receptors are bound.
[b] Number of case reports of NMS identified between 1980 and 1984 (total of 54).
[c] Ki 5-HT_{2A} serotonin/D_2 dopamine ratio.
[d] Number of total case reports of NMS identified by MEDLINE database search in January 2003. Note that data are biased by number of prescriptions for each antipsychotic with haloperidol being the most commonly prescribed antipsychotic in 1985. Adapted from Brunton et al. 2006 [12], Levenson, 1985 [6], and Ananth et al. 2004 [11].

However, the dopamine receptor theory alone is insufficient to explain NMS in its entirety. Some additional mechanism is theorized that results in up-regulation of the sympathetic-adrenal axis and promotes an inflammatory acute phase reaction [17]. On a cellular level, the acute phase reaction and increased sympathetic tone cause membrane instability and mitochondrial breakdown, especially in the basal ganglia and cerebellar hemispheres (Figure 26.1). Clinically, this manifests as further autonomic instability. Evidence for this is a measurable increase in serum levels of acute phase reactants and cerebrospinal fluid (CSF) levels of norepinephrine in NMS patients, although the exact underlying mechanism remains to be elucidated [18].

Some researchers propose that this hyperactive noradrenergic state is believed to be a common final pathway in both NMS and the serotonin syndrome (SS) [19]. In fact, serotonin receptors (5-HT_{2A}) that inhibit the release of dopamine have been found on axonal terminals of dopaminergic neurons.

At the gross anatomic level, prolonged hyperthermia can result in damage to the basal ganglia and cerebellar hemispheres. T2-weighted magnetic resonance imaging (MRI) of patients with NMS show restricted diffusion in the basal ganglia and cerebellar hemispheres [20]. Given the similar pattern of injury to that found in patients with hyperthermic brain injury, it is hypothesized that this pattern of injury is due to the breakdown of membrane lipids, protein denaturation, and mitochondrial damage due to extreme temperatures (>39.5–40°C). The cerebellum is especially sensitive to hyperthermic damage and the degree of injury correlates with temperature [21,22].

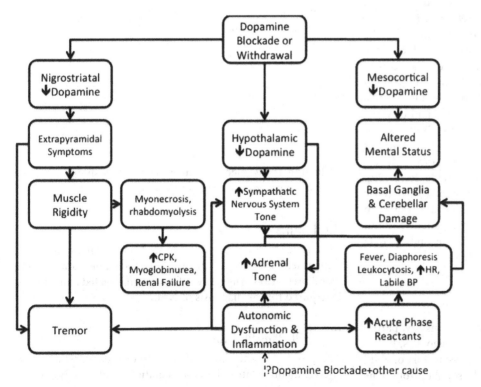

Figure 26.1. Basic pathophysiology of neuroleptic malignant syndrome. CPK, creatinine phosphokinase; HR, heart rate; BP, blood pressure.

Diagnosis

The patient with NMS classically develops worsening altered mental status over the course of several days after, or during, treatment with an antipsychotic medication. The patient becomes acutely febrile, diaphoretic, tachypneic, tachycardic; and demonstrates unexplained fluctuation in blood pressure. The patient develops a significantly decreased level of responsiveness, oftentimes bordering on complete unresponsiveness or catatonia. The patient may have generalized tremors but, on examination, will have whole-body lead-pipe rigidity. Laboratory tests will demonstrate leukocytosis and rhabdomyolysis, while the workup for infection and other causes of altered mental status will remain negative.

NMS should be considered in any patient who develops muscular rigidity, fever, altered mental status, or autonomic instability after the administration of a dopamine antagonist or withdrawal of a dopamine agonist [23]. A syndrome similar to NMS has also been described after the withdrawal of baclofen [24]. All four classic signs and symptoms of NMS are not always present (Table 26.2) [6]. Neurologic symptoms and changes in mental status precede systemic signs in 80% of cases of NMS [25]. The onset is generally insidious and occurs over several days, although fulminant cases are described. Most cases of NMS (66%) develop within 1 week of initiating a new antipsychotic, 16% within 24 hours, and a small minority occur after a change in medication dosage or addition of an additional dopamine antagonist [10]. NMS can occur with longstanding administration of an antipsychotic, but such cases are uncommon.

A multitude of diagnostic criteria for the diagnosis of NMS have been developed [23,26,27]. Sets of criteria only demonstrate modest agreement with one another for the diagnosis of NMS, and no one set is preferable [28]. One commonly used set of diagnostic criteria for the diagnosis of NMS is the Diagnostic and Statistical Manual of Mental Disorders, 4th Edition, Text Revision (DSM-IV-TR) criteria set, which requires both severe muscle rigidity and elevated temperature after administration of an antipsychotic as well as two associated signs, symptoms, or laboratory findings that are not better accounted for by a substance-induced, neurologic, or general medical condition (Table 26.3) [29]. The DSM-IV-TR criteria are the American Psychiatric Association's accepted diagnostic criteria, but are subject to criticism as they will not diagnose the rare patient without fever or rigidity, and are created by the secondary data analysis of work groups subject to bias [30].

History

A detailed history should focus on medication history, particularly exposure to neuroleptics, dopamine antagonists, baclofen, or withdrawal of dopamine agonists. A past history of NMS also makes NMS more likely and should be sought through the

Table 26.2. Diagnostic criteria for NMS as described in DSM-IV TR (strict research criteria)

A. Development of severe muscle rigidity and elevated temperature associated with use of a neuroleptic

B. Two (or more) of the following:
1. Diaphoresis
2. Dysphagia
3. Tremor
4. Incontinence
5. Changes in level of consciousness ranging from confusion to coma
6. Mutism
7. Tachycardia
8. Elevated or labile blood pressure
9. Leukocytosis
10. Laboratory evidence of muscle injury (e.g., elevated creatinine phosphokinase)

C. The symptoms in A and B are not due to another substance or a neurological or other general medical condition (e.g., encephalitis)

D. The symptoms in A and B are not better accounted for by a mental disorder (e.g., Mood Disorder with Catatonic Features)

Table 26.3. Frequency of clinical and laboratory signs in NMS

Clinical/laboratory sign	% of Patients with sign
Fever	98
Elevated serum creatinine	
Phosphokinase level	97
Tachycardia	91
Rigidity	89
Altered consciousness	84
Leukocytosis	79
Abnormal blood pressure	74
Tachypnea	73
Diaphoresis	67
Tremor	45
Incontinence	21

Adapted from Levenson, 1985 [6]

evaluation of past medical history. The history should also help to rule out other differential diagnoses.

Vital signs

Vital signs that suggest autonomic dysfunction or increased sympathetic tone such as tachycardia, tachypnea, and a labile blood pressure are suggestive of NMS. An elevated temperature is required for the diagnosis of NMS.

Physical examination

The physical exam should demonstrate muscle rigidity and altered mental status. Tremor, agitation, mutism, dysarthria, dysphagia, hypersecretion, and urinary incontinence are potential nonspecific findings that are suggestive of NMS.

Laboratory studies

Many nonspecific laboratory findings are found in NMS. A leukocytosis with or without a left shift is common. Muscle rigidity can result in rhabdomyolysis, leading to increased serum creatinine kinase, aldolase, transaminases, lactic acid dehydrogenase, and myoglobinuria. Rhabdomyolysis may lead to subsequent renal failure and a resultant increase in creatinine, potassium, and phosphate. Serum iron levels are generally low [31]. Lumbar puncture and standard CSF analysis is normal in over 95% of cases.

Other potentially useful laboratory tests include liver enzymes and serum iron levels. Thyroid function studies can be considered to rule out thyrotoxicosis. A urine toxicology screen, salicylate level, and acetaminophen level can be considered to rule out sympathomimetic abuse, salicylate toxicity, or elevated liver enzymes as a result of acetaminophen toxicity.

Additional tests and imaging

An electrocardiogram is useful for helping to rule out certain toxic ingestions or a cardiac etiology for altered mental status. The electrocardiogram in NMS will most likely demonstrate sinus tachycardia. Most patients will require a head CT and lumbar puncture to rule out infection, cerebrovascular accident, or mass lesions. MRI can be used if there is concern for ischemic cerebrovascular accident or demyelinating disease. Electroencephalogram (EEG) is not required but may be helpful if subclinical status epilepticus is considered a possibility.

Differential diagnosis

NMS is a diagnosis of exclusion and, therefore, the differential diagnosis is an important consideration (Table 26.4) [9]. Advanced psychosis with catatonia (malignant or lethal catatonia) is one of the most important diagnoses to consider. This diagnosis may be difficult to differentiate from NMS because, similar to NMS, it can also result in hyperthermia and autonomic instability in its late stages. Characteristics that may be used to distinguish the two include a temporal relationship with medications known to cause NMS and the degree of hyperthermia (generally smaller elevations in temperature accompany catatonia). Despite the diagnostic clues provided by potential exposure to NMS-associated medications and differences in temperature elevation, the exact diagnosis of NMS versus malignant catatonia is uncertain in up to 20% of cases of malignant catatonia [32]. However, the treatment for NMS and malignant catatonia is similar; therefore, the precise diagnosis should not influence patient treatment. Supportive care is the primary treatment for both NMS and lethal catatonia. Antipsychotics are ineffective in malignant catatonia and should be discontinued in NMS.

Table 26.4. Differential diagnosis of neuroleptic malignant syndrome

Psychiatric or neurologic
Malignant catatonia
Agitated delirium
Other extrapyramidal side effects
Nonconvulsive status epilepticus
Cerebrovascular accident or other structural lesion
Paraneoplastic syndrome
Pharmacologic or toxic
Malignant hyperthermia
Serotonin syndrome
Salicylate poisoning
Anticholinergic toxicity
Sympathomimetic toxicity
Hallucinogenic toxicity
Withdrawal from alcohol or sedative-hypnotic
Infectious
Meningitis or encephalitis
Brain abscess
Sepsis
Postinfectious encephalomyelitis syndrome
Endocrine
Thyrotoxicosis
Pheochromocytoma
Environmental
Heatstroke

Adapted from Strawn et al. 2007 [9].

Despite theories that SS and NMS have a similar final pathway, the two are considered distinct entities. SS is precipitated by serotonergic medications including selective serotonin reuptake inhibitors, monoamine oxidase inhibitors (including linezolid), tricyclic antidepressants, triptans, and combinations of medications that can cause excess serotonin agonism (meperidine, dextromethorphan, several opioids especially tramadol and psychedelics). SS has a more rapid onset than NMS, is often distinguishable by a history of medication administration or intoxication, and presents with hyperkinesia and clonus rather than the bradykinesia and lead-pipe rigidity found in NMS.

Malignant hyperthermia (MH) shares much of its pathophysiology with NMS. However, MH often occurs intraoperatively or after rapid sequence intubation and arises as a result of the use of volatile anesthetics or succinylcholine in susceptible patients. Patients with MH may have a known myopathy or family history of myopathy or MH [33].

The illicit abuse of multiple substances taken alone, or in combination, can result in presentations similar to NMS. Intoxication with sympathomimetic (e.g., cocaine or amphetamines), hallucinogenic (i.e., phencyclidine) or anticholinergic agents; or withdrawal from alcohol or sedative-hypnotic substances can present with symptoms similar to NMS, such as fever, altered mental status, and autonomic instability. These toxidromes are distinguished primarily based on history and physical examination. Patients with anticholinergic delirium often present with dry skin and mucous membranes compared to the diaphoretic patient with NMS or sympathetic toxicity. Salicylate toxicity must also be considered in the hyperthermic, delirious patient with an unclear ingestion history [34,35].

Heatstroke can present similarly to NMS. The diagnosis can be ascertained based on history. Elderly patients with heatstroke may not be able to provide a salient history, but classically have dry skin due both to dehydration and the use of anhydric medications while younger patients tend to present with pronounced diaphoresis and a history of prolonged heat exposure. Neither type of patient will have muscular rigidity [36].

Thyrotoxicosis and pheochromocytoma should also be considered as part of the differential diagnosis. Laboratory results may aid in the diagnosis of both thyrotoxicosis (decreased thyroid stimulating hormone with increased levels of thyroid hormones) and pheochromocytoma (increased catecholamines and metanephrines). Patients with thyrotoxicosis may have a history of thyroid disorder, and patients with pheochromocytoma may have a history of previous symptomatic episodes [37,38].

Subclinical or nonconvulsive status epilepticus is a possible cause of altered mental status, and rigidity. However, elevations in creatinine kinase are minimal and fever is not generally seen.

The most common causes of altered mental status with fever should also be eliminated using basic laboratory studies, urinalysis, lumbar puncture, and radiologic imaging including chest radiograph, and when appropriate based on history and physical examination, cerebral computed tomography or magnetic resonance imaging. These common causes of altered mental status include sepsis from any source, meningitis or brain abscess, encephalitis, or cerebrovascular accident. Post-infectious encephalomyelitis and paraneoplastic syndromes are also in the differential but are less common.

Treatment

The most important aspect of treatment for NMS is the discontinuation of the offending medication (or restarting a previously held dopamine agonist) followed by supportive care. Anticholinergic medications should also be discontinued as they may inhibit the diaphoresis necessary for physiologic compensation during hyperthermia. Supportive care should include passive cooling and antipyretics to maintain a body temperature below 39.5–40°C, as well as intravenous rehydration. Dehydration is a risk factor for NMS, and most patients will be intravascularly depleted both before and after the onset of disease. Intravenous hydration and sodium bicarbonate can be used to treat rhabdomyolysis. Renal failure with volume overload, significant electrolyte abnormalities, or acidosis will require continuous hemofiltration or dialysis.

Benzodiazepines should be used as a component of supportive care in patients with increased sympathetic tone. Benzodiazepine use in the treatment of NMS has been linked to decreased mortality in a retrospective analysis demonstrating 0% mortality in 17 NMS patients treated with benzodiazepines compared to 15% mortality in 19 patients not treated with benzodiazepines [8]. The benefit of γ-aminobutyric acid (GABA) receptor agonism by benzodiazepines is further supported by decreased levels of GABA in the CSF of patients with NMS [16].

Other treatments for NMS have been suggested, but their use is controversial. These treatments include dantrolene sodium, dopamine agonists, and electroconvulsive therapy. Due to the low incidence of NMS, randomized controlled double-blind prospective studies are nearly impossible to achieve. Therefore, all studies of pharmacologic treatment in NMS are restricted to case reports, case series, and retrospective analyses.

Dantrolene sodium use was first recommended for treatment of NMS in 1981 [39] and has since been considered the first line of pharmacologic treatment. It is the hallmark treatment for malignant hyperthermia and is recommended in NMS due to the similarities between MH and NMS. Dantrolene acts as a peripheral muscle relaxant by inhibiting intracellular calcium release from the sarcoplasmic reticulum. By relaxing skeletal muscle, dantrolene is believed to decrease muscle rigidity and resultant rhabdomyolysis. Dantrolene is given intravenously with 1–2.5 mg/kg body weight administered initially followed by 1 mg/kg every 6 hours if symptom improvement is seen. Dantrolene can then be given orally and down-titrated gradually over the course of days. Side effects of dantrolene include respiratory depression and impairment of hepatic function.

Initial reports demonstrated superior results with the use of dantrolene compared to supportive care alone [40]. These reports described rapid improvement in symptoms in nearly 80% of patients, and mortality was decreased by half. However, the largest and most recent study seemed to challenge the benefits of dantrolene. The analysis of 271 case reports by Reulbach et al. showed that, while dantrolene use led to increased effectiveness of therapy at 24 hours compared to other medications or supportive care alone, it was also associated with higher mortality than supportive care alone [41]. However, it is important to note that the study was a retrospective analysis, and it is possible that patients receiving dantrolene were more ill or had already failed supportive care.

Dopamine agonists such as bromocriptine and amantadine have been advocated as possible therapies based on a theory that NMS is primarily caused by dopamine blockade. Bromocriptine is the most studied dopamine agonist used in NMS. Retrospective analyses of bromocriptine use have found a statistically significant decrease in time to recovery and a 0 (no statistically significant difference) to 50% decrease in mortality compared to supportive care alone [42]. Amantadine is administered in doses of 100–200 mg orally or by nasogastric tube twice a day. Bromocriptine is started at a dose of 2.5 mg orally or by nasogastric tube three to four times a day and increased to a maximum total daily dose of 45 mg. The dose is continued for 7–10 days and then tapered over several days. Premature discontinuation of bromocriptine may result in rebound symptoms. Side effects of bromocriptine include psychosis, hypotension, and vomiting.

While it is out of the scope of the Emergency Physician, electroconvulsive therapy (ECT) has been shown to be effective therapy, even in patients with symptoms refractory to supportive or pharmacologic treatment [43,44].

Disposition

Patients with NMS should be admitted to an intensive care unit (ICU) for close monitoring of neurologic status, electrolyte imbalance, and renal failure from rhabdomyolysis.

The mortality rate for NMS is approximately 10% [4]. The remainder of patients will have a self-limited course with a mean recovery time of 7–10 days. Sixty-three percent of patients will recover by 1 week and nearly all will recover by 30 days (10).

There are reports of residual catatonia and Parkinsonian symptoms in patients with NMS, however, the majority will recover completely and can have antipsychotics safely reintroduced several months after a full recovery [45].

References

1. Delay JPP, Lempériére T, Elissde B, Peigne F. Un neuroleptique majeur non-phénothiazine et nonréserpinique, l'halopéeridol, dans le traitement des psychoses. *Ann Méd Psychol (Paris)* 1960;**118**:145–52.

2. Stubner S, Rustenbeck E, Grohmann R, et al. Severe and uncommon involuntary movement disorders due to psychotropic drugs. *Pharmacopsychiatry* 2004;**37** (Suppl 1):S54–64.

3. Keck PE Jr, Pope HG Jr, McElroy SL. Declining frequency of neuroleptic malignant syndrome in a hospital population. *Am J Psychiatry* 1991;**148**:880–2.

4. U.S. Department of Health & Human Services. HCUPnet. Rockville, Maryland 2009. Available at: http://hcupnet.ahrq.gov/ (Accessed 2011).

5. Addonizio G, Susman VL, Roth SD. Neuroleptic malignant syndrome: review and analysis of 115 cases. *Biol Psychiatry* 1987; **22**:1004–20.

6. Levenson JL. Neuroleptic malignant syndrome. *Am J Psychiatry* 1985;**142**:1137–45.

7. Keck PE Jr, Pope HG Jr, Cohen BM, McElroy SL, Nierenberg AA. Risk factors for neuroleptic malignant syndrome. A case-control study. *Arch Gen Psychiatry* 1989;**46**:914–18.

8. Tural U, Onder E. Clinical and pharmacologic risk factors for neuroleptic malignant syndrome and their association with death. *Psychiatry Clin Neurosci* 2010;**64**:79–87.

9. Strawn JR, Keck PE Jr, Caroff SN. Neuroleptic malignant syndrome. *Am J Psychiatry* 2007;**164**:870–6.

10. Caroff SN, Mann SC. Neuroleptic malignant syndrome. *Psychopharmacol Bull* 1988;**24**:25–9.

11. Ananth J, Parameswaran S, Gunatilake S, Burgoyne K, Sidhom T. Neuroleptic malignant syndrome and atypical antipsychotic drugs. *J Clin Psychiatry* 2004;**65**:464–70.

12. Brunton LL, Parker KL, Lazo J, Buxton I, Blumenthal D. *Goodman and Gilman's the Pharmacological Basis of Therapeutics*, (11th Edition). New York: Mcgraw-Hill; 2006.

13. Shalev A, Hermesh H, Munitz H. The role of loading rate in neuroleptic malignant syndrome. *Am J Psychiatry* 1986;**143**:1059.

14. Susman VL, Addonizio G. Reinduction of neuroleptic malignant syndrome by lithium. *J Clin Psychopharmacol* 1987;**7**:339–41.

15. Goldney RD, Spence ND. Safety of the combination of lithium and neuroleptic drugs. *Am J Psychiatry* 1986;**143**:882–4.

16. Nisijima K, Ishiguro T. Neuroleptic malignant syndrome: a study of CSF monoamine metabolism. *Biol Psychiatry* 1990;**27**:280–8.

17. Gurrera RJ. Sympathoadrenal hyperactivity and the etiology of neuroleptic malignant syndrome. *Am J Psychiatry* 1999;**156**:169–80.

18. Nisijima K, Ishiguro T. Cerebrospinal fluid levels of monoamine metabolites and gamma-aminobutyric acid in neuroleptic malignant syndrome. *J Psychiatr Res* 1995;**29**:233–44.

19. Steele D, Keltner NL, McGuiness TM. Are neuroleptic malignant syndrome and serotonin syndrome the same

syndrome? *Perspect Psychiatr Care* 2011;**47**:58–62.

20. Lyons JL, Cohen AB. Selective cerebellar and basal ganglia injury in neuroleptic malignant syndrome. *J Neuroimaging* 2011 [Epub ahead of print].

21. Park JW, Choi YB, Park SK, Kim YI, Lee KS. Magnetic resonance imaging reveals selective vulnerability of the cerebellum and basal ganglia in malignant hyperthermia. *Arch Neurol* 2004;**61**:1462–3.

22. Lee S, Merriam A, Kim TS, et al. Cerebellar degeneration in neuroleptic malignant syndrome: neuropathologic findings and review of the literature concerning heat-related nervous system injury. *J Neurol Neurosurg Psychiatry* 1989;**52**:387–91.

23. Gurrera RJ, Caroff SN, Cohen A, et al. An international consensus study of neuroleptic malignant syndrome diagnostic criteria using the delphi method. *J Clin Psychiatry* 2011;**72**:1222–8.

24. Turner MR, Gainsborough N. Neuroleptic malignant-like syndrome after abrupt withdrawal of baclofen. *J Psychopharmacol* 2001;**15**:61–3.

25. Velamoor VR, Norman RM, Caroff SN, et al. Progression of symptoms in neuroleptic malignant syndrome. *J Nerv Ment Dis* 1994;**182**:168–73.

26. Mathews T, Aderibigbe YA. Proposed research diagnostic criteria for neuroleptic malignant syndrome. *Int J Neuropsychopharmacol* 1999;**2**:129–44.

27. Pandya M, Pozuelo L. A malignant neuroleptic spectrum: review of diagnostic criteria and treatment

implications in three case reports. *Int J Psychiatry Med* 2004;**34**:277–85.

28. Gurrera RJ, Chang SS, Romero JA. A comparison of diagnostic criteria for neuroleptic malignant syndrome. *J Clin Psychiatry* 1992;**53**:56–62.

29. American Psychiatric Association. *Diagnostic and Statistical Manual of Mental Disorders*, (4th Edition). Washington, DC; American Psychiatric Association; 2004.

30. Widiger TA, Sankis LM. Adult psychopathology: issues and controversies. *Annu Rev Psychol* 2000;**51**:377–404.

31. Rosebush PI, Mazurek MF. Serum iron and neuroleptic malignant syndrome. *Lancet* 1991;**338**:149–51.

32. Mann SC, Caroff SN, Bleier HR, et al. Lethal catatonia. *Am J Psychiatry* 1986;**143**:1374–81.

33. Litman RS, Rosenberg H. Malignant hyperthermia: update on susceptibility testing. *JAMA* 2005;**293**:2918–24.

34. Anderson RJ, Potts DE, Gabow PA, Rumack BH, Schrier RW. Unrecognized adult salicylate intoxication. *Ann Intern Med* 1976;**85**:745–8.

35. Candy JM, Morrison C, Paton RD, Logan RW, Lawson R. Salicylate toxicity masquerading as malignant hyperthermia. *Paediatr Anaesth* 1998;**8**:421–3.

36. Bouchama A, Knochel JP. Heat stroke. *N Engl J Med* 2002;**346**:1978–88.

37. Hennessey JV. Diagnosis and management of thyrotoxicosis. *Am Fam Physician* 1996;**54**:1315–24.

38. Barron J. Phaeochromocytoma: diagnostic challenges for biochemical screening and diagnosis. *J Clin Pathol* 2010;**63**:669–74.

39. Delacour JL, Daoudal P, Chapoutot JL, Rocq B. [Therapy of neuroleptic malignant syndrome with dantrolene]. *Nouv Presse Med* 1981;**10**:3572–3.

40. Shalev A, Munitz H. The neuroleptic malignant syndrome: agent and host interaction. *Acta Psychiatr Scand* 1986;**73**:337–47.

41. Reulbach U, Dutsch C, Biermann T, et al. Managing an effective treatment for neuroleptic malignant syndrome. *Crit Care* 2007;**11**:R4.

42. Rosenberg MR, Green M. Neuroleptic malignant syndrome. Review of response to therapy. *Arch Intern Med* 1989;**149**:1927–31.

43. Davis JM, Janicak PG, Sakkas P, Gilmore C, Wang Z. Electroconvulsive therapy in the treatment of the neuroleptic malignant syndrome. *Convuls Ther* 1991;**7**:111–20.

44. Pelonero AL, Levenson JL, Pandurangi AK. Neuroleptic malignant syndrome: a review. *Psychiatr Serv* 1998;**49**:1163–72.

45. Levenson JL, Fisher JG. Long-term outcome after neuroleptic malignant syndrome. *J Clin Psychiatry* 1988;**49**:154–6.

Chapter 27

Treatment of psychiatric illness in the emergency department

Kimberly Nordstrom

Introduction

Treating the psychiatric patient in the emergency department means being aware of and possibly treating a disorder other than the primary complaint. In patients with known psychiatric illness, it is important to be aware of the underlying psychiatric disorder as it may affect how a patient is able to relay information, how a patient may receive medical information, and how a patient may be affected by the experience. In a patient with no known psychiatric history, a medical differential will need to be considered.

The psychiatric patient is more complicated in that treatment for the chief complaint and treatment of the underlying psychiatric condition may need to be concurrent. Reviewing common forms of psychiatric illness and presentations may be useful in considering a treatment plan.

This chapter will review the acute treatment process from evaluation and determination of the disease, which may or may not have a psychiatric origin, to stabilization. The chapter will conclude with thoughts around dispositional planning.

Acute treatment

It is necessary to have a broad knowledge of medical illnesses that can present with psychiatric symptoms as well as vice versa. It is difficult to determine the appropriate steps in the evaluation and treatment of a patient without this working knowledge.

Determination of disease process

Medical causes of psychiatric symptoms

A person presenting with a psychiatric symptom may or may not have a primary psychiatric illness. An example of this is agitation, which is commonly caused by intoxication on a substance or delirium. A thorough history and physical exam, as with any patient presenting to the emergency department (ED), can give vital clues to etiology. Common psychiatric presentations in the ED include agitation, psychosis, anxiety, mania, and depressed mood. Each symptom has its own differential of possible causes. A medical differential for psychiatric

presentations is listed in Table 27.1. Evaluating for symptoms and signs of the possible medical causes for the psychiatric presentation is necessary to determine appropriate care and disposition.

Agitation is actually a cluster of symptoms with core characteristics of irritability, restlessness, with excessive or semi-purposeful motor activity, heightened responsiveness to internal or external stimuli, and an unstable course [1]. Agitation is a cardinal symptom of delirium [2], intoxication, head injury [3] or neurological disease, metabolic dysregulation [2], and other life-threatening medical states. The agitated patient needs to be considered medical until determined to be otherwise. The exception would be the patient with known psychiatric illness who has had similar presentations. There are multiple agitation scales used in research settings, with little use clinically. Of note, however, is the finding of Damsa and colleagues. The routine use of the Positive and Negative Syndrome Scale – Excited Component (PANSS-EC) reduced the use of restraints in an emergency department from 8.6 to 6.3%, a reduction of 27% [4]. The use of scales can help the medical team determine the level of agitation and possibly cause the team to be more proactive early in the course. Severe agitation can become dangerous, as the patient may become frankly violent. If the patient's level of agitation is high and de-escalation techniques are not helpful, medication treatment may need to begin before understanding the underlying cause.

Psychosis in a patient with no history of mental illness clearly needs to be evaluated medically. In the elderly, delirium or worsening of dementia should be considered. In younger patients, especially those with a history of drug or alcohol issues, drug/alcohol intoxication or withdrawal might be the issue. The differential diagnosis for psychosis includes auto-immune diseases, neurologic diseases, such as specific forms of seizures [5], brain tumors, parkinsonism [6], use of corticosteroids [7], intoxication on several recreational drugs (many not screened on routine drug testing) [8], withdrawal from alcohol [2] or benzodiazepines, and delirium.

Anxiety may be severe and manifest as significant agitation. The patient may be unable to verbally express their symptoms in any other terms. Or, the patient may present with a myriad of

Behavioral Emergencies for the Emergency Physician, ed. Leslie S. Zun, Lara G. Chepenik, and Mary Nan S. Mallory. Published by Cambridge University Press. © Cambridge University Press 2013.

Table 27.1. Medical causes of psychiatric symptoms

Differential diagnoses	
Agitation	Acute pain
	Head trauma
	Infection
	Encephalitis or Encephalopathy
	Exposure to environmental toxins
	Metabolic derangement
	Hypoxia
	Thyroid disease or other hormone irregularity
	Neurological disease
	Toxic levels of medications
	Alcohol or recreational drugs: intoxication or withdrawal
	Exacerbation of a primary psychiatric illness
Psychosis	Delirium
	Chronic neurological disease (dementia, seizures, parkinsonism, brain tumors)
	Steroid use, other medications
	Alcohol or recreational drugs: intoxication or withdrawal
Mania	Delirium
	Thyrotoxicosis
	Alcohol or recreational drugs: intoxication or withdrawal
Anxiety	Respiratory disease
	Cardiac disease
	Thyroid disease
	Toxic levels of medications
	Alcohol or recreational drugs: intoxication or withdrawal
Depression	Reaction to medication
	Chronic disease or chronic pain
	Hormonal variations
	Subclinical/clinical hypothyroidism
	Alcohol or recreational drugs: intoxication or withdrawal

other symptoms such as chest pain, shortness of breath, dizziness, and nausea. If a patient does not have a history of an anxiety disorder, other causes for the symptoms should be considered. Historically, women presenting to emergency departments with these symptoms were not referred as often as men for appropriate diagnostic procedures [9]. Other causes for anxiety and associated symptoms could include hyperthyroid illness [10], drug intoxication [8], and neurological disease [6].

Manic symptoms can be caused by multiple medical issues. One symptom of mania is restlessness or feeling overly energized. The person with akathisia, a side effect of numerous psychotropic and phenothiazine-related anti-emetic medicines, will have similar complaints of internal restlessness. Both the akathitic and manic patient can also appear overtly agitated. Severe caffeine intoxication and intoxication on other stimulants can cause increased energy, decreased need for sleep, mood lability, and even psychosis [8].

Depressed mood has been found to be related to many chronic and acute medical illnesses. Historically, it has been thought that beta-blockers and centrally acting antihypertensives (clonidine,

methyldopa, reserpine) were directly related to depressed mood but that is now questioned [11]. The same study questioning antihypertensives, found a correlation between corticosteroids and depression [11]. Chronic illnesses [12], hormonal variations, especially women's gonadal steroid hormones [13], and hypothyroidism [10] have all been found to be related to depression. In this case, the primary illness needs to be treated but the depressed mood also needs consideration. If it is severe, the patient may be having suicidal thoughts or unable to care for self.

Psychiatric medication side effects or drug–drug interactions as causes of psychiatric symptoms

Delirium

A person with established psychiatric illness may present without any of the major symptoms of the primary illness but appear disoriented, confused, agitated, or even somnolent. Medications, in overdose, or in the form of drug–drug interactions, can cause delirium as well as other serious medical concerns.

Serotonin syndrome can be caused by both an overdose of a single agent or therapeutic doses of multiple medications that increase serotonin levels in the brain; this includes both direct and indirect serotonergic agonists [14]. Caution should be used in prescribing these medications, in the form of polypharmacy, especially in elderly patients [14]. Serotonin syndrome should be considered in the differential of elderly patients, taking serotonergic agents, presenting with severe myoclonus [15]. This syndrome features: hyperthermia, rigidity, autonomic instability, myoclonus, delirium, and if left untreated can cause rhabdomyolysis, renal failure, and coma [15].

Neuroleptic malignant syndrome (NMS) can be caused by recent dopamine antagonist exposure [16] or dopamine agonist withdrawal [17]. Although there are often many symptoms that are suggestive of NMS, a recent international consensus study supports the following symptom cluster for diagnosis: "recent dopamine antagonist exposure or dopamine agonist withdrawal, hyperthermia, rigidity, mental status alteration, creatinine kinase elevation, sympathetic nervous system lability, tachycardia plus tachypnea, and a negative workup for other causes" [18]. Serotonin syndrome and NMS have many overlapping symptoms. It is important to differentiate the two, as treatment is different and offending agents need to be identified and either discontinued or restarted, as in the case of bromocriptine.

Serotonin discontinuation syndrome, while not a medical emergency, may lead patients into the ED. Various symptoms have been reported after both abrupt and tapered withdrawal of serotonergic agents. The onset of symptoms is usually from 1 to 3 days after discontinuation and usually lasts up to 2 weeks [19]. Symptoms can include: mood change, dizziness, paresthesia (numbing, tingling, "electric shock"), nausea, and flu-like symptoms such as headache, lethargy, or diffuse muscle ache [19]. Hallucinations have also been reported after discontinuation with paroxetine [20]. In most cases, the symptoms are mild to moderate and will resolve on their own. Patient education and reassurance may be all that is needed; if the symptoms are particularly troublesome, focused symptomatic treatment can be used. For more severe symptoms, reintroduction of the original medication will alleviate symptoms [21]. A more gradual taper may be indicated.

Recreational drug, alcohol, or benzodiazepine intoxication or withdrawal as a cause for psychiatric symptoms

Drug and alcohol intoxication and withdrawal can complicate a medical issue or may be the primary cause of a medical presentation. It is important to keep this in mind, as treatment may be considerably different.

The signs and symptoms related to intoxication and withdrawal on substances should be reviewed, as there is much overlap with presentations of psychiatric illness. Anxiety, paranoia, and hallucinations may be related to use of hallucinogens and stimulants. Dysphoria and anxiety are common after intoxication on stimulants and alcohol. The specifics of each recreational drug are detailed elsewhere.

Psychiatric causes of symptoms

If a patient with a known psychiatric illness presents similarly to previous presentations, usual diagnosis and treatment would be the standard. If a patient with a psychiatric illness presents with a symptom that is inconsistent with the diagnosis, medical causes for the symptom should be considered.

Per the Diagnostic and Statistical Manual of Mental Disorders, 4th Edition, Text Revision (DSM-IV-TR), a person can only have a psychiatric diagnosis if medical, medication, and recreational drug causes have been first ruled out [22]. With that being said, it is not always feasible to get an exact diagnosis in the ED setting. If a person has depressive symptoms, a family history of depression, multiple psychosocial stressors, has recently stopped using alcohol, and is also hypothyroid, a not otherwise specified (NOS) diagnosis (for example, depressive disorder, NOS) is sufficient and referral can aid in determining a further direction in care.

Psychosis

Psychosis is disruption in perception, organization of speech and/or organization of behavior. There are several disorders related to psychosis: brief psychotic disorder, schizophreniform, schizophrenia, severe mood disorders (depression or mania) with psychosis, schizoaffective disorder, delusional disorder, and shared psychotic disorder. Presentations to the ED, for a non-medical or non–substance-related psychotic episode, might include first-break psychosis, exacerbation of psychotic symptoms secondary to noncompliance with treatment or symptoms of a severe mood disorder (depression or bipolar). Many times, the history will give clues as to the underlying reason for the presentation. If a patient has stopped home medication, first try to understand the reasoning for this (information is usually from family or close friends). It is helpful to

know if the patient was reacting poorly to the medication, in the form of an allergy or side effect. Otherwise reinitiating a medication that a patient could not tolerate will not be successful long term.

Bipolar disorder

Patients with bipolar disorder have suicide rates of approximately 1% annually; in 2006, this was up to 60 times greater than the international population rate of suicide [23]. Suicidal acts tend to occur early in the course of bipolar illness and typically happen in the depressed or mixed phase of illness. There is little evidence for long-term effectiveness of treatment to aid in the prevention of suicide attempts, with the one exception of lithium. Lithium has been found to cause a reduction in risk of suicide attempts and this medication is also associated with lower lethality of attempts [23]. The presentation for mania tends to have similar underlying reasons as that for schizophrenia. Many times it is the (known) bipolar patient who is either off of medications, on recreational drugs, or both. Again, understanding the reasoning for noncompliance tends to be important. Without understanding this reasoning, restarting the medication will probably not have lasting benefit. For mania and psychosis, treatment should begin in the ED. In most cases, the treatment is first focused on agitation but then should become more focused on the underlying disorder. In both cases, the patient is likely to be admitted into a psychiatric facility. Starting treatment right away, in the ED, may help the patient experience and may prevent heightening of agitation.

Anxiety disorders

Anxiety is a common cause of presentation to the ED. There are several different anxiety disorders. Generalized anxiety disorder (GAD), as based on DSM-IV criteria, has an estimated lifetime prevalence in community samples of 5% and panic disorder, as high as 3.5% [24]. In a study specific to patients with panic disorder, it was found that of the 97 patients with this disorder, 32% were initially diagnosed in the ED setting [25]. Many of the anxiety disorders, such as GAD, panic disorder, post-traumatic stress disorder, social phobia, and specific phobia, are comorbid with each other and panic attacks, different from panic disorder, can occur with any form of anxiety. It is important to have a general understanding of these disease states, as one study found that patients with a co-occurring anxiety and mood disorder had a greater likelihood of suicide attempt, than those with a mood disorder alone [26].

Depressive disorders

There are various psychiatric disorders that include the symptom of depression, such as major depressive disorder, bipolar disorder, dysthymic disorder, and substance-induced depressive disorder. The depressed person may or may not present to the ED with depressed mood. The patient may complain of persistent irritability, lack of interest or pleasure, sad mood, or various somatic symptoms. Studies have shown that people will seek some form of medical service within weeks before a suicide attempt; one study reports that up to 69% may present to an ED for non–suicide-related reasons before committing suicide [27]. Another study of the ED population found suicidal ideation in 11.6% and suicide intent in 2% of screened patients. Depression was most highly associated, 68% with ideation and 74% with intent, and panic attacks were also found to be closely associated, with 43% and 55%, respectively [28]. As noted previously, the depressed patient may have several factors relating to the presentation of depressed mood, such as medical conditions, use of recreational substances, and psychosocial issues, so a definitive diagnosis may be problematic. Also, patients with active depressed mood may have less energy and motivation. This is an important consideration as it may affect follow through of instructions given at discharge.

Somatoform disorders

A patient presenting with somatic issues with a negative medical workup may actually be anxious or depressed. Somatoform disorders, such as somatization disorder, conversion disorder, and hypochondriasis, are syndromes where one or more physical symptoms are prominent and cause impairment to the patient but the medical workup fails to find a cause. These disorders are not intentional, which separate them from malingering and factious disorders. Usage of services tend to be high, independent of comorbidity, raising healthcare costs [29]. There is a strong correlation between somatoform disorders and anxiety and depression [30], as well as certain personality characteristics. The reasoning behind this connection is unclear and may be multi-factorial. Because there is a high association between them, screening for depression and anxiety should be considered when a patient presents with strictly somatic complaints. One large, multicenter study found that 69% of those that had major depressive disorder presented initially with somatic symptoms only [31].

Malingering and factitious disorders

Unfortunately in the ED, clinicians also have to determine which patients have disease and which may be purposefully feigning symptoms for another reason. There are two disorders that may present similarly in the ED: malingering and factitious disorder. The malingerer may be quite good at manipulation for a secondary (external) gain: medications (opioids, benzodiazepines – related to addiction or for resale), housing, and disability claims are common. The person with factitious disorder tends to feign symptoms for an internal gain, such as the need to be cared for, feelings of loneliness, and isolation in current home situation, etc. The person with a somatoform disorder may present similarly but these patients are not considered to be purposefully manipulating. Also, schizophrenics may present with vague somatic complaints when becoming symptomatic with their mental illness and, as noted previously,

some depressed patients are better able to describe physical, rather than emotional, needs.

Evaluation

Knowledge of the symptoms and signs related to medical and psychiatric diagnoses is key to formulating a thorough differential relating to the patient's chief complaint or presentation. Unless the patient needs to be quickly stabilized (medically) or de-escalated (psychiatrically), the evaluation process is the same as with any patient. The medical workup for a patient presenting with a psychiatric symptom starts first with attending to vital signs, completing a history and physical exam, and determining the differential diagnosis for the symptom or symptom clusters. The history should be obtained from whatever sources are available, including the patient, paramedics, bystanders, family, friends, and hospital records. If the patient is frankly psychotic, highly anxious, or agitated, he or she may only be able to supply limited information. Abnormal vital signs can be helpful in pointing to a medical cause, although patients who are anxious or intoxicated on recreational drugs or alcohol may also have abnormal vital signs. The physical exam should be a focused, unclothed, but gowned, examination of the patient. All major systems should be examined; including a neurological and mental status examination. Laboratory and other studies should be directed by the differential diagnoses for the patient. Completing universal lab studies when not indicated tend to yield very little [32].

Stabilization of the patient

Stabilization of the psychiatric patient in the ED depends largely on the presenting symptoms but can be thought of as having three main components: de-escalation, treatment, and evaluation of safety.

De-escalation

De-escalation is needed for the agitated patient, to ensure safety. As discussed previously, there are different levels of severity of agitation and focusing on de-escalation early may prevent the need for physical and chemical restraints. The literature supports training in de-escalation techniques to aid in violence prevention [33]. This is for the protection of the staff, as well as the patient. An expert consensus of 50 expert emergency psychiatrists supported verbal interventions, offering food and other assistance, voluntary medications, and a show of force as first-line interventions; saving involuntary medications, seclusion, and restraints for only when first-line management proved ineffective [34]. Legal consideration around the use of restraints is different in many states. Most states allow for use of restraints in emergency departments for "medical emergencies." Patient-centered consideration looks at this from a very different perspective. In a report summarizing a multi-centered consumer survey and related focus groups, consumers (patients) strongly supported having a say in their treatment and wanting treatment to be more collaborative. They noted verbal interventions and offering of appropriate medications as desirable means of de-escalation [35]. Another consideration is that victims of sexual assault have explained that being in restraints caused traumatic feelings, becoming a form of re-victimization [36].

Treatment

Treatment depends largely upon presentation. When treatment is immediately necessary is in the case of agitation. As noted above and in Table 27.1, agitation can be caused by various sources, medical and psychiatric. The basic goal of treatment is to calm the patient, rather than sedate, so that the patient can participate in the assessment and treatment [37]. Other forms of treatment are more related to the presenting symptoms and underlying conditions. As discussed previously, agitation should be treated but so should the underlying cause. An expert consensus of 48 experts in the field of psychiatric emergencies recommended the use of benzodiazepines in three situations: when no data were available, when there is no specific treatment, or when benzodiazepines confer a specific benefit, as in the case of alcohol withdrawal [38]. If the agitated patient has a history of psychosis, is presenting with psychosis, or is not responding to the benzodiazepines, antipsychotics are warranted. Haloperidol, as well as second-generation antipsychotics, are commonly used. The consensus guidelines suggest that clinicians possibly feel more comfortable using one medication over another in situations where a medication has been specifically studied [38].

Another consideration for choice of medication would be medication form. There are now antipsychotics available in tablet/capsule form, rapid-dissolving tablet, intramuscular (IM) injection and intravenous (IV) injection. The choice is largely made by the level of cooperation of the agitated patient in the process. A mildly to moderately agitated patient, who sees himself in distress, may cooperate with treatment and accept a standard oral medication. On the other hand, a mildly to moderately agitated patient who is not cooperative may accept a medication with the plan to divert the tablet (commonly referred to as "cheeking"). In this case, a rapidly dissolving tablet, such as Zyprexa, Zydis, or Risperdal M-tab, might prove most useful. When a patient is highly agitated, a tablet may not be feasible and an IM or IV formulation may be considered necessary. A patient may ask for an IM form or may be given it emergently if considered dangerous. There are now several options to choose from for IM antipsychotics; the main restriction will be the institutional formulary, as to what is available for use. The more commonly used IM antipsychotic medications include haloperidol, ziprasidone, olanzapine, and aripiprazole. There are possible drawbacks to using the atypical antipsychotics as ziprasidone has a slightly greater likelihood of prolonging QTc and IM olanzapine has caused several adverse events (including eight fatalities) when used with other CNS depressants [39]. Also of concern, aripiprazole tends to be activating. As noted above, benzodiazepines are commonly used for agitation and come in oral, IM, and IV formulations.

Table 27.2. General treatments of agitation with suggested dosage range

Treatment of agitation	
Severe agitation	Treat underlying cause, if known Lorazepam IM/IV Haldol IM/IV Ziprasidone IM[a,b] (10–20 mg) Olanzapine IM[b,c] (5–10 mg) Aripiprazole IM[b] (9.75 mg)
Moderate agitation	Treat underlying cause, if known Above IMs or consider oral (dissolving) Risperdal M-Tab[b] (0.5–2 mg) Zyprexa Zydis[b] (5–15 mg)
Mild agitation	Treat underlying cause, if known Consider dosing of home psychiatric medication Oral dosing of typical or atypical[b] antipsychotics Oral benzodiazepines

[a] Ziprasidone is associated with a greater propensity to cause prolongation of the QT interval [1].
[b] Studies for use of atypicals in acute agitation were related to agitation from schizophrenia or bipolar mania [3].
[c] Olanzapine IM should not be used with other CNS depressants [2].

When it comes to best practices for IM antipsychotic use, the literature is instructive for specific populations but because of regulatory guidelines, each patient must consent to research and therefore the studies do not capture the more extremely agitated patients. Also, the Food and Drug Administration considers agitation to be a symptom of underlying disease processes so specific diseases, such as schizophrenia and bipolar, have been the target of registration trials. This raises the question of the ability to generalize from mildly to moderately agitated patients in specific disease states to severely agitated patients with unknown etiology. Because of this, the American College of Emergency Physicians (ACEP) has considered all the available literature of second-generation antipsychotics to be no better than class II. Table 27.2 lists options in treatment in the differing levels of severity of agitation. The actual dose of medications is broad as literature supports a broad range, with the example of lorazepam being dosed from 1 to 4 mg in studies.

Emergency physician-derived consensus recommendations for the specific treatment of the acutely agitated patient suggest using a benzodiazepine or conventional antipsychotic in the patient with undifferentiated agitation [32]. Psychiatrists agree [40]. Atypical antipsychotics should be used in patients with agitation caused by a psychiatric illness for which the drug is indicated [32].

For initial treatment of the psychotic, non-agitated patient, thought should be given to patient preference. A psychotic patient has decision-making capacity unless, on exam, the patient is found not to have capacity for treatment decisions. This is an important concept, as psychotic patients should be afforded autonomy and allowed to participate in treatment decisions. There are various treatment strategies for psychosis; the decision is based on several factors, such as patient preference, cost, and access to care. In the ED, an antipsychotic may be initiated but thought to follow-up care is necessary, as some psychotic disorders may be chronic in nature, such as schizophrenia and a persistent substance-induced psychosis. The other major consideration is side-effect profile. The typical antipsychotics have a greater rate of extrapyramidal effects, whereas the atypical antipsychotics have a higher propensity toward metabolic effects. Within the atypical class, some medications are linked more to weight gain, diabetes, and cholesterol elevation than others, although all of the medications in the class have risk.

If the psychotic patient has a long history of noncompliance, the usual, home medications may be able to be restarted. Beware, as some medications must be re-titrated for both tolerance and safety, most notably clozapine (Clozaril). The hospital pharmacist may be consulted.

The manic patient, like the psychotic patient, may need immediate treatment initiation, for agitation. See Table 27.2 for treatment suggestions. All of the atypical (second-generation) antipsychotics have been approved for treatment in acute mania as monotherapy or as an adjunct with lithium or divalproate, except for paliperidone (Invega) and iloperidone (Fanapt). One could also consider treatment with mood stabilizers valproic acid/divalproate, carbamazepine, and lithium. Valproic acid can be oral-loaded in the ED at 20–30 mg/kg/day in a healthy person, with normal liver function [41]. Carbamazepine needs titration and has multiple drug–drug interactions, making it less attractive in the ED setting. Lithium, while also requiring titration, can be initiated in the ED. The advantage of the mood stabilizers is that there is extensive history with these medications and therapeutic target dosing is known. The "rule of 8's" is a helpful pneumonic for target therapeutic levels for maintenance treatment: 0.8 for lithium, 8 for carbamazepine, and 80 for valproic acid. The major disadvantage of the mood stabilizers, especially lithium, is that they can be fatal in overdose. In the case of lithium, the therapeutic window is narrow, with toxicity beginning at blood levels just outside of this window. A recent meta-analysis of all of the atypical antipsychotics used in treatment of acute mania, except for asenapine, as well as lithium, carbamazepine, oxcarbazepine, divalproex, and haloperidol found that patients had an increased chance of response and remission (expect for oxcabazepine) than placebo but also had a higher risk of discontinuation due to adverse events [42].

For patients presenting with anxiety or depression, caution should be used before discharging the patient with a prescription for benzodiazepines or any antidepressant, even with the selective serotonin reuptake inhibitors (SSRIs) or serotonin norepinephrine reuptake inhibitors (SNRIs). Patient education regarding multi-disciplinary treatment methods, medication limitations, and coordination with the follow-up physician are paramount. First, it is well understood that benzodiazepines should not be used chronically, if at all possible [43]. If a patient

does not have follow-up to see a primary care physician or psychiatrist for treatment of anxiety, the patient discharged with a 1-week prescription for a benzodiazepine is likely to return to the ED requesting a refill. The patient may be erroneously labeled a "drug-seeker" when, in fact, the benzodiazepine was temporarily effective and ongoing symptom management is desired. While benzodiazepines may be effective for treating anxiety in the short-term, SSRIs and SNRIs are considered better long-term agents. Despite their efficacy, however, timely follow-up is still important. SSRIs are known to have a myriad of side effects that lead many to premature treatment discontinuation [44]. They can be initially activating, increasing anxiety. For the anxious patient, initiating an SSRI at half the normal starting dose for 1–2 weeks may mitigate this activation. Some side effects, such as sexual difficulties, are extremely worrisome for patients and may lead to discontinuation of the medication as well as treatment, generally. An increase in suicidal behavior has long been a concern. The depressed patient is thought to be more likely to attempt suicide after the initiation of treatment, when energy and motivation is stronger. A recently published, 27-year longitudinal, observational study refutes this belief. Despite noting that antidepressants were more likely to be used in participants with greater symptom severity or symptom worsening an overall reduction in the risk of suicidal behavior after antidepressant initiation was observed [45].

The acute treatment of bipolar depression also requires caution. At best, typical antidepressants have been found to lack efficacy [46]. Of more concern is their potential role in manic relapse [47]. In the meta-analysis mentioned above, lamotrigine, aripiprazole, olanzapine, and quetiapine were included to determine efficacy as monotherapy. Only quetiapine and, to a lesser degree, olanzapine showed efficacy as monotherapy for acute bipolar depression [42].

Safety evaluation

Assessing patient safety is important, not just for determination of discharge but also to make sure safety issues in the ED are explored. In fact this usually starts at the outset; many EDs require patients to walk through a metal detector before being seen, and triage nurses to inquire about suicidality, plans, and opportunity. The impulsive, suicidal patient may try to cut themselves or overdose on medications while in triage or the ED examination room. Sharp objects and medications should be secured at all times, including home medications. Bedside sitters may be necessary to ensure safety.

Patients who have suicidal thoughts or intention often seek out medical services before an attempt. Inquiry about suicidal ideation is imperative for any patient presenting with a psychiatric chief complaint, who has an alcohol- or drug-related issue, expresses multiple somatic complaints, or appears to be depressed or anxious on evaluation. There is no validity to the common misgiving that asking about suicide creates an intention in someone not thinking of suicide. Safety reassessment is indicated for those patients with prolonged ED stays, who have been medicated, or who have mood or affect changes during their visit. A safety assessment includes considering protective and risk factors, as well as identifying those risk factors that can be modifiable. Some common protective factors include: certain religious beliefs, supportive system of family and friends, having a family pet that the patient is particularly fond of, access to medical care, hopefulness and future-orientation, and willingness to participate in care. Risk factors include: demographics (older, single, male), owning a gun, presence of a major psychiatric disorder or severe anxiety, history of suicide attempts and self-harm behaviors, history of violence, family history of suicide, history of physical or sexual abuse, history of impulsivity or traumatic brain injury, presence of a substance disorder or current intoxication, and serious medical conditions or chronic pain [48]. To modify risk factors, one must determine what is currently affecting the patient. An example of this is allowing an intoxicated suicidal patient to sober and offering support around long-term treatment. This may be in the form of a community detox (where safety is monitored) and offering of alcohol rehabilitation treatment. It is helpful to have a running knowledge of community resources, in these cases. Another example of intervening would be getting social work support for an abused spouse or eliciting family support if this would help a psychosocial stressor. All of this takes understanding why the patient currently feels suicidal. In any case, if during the assessment, the patient appears to be at imminent risk for suicide, inpatient hospitalization will be necessary. This is not usually the question, though. Where it is difficult is when a patient presents with suicidal ideation and has several risk, as well as protective factors. It may be difficult to discern the "at risk" patient and a psychiatric consult may be necessary.

Disposition

Disposition is largely determined on severity of illness. If a patient is deemed unsafe or unable to care for self because of a psychiatric condition, admission to an inpatient psychiatric unit is necessary. The patient sometimes, because of severe medical issues, needs to be admitted medically, with psychiatric consultation. In the case where emergent psychiatric hospitalization is not necessary for safety, it may still be determined that hospitalization can be largely beneficial and may be best treatment. When making a determination to discharge a psychiatric patient, a safety evaluation needs to be documented and referrals for follow-up treatment are a helpful piece of care. Sometimes discharge can be aided if the psychosocial stressors of the patient are addressed.

"Boarding" of patients awaiting admission

Although immediate admission to a psychiatric facility is often the goal, it is not always an option. In many states, inpatient psychiatric beds are at an all-time low and patients who have been assessed, stabilized, and deemed appropriate for inpatient care by the emergency physicians and psychiatrists must remain in the ED for hours to days awaiting an appropriate inpatient bed.

Termed "boarding" this queuing of inpatients in the ED is not uncommon. Understandably, acute and intermediate-term care have different goals. Acute care focuses mainly on stabilization, whereas intermediate care approaches the disease process in a more comprehensive way. Coordination of care for these patients so that intermediate care may begin during their ED stay should benefit patients.

In some facilities the consult-liaison psychiatrist or the inpatient psychiatric team member can be called to take a direct role in patient care. Staff psychiatrists may provide useful phone consultation even if unable to initiate direct care for the patient. For the established patient, contacting the patient's psychiatrist or therapist may help define treatment goals and effective therapy. Pre-determined order sets that can be tailored for each patient are used in the management of medical and surgical patients who are "boarding" in the ED and may be of use during the transition to intermediate psychiatry care.

Care focuses on the underlying illness. For the psychotic and manic patient, re-starting and/or re-titrating home medications while covering for break-through symptoms can be considered. Familiarity with side-effect profiles of psychotropics as well as titration nuances of clozapine (Clozaril) and lithium are important. For example, re-titrating lithium while also using an atypical antipsychotic and benzodiazepine is an effective bridge between acute stabilization and intermediate care. Akathisia and orthostatic hypotension are anticipated with some antipsychotics, particularly when restarting the home dose. Both can be managed easily in the ED. Use of fall precautions and urinals might be helpful for orthostasis. Propranolol and benzodiazepines [49], as well as low-dose mirtazepine [50], have been found to be helpful for akathisia. In the event of akathisia, the antipsychotic dose is tapered, and repeat doses of the effective reversal agent are given as needed.

The newly diagnosed psychotic patient is more complicated. Best efforts in attaining collateral history, review of the initial medical presentation and toxicological screens, and patient demographics may assist in developing a differential diagnosis to guide further treatment. The psychotic patient should be started or continued on an antipsychotic of either class, noting side effects. Atypical antipsychotics are commonly chosen in the acute setting because they are less likely to cause dystonia or dyskinesia. Reassessment is important. As soon as the patient is able to understand concepts of disease, further therapeutic history can be obtained and risks and benefits of medication can be discussed. Several options for the newly diagnosed manic patient are available. Of the mood stabilizers, lithium, valproic acid, and carbamazepine are the best studied. Any one of these may be added to the atypical antipsychotic and/or benzodiazepine likely already initiated for control of acute agitation on presentation. Titration is imperative. Serum creatinine and TSH should be tested before starting lithium. For valproic acid and carbamazepine, baseline AST and ALT are indicated as both medications can cause a toxic effect with regard to hepatitis.

The depressed suicidal patient should be started on an antidepressant. The primary antidepressant selection determinants are cost, side-effect profiles, and compliance likelihood. Most of the SSRIs are now generic. If the patient has never had an adequate trial (defined by most as at least 6–8 weeks) on an SSRI this is a good choice. Because there are serotonin receptors in the gastrointestinal system, any SSRI can cause nausea. On the spectrum of activation, fluoxetine tends to be the most activating, with paroxetine the least activating. These two medications are also on each side of the spectrum for half-life. Fluoxetine has a very long half-life. With paroxetine having a short half-life, serotonin discontinuation syndrome can be seen after missing just one dose of this medication.

Basic non-medication therapies can be initiated in the ED setting. At its simplest form, supportive therapy is listening and encouraging the patient. This can be very helpful in calming the patient who is overwhelmed. Solution-focused therapy basically helps the patient problem-solve. This is particularly helpful for the depressed or anxious patient. The idea is not to problem-solve for the patient, but rather to create an environment and gently question the patient to help the patient become more goal-directed.

Care coordination

Many patients who present with psychiatric complaints have psychosocial issues that may relate to the complaint. It is often helpful to use social work services while the patient is in the ED. If social work is not available, knowing the resources in the community and giving the patient appropriate referrals can help in problem-solving and may reduce anxiety for the patient. Knowledge about alcohol and drug detoxification and rehabilitation programs, resources for the homeless, domestic violence resources, and indigent care programs is helpful. Nurses and social workers can also help in eliciting information from families when abuse or neglect is suspected, and identifying and enlisting the emotional support system available to the patient.

Referrals

If a medication is started in the ED, a referral and/or consultative call should be made to a primary care physician (or group), a psychiatrist, or community mental health clinic. It is helpful to give the patient a list of these providers and the insurances they accept, as well as indigent care programs, to the patient at discharge. Social workers are a source for referrals that may meet the patient's psychosocial needs. When indicated, refer patients to dedicated treatment programs, such as dual diagnosis clinics where the patient's primary psychiatric illness plus substance abuse can be treated. The goal is to provide a coordinated "hand off" so that the patient does not have to continue to use the ED for psychiatric care.

References

1. Lindenmayer JP. The pathophysiology of agitation. *J Clin Psychiatry* 2000;**61**:5–10.

2. Caplan LR. Delirium: a neurologist's view-the neurology of agitation and overactivity. *Rev Neurol Dis* 2010;**7**:111–18.

3. Ciurli P, Formisano R, Bivona U, et al. Neuropsychiatric disorders in persons with severe traumatic brain injury: prevalence, phenomenology, and relationship with demographic, clinical, and functional features. *J Head Trauma Rehabil* 2011;**26**:116–26.

4. Damsa C, Ikelheimer D, Adam E, et al. Heisenberg in the ER: observation appears to reduce involuntary intramuscular injections in a psychiatric emergency service. *Gen Hosp Psychiatry* 2006;**2**:431–3.

5. de Araujo Filho GM, da Silva JM, Mazetto L, Marchetti RL, Yacubian EM. Psychoses of epilepsy: a study comparing the clinical features of patients with focal versus generalized epilepsies. *Epilepsy Behav* 2011;**20**:655–8.

6. Weintraub D, Burn DJ. Parkinson's disease: the quintessential neuropsychiatric disorder. *Mov Disord* 2011;**26**:1022–31.

7. Benyamin RM, Vallejo R, Kramer J, Rafeyan R. Corticosteroid induced psychosis in the pain management setting. *Pain Physician* 2008;**11**:917–20.

8. Leikin JB, Krantz AJ, Zell-Kanter M, et al. Clinical features and management of intoxication due to hallucinogenic drugs. *Med Toxicol Adverse Drug Exp* 1989;**4**:324–50.

9. Lehmann JB, Wehner PS, Lehmann CU, Savory LM. Gender bias in the evaluation of chest pain in the emergency department. *Am J Cardiol* 1996;**77**:641–4.

10. Melish JS. Thyroid disease. In: Walker HK, Hall WD, Hurst JW, (Eds.). *Clinical Methods: the History, Physical, and Laboratory Examinations*, (3rd Edition, Chapt. 135). Boston: Butterworths; 1990.

11. Patten SB, Lavorato DH. Medication use and major depressive syndrome in a community population. *Compr Psychiatry* 2001;**42**:124–31.

12. Millan-Calenti JC, Maseda A, Rochette S, et al. Mental and psychological conditions, medical comorbidity and functional limitation: differential associations in old adults with cognitive impairment, depressive symptoms and co-existence of both. *Int J Geriatr Psychiatry* 2011;**26**:1071–9.

13. Ostlund H, Keller E, Hurd YL. Estrogen receptor gene expression in relation to neuropsychiatric disorders. *Ann N Y Acad Sci* 2003;**1007**:54–63.

14. Poeschla BD, Bartle P, Hansen KP. Serotonin syndrome associated with polypharmacy in the elderly. *Gen Hosp Psychiatry* 2011;**33**:301.e9–11.

15. Yee AH, Wijdicks EF. A perfect storm in the emergency department. *Neurocrit Care* 2010;**12**:258–60.

16. Caroff SN, Hurford I, Lybrand J, Campbell EC. Movement disorders induced by antipsychotic drugs: implications of the CATIE schizophrenia trial. *Neurol Clin* 2011;**29**:127–48.

17. Wu YF, Kan YS, Yang CH. Neuroleptic malignant syndrome associated with

bromocriptine withdrawal in Parkinson's disease – a case report. *Gen Hosp Psychiatry* 2011;**33**:301.e7–8.

18. Gurrera RJ, Caroff SN, Cohen A, et al. An international consensus study of neuroleptic malignant syndrome diagnostic criteria using the Delphi method. *J Clin Psychiatry* 2011;**72**:1222–8.

19. Black K, Shea C, Dursun S, Kutcher S. Selective serotonin re-uptake inhibitor discontinuation syndrome: proposed diagnostic criteria. *J Psychiatry Neurosci* 2000;**25**:255–61.

20. Yasui-Furukori N, Kaneko S. Hallucination induced by paroxetine discontinuation in patients with major depressive disorders. *Psychiatry Clin Neurosci* 2011;**65**:384–5.

21. Haddad P. Antidepressant discontinuation syndromes. Clinical relevance, prevention and management. *Drug Saf* 2001;**24**:183–97.

22. American Psychiatric Association. *Diagnostic and Statistical Manual of Mental Disorders*, (4th Edition), Text Revision. Washington, DC: American Psychiatric Association; 2000.

23. Baldessarini RJ, Pompili M, Tondo L. Suicide in bipolar disorder: risks and management. *CNS Spectr* 2006;**11**:465–71.

24. American Psychiatric Association. *Diagnostic and Statistical Manual of Mental Disorders*, (4th Edition), Text Revision. Washington, DC: American Psychiatric Association; 2000:436, 474.

25. Katerndahl DA, Realini JP. Where do panic attack sufferers seek care? *J Fam Pract* 1995;**40**:237–43.

26. Sareen J, Cox BJ, Afifi TO, et al. Anxiety disorders and risk for suicidal ideation and suicide attempts: a population-based longitudinal study of adults. *Arch Gen Psychiatry* 2005;**62**:1249–57.

27. Gairin I, House A, Owens D. Attendance at the accident and emergency department in the year before suicide: a retrospective study. *Br J Psychiatry* 2003;**183**:28–33.

28. Claassen CA, Larkin GL. Occult suicidality in an emergency department population. *Br J Psychiatry* 2005;**186**:352–3.

29. Barsky AJ, Orav EJ, Bates DW. Somatization increases medical utilization and costs independent of psychiatric and medical comborbidity. *Arch Gen Psychiatry* 2005;**62**:903–10.

30. Lowe B, Spitzer RL, Williams JB, et al. Depression, anxiety and somatization in primary care: syndrome overlap and functional impairment. *Gen Hosp Psychiatry* 2008;**30**:191–9.

31. Simon GE, VonKorff M, Piccinelli M, et al. An international study of the relation between somatic symptoms and depression. *N Engl J Med* 1999;**341**:1329–35.

32. Lukens TW, Wolf SJ, Edlow JA, et al. Clinical policy: critical issues in the diagnosis and management of the adult psychiatric patient in the emergency department. *Ann Emerg Med* 2006;**47**:79–99.

33. Brasic J, Fogelman D. Clinician safety. *Psychiatr Clin North Am* 1999;**22**:923–40.

34. Allen MH, Currier GW, Hughes DH, Docherty JP, et al. Treatment of behavioral emergencies: a summary of the expert consensus guidelines. *J Psychiatr Pract* 2003;**9**:16–38.

35. Allen MH, Carpenter D, Sheets JL, et al. What do consumers say they want and need during a psychiatric emergency? *J Psychiatr Pract* 2003;**9**:39–58.

36. Smith SB. Restraints: retraumatization for rape victims? *J Psychosoc Nurs Ment Health Serv* 1995;**33**:23–8.

37. National Collaborating Centre for Mental Health. *Schizophrenia: Core Interventions in the Treatment and Management of Schizophrenia in Primary and Secondary Care*. London: National Institute for Clinical Excellence (NICE); 2002.

38. Allen MH, Currier GW, Carpenter D, et al. The expert consensus guideline series. Treatment of behavioral emergencies 2005. *J Psychiatr Pract* 2005;**11**:5–108.

39. Battaglia J. Pharmacological management of acute agitation. *Drugs* 2005;**65**:1207–22.

40. Allen MH, Currier GW, Carpenter D, et al. The expert consensus guideline series. Treatment of behavioral emergencies 2005. *J Psychiatr Pract* 2005;**11**:5–108.

41. Hirschfeld RM, Baker JD, Wozniak P, et al. The safety and early efficacy of oral-loaded divalproex versus standard-titration divalproex, lithium, olanzapine, and placebo in the treatment of acute mania associated with bipolar disorder. *J Clin Psychiatry* 2003;**64**:841–6.

42. Tamayo JM, Zarate CA, Vieta E, et al. Level of response and safety of pharmacological monotherapy in the treatment of acute bipolar I disorder phases: a systematic review and meta-analysis. *Int J Neuropsychopharmacol* 2010;**13**:813–32.

43. Vicens C, Socias I, Mateu C, et al. Comparative efficacy of two primary care interventions to assist withdrawal from long term benzodiazepine use: a protocol for a clustered, randomized clinical trial. *BMC Fam Pract* 2011;**12**:23.

44. Warden D, Madhukar H, Trivedi MD, et al. Early adverse events and attrition in SSRI treatment: a suicide assessment methodology study. *J Clin Psychopharmacol* 2010;**30**:259–66.

45. Leon AC, Solomon DA, Li C, et al. Antidepressants and risks of suicide and suicide attempts: a 27-year observational study. *J Clin Psychiatry* 2011;**72**:580–6.

46. Sachs GS, Nierenberg AA, Calabrese JR, et al. Effectiveness of adjunctive antidepressant treatment for bipolar depression. *N Engl J Med* 2007;**356**:1711–22.

47. Lewis J, Winokur G. The induction of mania: a natural history study with controls. *Arch Gen Psychiatry* 1982;**39**:303–6.

48. Gelenberg AJ, Freeman MP, Markowitz JC, et al. Practice guideline for the treatment of patients with major depressive disorder, (3rd Edition). American Psychiatric Association. *Am J Psychiatry* 2010;**167**:23–4.

49. Miller CH, Fleischhacker WW. Managing antipsychotic-induced acute and chronic akathisia. *Drug Saf* 2000;**22**:73–81.

50. Poyurovsky M, Pashinian A, Weizman R, et al. Low-dose mirtazapine: a new option in the treatment of antipsychotic-induced akathisia. A randomized, double-blind, placebo- and propranolol-controlled trial. *Biol Psychiatry* 2006;**59**:1071–7.

Chapter 28

Rapidly acting treatment in the emergency department

Ross A. Heller and Laurie Byrne

Introduction

Psychiatric patients in the emergency department (ED) present unique and difficult challenges for the emergency medicine physician. Patients may present with new, undifferentiated behavioral symptoms such as agitation, confusion, combativeness, agitated delirium, or hallucinations. Patients with known psychiatric disorders may present similarly or with specific exacerbations of their symptoms. To a reasonable degree, based upon the presentation, exam, and indicated ancillary testing, the ED physician must use methods to decrease patient symptoms and improve behavioral control while managing potential underlying medical issues. Thus, the evaluation and treatment of the psychiatric patient is often not done in a linear manner.

The initial management of any psychiatric patient is to assure their safety and health, as well as the safety of others in the ED. A calm, quiet patient with a history of depression who presents to the ED with complaints of their typical depression and feeling of hopelessness is a fairly routine patient to evaluate. However, patients who are acutely agitated, hostile, aggressive, psychotic, altered in sensorium, or aggressively homicidal or suicidal present an entirely different challenge. Because of potential imminent danger to the physician, the staff and the patient, restraint measures may be necessary to rapidly treat or "lyse" the patient's symptoms to facilitate rapid and effective medical and psychiatric assessment. This chapter will review current therapies, as well as newer and investigational treatment options useful to diminish acute psychiatric symptoms.

Treatment of the acute psychotic, aggressive, and violent patient

The Diagnostic and Statistical Manual of Mental Disorders, 4th Edition, Text Revision (DSM-IV-TR) describes a brief psychotic episode as one or more of the following: delusions, hallucinations, disorganized speech, or grossly disorganized behavior. These patients may also have a rapidly changing mood, disorientation, and impaired attention, and can have emotional volatility, outlandish behavior, and rampant screaming. A careful mental status examination is required to distinguish this from delirium, dementia, organic brain syndrome, or another medical condition.

Immediate medical assessment and intervention

While it is incumbent on the ED physician to ensure that a patient exhibiting psychiatric symptoms is medically assessed, often the patient must be treated acutely with medications to prevent aggressive and agitated symptoms from progressing and to allow for an effective medical examination process. This requires a flexible and simultaneous combination of pertinent medical assessment and stabilization along with the use of restraints, both physical and pharmacologic, as indicated. Particular attention to abnormal vital signs, including the blood pressure, pulse, respiratory rate, pulse-oximetry, and temperature, and the bedside glucose measurement are important for any patient with an altered sensorium. Appropriate interventions are made as abnormalities are identified.

Restraint

During early stabilization and evaluation and before an understanding of the underlying cause of the altered sensorium, restraint of the patient may be necessary. All ED staff involved in the use of restraints must be well versed in criteria for use of restraints and their proper and appropriate application [1]. Studies have found that the application of restraints in and of themselves can increase agitation. Techniques for de-escalation should also be applied when time permits to avoid the use of restraints as there are well-recognized risks involving restraints including serious injury and death to the patient. The use of restraints must be minimal in duration and appropriate in application [1]. Physical restraint may be necessary so that the staff can safely administer medications to extremely agitated patients. Early initiation of medications to rapidly "lyse" agitation can assist in reducing seclusion and physical restraint use and improve safety of patients and staff.

Chemical restraint

Rapid treatment to stop acute psychotic symptoms should be initiated whenever the patient is out of control or escalating in

Behavioral Emergencies for the Emergency Physician, ed. Leslie S. Zun, Lara G. Chepenik, and Mary Nan S. Mallory. Published by Cambridge University Press. © Cambridge University Press 2013.

such a manner as to put them or staff at risk of injury. Traditionally, the acute psychotic state was treated with "typical" antipsychotics [2]. These agents have been used for many decades and have a well-known therapeutic range as well as known risks. In the past decade a group of drugs known as atypical antipsychotics have shown increasing use in the management of the psychotic patient [3]. There has been extensive evaluation in the management of the acutely psychotic patient's symptoms in the emergency department setting using these agents [4,5,6,7,8]. The key for the emergency physician is to be knowledgeable about the risks and benefits, of all of the medications used for rapid "lysis" of acute psychosis as well as knowing which drugs to use in specific subsets of patients.

Typical antipsychotics

The typical antipsychotics have been shown to provide rapid, predictable, and effective sedation in the management of patients who are acutely psychotic [9]. The most used typical antipsychotics in the emergency department for rapid lysis of acute psychosis have been haloperidol (Haldol) and droperidol (Inapsine). Intramuscular (IM) Haldol in typical doses of 5–10 mg works well to eliminate thought disorder, hallucinations and delusional activity in patients treated for acute psychosis [9]. It can be given both orally and IM in the emergency department setting at 2- to 5-mg doses repeated up to three times. A study looked at treating patients with active functional psychosis using pulse doses of haloperidol intramuscularly over a 3-hour period [10]. The dose range over the 3 hours was a low of 13 mg IM up to a high of 33 mg IM. Approximately 35% of the patients suffered the major side affect of acute dystonia and extrapyramidal symptoms (EPS) [9,10]. The EPS side effects are known to be dose dependent which limits the use of high dose haloperidol.

The EPS side effect as well as the discovery that haloperidol can cause neuroleptic malignant syndrome (NMS) has caused scientists to look for other modalities in treating this patient population. Giving haloperidol in combination with lorazepam showed superior results in both sedation and decreased side effects [10]. However, those patients who show signs of dystonia or movement disorder may still need treatment with cogentin or diphenhydramine (Benadryl) [10].

Droperidol is another typical antipsychotic that was long used to treat acutely psychotic patients in the emergency room. Droperidol has many benefits as an antipsychotic and an antiemetic. However, in 2001 the FDA placed a "black box" warning on this drug, due to a concern that it may result in sudden death in patients with QT interval prolongation causing sudden life-threatening arrhythmias such as torsades de pointes [11]. As a result, the use of droperidol for antipsychotic treatment in the emergency department setting drastically declined. However, recent studies have found that while droperidol does appear to cause QT interval prolongation, there is lack of convincing evidence of a causal relation linking droperidol to life-threatening cardiac events [11]. Furthermore, studies have shown that lower dosages (< 5 mg) are very safe and effective [12].

Benzodiazepines and combination therapy

Benzodiazepine, such as lorazapam (Ativan) at 1–2 mg IM or orally, or clonazepam (Klonopin) at 1–2 mg IM, can be given alone [13,14]. It is a reasonable alternate or adjunct to antipsychotics to avoid typical antipsychotic toxicity. It has been found that given by itself lorazepam has better effect in the management of aggression, although is more sedating than haloperidol [10]. There are no EPS side effects with lorazepam, however, its use can lead to serious complications including excessive sedation, confusion, disinhibition, ataxia, and respiratory depression, therefore requiring patients be monitored continuously [10]. Due to the potential for extrapyramidal symptoms developing hours or days after a single dose of haloperidol, lorazepam may provide an excellent alternative for the management of the acutely agitated psychotic patient in the emergency department [13,14]. It is suggested that benzodiazepines are very effective with manic patients and may lower the total dose of antipsychotics required. It should be considered in the control of acute exacerbations in schizophrenia, mania, and substance abuse [15].

Atypical antipsychotics

The advent of the atypical antipsychotics was promising with the suggestion that patients would be treated for their symptoms with much less concern for the EPS and other side effects of typical antipsychotics. These medications have been studied directly and in comparison to both typical antipsychotics and benzodiazepines for the treatment of acute psychosis and agitation. The atypical antipsychotics (see Table 28.1) such as risperidone (Risperdal), olanzapine (Zyprexa), quetiapine (Seroquel), and ziprasidone (Geodon) have a pharmacologic profile that is favorable. They effectively control a broad range of symptoms associated with psychosis including agitation and aggression with a much reduced side-effect profile [2,5,6,7,16,17,18]. These agents are believed to work through the D2 (dopamine) receptors and/or they inhibit serotonin reuptake. Specifically as a group, these drugs appears to work with greater efficacy against the acute psychosis symptoms with a reduction in the side effects seen with the typical antipsychotics. It is important to be aware that these agents do have some of the side effects seen with the typical antipsychotics, although significantly less. Although the uses of these agents have a predictable pattern of benefits and risks, one of the severe risks is the development of neuroleptic malignant syndrome [3,19]. These drugs can be used alone or in combination with benzodiazepines and come in both oral and IM formulations. Both ziprasidone (Geodon) and olanzapine (Zyprexa) have been shown to have a more rapid onset and effect in reducing acute psychotic symptoms than halperidol [4,16]. Olanzapine (initiated at 15 to 20 mg/day) was a safe and effective medication for rapidly calming the agitation of acutely agitated psychotic patients with less side effects of the typical antipsychotics [18].

A double-blinded study showed that risperidone (Risperdal) was more effective in reducing hostility in schizophrenics than

Table 28.1. Medications useful for the "lysis" of acute psychiatric symptoms in the ED

Drug	Indication	Dosage	Primary side effects	Secondary side effects	Warnings
Haloperidol[a] (Haldol)	Acute psychosis and agitation	2–5 mg IM may repeat	EPS, movement disorders	NMS	Has been reported to be a problem in prolonged QTC
Droperidol[a]	Acute psychosis/agitation Typicals are regarded as better than atypicals in dementia patients with agitation	2.5–5 mg IM	Sedation	EPS	Not safe in patients with prolonged QT or arrhythmias
Ziprasidone (Geodon)[b]	Acute psychosis/agitation	10–20 mg IM up to 40 mg	Sedation, EPS, orthostatic hypotension	NMS	Can cause increased QTC – do not use in patients with known QTC prolongation. Do not use in patients with dementia
Olanzapine (Zyprexa)[b]	Acute psychosis/agitation	10 mg IM or oral dissolving tablet	Sedation, EPS, Orthostatic hypotension	NMS	Do not use with other CNS depressants. Do not use in patients with dementia
Quetiapine (Seroquel)[b]	Acute psychosis/agitation but primarily shown in bipolar/ schizophrenia and ICU Delirium	25–50 mg PO starting dose BID	Sedation, EPS, orthostatic hypotension	NMS	Can cause increased QTC – do not use in patients with known QTC prolongation. Do not use in patients with dementia
Risperidone (Risperdal)[b]	Acute psychosis/agitation but primarily shown in bipolar/ schizophrenia	1–2 mg PO or ODT	Sedation, EPS, orthostatic hypotension	NMS	Do not use in dementia patients
Lorazepam (Ativan)	Rapid tranquilization of the agitated patient	1–2 mg IM or PO may repeat	Sedation and respiratory depression	CNS depression	Can cause respiratory arrest, must monitor

[a] Typical antipsychotic.
[b] Atypical antipsychotic.

haloperidol. In addition, risperidone was found to be effective in reducing aggression in patients with dementia and mental retardation [13,14,15,17]. However, risperidone is only available in an oral preparation thus its use in the uncooperative patient may be limited. Quetiapine (Seroquel) is effective in alleviating aggression in elderly psychotic patients. However, this medication requires titration for optimal effect; thus, it is not an ideal agent for use in the emergency department setting [20].

Rapid lysis of acute depression with suicide ideation

The acute management of the depressed and suicidal patient requires a comprehensive approach. Disposition of these patients can be difficult and fraught with potential hazards. Whereas it is impractical to admit all patients with suicide ideation, suicide gesture, and self-injury, the use of a high-risk screen is not a panacea. Such techniques as a no harm contract, a joint safety plan with the patient's family, or the patient's commitment to treatment may be of benefit but are not proven to reduce the risk of suicide attempt [21]. Collaboration with a mental health clinician is necessary to develop a treatment plan, especially if the patient is to be discharged from the ED. The prescribing of antidepressant medications is typically not performed in the ED and not considered standard care [21]. Most of these medications do not have a clinical effect for at least 2 weeks after initiation of treatment. Some antidepressants

have been associated with an initial increase risk for suicidal behavior, particularly the SSRI class.

An agent that would provide the acute "lysis" of suicide thoughts and provide for a "cooling off period" for patients while they achieve therapeutic benefit from antidepressant therapy and receive outpatient therapy would be quite useful in the ED setting. Ketamine, a well-known agent used as an anesthetic and for pain management, has been recently studied for this purpose. Its use in treating acute depression with relief of symptoms such as depression, anxiety, and hopelessness is relatively new, with many small size studies, and is not considered standard care [23]. However, these early studies are showing promise for stopping the suicidal thoughts in patients for approximately 7–10 days. If proven effective, ketamine therapy may allow discharge and follow-up for some patients, without the need for emergency psychiatric hospitalization from the ED. The dose of ketamine used in these studies varied from 0.2 to 0.5 mg/kg. An NIH sponsored study continues to look at patients with major depressive disorder and the usage of ketamine as a temporizing treatment [21,22,23].

In conclusion, acute psychiatric conditions that present to the ED often require a multifaceted approach. Underlying medical conditions must be evaluated, treated, or excluded. To assist in the process, "lysing" psychotic symptoms is useful. Understanding the available medication armamentarium for the rapid control of the acutely agitated, psychotic, or depressed patient is mandatory for the safe evaluation, treatment, and disposition. These medications not only stabilize the patient from immediate harm to self and others, but also facilitate further psychiatric intervention when needed, and potentially reduce the patient's symptoms enough to allow for safe discharges from the ED. The future of mental health care and its dwindling resources require additional research to achieve safe treatment alternatives for appropriate disposition of patients.

References

1. Zun LS, Downey LA. Level of agitation of psychiatric patients presenting to an emergency department. *Prim Care Companion J Clin Psychiatry* 2008;**10**:108–13.

2. Hirayasu Y, Korn M. *Management of Patients with Acute Psychosis*. Available at: www.medscape.org/viewarticle/420241 (Accessed October 2011).

3. Zimbroff DL. Management of acute psychosis: from emergency to stabilization. *CNS Spectrum* 2003;**8** (Suppl 2):10–15.

4. Mendelowitz AJ. The utility of intramuscular ziprasidone in the management of acute psychotic agitation. *Ann Clin Psychiatry* 2004;**16**:145–54.

5. Zimbroff DL, Allen MH, Battaglia J, et al. Best clinical practice with ziprasidone IM: update after 2 years of experience. *CNS Spectr* 2005;**10**:1–15.

6. Karagianis JL, Dawe IC, Thakur A, et al. Rapid tranquilization with olanzapine in acute psychosis: a case series. *J Clin Psychiatry* 2001;**62**(Suppl 2):12–16.

7. Bartko G. New formulations of olanzapine in the treatment of acute agitation. *Neuropsychopharmacol Hung* 2006;**8**:171–8.

8. Battaglia J. Pharmacological management of acute agitation. *Drugs* 2005;**65**:1207–22.

9. Anderson WH, Kuehnle JC. Rapid treatment of acute psychosis. *Am J Psychiatry* 1976;**133**:1076–8.

10. Battaglia J, Moss S, Rush H, et al. Haloperidol, lorazepam or both for psychotic agitation? A multicenter, prospective, double-blind, emergency department study. *Am J Emerg Med* 1997;**15**:335–40.

11. Kao LW, Kirk MA, Evers SJ, Rosenfeld SH. Droperidol, QT prolongation and sudden death. What is the evidence? *Ann Emerg Med* 2003;**41**:546–58.

12. Gan TJ. "Black box" warning on droperdol: report of the FDA convened expert panel. *Anesth Analg* 2004;**98**:1809.

13. Currier GW, Simpson GM. Risperidone liquid concentrate and oral lorazepam versus intramuscular haloperidol and intramuscular lorazepam for treatment of psychotic agitation. *J Clin Psychiatry* 2001;**62**:153–7.

14. Currier GW, Chou JC, Feifel D, et al. Acute treatment of psychotic agitation: a randomized comparison of oral treatment with risperidone and lorazepam versus intramuscular treatment with haloperidol and lorazepam. *J Clin Psychiatry* 2004;**65**:386–94.

15. Veser FH, Veser BD, McMullan JT, Zealberg J, Currier GW. Risperidone versus haloperidol in combination with lorazepam, in the treatment of acute agitation and psychosis: a pilot randomized, double blind placebo controlled trial. *J Psychiatr Pract* 2006;**12**:103–8.

16. Brook S, Lucey JV, Gunn KP. Intramuscular ziprasidone compared with intramuscular haloperidol in the treatment of acute psychosis. Ziprsidone I.M. Study Group. *J Clin Psychiatry* 2000;**61**:933–41.

17. Lim HK, Kim JJ, Pae CU, et al. Comparison of risperidone orodispersible tablet and intramuscular haloperidol in the treatment of acute psychotic agitation: a randomized open, prospective study. *Neuropsychobiology* 2010;**62**:81–6.

18. Hsu WY, Huang SS, Lee BS, Chiu NY Comparison of intramuscular olanzapine, orally disintegrating olanzapine tablets, oral risperidone solution and intramuscular haloperidol in the management of acute agitation in an acute care psychiatric ward. *J Clin Psychopharmacol* 2010;**30**:230–4.

19. McAllister-Williams RH, Ferrier IN. Rapid tranquilization: time for a reappraisal of options for parenteral therapy. *Br J Psychiatry* 2002;**180**: 485–9.

20. Mohr P, Pecenak J, Svestka J, Swingler D, Treueer T. Treatment of acute agitation in psychotic disorders. *Neuro Endocrinol Lett* 2005;**26**:327–35.

21. Larkin GL, Beautrais AL. A preliminary naturalistic study of low-dose ketamine for depression and suicide ideation in the emergency department. *Int J Neuropsychopharmacol* 2011:**14**; 1127–31.

22. DiazGranados, N, Ibrahim LA, Brutsche NE, et al. Rapid resolution of suicidal ideation after a single infusion of an NMDA antagonist in patients with treatment-resistant major depressive disorder. *J Clin Psychiatry* 2010;**71**:1605–11.

23. Price R, Nock MK, Chamey DS, Mathew SJ. Effects of intravenous ketamine on explicit and implicit measures of suicidality. *Biol Psychiatry* 2009;**66**: 522–6.

Chapter

29

Pediatric psychiatric disorders in the emergency department

Margaret Cashman and Jagoda Pasic

Introduction

Children and adolescents who come to the emergency department (ED) with a psychiatric crisis are a concern for all ED professionals. Their visits tend to absorb more prehospital and ED resources than other classes of pediatric patient, as well as leading to higher rates of admission from the ED [1,2]. Some studies suggest their numbers may be growing [3,4].

Children and adolescents present to the ED with certain predictable crises involving mental health problems. One set of concerns arises from *deliberate self-injury* or the *imminent threat of such injury*. Another set of concerns arises from the acute emergency of *psychosis*. Children and adolescents may have become *out of control*, directing hostility and aggression at the people in their lives. Some youth may be brought in with *"internalizing" conditions such as depression or anxiety*, in which the youngster's distress is turned "inward" rather than being expressed through acting out on the child's environment or family. *Substance abuse* creates several scenarios which may bring a teen or a child into the ED.

Some conditions are beyond the scope of this chapter. For example, *eating disorders* can cause a medical crisis leading to an adolescent or child to be brought to the ED. (See Chapter 19 on emergency management of eating disorders for more information.) Some children and teens come to the ED because they've been the *victims of abuse or neglect*. Most emergency departments have established protocols for identifying and managing these youngsters. Additionally, some children and adolescents arrive at the ED with acute and serious physical injury or illness but are at high risk to develop a *secondary acute stress disorder* from their experience. These youngsters, too, may require emergency psychiatric assessment (Table 29.1).

Psychiatric evaluation of the child or adolescent patient requires particular emphasis on gathering information from multiple sources. Collection and integration of these collateral sources of information frequently leads to longer lengths of stay in the ED for pediatric behavioral health visits, compared with adult psychiatric ED visits.

The emergency department setting available to children and adolescents varies substantially from facility to facility. Children's hospitals may or may not have a specific section

dedicated to mental health emergencies with environmental adaptations appropriate for this purpose. General hospital emergency departments similarly may or may not have a dedicated psychiatric emergency service section, let alone a dedicated pediatric psychiatric emergency service section. As much as possible, try to limit the young patient's exposure to the overwhelming sights, sounds, and odors of the busy adult ED, as these stimuli can become associated with a stressful and potentially traumatizing ED experience.

The sequence in which interviewing is conducted is arbitrary. Some experts suggest speaking before the child interview with parents or guardians in the case of the *prepubertal child*, while speaking initially to *adolescents* before talking with their parents, guardians, or accompanying staff. However, you may choose to conduct an initial interview with both patient and adults present, in some circumstances. Bear in mind the importance of interviewing the young patient individually at some point, in case sensitive information needs to be shared which the adults' presence might squelch.

Hospitals typically will have protocols in place determining the handling of pediatric psychiatric patients in EDs. States vary in the regulations pertaining to such issues as age of consent, privacy of clinical information from parents or guardians, and involuntary treatment practices. Fortunati and Zonana have provided a helpful discussion of the legal concepts pertinent to addressing this population's needs in the ED [5]. The availability of specialty care, such as inpatient child psychiatric units, also varies from one locality to another. Some counties provide a backup level of crisis-based resources, which either can or must be used before considering psychiatric hospitalization.

The wild child: out-of-control children and adolescents

The child or teen who is aggressive, hostile, and disruptive may be brought to the ED at any hour of day or night. Establish how the current offending behavior fits into the young patient's typical behavior patterns. Collateral information is essential in such a case. The more convergence there is in information from

Behavioral Emergencies for the Emergency Physician, ed. Leslie S. Zun, Lara G. Chepenik, and Mary Nan S. Mallory. Published by Cambridge University Press. © Cambridge University Press 2013.

Table 29.1. Common presentations of the child or adolescent in the psychiatric ED

- Self-injury or threat of self-injury – suicidal or non-suicidal
- Psychosis
- Out of control – the wild child
- Internalizing disorders – depression, anxiety, OCD
- Substance abuse
- Eating disorders
- Traumatization – by abuse, accident, or medical/surgical interventions

different sources, the more confident you can be in the current assessment. Try to obtain immediate history from the child or teen individually, and observe how reactive the young patient is to the people who brought the child or teen in. Most often, the wild teen will be a male [6].

The raging child may arrive in an uncooperative state of mind, but collateral information can be sought during this stage of the visit. Children's aggression can be characterized as proactive or reactive, with differing trajectories for subsequent behavior [7,8]. The *proactively aggressive* child deliberately engages in aggression for identifiable external goals. Youngsters with conduct disorders typically use proactive aggression on a frequent basis [9].

In contrast, youngsters with *reactive aggression* have difficulties with emotional dysregulation, peer rejection, and peer victimization [10]. Reactively aggressive girls, in particular, are at heightened risk for suicidal behavior, especially if they also are depressed. Reactive aggression can erupt when developmentally disabled youth, who already have increased vulnerability toward becoming overwhelmed, face changing environmental demands. Children and adolescents with bipolar disorder display elevated levels of reactive aggression and verbal aggression [11]. Delaney suggests reducing the youth's reactive aggression in the hospital by addressing the emotional dysregulation from which this aggression stems: (1) provide structure; (2) buffer unexpected changes to reduce frustration; (3) maintain a positive tone to interactions; (4) reduce perceived threat by establishing ground rules which elicit cooperation and encourage choice; (5) set expectations appropriate to the youngster's information-processing capacities [12].

The ED tasks with such children include the following:

1. *Establish current safety for the youngster and those around the youngster.* If the child or teen is agitated or menacing in the ED setting, first use verbal and behavioral interventions to reassure the youngster. For example, establish basic expectations and reduce aversive or excessive environmental stimuli. Orient the youngster to the ED environment and make it clear that you will obtain the youngster's side of the story as part of the evaluation [13].

   a. If the young patient continues to be out of control, some degree of seclusion, physical restraint, or chemical restraint may be necessary. Numerous practice

guidelines as well as institutional guidelines are available to guide (and restrict) the use of seclusion and restraint in children and adolescents [14–16].

   b. As with much of child psychiatric practice, medication use in such circumstances is largely "off-label." See Table 29.2 for a list of commonly used medications for the child and adolescent psychiatric emergency patient [17].

2. *Establish the narrative of what led to the out-of-control behaviors which precipitated a trip to the ED, using multiple sources of information.* What has happened in the past when similar behaviors erupted? What made today's events different from past events which did not lead to an ED visit?

3. *Establish whether important comorbid conditions are present (and if these are, address accordingly):*

   a. Drug or alcohol intoxication
   b. Psychosis
   c. Mood disorder or anxiety disorder
   d. Established pattern of oppositional-defiant behavior or conduct disorder
   e. Significant level of intellectual disability and a recent overwhelming challenge the youngster cannot master
   f. Acute traumatization (e.g., sexual assault)

4. *Determine if there is significant acute risk for this youngster to harm self or others.* This will influence the type of disposition plan which is appropriate (i.e., whether hospitalization is indicated).

5. *If available, consider enlisting a child crisis intervention response team at this point.* Such teams can provide options for emergency temporary placement or rapid intensive outreach to the home. When out-of-control children go home, the family will need assistance with how to manage future behavior problems.

Use of restraints (physical, pharmacologic, or both) with children and adolescents undergoing psychiatric evaluation in the ED is associated with the symptoms of visual hallucinations, out-of-control behavior, and hyperactivity, and with the outcome of hospitalization [18].

Self-injury and suicidality

Interestingly, patients 9–17 years of age at pediatric EDs are least likely to be engaged in current mental health treatment if their current problem is a suicide attempt, compared with young patients who present with behavior problems. Children and teens who present with both existing behavior problems and a suicide attempt fall into an intermediate group, in terms of their likelihood already to be engaged in care [19]. The squeaky wheel of the out-of-control child tends to demand attention more compellingly.

Always ask

Self-injury in the young patient can arise out of a spectrum of intention, ranging from pure accident with no intent to kill

Table 29.2. Suggested medication options in child and adolescent psychiatric emergencies

Medication	Dose range	Target symptoms	Comments	Adverse effects
Aripiprazole (Abilify)	< 25 kg, 1 mg/day 25–50 kg, 2 mg/day 51–70 kg, 5 mg/day >70 kg, 10 mg/day	Severe irritability; psychosis; mania	An injectable form is available	Sedation, akathisia, NMS. Lower risk of metabolic adverse effects than most atypical antipsychotics
Clonazepam (Klonopin)	<30 kg or age 10, 0.01–0.03 mg/kg/day, divided into 2–3 doses. Do not exceed 0.05 mg/kg/day	Panic and severe anxiety; extreme agitation	Can use as adjunct with antipsychotic	Sedation, confusion, ataxia, paradoxical agitation, respiratory depression
Diazepam (Valium)	Oral: 1–2.5 mg 3–4 times a day	Panic and severe anxiety; extreme agitation	An oral liquid is available	Sedation, confusion, ataxia, paradoxical agitation, respiratory depression
Haloperidol (Haldol)	Oral: Initial dose 0.5 mg/day, divided into 2–3 doses Target dose for psychosis: 0.05–0.15 mg/kg/day Target dose for nonpsychotic disorders: 0.05–0.075 mg/kg/day	Extreme agitation, psychosis, mania, irritability	Considered second-line to atypical antipsychotic medications	Extrapyramidal symptoms (dystonia, akathisia), hypotension, NMS, QTc prolongation
Hydroxyzine (Vistaril, Atarax)	Under age 6: 50 mg/day, divided into 4 doses Age 6 and older: 50–100 mg/day, divided into 4 doses	Anxiety, pruritis		Sedation, anticholinergic symptoms
Lorazepam	0.05–0.1 mg/kg/day, divided into 3–4 doses PO, IM, and IV administration routes	Panic and severe anxiety; extreme agitation	Can use as adjunct with antipsychotic	Sedation, confusion, ataxia, paradoxical agitation, respiratory depression
Olanzapine (Zyprexa)	5–20 mg/day, divided into 2 doses	Extreme agitation, psychosis, mania, irritability Approved for schizophrenia and manic/mixed episodes (ages 13 and older)	IM formulation not yet studied in children Separate IM olanzapine dose from benzodiazepine dose by at least 90 minutes	Hypotension, bradycardia, NMS
Quetiapine (Seroquel)	Schizophrenia: Start at 50 mg/day, divided into 2 doses. May increase daily dose by 25–50 mg each day until at 400 mg/day. Bipolar mania: Start at 100 mg/day, divided into 2 doses. May increase daily dose by 100 mg each day until at 400–800 mg/day.	Extreme agitation, psychosis, mania, irritability Approved for schizophrenia (age 13 and older) and manic/mixed episodes (ages 10 and older)	Oral. Lower dose range can be more sedating than mid-dose range	Sedation, NMS
Risperidone (Risperdal)	Oral: 0.5 – 4.0 mg/day, divided into 2 doses	Approved for schizophrenia (ages 13 and older), mania/ mixed episodes (ages 10 and older), and irritability associated with autism (ages 5–16)	Most commonly used atypical antipsychotic in children and adolescents, in U.S.	Dystonia, akathisia, hyperprolactinemia, NMS
Ziprasidone (Geodon)	Oral: Initially, 80 mg/day, divided into 2 doses; on day 2, may increase to 120 mg/day, divided into 2 doses. Give oral doses with food IM: 5 mg IM, may repeat after 90 min	Not approved for patients under 18, but clinical data suggest it appears safe and effective in children and adolescents	For agitation target, IM takes effect within 30 minutes. Lower doses are often more activating than higher doses	Nausea, QTC prolongation, NMS. Lower risk of metabolic adverse effects than most atypical antipsychotics

oneself at one extreme, to clear and planned intent to kill oneself at the other extreme. Ask the child or teen with self-injury whether the injury represents the result of an effort to harm or kill himself or herself. Inquire about the degree of suicidality without the parent or guardian being present, at some point in the evaluation. Ask the young patient if he/she has made a suicide attempt in the past or has contemplated suicide. Positive responses should be explored further. To date, there is no evidence that asking a young person about suicide heightens subsequent risk of a suicide attempt, "putting it into the mind" of the patient. The only way to discover which children or teens are at heightened present risk for suicide is to ask directly. One can start with a lead-in query such as, "Sometimes kids just don't want to be alive anymore. Do you feel that way sometimes?" and move into greater specificity from there. Wintersteen and colleagues suggest a two-question algorithm to identify adolescents with imminent risk for a suicide attempt: (1) In the past week, including today, have you felt like life is not worth living? (2) In the past week, including today, have you wanted to kill yourself? Follow-up screening questions for youngsters endorsing recent suicidal ideation include: (3) Have you ever tried to kill yourself? (4) In the past week, including today, have you made plans to kill yourself [20]?

Much is made of risk factors for suicidality. These aid in knowing when to suspect heightened suicide risk. However, only direct inquiry will tell you if the teen or child you're dealing with in the ED is suicidal.

Establish the behavioral chain

As with the adult patient, one can learn much by inquiring into the concrete events, thoughts, and feelings which immediately preceded the injurious act, such as"And what was happening just before that?" Take the events back in time, stepwise, and then forward from the self-injury's occurrence, until a clear picture emerges of (1) the context for the self-injury, (2) the degree of planning (and intent) involved, and (3) the young patient's expectations for what would happen next. Decide where to place the current suicidal act along the continuum from ambivalent rolling-of-the dice to clearly lethal intent.

Focus on means restriction as part of making a safety plan, and use this as an opportunity to educate the family

Presence of firearms in the home clearly represents a risk for subsequent completion of a suicide attempt and one *must* inquire about the presence of firearms in the homes which the patient will frequent after discharge from the ED [21,22]. The guns used in four fifths of adolescent suicides by firearm were found in the victims' homes, and most of these were owned by their parents [23]. If weapons are present, a plan for their safe removal should be explored. Decreasing access to firearms clearly decreases rates of suicide among adolescents [24,25]. Similarly, review the degree to which family members' medications are secure and address this accordingly. Explore with the patient and adults how to make the suicide method's paraphernalia unavailable. *Means restriction* does not prevent a subsequent attempt, but it affords the patient an opportunity to revisit the question of suicidal intent (whether the suicide act really is what the patient wants to enact): barriers provide thinking time.

The disposition plan for the suicidal child or teen should include mental healthcare referral. Often, this may mean psychiatric hospitalization. If an outpatient treatment disposition

was made, the risk of subsequent suicidal behavior may be reduced by such measures as a follow-up call to verify that the youngster has connected with care [26].

Nonsuicidal self-injury

It has become clear that, by adolescence, several young people engage in non-suicidal self-injuring behavior. This usually represents a maladaptive effort to modulate internal emotional states, rather than being an interpersonal message aimed at coercing desired responses from the people around them. A typical nonsuicidal, self-injuring behavior is superficial self-cutting, initiated to shift from one emotional state to another. There is a self-reinforcing aspect to such behavior which makes it "habit-forming." Specific types of psychotherapy, including specialized cognitive–behavioral therapy (CBT) and dialectical behavioral therapy (DBT) appear to be effective in treating repetitive nonsuicidal self-injury. A challenge for the ED clinician is to avoid indulging in undue frustration toward the young patient who comes in with the results of nonsuicidal self-injury. It is helpful to address the injury and its commission with a matter-of-fact approach, steering the patient toward appropriate treatment.

Management of the nonsuicidal self-injuring patient is complicated by the fact that this group of patients does overlap the group of young patients who harbors suicidal ideation and engages in suicidal action as well; these are not mutually exclusive groups [27].

Substance use

By adolescence, drug and alcohol use is common. In one urban psychiatric emergency service, 28% of the adolescents seen had a substance use disorder [28]. Recurrent substance use often is a comorbid condition with other behaviors of concern, such as conduct problems and risky sexual behavior [29–31]. As such, it can serve as a flag indicating a young patient who may be more likely to have been exposed to traumatic experiences. The substance use may represent an incidental finding in the ED, or the substance use can cause directly a youth's presentation in the ED due to symptoms of intoxication. The substance use also can be a secondary part of the clinical picture when, for example, an intoxicated teen has a motor vehicle accident and the resulting injuries lead to ED presentation.

Boys are more likely to engage in illicit substance use, with the exception of ecstasy (MDMA), which girls more frequently use, particularly the younger adolescent age group [32]. It may be that girls also are more vulnerable to hallucinosis while intoxicated with ecstasy, compared with boys [33].

Some experts note that youths with substance use who have dropped out of school before graduation are particularly prone to risky sexual behavior, so that both the substance use and the risky sexual behavior should be addressed [34].

Some clinicians argue against the clinical utility of routinely using an emergency qualitative urine drug screen in pediatric ED patients who have a psychiatric presentation. The drug screen rarely appears to impact ED management of the patient [35,36].

Refer to the chapter on substance abuse emergencies for a broader discussion of assessment and emergency treatment of the substance-abusing patient.

Psychosis

Schizophrenia and bipolar disorder, two common and severe psychiatric disorders arising in young adulthood, can occur with an earlier onset if there is strong familial genetic loading for the condition. Depression associated with psychotic features appears more likely to represent a bipolar form of depression in adolescence compared to adulthood.

The psychotic child or adolescent may or may not show paranoia. The degree of disorganization in thinking may be subtle, so that the child simply hasn't been able to process information as effectively in school and the child's grades have dropped. The degree of thought disorganization may also be so florid that the child cannot express ideas clearly in the ED. Inquire about the child's baseline level of function and note the degree of current deviation from that baseline. If the child suddenly stops in mid-sentence and appears blank, inquire about the child's thoughts: is this an ictal event, or an instance of thought "blocking" where the mind was blank, or was the child's train of thought "derailed" by the intrusion of bizarre or irrelevant other thoughts?

Hallucinations in the prepubertal child may represent normative experiences (including the familiar "imaginary friend") [37]. Visual hallucinations are often present in youngsters with childhood-onset schizophrenia [38]. Just as with adult ED patients, hallucinations can arise from an array of toxidromes as well as from primary psychiatric disorders. Edelsohn provides a practical discussion of evaluating this symptom in children and adolescents [39].

Always explore the presence of suicidal and homicidal ideation in the psychotic child or teen.

Bipolar disorder

A definitive diagnosis of pediatric bipolar disorder may occur after initial contact in the ED so as to allow for additional examination of the pattern of symptoms over months and across various settings. Most children and adolescents with rapidly shifting moods and high energy turn out to have conditions other than bipolar disorder [40]. Complicating diagnosis further, attention-deficit/hyperactivity disorder (ADHD) can be a comorbid condition with bipolar disorder, and it can be challenging to distinguish symptoms generated by the one from the other. Doerfler and colleagues note that manic children and adolescents without ADHD are more verbally aggressive and argumentative and more prone to reactive aggression (angry responses when frustrated), compared with ADHD children and adolescents without bipolar disorder [11].

Children and teens with bipolar disorder appear to be more responsive to atypical antipsychotic medications than to lithium and other mood stabilizing agents compared with bipolar adults [41,42]. The choice and titration of a mood stabilizer may be deferred until the patient is in an appropriate inpatient psychiatric treatment setting. Therefore, ED management of the acutely psychotic or bipolar manic child or teen should consist of the following tasks:

- Ensure immediate safety of the patient
- Reduce environmental stimulation
- Evaluate for other conditions (substance abuse mimicking psychosis; metabolic abnormalities)
- Initiate an atypical antipsychotic, which can be augmented by a benzodiazepine (see Table 29.2)
- Establish a disposition plan (either hospitalization or discharge home with timely and intensive outpatient support).

Internalizing disorders in the ED

Anxiety disorders

Anxiety-related visits to the ED by children younger than 15 years have increased in recent years [43]. Youngsters with early-onset anxiety and mood disorders suffer significant disability as well as psychological distress [44]. The child with severe separation anxiety may manifest impressive rages when forced to experience the separation (e.g., leaving home for school) which the child is dreading and wishing to avoid. Such children should be directed rapidly into outpatient treatment which includes intensive behavioral or cognitive–behavioral treatment. Similarly, the child or adolescent who is paralyzed functionally by severe obsessive-compulsive disorder should receive appropriately intensive and specific cognitive–behavioral treatment as soon as possible. In both conditions, antidepressants (rather than anxiolytic medications) play an adjunctive role in treatment, but medications alone do not treat the conditions adequately.

Simple phobias are fairly common during childhood, yet rarely do these precipitate emergency room visits. Panic attacks can begin during childhood and youngsters suffering from these may arrive in the ED. Just as with adults, one often can provide some immediate relief with behavioral interventions in the ED visit. This can provide an empowering sense that there are tools the child (and supportive caregivers, as coaches) can use. The youngster with panic disorder should be referred to outpatient treatment which includes a cognitive–behavioral intervention. The role of medication in the ED should be secondary, but in severe cases a modest lorazepam dose can be of help so that the young patient can focus on the behavioral intervention.

Depression

Children with depression may go substantially longer than adult-onset depressed people between onset of major depressive disorder and entry into treatment [45]. Compared with the adult-onset form of major depression, children have longer episodes, higher rates of comorbid psychiatric disorders, and increased suicidality. Case-finding for these young depressed patients must be a priority in the ED, so that appropriate referral into treatment can commence and the protracted morbidity associated with this condition can be reduced. Rutman and colleagues suggest that a two-question screen for depression is feasible in a busy ED to identify youth who should be evaluated more extensively for depression: (1) "During the past month, have you often been bothered by feeling down, depressed, or hopeless?" and (2) "During the past month, have you often been bothered by little interest or pleasure in doing things [46]?"

As mentioned previously, the presence of psychotic symptoms in a depressed child or adolescent is suggestive, although not firmly diagnostic, of the possibility that the depression is secondary to bipolar disorder. Particular care should be taken in exposing such patients to antidepressants without first prescribing an atypical antipsychotic or mood stabilizer.

It rarely is appropriate to initiate antidepressant medication treatment in the ED. Most children and adolescents with depression should receive a trial of appropriately specific and intensive psychotherapy for depression (cognitive–behavioral or interpersonal therapy for depression) if they have no prior history of treatment. Children and adolescents who do go on antidepressant treatment must be monitored frequently (e.g., weekly) in the first month of treatment to monitor for signs of untoward activation or suicidality. Therefore, decisions regarding medication choice usually are deferred to the outpatient prescriber who will monitor the patient.

Trauma

Post-traumatic stress may emerge in children and teens who are exposed to overwhelming experiences: accidental trauma; physical or sexual abuse; repeated or prolonged medical or surgical hospitalizations with difficult procedures to endure. At ED presentation, the young person who just experienced such trauma will not have developed post-traumatic stress disorder (PTSD), but may be manifesting acute stress. The National Child Traumatic Stress Network (at www.nctsn.org/) and the National Center for PTSD have developed a terrific resource which is available online: Psychological First Aid: Field Operations Guide (2nd Edition), at www.ptsd.va.gov/professional/manuals/psych-first-aid.asp. Although the guide is directed toward helping people in the immediate aftermath of disaster or terrorism, many of its principles apply to more individually experienced traumas, as well. The chief intervention for post-traumatic stress disorder is a specialized form of cognitive–behavioral therapy for trauma. Typically, there will be a family component as well as a child-specific component to the treatment.

EDs often must provide the initial screening and evaluation of young people whose trauma will require forensic investigation. The U.S. Department of Justice's Office for Victims of Crime website provides helpful resources (www.ojp.usdoj.gov/ovc/publications/infores/sane/saneguide.pdf) for the sexual assault nurse examiner (SANE) and the sexual assault response team (SART) models which have become prominent over the past forty years. The ChildAbuseMD.com website, at www.childabusemd.com/index.shtml, provides an efficient resource for reviewing the evaluation and management of child and adolescent abuse. One must remember that, along with providing assessment in the ED, reporting the suspected abuse to the state child abuse hotline or to the police is mandatory.

Class and ethnicity issues

Cultural diversity adds complexity and challenge to an already lengthy process of pediatric psychiatric care in the ED. Minority and immigrant individuals are particularly vulnerable to the effects of poverty and acculturation. Some ethnic and racial minority patients are at increased risk for traumatic experiences, including child abuse [47]. Culture also can have a profound effect on the expression of psychiatric illness, so it is vital for clinicians to recognize, understand, and respond to cultural elements when treating pediatric patients [48].

In adults, the patient's race appears to predict a more likely diagnosis of psychosis. Muroff and colleagues found that these patterns apply to children and adolescents with psychiatric problems who are evaluated in the ED as well: African-American and Hispanic-American youngsters were more likely to receive diagnoses of psychotic disorders and behavioral disorders compared with Caucasian youngsters [49]. African-American children and teens also were less likely, compared with Caucasian youth, to receive mood disorder (depression or bipolar) or alcohol/substance abuse diagnoses [49]. Culturally adaptive restricted affect in children of some ethnic groups can be misinterpreted as mood disorder.

There are high rates of PTSD among some refugee populations with past exposure to chronic warfare and civil disruption, such as Somali-American families. Clinicians also need to be aware of specific issues in treating children of Muslim origin. Cultural issues of particular relevance include: gender relations within the patient–doctor relationship; dress code; and, for adolescents, birth control, to name a few. Finally, in many cultures, patients avoid mental health treatment due to cultural stigma of mental illness and fear of institutionalization. Snowden and colleagues found racial and ethnic differences in children and adolescents who receive psychiatric emergency services [50]. Asian-American/Pacific Islander and American Indians/Alaska Native children rarely visited such services and even more rarely revisited. African-American children were more likely to use crisis services compared with other groups. Goldstein and colleagues also noted that some groups, such as African-Americans, also are more likely to use the ED for revisits as part of the continuum of psychiatric care, even if they are engaged in outpatient services [51]. This is particularly likely to occur if the youngster has a disruptive behavior problem.

Ethnomed (ethnomed.org) is an example of a continually updated resource for integrating cultural information into clinical practice. The website addresses cultural beliefs, medical issues, and related topics pertinent to the health care of immigrants. Two videos available through the website address understanding and managing the stigma of mental illness in Asian-Americans and Hispanic-Americans.

Conclusion

Youngsters in the ED with psychiatric difficulties can be managed safely, with attention to reducing ED environmental demands which challenge their capacity for emotional regulation. The assessing clinician *must* obtain collateral information beyond what is available from the young patient directly, a suggestion which could benefit the evaluation of patients of any age. A systematic approach to conceptualizing the youth's presenting problems, considering the seven categories listed in Table 29.1, enables the ED clinician to focus more efficiently on the essential concerns demanding attention during the current ED visit.

References

1. Majahan P, Alpern ER, Grupp-Phelan J, et al. Pediatric Emergency Care Applied Research Network (PECARN). Epidemiology of psychiatric-related visits to emergency departments in a multicenter collaborative research pediatric network. *Pediatr Emerg Care* 2009;**25**:715–20.

2. Santiago LI, Tunik MG, Foltin GL, Mojica MA. Children requiring psychiatric consultation in the pediatric emergency department: epidemiology, resource utilization, and complications. *Pediatr Emerg Care* 2006;**22**:85–9.

3. Newton AS, Ali S, Johnson DW, et al. A 4-year review of pediatric mental health emergencies in Alberta. *CJEM* 2009;**11**:447–54.

4. The Committee on Pediatric Emergency Medicine. Pediatric and adolescent mental health emergencies in the emergency medical services system. *Pediatrics* 2011;**127**:e1356–66.

5. Fortunati FG Jr, Zonana HV. Legal considerations in the child psychiatric emergency department. *Child Adolesc Psychiatr Clin N Am* 2003;**12**:745–61.

6. Kennedy A, Cloutier P, Glennie JE, Gray C. Establishing best practice in pediatric emergency mental health: a prospective study examining clinical characteristics. *Pediatr Emerg Care* 2009;**25**:380–6.

7. Greening L, Stoppelbein L, Luebbe A, Fite PJ. Aggression and the risk for suicidal behaviors among children. *Suicide Life Threat Behav* 2010;**40**:337–45.

8. Fite P, Stoppelbein L, Greening L. Proactive and reactive aggression in a child psychiatric inpatient population. *J Clin Child Adolesc Psychology* 2009;**38**:199–205.

9. Card NA, Little TD. Proactive and reactive aggression in childhood and adolescence: a meta-analysis of differential relations with psychosocial adjustment. *Int J Behav Dev* 2006;**30**:466–80.

10. Dodge KA, Coie JD. Social information-processing factors in reactive and proactive aggression in children's peer groups. *J Pers Soc Psychol* 1987;**53**:1146–58.

11. Doerfler LA, Connor DF, Toscano PF Jr. Aggression, ADHD symptoms, and dysphoria in children and adolescents diagnosed with bipolar disorder and ADHD. *J Affect Disord* 2011;**131**:312–19.

12. Delaney KR. Reducing reactive aggression by lowering coping demands and boosting regulation: five key staff behaviors. *J Child Adolesc Psychiatr Nurs* 2009;**22**:211–19.

13. Hilt RJ, Woodward TA. Agitation treatment for pediatric emergency patients. *J Am Acad Child Adolesc Psychiatry* 2008;**47**:132–8. Erratum in *J Am Acad Child Adolesc Psychiatry* 2008;**47**:478.

14. Hamm MP, Osmond M, Curran J, et al. A systematic review of crisis interventions used in the emergency department: recommendations for pediatric care and research. *Pediatr Emerg Care* 2010;**26**:952–62.

15. Master KJ, Bellonci C, Bernet W. Practice parameter for the prevention and management of aggressive behavior in child and adolescent psychiatric institutions, with special reference to seclusion and restraint. *J Am Acad Child Adolesc Psychiatry* 2002;**41** (Suppl 2):4S–25S.

16. Azeem MW, Aujla A, Rammerth M, Binsfeld G, Jones RB. Effectiveness of six core strategies based on trauma informed care in reducing seclusions and restraints at a child and adolescent psychiatric hospital. *J Child Adolesc Psychiatr Nurs* 2011;**24**:11–15.

17. Adimondo AJ, Poncin YB, Baum CR. Pharmacological management of the agitated pediatric patient. *Pediatr Emerg Care* 2010;**26**:856–60.

18. Dorfman DH, Mehta SD. Restraint use for psychiatric patients in the pediatric emergency department. *Pediatr Emerg Care* 2006;**22**:7–12.

19. Frosch E, McCulloch J, Yoon Y, DosReis S. Pediatric emergency consultations: prior mental health service use in suicide attempters. *J Behav Health Serv Res* 2011;**38**:68–79.

20. Wintersteen MB, Diamond GS, Fein JA. Screening for suicide risk in the pediatric emergency and acute care setting. *Curr Opin Pediatr* 2007;**19**:398–404.

21. Brent DA. Firearms and suicide. *Ann N Y Acad Sci* 2001;**932**:225–40.

22. Brent DA, Perper JA, Goldstein CE, et al. Risk factors for adolescent suicide: a comparison of adolescent suicide victims with suicidal inpatients. *Arch Gen Psychiatry* 1988;**45**:581–8.

23. Johnson RM, Barber C, Azrael D, Clark DE, Hemenway D. Who are the owners of firearms used in adolescent suicides? *Suicide Life Threat Behav* 2010;**40**:609–11.

24. Lubin G, Werberloff N, Halperin D, et al. Decrease in suicide rates after a change of policy reducing access to firearms in adolescents: a naturalistic epidemiological study. *Suicide Life Threat Behav* 2010;**40**:421–4.

25. Grossman DC, Mueller BA, Riedy C, et al. Gun storage practices and risk of youth suicide and unintentional firearm injuries. *JAMA* 2005;**293**:707–14.

26. Newton AS, Hamm MP, Bethell J, et al. Pediatric suicide-related presentations: a systematic review of mental health care in the emergency department. *Ann Emerg Med* 2010;**56**:649–59.

27. Cloutier P, Martin J, Kennedy A, Nixon MK, Muehlenkamp JJ. Characteristics and co-occurrence of adolescent non-suicidal self-injury and suicidal behaviours in pediatric emergency crisis services. *J Youth Adolesc* 2010;**39**:259–69.

28. McDonald MG, Hsiao RC, Russo J, Pasic J, Ries RK. Clinical prevalence and correlates of substance use in adolescent psychiatric emergency patients. *Pediatr Emerg Care* 2011;**27**:384–9.

29. Wu J, Witkiewitz K, McMahon RJ, Dodge KA. A parallel process growth mixture model of conduct problems and substance use with risky sexual behavior. *Drug Alcohol Depend* 2010;**111**:207–14.

30. Moffitt TE, Arseneault L, Jaffee SR, et al. DSM-V conduct disorder: research needs for an evidence base. *J Child Psychol Psychiatry* 2008;**49**:3–33.

31. Armstrong TD, Costello EJ. Community studies on adolescent substance use, abuse, or dependence and psychiatric comorbidity. *J Cons Clin Psychol* 2002;**70**:1224–39.

32. Wu P, Liu X, Pham TH, et al. Ecstasy use among US adolescents from 1999 to 2008. *Drug Alcohol Depend* 2010;**112**:33–8.

33. Wu LT, Ringwalt CL, Weiss RD, Blazer DG. Hallucinogen-related disorders in a national sample of adolescents: the influence of ecstasy/MDMA use. *Drug Alcohol Depend* 2009;**104**:156–65.

34. Latkin C, Sonenstein F, Tandon SD. Psychiatric disorder symptoms, substance use, and sexual risk behavior among African-American out of school youth. *Drug Alcohol Depend* 2011;**115**:67–73.

35. Tenenbein M. Do you really need that emergency drug screen? *Clin Toxicol (Phila)* 2009;**47**:286–91.

36. Fortu JM, Kim IK, Cooper A, et al. Psychiatric patients in the pediatric emergency department undergoing routine urine toxicology screens for medical clearance: results and use. *Pediatr Emerg Care* 2009;**25**:387–92.

37. Askenazy FL, Lestideau K, Meynadier A, et al. Auditory hallucinations in pre-pubertal children: a one-year follow-up, preliminary findings. *Eur Child Adolesc Psychiatry* 2007;**16**:411–15.

38. David CN, Greenstein D, Clasen L, et al. Childhood onset schizophrenia: high rate of visual hallucinations. *J Am Acad Child Adolesc Psychiatry* 2011;**50**:681–6.

39. Edelsohn GA. Hallucinations in children and adolescents: considerations in the emergency setting. *Am J Psychiatry* 2006;**163**:781–5.

40. Findling RL, Youngstrom EA, Fristad MA, et al. Characteristics of children with elevated symptoms of mania: the Longitudinal Assessment of Manic Symptoms (LAMS) study. *J Clin Psychiatr* 2010;**71**:1664–72.

41. Pfeifer JC, Kowatch RA, DelBello MP. Pharmacotherapy of bipolar disorder in children: recent progress. *CNS Drugs* 2010;**24**:575–93.

42. Scheffer RE, Tripathi A, Kirkpatrick FG, Schultz T. Guidelines for treatment-resistant mania in children with bipolar disorder. *J Psychiatr Pract* 2011;**17**:186–93.

43. Smith RP, Larkin GL, Southwick SM. Trends in U.S. emergency department visits for anxiety-related mental health conditions, 1992–2001. *J Clin Psychiatry* 2008;**69**:286–94.

44. Naismith SL, Scott EM, Purcell S, Hickie IB. Disability is already pronounced in young people with early stages of affective disorders: data from an early intervention service. *J Affect Disord* 2011;**131**:84–91.

45. Korczak DJ, Goldstein BI. Childhood onset major depressive disorder: course of illness and psychiatric comorbidity in a community sample. *J Pediatr* 2009;**155**:118–23.

46. Rutman MS, Shenassa E, Becker BM. Brief screening for adolescent depressive symptoms in the emergency department. *Acad Emerg Med* 2008;**15**:17–22.

47. Harris TB, Carlisle LL, Sargent J, Primm AB. Trauma and diverse child populations. *Child Adolesc Psychiatr Clin N Am* 2010;**19**:869–87.

48. Pumariega AJ, Rothe E. Cultural considerations in child and adolescent psychiatric emergencies and crisis. *Child Adolesc Psychiatr Clin N Am* 2003;**12**:723–44.

49. Muroff J, Edelsohn GA, Joe S, Ford BC. The role of race in diagnostic decision making in a pediatric psychiatric emergency service. *Gen Hosp Psychiatry* 2008;**30**:269–76.

50. Snowden LR, Masland MC, Libby AM, Wallace N, Fawley K. Racial/ethnic minority children's use of psychiatric emergency care in California's public mental health system. *Am J Public Health* 2008;**98**:118–24.

51. Goldstein AB, Frosch E, Davarya S, Leaf PJ. Factors associated with a six-month return to emergency services among child and adolescent psychiatric patients. *Psychiatr Serv* 2007;**58**:1489–92.

Chapter 30

Geriatric psychiatric emergencies

Michael A. Ward and James Ahn

Introduction

2011 marks the induction of the baby boomer generation into the geriatric population; this population is anticipated to rapidly expand the number of individuals with psychiatric conditions over the age of 65. The psychiatric workforce is poorly positioned to manage this burgeoning demand for mental health services. Currently, the number of appropriately trained professionals are decreasing in number with an estimated 0.9 geriatric psychiatrists for every 10,000 Americans over the age of seventy-five [1]. As has been the trend with other deficiencies in medical care, emergency physicians (EPs) will have the opportunity to bridge the gap in mental health care for our increasingly senescent population.

Geriatric patients represent a disproportionately small number of emergency psychiatric visits. However, these patients present a larger portion of admissions compared to their younger counterparts, highlighting the relative complexity of these patients [2]. Mental status in elderly patients can be acutely affected by several factors, including organic illness, polypharmacy, cognitive disorders, psychosis, substance abuse, and elder abuse. The complex nature of elderly patients makes it often difficult to discern organic versus psychiatric etiologies of mental status changes. Furthermore, EPs may consider signs of depression as a normal response in elderly patients who may have experienced a recent medical illness, death of a loved one, retirement, increasing dependency needs, or removal from their home, instead of recognizing the presentation as abnormal and an opportunity for important interventions.

Behavioral emergencies in the elderly carry significant morbidity and mortality. Psychiatric emergencies in this age group, as compared to younger patients, are rarely isolated to a specific psychiatric condition. Rather, when considering evaluation, treatment, and disposition, EPs need to navigate through a sophisticated interplay of psychiatric, medical, and social factors. This chapter will cover key emergent geriatric psychiatric conditions including depression, suicide, psychosis, substance abuse, and elder abuse and will provide guidelines for diagnosis, assessment, and management for these conditions.

Depression

Geriatric individuals suffering from depression are at increased risk for significant morbidity and mortality. Studies demonstrate that the depressed elderly present to emergency departments (EDs) more frequently and have longer lengths of stay once hospitalized [3,4]. Depression is associated with marked disability, hastened functional decline, increased risk of hospitalization, diminished quality of life, and an increase in non-suicidal mortality [5–7]. Furthermore, the elderly have the highest rate of suicide compared to any other segment of the population with depression being the most common psychiatric comorbidity [8]. One in four geriatric patients presenting to the ED are positively screened for major depression [9,10]. When coupling this finding with the high risk for death and disability associated with a depression diagnosis, it is imperative that EPs remain vigilant for the signs and symptoms of depression and be prepared to effectively evaluate and manage this disease [11].

Psychiatric and medical conditions in the geriatric patient demonstrate significant overlap in clinical features: fatigue, insomnia, lack of appetite, and somatic complaints, including change in mental status. Additionally, older, depressed patients present with more somatic and cognitive symptoms than affective symptoms [11]. As a result, EPs miss depression in the elderly and, subsequently, fail to manage the majority of patients with this condition [9,10,12]. Multiple studies show that despite EPs knowledge of a patient's active signs and symptoms of depression, EPs are reticent to provide referrals or other interventions specific to depression [9,10,12]. Hustey and Smith list several factors which may contribute to the poor referral rate by EPs: (1) EPs fail to understand the magnitude for which depression affects healthcare outcomes, (2) the rapid pace of the ED only allows for EPs to focus on the chief complaint, and (3) EPs may assume that the patient's primary provider is already managing these complaints [10].

Several risk factors for development of depression are identified in the elderly. Disability, poor social support, new medical illness, poor health status, sleep disturbance, prior depression, bereavement, and cognitive impairment are all risk factors for late life depression and may aid in recognition and treatment of

Behavioral Emergencies for the Emergency Physician, ed. Leslie S. Zun, Lara G. Chepenik, and Mary Nan S. Mallory. Published by Cambridge University Press. © Cambridge University Press 2013.

this disease [13]. Interestingly, functional disability and medical illness possess a bidirectional relationship with depression. Both disability and medical illness place a patient at risk for depression. Furthermore, a depressed patient is at increased risk for developing medical illness and disability. Specifically, depression is strongly linked with coronary artery disease, cerebrovascular disease, dementia, and in residents of nursing homes [14].

The Diagnostic Manual of Mental Disorders, 4th Edition, Text Revision (DSM-IV-TR) provides a list of criteria to make a clinical diagnosis of major depression irrespective of age. A patient must possess at least five of the listed symptoms for two or more weeks, with at least one of the symptoms being 1) depressed mood or 2) loss of interest or pleasure: depressed mood, diminished interest or pleasure, decreased appetite or weight loss, sleep disturbances, psychomotor agitation or retardation, fatigue, feelings of guilt or worthlessness, impaired

Table 30.1. Emergency department depression screening instrument (ED-DSI)[a] [16]

1. Do you often feel sad or depressed?	Yes	No
2. Do you often feel helpless?	Yes	No
3. Do you often feel downhearted or blue?	Yes	No

[a] A "Yes" response to any of the three questions is considered a positive screen. Table 30.2 should be referenced for all negative screens. Substance abuse, elder abuse, medication side effects, living situation, functional status, and other psychosocial factors can contribute to symptoms and disposition and should be assessed. This scale should be limited to elderly patients without acute medical illness, dementia, or acute changes in mental status.

concentration, or suicidal ideation [15]. An emergency department-depression screening instrument (ED-DSI) has been developed as a quick tool to identify elderly patients with depression in the ED setting (Table 30.1) [16]. The ED-DSI has significant limitations as the tool has 79% sensitivity and excludes patients who were too ill to participate, were afflicted with dementia, or possessed acute changes in mental status. Because of these limitations, the ED-DSI may not be applicable in a significant portion of geriatric patients presenting to the emergency department.

The DSM-IV and ED-DSI do capture some aspects of a geriatric mood disorder, but do not identify distinctive clinical features of the condition. Many depression scales specific to the elderly exist, including the geriatric depression scale (GDS) and the Center for Epidemiological Studies Depression (CES-D). However, these scales can require up to 15 minutes to perform, making them impractical for use in a busy ED [17]. As previously mentioned, depressed geriatric patients express fewer affective symptoms, which has led to the concept of "depression without sadness"[11]. Therefore, EPs should inquire whether their elderly patients suffer from apathy, loss of interest, fatigue, and insomnia to fully screen for depressive symptoms. Importantly, signs and symptoms of depression in the elderly may not fall under the formal diagnosis of major depressive disorder and other special considerations should exist, including subsyndromal depression (minor depression), medical illness, and cognitive disorders (Table 30.2).

Minor depression occurs in patients with clinically significant depressive symptoms but who do not meet full criteria for major depression. This disease is not described in the DSM-IV,

Table 30.2. Special considerations in assessing geriatric patients for depression: minor depression; medical illness; dementia[a]

	Comparison to major depression[b]	Special considerations
Minor depression	– Increased somatic complaints: fatigue; sleep issues; vague pain; psychomotor retardation; weight loss – Irritability, social withdrawal, apathy, and diminished self-care are increased.	– Often without affective symptoms: "depression without sadness" – Similar incidence of morbidity and many progress to major depression – Should be treated similarly to major depression – Poorly recognized by EPs
Medical illness	– Depressive signs and symptoms are worsened by medical illness and medical illness is worsened by depression – Similar to minor depression: increased somatic complaints, etc. – Symptoms common to medical illness are very similar to that of depression	– Given misattribution of depressive symptoms as medically related, an inclusive approach is recommended: medical symptoms overlapping with depressive symptoms should at least partially be considered to be secondary to depression – Vitamin B_{12}, folate, thyroid dysfunction, corticosteroid use and interferon use are known to be associated with depression
Dementia	– PDC-dAD more sensitive and specific for depression in demented patients: fewer criteria and for less period of time; given poor ability to communicate, substitutes decreased positive affect for loss of pleasure and tearfulness for depressed mood; includes social isolation and irritability as novel criteria [21] – Motivational symptoms (social isolation) and delusions more prevalent than core symptoms	– EPs should consider decreased positive affect, tearfulness, social isolation, and delusions as hallmark signs and symptoms of depression in the demented patient – Up to 50% of patients with cognitive disorders will develop depression – Care takers of demented patients have an increased risk of depression

[a] The table compares and isolates differences between the diagnosis of major depression by DSM-IV and various scenarios typical of geriatric patients. The table also includes special considerations for each scenario: minor depression; medical illness; dementia.
[b] Differences are compared to DSM-IV criteria for major depression [15].
EPs, emergency physicians; PDC-dAD, Provisional Diagnostic Criteria for Depression in Alzheimer's Disease; DSM-IV-TR, *The Diagnostic Manual of Mental Disorders-IV-TR*.

but exists as the most common form of depressive disorder in the elderly [18]. Minor depression is associated with significant morbidity and disability, as approximately 25% of cases progress to major depression within two years [19]. Studies show that minor depression contributes negatively to patient well-being and disability as much as major depression [19,20]. Given the frequency and morbidity attributed to minor depression, this disease should be treated similarly to major depression.

There are several medical disorders (thyroid dysfunction and vitamin B12 and folate deficiency) and medications (corticosteroids and interferon) with well-established causal and reversible links to depression. However, EPs may misattribute signs and symptoms of depression to medical etiologies and miss the diagnosis of depression. Alexopoulos et al. describe four approaches that help a physician account for symptoms caused by both medical illness and depression: (1) exclusive approach, excludes symptoms as part of a depression syndrome that are thought to be commonly part of a medical syndrome; (2) substitutive approach, ignores symptoms such as changes in sleep, energy, appetite, and weight, that may be typical of a medical syndrome and substitutes other cognitive symptoms (i.e., hopelessness); (3) best estimate approach, requires the physician to make a clinical judgment as to whether the symptom is more likely secondary to depression or a medical syndrome; (4) inclusive approach, assumes that all depressive symptoms contribute to the depression syndrome regardless of the underlying medical illness [11]. Given the poor rate of recognition and intervention by EPs, the inclusive approach to assess for depression should be used [11]. This approach should improve the detection rate of depression in the elderly.

Up to 50% of patients with a cognitive disorder (dementia) may develop depression, which also places their caretakers at increased risk for depression, regardless of the caretaker's age [17]. Depression in individuals with cognitive disorders like Alzheimer's disease (AD) presents more typically with motivational symptoms and delusions, and less commonly with core symptoms of depression such as sadness, sleep disturbances, and appetite loss. The Provisional Diagnostic Criteria for Depression in Alzheimer's Disease (PDC-dAD) is similar to the DSM-IV criteria for major depression but provides a less restrictive set of criteria and is more specific to the presenting symptoms of a demented patient afflicted with depression. These criteria require three or more matching criteria for a diagnosis of Depression of AD versus the five required for the DSM-IV for Major Depressive disorder. The PDC-dAD substitutes affective symptoms for verbally expressive symptoms: decreased positive affect substitutes for loss of pleasure and tearfulness substitutes for depressed mood. Social isolation and irritability are included as novel criteria [21]. The PDC-dAD is validated through numerous studies as a more sensitive and specific criteria for detection of depression in AD and, thus, should be strongly considered for use by EPs [22,23].

The function of an EP is not to make a definitive diagnosis and treatment plan for geriatric depression. Rather the EP needs to identify patients who may meet criteria, initiate a reasonable work up while considering interplay with acute medical illness, and create a disposition that will ultimately allow the patient to obtain appropriate treatment. EPs often are inundated in a chaotic environment and a complete assessment for depression is often neither realistic nor prudent for the well-being of the emergency department as a whole. A reasonable approach is to apply the ED-DSI (Table 30.1) for the relatively healthy, nondemented geriatric patients and to strongly consider other factors related to depression in the healthy/nondemented, medically ill, or demented geriatric patients summarized in Table 30.2. Substance abuse, elder abuse, medication side effects, living situation, functional status, and other psychosocial factors can largely contribute to symptoms while affecting the disposition, and should be included in the history. These factors will be covered in increased depth in subsequent sections.

Untreated depression in the elderly is costly to society (increased ED visits, hospital admissions, and length of stay), to families (increased suicidal and nonsuicidal mortality), and most importantly to the patient (functional decline and decreased quality of life) [3–8]. Numerous cost–benefit analyses show the effectiveness of treatment based on a multifaceted and synergistic approach [24,25]. The role of the EP is not to provide counseling or medical therapy but to effectively detect depression in the elderly, ensure a safe disposition, and then refer the patient to effective treatment methodologies.

As previously discussed, the assessment of depression in the ED for elderly patients includes a strong consideration for medical illness as an etiology for the patient's signs and symptoms. No definitive guidelines exist for the evaluation of the depressed elderly patient. A thorough history and physical will dictate the need for further diagnostic tests. Commonly, patients admitted to inpatient psychiatric units require "medical clearance," needing, at a minimum, a specific panel of laboratory tests. The minimum requirement for medical clearance is state and institution specific and should be determined before admission or transfer. Furthermore, medical clearance is meant to differentiate organic etiology from functional disorders to determine whether serious underlying medical illness would render admission to a psychiatric facility unsafe, and to identify medical conditions that may need treatment while in a psychiatric facility [26]. Additionally, while mental status is invaluable in differentiating medical versus psychiatric disease, studies demonstrate that few EPs perform an appropriate mental status examination [26]. For example, it would be important to ensure that an elderly patient with altered mental status (AMS) secondary to encephalitis from either infectious or profound metabolic derangement was not sent to a psychiatric facility with limited medical capabilities. The Brief Mental Status Examination has been validated as an effective tool for mental status assessment and may allow for a rapid evaluation by the EP. Patients will undoubtedly have ongoing comorbid medical issues, but the EP should be cognizant of the psychiatric facility's capabilities and exclude admission for

Table 30.3. Indications for inpatient admission for depression in elderly patients [27][a]

1. Attempted suicide or expressed suicidal ideations with intent

2. Compliance issues leading to insufficient management and decompensation of depression

3. Depression with new-onset psychotic features

4. Self-neglect to the degree that patient is inadequately cared for

5. Need for removal from hostile environment

6. Medical illness that would complicate the outpatient treatment of depression

7. Distress or agitation that requires skilled nursing

[a] This table lists specific indications for inpatient admission for elderly patients with depression. This table was developed based on recommendations listed by Macdonald but includes several modifications.

patients with medical conditions beyond what may be safely managed [26].

A proper disposition is paramount for the depressed elderly patient and may be the most important intervention or treatment offered by the EP. As previously mentioned, EPs are suboptimal at recognizing depression in the elderly and even when recognized are poor at initiating referrals [9,10,12]. The pathway for management is essentially 2-fold: inpatient or outpatient. A set of developed criteria is generally accepted for either inpatient hospitalization or psychiatric admission of the depressed elderly (Table 30.3): (1) the patient attempted suicide or has expressed suicidal ideations with suicidal intent; (2) poor treatment compliance leading to insufficient management and decompensation of depression; (3) the presence of depression with new-onset psychotic features; (4) self-neglect to the degree that the patient is unable to adequately be cared for either by themselves or their caregiver/s; (5) removal of the patient from a hostile social environment; (6) presence of medical illness that would complicate the outpatient treatment of their depression; (7) the patient demonstrates distress or agitation which requires skilled nursing [27]. All other patients should be referred to their primary doctor, psychiatric professionals, or partial hospitalization programs. A direct conversation stating the intended referral to the eventual medical provider is optimal.

Suicide

Compared to other age groups, elderly patients are at the greatest risk for completed suicide [8]. Specifically, white males over the age of 85 have the highest risk of suicide. Suicide attempts are more lethal in this age group with an estimated ratio of 4:1 attempts to completed suicide versus a ratio of 8–40:1 in the general population. The high lethality of suicide attempts are hypothesized to be secondary to the combination of the following factors: self-inflicted injuries are more lethal due to the frailty of the elderly patient, timely rescue is less likely because of the increased number of elderly patients living alone, and

finally, the more lethal means by which the elderly attempt suicide. Making matters increasingly difficult, elderly patients are more reluctant to talk about their emotional problems and less likely to report suicidal ideations [28].

EPs are likely to see a significant number of elderly patient visits shortly before their eventual suicide. Many geriatric patients live on a fixed income and Medicare recipients are required to pay 50% of their medical health services bill compared to the 20% copay for physical health conditions. Because of this significant financial barrier, older patients tend to rely on primary care providers during times of great psychiatric need [28]. Retrospective studies indicate that 43% to 70% of elderly suicide victims visit primary physicians within 1 month of death. This represents a critical observation: prevention may be possible in the time immediately preceding the development of the suicidal state [29]. In conclusion, psychiatric illness in the elderly represents a very high risk of suicide and portends the need for early recognition coupled with aggressive and timely intervention.

Risk factors for suicide are unfortunately common among the elderly, with advanced age as one the strongest predictors – a rather inherent trait in the geriatric population. Additionally, psychiatric illnesses play a substantial role in suicide. Between 71% and 95% of elderly suicide victims had a diagnosable Axis I condition – major depression being the most common disorder. Substance abuse, although less frequent, is an independent risk factor for elderly suicide and is a potent risk factor when coupled with depression [28]. Conwell et al. determined that older suicide victims suffer from a single episode of major depression before death, notably, the type of depression often responsive to standard therapies [30]. Psychotic illness, while a significant risk factor for elderly suicide, plays a much smaller role [28].

Medical illness is an independent risk factor for elderly suicide, but, surprisingly, when compared to psychiatric illness, the additive risk is small. Predictably, an increased severity of medical illness, disability associated with the illness, and medical comorbidities contribute additive risk for suicide. Studies demonstrate an association between increased risk of suicide and HIV/AIDS, Huntington's disease, multiple sclerosis, renal disease, spinal cord injury, and malignant neoplasms [28]. Untreated or undertreated pain, anticipatory anxiety regarding progression of an illness, fear of dependence, and fear of burden on families are the major contributing factors for suicide in elderly patients with medical illness [14]. However, psychiatric illnesses often precede suicide in the elderly patient with medical illness and tend to occur as a first time, single episode of major depression. Therefore, EPs should maintain a high index of suspicion assessing for new-onset psychiatric illness in the elderly patient with medical illness.

Elderly patients endure life event stressors that can increase their risk for suicide. Bereavement, retirement, financial stressors, and family discord are all associated with increased risk of suicide in the elderly population. Living alone is an additional risk factor for suicide but having a greater number of friends and family to confide with is a protective factor for suicide in the elderly [28]. Duberstein et al. analyzed the risk of suicide shortly after the death of a spouse and determined that the suicide victim often developed psychiatric illnesses. These same victims are more apt to visit a physician before death, again, emphasizing a high priority for recognition and an opportunity for intervention [31].

The assessment for suicide in the elderly requires the EP to perform a comprehensive history and examination, assess for risk factors, and to constantly maintain a high index of suspicion. As previously mentioned, elderly patients are reluctant to initiate a discussion about suicidal ideations and possess atypical signs and symptoms of psychiatric illness that are proven to be subtle to EPs. Fortunately, Waern et al. demonstrated that elderly patients will often admit their suicidal thoughts when the topic is broached by physicians [32]. The EP should ask questions pertaining particularly to signs and symptoms of depression and other psychiatric illness, previous suicide attempts, substance abuse, social situation, recent stressful life events, and medical illness and how this has impacted their quality of life and functionality. Specifically, the patient needs to be asked about death wishes, thoughts of suicide, intent to harm self, and access to weapons or medications that could be of potential harm [14].

Outside of extremely rare exceptions, elderly patients admitting to suicidal ideation with intent require inpatient evaluation and treatment (Table 30.3). Before death, suicide victims often share their ideations with a significant other despite occasionally denying this fact to their physician [32]. Therefore, an attempt should be made to contact caretakers for patients in which suicidal ideation is suspected. During the evaluation of the suicidal patient, the EP should consider and examine for intentional overdoses, toxic ingestions, or self-inflicted wounds as potential avenues for suicide attempts. After close inspection of the patient's medication list, EPs should judiciously order drug levels in suspected toxicities.

In the rare exception an elderly patient with suicidal ideation is discharged, the EP should attend to a few key items. First, this decision for discharge should always be made in conjunction with the patient's primary mental health provider with follow-up planned within several days. No-suicide contracts have been used to contract for safety; however, upward of 41% of clinicians who have used no-suicide contracts have had patients die by means of suicide or made very serious attempts while under contract [33]. Because of the high variability of success, no-suicide contracts are not recommended. A double-blind study revealed that psychiatrists recommended discharge for approximately 19% of patients who EPs felt required admission and declared 11% of patients non-suicidal that EPs assessed as suicidal [34]. EPs must actively participate in the discussion regarding disposition with the other mental health professionals and advocate for admission in appropriate situations. Second, older adults tend to act on suicidal thoughts with greater lethality; therefore, the EP must assess the ability to access weapons. One study comparing suicide victims to controls showed no difference in the proportion of men who possessed a firearm, but did note a significant proportion of the suicide victims obtained their firearm within a week before their death [28]. Lastly, the elderly patient must have adequate monitoring upon being discharged home, e.g., a patient living alone and with poor social support may not be safe for discharge to home. All of these factors need to be closely considered before discharge and the EP should be actively involved with a mental health professional in this decision.

Psychosis

Psychosis is defined as the disorganization of an individual's mental capacity characterized by defective contact with reality as evidenced by delusions, hallucinations, or disorganized speech and behavior. This general definition encompasses many specific conditions common to the geriatric population and includes diseases primary to psychiatric conditions. However, psychosis is more often secondary to medical illness, cognitive disorders, iatrogenic causes, and substance abuse. Approximately 23% of the elderly will experience psychotic symptoms that may be associated with aggressive or disruptive behavior [35]. Psychosis can prompt neglect or abuse by the patient's caregiver and is a risk factor for institutionalization. These disorders are reported in less than 5% of elderly patients, but are present in 10–63% of nursing home dwellers [36]. Similar to mood disorders, psychotic disorders in the elderly are often multifactorial and can present a significant diagnostic challenge. In an effort to simplify the assessment and management for this condition, we will describe three main categories for psychosis in the elderly: psychosis with dementia, psychosis without dementia, and psychosis secondary to age-related medical and social factors.

Dementia is the most common cause of psychosis in the elderly. Approximately 50% of AD patients experience delusions or hallucinations within the first 3 years of clinical onset and greater than 50% of demented patients develop paranoia or hallucinations throughout their lifetime [14,35]. Psychosis can be pathognomonic in some forms of dementia, e.g., Lewy body dementia, but can be present in all forms of dementia. AD with psychosis is a common subtype of AD that is associated with a more rapid cognitive decline and is often complicated by patients who become aggressive, difficult to manage, and a danger to themselves and others. Elderly patients with vascular dementia are also at high risk for developing psychotic symptoms and behavioral disturbances.

Primary psychiatric disorders make up a significant but less common cause of psychosis in the elderly. Schizophrenia typically develops in early adulthood but occasionally occurs as a late-onset variant with patients possessing mostly positive symptoms (delusions, hallucinations, and disorganized speech). The symptoms of brief psychotic episodes and schizophreniform disorder are similar to schizophrenia but often the onset is more acute and occurs with shorter disease time courses. Depression with psychotic features is most common in depressed patients whose first depressive episode occurs later in life. These patients often demonstrate somatic delusions such as the belief they have incurable or mistreated diseases. Depression with psychotic features incurs a higher risk of suicide compared to major depression without psychotic features [35].

Psychosis may commonly develop in the elderly secondary to medical illness, substance use, medication side effects, or exposure to a stressful situation. As individuals age, the brain, similar to the rest of the body, slowly deteriorates and atrophies causing individuals to possess less "cognitive reserve." Cognitive reserve, also known as brain reserve, refers to the ability of the brain to function appropriately while compensating for neuropathic insults. Decreased cognitive reserve inherent with the aging process provides a theoretical framework to explain the increased onset or exacerbation of dementia, risk for the development of schizophrenia and depression, and susceptibility for delirium in the setting of medical illness in elderly individuals [37]. Even with mild stressors, such as a urinary tract infection or medication change, the maladaptive brain may allow for confusion or development of psychotic features. Delirium is defined as an acute decline in cognition and attention and may be caused by medical illness, medication use, substance use or withdrawal, social stressors, or environmental change. This condition develops over the course of hours to days and is associated with altered consciousness, disturbances in sleep–wake cycle, confusion, disorientation, and psychotic symptoms [35]. Delirium is common among the elderly – approximately 56% of the elderly develop delirium during their hospital admission. This condition is associated with significant risk, including functional decline, nursing home placement, and death, with a 33% in-hospital mortality rate [37,38]. Furthermore, psychotic symptoms may also be present in substance intoxication and withdrawal [15]. Additionally, various medications commonly used by the elderly can cause psychosis, including corticosteroids, anti-inflammatories, angiotensin converting enzyme inhibitors, aspirin, opioids, dopamine agonists, anticholinergics, antihistamines, and antidepressants [38]. Lastly, psychosocial stress, which unfortunately is common among the elderly (in the form of functional decline, bereavement, etc.), increases the risk for the development of psychotic symptoms [39]. Taken together, the elderly possess inherent traits and risk factors that predispose them to the development of psychotic symptoms. A careful history and physical examination is paramount in determining the possible underlying cause/s.

The EP's role includes the stabilization of the patient's behavior, delineation of the etiology of the psychosis, initiation of treatment when appropriate, the arrangement of appropriate disposition [14]. To optimize care for the patient, the EP must unearth the etiology of the psychosis and initiate the correct therapy and disposition. Delirium is often confused with primary psychiatric disease and/or dementia secondary to the similarities that exists between all three processes. However, there are very distinct features that will assist in differentiating one from another highlighted in Table 30.4. Delirium, unlike psychiatric disease, causes disorientation or alterations in

Table 30.4. Presenting characteristics in the psychotic elderly patient to help differentiate underlying illness such as delirium, dementia, and/or primary psychiatric illness[a] [35]

Characteristics	Delirium	Dementia	Psychiatric illness
General traits	Acute onset of confusion with signs and symptoms of medical illness	History of dementia; commonly short-term memory deficit but also may include CVA and PD traits	Psychiatric history; commonly on psychotropic medications
Onset	Sudden	Insidious	Variable
Alertness	Fluctuating	Normal except in late or severe disease	Normal
Duration	Hours to weeks	Typically lifetime deficits	Variable depending on response to treatment
Orientation	Disoriented	Increasingly disoriented with worsening disease	Normal
Hallucinations	At onset	Usually only with late or severe disease or comorbid illness	Dependent on psychiatric illness and compliance with medications
"Sundowning"	Present	Present	Absent
Course	Usually reversible	Irreversible	Usually partially to fully reversible
Special considerations	Initiate workup and treatment; strongly consider encephalitis	Consider medical illness as precipitant for acute decompensation	Critical to assess for suicidal ideation; consider medical illness as exacerbating factor

[a] This table summarizes the characteristics of delirium, dementia, and primary psychiatric illness in the psychotic, elderly patient. This table is adapted and modified in reference to the original table by Khouzam and Emes [35]. It should be noted that the patient may carry traits and underlying illness from one or more of the categories covered above. All patients should be appropriately screened for medical illness. It is important to consider substance abuse, elder abuse, medication changes, and psychosocial conditions as comorbid factors.
CVA, cerebrovascular accident; PD, Parkinson's disease.

consciousness. Dementia may prove more difficult to discern, as most demented patients with psychotic features have severe cognitive illness. Many of the temporal traits that differentiate dementia from delirium may be difficult to distinguish in this particular situation. However, typically with information obtained through the patient's medical history an EP may differentiate dementia from delirium. Dementia, by itself, has an insidious onset and an alert patient versus delirium which has an acute onset and demonstrates a fluctuating level of alertness [35]. Elderly patients are more susceptible to multiple comorbidities, therefore, this patient population may exhibit traits from more than one category. This is especially relevant with elderly patients possessing psychiatric illness presenting with acute decompensation. Therefore, the EP should consider delirium, dementia, and psychiatric illness in the evaluation and management of their patient and should inquire regarding substance abuse, elder abuse, medication changes, and psychosocial conditions.

The assessment of psychosis in the ED for elderly patients should include a medical clearance with special attention to a neurologic evaluation, including consideration of head trauma, malignancy, infection, and seizures [35]. EPs should have a very low threshold for neuroimaging in elderly patients with acute psychosis, particularly patients without a history of pre-existing psychotic features. A routine screen for new-onset psychosis may include a complete blood count, comprehensive metabolic panel, vitamin B12 and folate levels, thyroid function tests, urinalysis, electrocardiogram, and neuroimaging studies [14,38]. For the patients in which infection is probable and a primary source cannot be discerned, a lumbar puncture and testing for HIV should be strongly considered. The elderly are susceptible to central nervous system infections and have a high risk of death if not appropriately managed [40]. Furthermore, EPs should consider checking medication levels when appropriate (e.g., lithium, digoxin, and antiepileptics); medication changes, polypharmacy, confusion with dosing of medications, and renal insufficiency may cause erratic changes in drug levels [38]. Lastly, elderly individuals are more sensitive to the psychotropic effects of drugs of abuse and therefore, a drug screen, including an ethanol level, may help differentiate a toxicologic cause for psychosis [35,38].

The disposition of the psychotic elderly patient will likely depend on the etiology of their condition. With rare exceptions, the high mortality risk associated with delirium should warrant a medical admission. The threshold for admission should be particularly low for those patients without a previous history of altered mental status or cognitive disorder. For the elderly with dementia or primary psychiatric illness, EPs should review the criteria listed in Table 30.3, as well as assess the patient for homicidal ideation when considering admission to a psychiatric facility [27]. As previously mentioned, medical clearance and stabilization is mandatory by law before psychiatric admission or transfer [41]. Similar to mood disorders, psychosis in the elderly carries very

significant morbidity and mortality regardless of etiology and, therefore, EPs should proceed with caution with disposition of patients.

Agitation

Agitation is a common manifestation of psychosis in the elderly and commonly includes hyperactivity, assaultiveness, verbal abuse, threatening gestures, physical destructiveness, vocal outbursts, and excessive verbalizations of distress [14]. Zun (2005) highlights three main reasons to initiate treatment of the elderly patient suffering from psychiatric illness: (1) improve patient cooperation; (2) reduce patient agitation in an effort to reduce the risk of injury to the patient and to the staff; (3) begin the therapeutic process [42]. The management of agitation, especially in severe cases, will be essential to move forward with any disposition in the elderly psychiatric patient. Before the transfer of psychiatric patients, EMTALA mandates stabilization. Stabilization means that no deterioration of the condition is likely to result from or occur during transfer, within a reasonable medical probability [41]. Severe agitation and combativeness may put both the patient and transporters at increased risk for harm. Multiple strategies and treatments exist for the management of agitation and may need to occur in combination. However, certain pitfalls need to be considered: (1) treating the agitated behavior without adequate consideration of the underlying cause; (2) as needed or PRN dosing in the ED, which may lead to either underdosing or overdosing; (3) aggressive sedation leading to complications such as falls, respiratory depression, pneumonia, dehydration, or death [43]. Agitation in the elderly is best treated first with simple and noninvasive techniques.

Noninvasive strategies may greatly improve agitation of an elderly patient and may reduce the need, and subsequent risks, of chemical or physical restraints. First, EPs should consider potentially reversible medical factors such as dehydration, pain, hypoxia, hypercarbia, or electrolyte derangements [43]. Second, environmental modifications may significantly improve the safety of the patient and others, including: (1) involvement of family members in the management of the patient will provide a familiar face and may reduce the patient's fears and agitation; (2) movement of the patient to a location of best observation; (3) prevent the patient access to means that may harm them or others, such as open windows, balconies, stairwells, hand hoists over beds, cords, and coat hangers; (4) use fall prevention strategies; (5) place devices and catheters in areas that are either inaccessible to the patient or not readily noticeable; (6) consider a one-to-one sitter [43]. Lastly, EPs should attempt to communicate with the elderly patient in a calming voice and redirect them away from agitating topics or factors.

Chemical restraint is a common approach in the management of the agitated patient. Scant ED specific evidence supports the use of chemical restraint, but recommendations include the use high-potency antipsychotics, benzodiazepines (especially in the setting of alcohol withdrawal), or the combination of both [43,44]. Typical antipsychotics, including haloperidol and droperidol, have showed efficacy in reducing agitation and/or aggression during episodes of agitation in the elderly. However, these medications may have significant side effects, including dystonia and extrapyramidal symptoms. Therefore, atypical antipsychotics have been recommended in the elderly over typical antipsychotics [14,38,44]. Atypical antipsychotics have fewer complications with dystonia and extrapyramidal symptoms and have shown efficacy equivalent to typical antipsychotics and benzodiazepines [43]. However, black box warnings exist for both typical and atypical antipsychotics secondary to studies showing increased mortality with use in the demented elderly [45]. It should be noted that these studies analyzed this risk after several weeks and in most cases after several months of use [46]. No reports exist on safety with single doses. Benzodiazepines have also shown efficacy in decreasing agitation and are not associated with extrapyramidal symptoms. Studies have shown increased efficacy when used in combination with haloperidol. However, benzodiazepines are associated with respiratory depression, excess sedation, and occasionally paradoxical increase in agitation. Because of these adverse effects, it is recommended to start at lower doses with cautious intravenous use [43,44].

Physical restraints should be considered when the patient becomes a danger to themselves or to the hospital staff after pharmacologic and non-pharmacologic methods have failed or are not available. Limb, wrist, and vest restraints should be available in addition to mittens and bed rails as methods to restrain the patient [43]. Conclusive studies do not exist in regards to use of physical restraints in elderly patients. However, anecdotal evidence has shown that restraints are fraught with complications, including aspiration pneumonia, circulatory obstruction, cardiac stress with cardiovascular collapse, dehydration, and skin breakdown [42]. Seclusion in which a patient is typically placed in a locked room has been used in substitution for physical restraints for patients who are imminently violent. Complications with seclusion include assaultiveness toward staff, self-injury, destruction of seclusion room, and deterioration of physical and mental status [42].

Substance abuse

The impending flux of elderly individuals in the population will undoubtedly carry an increase in the absolute number of geriatric patients with substance abuse. In fact, substance abuse and dependence in the elderly population has been identified as the fastest growing health problem in the United States [14]. Specifically, studies on alcohol misuse and dependence show rates between 2% and 4% in the elderly population. When less stringent criteria are used, 17% of elderly men and 7% of elderly women were found to have excessive alcohol use [47]. Illicit drug use is relatively rare among elderly patients, with a rate between 1% and 2%, and twice the incidence in men with respect to women. This rate is

expected to rise and is much higher in psychiatric patients and within urban areas. Additionally, one of every four elderly patients use prescribed psychoactive medications and approximately 11% of elderly women abuse these medications [48]. The misuse of alcohol, illicit drugs, and prescribed medications may have deleterious medical consequences and psychiatric effects and should be investigated by the EP evaluating elderly patients.

As previously mentioned, substance use in conjunction with depression is associated with very significant morbidity and mortality in the elderly, including increased risk of suicide [14,28]. Elderly patients are more susceptible to adverse effects of substance use secondary to decreased lean body mass, cognitive reserve, and hepatic and renal function [14,37,49]. Specifically, alcohol use is associated with mood disorders, anxiety, cognitive impairment, personality disorders, and schizophrenia. Furthermore, chronic alcohol use is a risk factor for the development of a host of medical conditions, including malignancy, osteoporosis, peripheral neuropathy, and cerebellar atrophy leading to increased falls and injuries, Wernicke's and/or Korsakoff's syndrome, gastrointestinal bleed, withdrawal complications including seizures, and many adverse medication interactions [14]. Commonly prescribed medications such as benzodiazepines may cause agitation, psychosis, depression, and worsening of an underlying cognitive impairment. Additionally, benzodiazepines may lead to dependency issues, drowsiness, fatigue, and unsteady gait. In fact, benzodiazepines are the psychotropic medication most associated with falls and hip fractures [49]. Opioid use is prevalent and may be associated with increased sedation, impairment of motor coordination, and constipation [48]. The adverse effects of cocaine use specific to the elderly are not well described but cardiovascular complications, seizures, agitation, anxiety, and psychosis have been well documented across all age groups [50].

As is the trend with geriatric psychiatric emergencies, substance abuse is underdetected by primary providers and EPs [14]. Multiple studies report elderly patients are under-sampled when assessing for incidence of substance abuse [14,48]. A study using a mock clinical scenario found that only 1% of primary physicians correctly identified substance abuse as the underlying issue for an elderly patient [48]. Comorbid conditions common in elderly patients, including psychiatric disorders, cognitive impairment, tremor, chronic pain, functional decline, and hepatic/renal disorders, may make detection of substance abuse quite difficult as many overlapping symptoms may exist [48]. The DSM-IV has specific criteria for both substance abuse and dependence regardless of age. Substance abuse is defined as one or more of the following signs recurring for greater than 12 months as a result of substance use: (1) failure to fulfill major obligations; (2) use in physically hazardous situations; (3) legal problems; (4) interpersonal/social issues. Substance dependence is defined as 3 or more of the following signs or symptoms for greater than 12 months in

Table 30.5. CAGE screening for alcohol and drug abuse in the elderly[a] [51]

1. Have you ever felt you needed to **c**ut down on your drinking or drug use?
2. Have people **a**nnoyed you by criticizing your drinking or drug use?
3. Have you ever felt **g**uilty about drinking or drug use?
4. Have you ever felt you needed a drink or to use drugs the first thing in the morning (**e**ye-opener) to steady your nerves or to get rid of hangover?

[a] This table contains a screening questionnaire for the detection of alcohol or drug abuse. The screen should be considered positive if the patient answers "yes" to any of the above questions. This screening questionnaire becomes more specific for abuse for each additional "yes" answer. This table is adapted from Hinkin et al. [51].

CAGE = acronym using the bolded, capitalized letters from the above four questions

regards to a specific substance: (1) tolerance; (2) withdrawal symptoms; (3) taken in larger amounts than intended; (4) repeated, unsuccessful attempts to quit; (5) significant time spent obtaining the substance; (6) important activities/responsibilities are given up or reduced; (7) continued use despite known adverse consequences [15].

The establishment of precise diagnoses for substance abuse or dependence should not be considered the standard of practice for EPs. Rather, the objective should be to detect the potential for substance abuse or dependence, as it may have a significant impact on patient resuscitation, management, and disposition. The CAGE questionnaire, summarized in Table 30.5, has been adapted as a screening tool for both drug and alcohol abuse and has been validated in elderly patients [51]. This questionnaire does not assess for current drug use or drinking behavior, therefore a careful history including use, frequency, and amount of laboratory drug or alcohol use, in addition to a careful medication review, should be performed by the EP. A drug screen may be helpful in management and disposition of the undifferentiated patient, especially when a reliable history is not available [52]. However, the global use of a drug screen should be discouraged, as this information can typically be obtained with a good history and may not aid in management. Furthermore, routine drug screens may be financially costly to the patient or patient's family [53].

After the determination of abuse has been made, the appropriate management and disposition is vital to the safety of the patient. The type, amount, and frequency of the abused substance, co-ingestions including current prescriptions, and medical and psychiatric comorbidities will dictate the management. In the alcoholic patient, important historical components include prior complicated detoxifications, history of withdrawal seizures or delirium tremens, or other comorbid factors that would require hospital admission [14]. EPs should be aware of the kindling phenomenon where patients develop increasingly severe withdrawal symptoms with repeated alcohol detoxification attempts [54]. Benzodiazepines are the treatment of choice for alcohol withdrawal and for complications of acute cocaine intoxication [55,56]. Naltrexone is the well-known

antidote for opioid intoxication and may help differentiate drug intoxication versus other organic etiologies for the unresponsive elderly patient. Lastly, elderly patients with acute benzodiazepine intoxication may undergo reversal with flumazenil. However, caution should be used because life-threatening seizures may develop, especially in chronic benzodiazepine users. The chronic benzodiazepine abuser will benefit more from supportive care without antidote therapy [57]. The elderly patient not admitted for further medical or psychiatric management should receive a timely outpatient referral.

Elder abuse

The American Medical Association defines elder abuse and neglect as an act of omission that results in harm or threatened harm to the health or welfare of an elderly person. Its incidence is not known secondary to cognitive impairment of the victims, hesitancy to report for fear of worsening the situation, and reluctance to report by the physician because of skepticism, fear of angering the abuser, and lack of support from the patient [49]. Despite this, it is speculated that over two million elderly adults are mistreated in the United States each year with complications ranging from depression to injury to death [49].

Abuse or neglect may be in the form of physical abuse, psychological abuse, caregiver neglect, self-neglect, and financial exploitation [49]. The abusers of the elderly are most often family members. Adult children or spouses of the victims make up approximately two thirds of the perpetrators [14]. Additionally, nursing homes account for a significant portion of elder abuse -36% of nursing home staff reporting at least one witnessed incident of physical abuse. Risk factors for abuse include cognitive impairment, shared living space with the abuser, a high degree of dependence on caretakers, social isolation, and minority status [14].

Recognition of abuse or neglect will be a difficult task unless the diagnosis is considered by EPs. The diagnosis of abuse should be considered when an elderly patient presents with multiple injuries in various stages of healing or when injuries are unexplained. Neglect should be considered when an elderly person with adequate resources presents with negligence in hygiene, nutrition, and/or medical care [14]. The EP should interview the patient either alone or in the absence of the suspected abuser to increase the probability of detection of abuse or neglect [49]. Furthermore, the interview process should start with asking the patient for their perception of the safety within their home and neighborhood [14]. Lastly, a nonjudgmental and empathetic approach may help elicit more accurate information.

In the event that elder abuse is suspected, the EP is responsible for ensuring the safety of the elderly patient. The disposition should place the patient away from the suspected abuser(s), which may require an inpatient admission [58]. A careful assessment for comorbid psychiatric conditions and risk for suicide should be performed. Lastly, the EP is legally bound to report suspected elder mistreatment to adult protective services.

References

1. American Geriatrics Society and the Association of Directors of Academic Geriatric Center's Geriatric Workforce Policy Studies Center. 2010.

2. Walsh PG, Currier G, Shah MN, Lyness JM, Friedman B. Psychiatric emergency services for the U.S. elderly: 2008 and beyond. *Am J Geriatr Psychiatry* 2008;**16**:706–17.

3. Thienhaus OJ, Piasecki MP. Assessment of geriatric patients in the psychiatric emergency service. *Psychiatr Serv* 2004;**55**:639–40, 642.

4. Unutzer J, Patrick DL, Simon G, et al. Depressive symptoms and the cost of health services in HMO patients aged 65 years and older. A 4-year prospective study. *JAMA* 1997;**277**:1618–23.

5. Ganguli M, Dodge HH, Mulsant BH. Rates and predictors of mortality in an aging, rural, community-based cohort: the role of depression. *Arch Gen Psychiatry* 2002;**59**:1046–52.

6. Huang BY, Cornoni-Huntley J, Hays JC, et al. Impact of depressive symptoms on hospitalization risk in community-dwelling older persons. *J Am Geriatr Soc* 2000;**48**:1279–84.

7. Schulz R, Drayer RA, Rollman BL. Depression as a risk factor for non-suicide mortality in the elderly. *Biol Psychiatry* 2002;**52**:205–25.

8. Waern M, Runeson BS, Allenbeck P, et al. Mental disorder in elderly suicides: a case-control study. *Am J Psychiatry* 2002;**159**:450–5.

9. Meldon SW, Emerman CL, Schubert DS, Moffa DA, Etheart RG. Depression in geriatric ED patients: prevalence and recognition. *Ann Emerg Med* 1997;**30**:141–5.

10. Hustey FM, Smith MD. A depression screen and intervention for older ED patients. *Am J Emerg Med* 2007;**25**:133–7.

11. Alexopoulos GS, Borson S, Cuthbert BN, et al. Assessment of late life depression. *Biol Psychiatry* 2002;**52**:164–74.

12. Meldon SW, Emerman CL, Schubert DS. Recognition of depression in geriatric ED patients by emergency physicians. *Ann Emerg Med* 1997;**30**:442–7.

13. Cole MG, Dendukuri N. Risk factors for depression among elderly community subjects: a systematic review and meta-analysis. *Am J Psychiatry* 2003;**160**:1147–56.

14. Piechniczek-Buczek J. Psychiatric emergencies in the elderly population. *Emerg Med Clin North Am* 2006;**24**:467–90.

15. American Psychiatric Association. *Diagnostic and Statistical Manual of Mental Disorders*, (4th Edition). Washington, DC: American Psychiatric Association; 2000.

16. Fabacher DA, Raccio-Robak N, McErlean MA, Milano PM, Verdile VP. Validation of a brief screening tool to detect depression in elderly ED patients. *Am J Emerg Med* 2002;**20**:99–102.

17. Sharp LK, Lipsky MS. Screening for depression across the lifespan: a review of measures for use in primary care settings. *Am Fam Physician* 2002;**66**:1001–8.

18. Fischer LR, Wei F, Solberg LI, Rush WA, Heinrich RL. Treatment of elderly and other adult patients for depression in primary care. *J Am Geriatr Soc* 2003;**51**:1554–62.

19. Lyness JM, King DA, Cox C, Yoediono Z, Caine ED. The importance of subsyndromal depression in older primary care patients: prevalence and associated functional disability. *J Am Geriatr Soc* 1999;**47**:647–52.

20. Beekman AT, Deeg DJ, Braam AW, Smit JH, Van Tilburg W. Consequences of major and minor depression in later life: a study of disability, well-being and service utilization. *Psychol Med* 1997;**27**:1397–409.

21. Olin JT, Schneider LS, Katz IR, et al. Provisional diagnostic criteria for depression of Alzheimer disease. *Am J Geriatr Psychiatry* 2002;**10**:125–8.

22. Engedal K, Barca ML, Laks J, Selbaek G. Depression in Alzheimer's disease: specificity of depressive symptoms using three different clinical criteria. *Int J Geriatr Psychiatry* 2011;**26**:944–51.

23. Verkaik R, Francke AL, van Meijel B, Ribbe MW, Bensing JM. Comorbid depression in dementia on psychogeriatric nursing home wards: which symptoms are prominent? *Am J Geriatr Psychiatry* 2009;**17**:565–73.

24. Katon W, Unutzer J, Fan MY, et al. Cost-effectiveness and net benefit of enhanced treatment of depression for older adults with diabetes and depression. *Diabetes Care* 2006;**29**:265–70.

25. Agius M, Murphy CL, Zaman R. Does shared care help in the treatment of depression? *Psychiatr Danub* 2010;**22** (Suppl 1):S18–22.

26. Zun LS. Evidence-based evaluation of psychiatric patients. *J Emerg Med* 2005;**28**:35–9.

27. Macdonald AJ. ABC of mental health. Mental health in old age. *BMJ* 1997;**315**:413–17.

28. Conwell Y, Thompson C. Suicidal behavior in elders. *Psychiatr Clin North Am* 2008;**31**:333–56.

29. Conwell Y. Suicide in later life: a review and recommendations for prevention. *Suicide Life Threat Behav* 2001;**31** (Suppl):32–47.

30. Conwell Y, Duberstein PR, Cox C, et al. Relationships of age and axis I diagnoses in victims of completed suicide: a psychological autopsy study. *Am J Psychiatry* 1996;**153**:1001–8.

31. Duberstein PR, Conwell Y, Cox C. Suicide in widowed persons. A psychological autopsy comparison of recently and remotely bereaved older subjects. *Am J Geriatr Psychiatry* 1998;**6**:328–34.

32. Waern M, Beskow J, Runeson B, Skoog I. Suicidal feelings in the last year of life in elderly people who commit suicide. *Lancet* 1999;**354**:917–18.

33. Rudd MD, Mandrusiak M, Joiner TE Jr. The case against no-suicide contracts: the commitment to treatment statement as a practice alternative. *J Clin Psychol* 2006;**62**:243–51.

34. Douglass AM, Luo J, Baraff LJ. Emergency medicine and psychiatry agreement on diagnosis and disposition of emergency department patients with behavioral emergencies. *Acad Emerg Med* 2011;**18**:368–73.

35. Khouzam HR, Emes R. Late life psychosis: assessment and general treatment strategies. *Compr Ther* 2007;**33**:127–43.

36. Mintzer J, Targum SD. Psychosis in elderly patients: classification and pharmacotherapy. *J Geriatr Psychiatry Neurol* 2003;**16**:199–206.

37. Jones RN, Fong TG, Metzger E, et al. Aging, brain disease, and reserve: implications for delirium. *Am J Geriatr Psychiatry* 2010;**18**:117–27.

38. Patkar AA, Mago R, Masand PS. Psychotic symptoms in patients with medical disorders. *Curr Psychiatr Rep* 2004;**6**:216–24.

39. van Winkel R, Stefanis NC, Myin-Germeys I. Psychosocial stress and psychosis. A review of the neurobiological mechanisms and the evidence for gene-stress interaction. *Schizophr Bull* 2008;**34**:1095–105.

40. Mace SE. Central nervous system infections as a cause of an altered mental status? What is the pathogen growing in your central nervous system? *Emerg Med Clin North Am* 2011;**28**:535–70.

41. Moy MM, (Ed.). EMTALA and psychiatry. In: *The EMTALA Answer Book*, (2nd Edition). Gaithersburg, MD: Aspen Publishers; 2000.

42. Zun LS. Evidence-based treatment of psychiatric patient. *J Emerg Med* 2005;**28**:277–83.

43. Peisah C, Chan DK, McKay R, Kurrle SE, Reutens SG. Practical guidelines for the acute emergency sedation of the severely agitated older patient. *Intern Med J* 2011;**41**:651–7.

44. Yildiz A, Sachs GS, Turgay A. Pharmacological management of agitation in emergency settings. *Emerg Med J* 2003;**20**:339–46.

45. Yan J. FDA extends black-box warning to all antipsychotics. *Psychiatric News* 2008;**43**:1–27.

46. Jeste DV, Blazer D, Casey D, et al. ACNP White Paper: update on use of antipsychotic drugs in elderly persons with dementia. *Neuropsychopharmacology* 2008;**33**:957–70.

47. O'Connell H, Chin AV, Cunningham C, Lawlor B. Alcohol use disorders in elderly people–redefining an age old problem in old age. *BMJ* 2003;**327**:664–7.

48. Simoni-Wastila L, Yang HK. Psychoactive drug abuse in older adults. *Am J Geriatr Pharmacother* 2006;**4**:380–94.

49. Borja B, Borja CS, Gade S. Psychiatric emergencies in the geriatric population. *Clin Geriatr Med* 2007;**23**:391–400.

50. Devlin RJ, Henry JA. Clinical review: major consequences of illicit drug consumption. *Crit Care* 2008;**12**:202.

51. Hinkin CH, Castellon SA, Dickson-Fuhrman E, et al. Screening for drug and alcohol abuse among older adults using a modified version of the CAGE. *Am J Addict* 2001;**10**:319–26.

52. Fabbri A, Marchesini G, Morselli-Labate AM, et al. Comprehensive drug screening in decision making of patients attending the emergency department for suspected drug overdose. *Emerg Med J* 2003;**20**:25–8.

53. Perrone J, De Roos F, Jayaraman S, Hollander JE. Drug screening versus history in detection of substance use in ED psychiatric patients. *Am J Emerg Med* 2001;**19**:49–51.

54. Malcolm RJ. GABA systems, benzodiazepines, and substance dependence. *J Clin Psychiatry* 2003;**64** (Suppl 3):36–40.

55. Amato L, Minozzi S, Vecchi S, Davoli M. Benzodiazepines for alcohol withdrawal. *Cochrane Database Syst Rev* 2010;(**3**):CD005063.

56. McCord J, Jneid H, Hollander JE, et al. Management of cocaine-associated chest pain and myocardial infarction: a scientific statement from the American Heart Association Acute Cardiac Care Committee of the Council on Clinical Cardiology. *Circulation* 2008;**117**:1897–907.

57. Seger DL. Flumazenil–treatment or toxin. *J Toxicol Clin Toxicol* 2004;**42**:209–16.

58. Geroff AJ, Olshaker JS. Elder abuse. *Emerg Med Clin North Am* 2006;**24**:491–505.

Chapter 31

Disaster and terrorism emergency psychiatry

Michael S. Pulia

Introduction

In an ideal world, disasters would never occur. However, if recent events teach us anything, it is a matter of when, not if, the next large-scale disaster will occur. Whether natural occurrences, man-made accidents, or intentional acts of terrorism, these events are becoming more common and larger in scale [1]. According to the World Health Organization, a disaster is an event "which greatly exceeds the coping capacity of the affected community" [2]. For the emergency physician (EP), this means scores of victims could arrive at the emergency department (ED) and rapidly overwhelm capacity for medical and psychiatric care, as was seen following the Sarin gas terrorist attack in Tokyo [3].

Often unexpected, disasters promote chaos and panic among those facing injury, loss, and death [4]. In addition to expertise in handling victims with traumatic, biological, chemical, and radiation exposures, the EP must also be proficient in managing those suffering from psychological trauma. The vast majority of morbidity from disasters, especially terrorist acts, is psychological in nature [5]. As acute care providers, EPs will likely be the first physician contact for victims and this is an ideal opportunity to assess for psychiatric injuries [6]. Disaster mental health care is similar to physical first aid but with the goal of stabilizing "psychological hemorrhage" [7]. This chapter will focus on the essential elements of an immediate post-disaster assessment and treatment plan for EPs. Although preparedness is an essential precursor to any disaster response, a detailed description of how to set up a disaster mental health plan is beyond the scope of this chapter. Excellent summaries of this information can be found in comprehensive Disaster Psychiatry textbooks [8,9].

Terrorism and its impact

As its name reflects, terrorism is designed specifically to inflict fear. This form of psychological warfare aims to advance an agenda through fear-based behavioral changes in victims [10,11]. It is not surprising that these attacks are often large scale, come without warning, involve unconventional methods, and make no exception for innocent victims. The disrupted sense of security, uncertainty about the future, and intense exposures that accompany terrorist acts make them particularly high risk for inflicting psychological trauma [12,13]. Studies indicate the rate of post-traumatic stress disorder (PTSD) following the September 11th terrorist attacks in New York City ("9/11") may be increasing with time; decades may pass before we can fully appreciate the long-term mental health consequences of this disaster [13]. In the era of constant media coverage, terrorist acts can also have impact beyond direct victims. Post-9/11 research demonstrated that hours spent watching coverage of the attacks was a risk factor for the development of PTSD [14]. It is important for the EP working with terrorism victims to remember the unique aspects of these events and have a high index of suspicion for psychological sequelae.

Staged assessments

The immediate challenge of post-disaster care is differentiating normal stress responses from life-threatening medical conditions, which often have similar symptomatology. For a list of the normal psychological and physiologic responses to acute trauma see Table 31.1 [15]. This distinction is crucial as pathologizing a normal response can further traumatize and alienate the victim [6]. Avoiding the use of terminology like "symptoms" and "diagnosis," to describe acute reactions, is recommended [16]. Conversely, assuming the symptoms are somatic in nature can delay definitive treatment of any underlying medical conditions.

Medical assessment

Dissociation in disaster victims can also be difficult to distinguish from delirium due to medical causes [17]. Although confusion is on the spectrum of normal stress responses, in a disaster scenario, it becomes a diagnosis of exclusion [18]. These patients must be evaluated for delirium due to traumatic brain injury, hypoxia, sepsis, metabolic derangements, intoxication, and withdrawal states. Medications they may have received on scene from first responders, such as

---

Behavioral Emergencies for the Emergency Physician, ed. Leslie S. Zun, Lara G. Chepenik, and Mary Nan S. Mallory. Published by Cambridge University Press. © Cambridge University Press 2013.

Table 31.1. Acute traumatic stress reactions [15]

Emotional effects	Cognitive effects
• Shock	• Impaired concentration
• Terror	• Impaired decision-making ability
• Irritability	• Memory impairment
• Blame	• Disbelief
• Anger	• Confusion
• Guilt	• Decreased self-efficacy
• Grief or sadness	• Intrusive thoughts/memories
• Emotional numbing	• Dissociation (e.g., tunnel vision,
• Helplessness	dreamlike or "spacey" feeling)

Physical effects	Interpersonal effects
• Fatigue, exhaustion	• Increased relational conflict
• Insomnia	• Social withdrawal
• Cardiovascular strain	• Alienation
• Startle response	• Distrust
• Hyper-arousal	• Externalization of blame
• Increased physical pain	• Externalization of vulnerability
• Headaches	• Feeling abandoned/rejected
• Gastrointestinal upset	• Overprotectiveness
• Decreased appetite	

atropine, epinephrine, and morphine, can also impair mental status. Anxiety, another common stress response, can also be a symptom of serious medical pathologies such as hypoglycemia, cardiac arrhythmias, hypotension, pulmonary embolus, internal hemorrhage, seizure, postconcussive syndrome, and myocardial infarction [4]. One helpful way to distinguish psychogenic from medical symptoms is to appreciate that dissociating patients should be easier to re-orient, improve with time, and not have the dramatic fluctuations in level of consciousness seen with delirium [17,18]. A quick history and physical combined with some rapid diagnostic tests (e.g., electrocardiogram [ECG], fingerstick glucose) should be able to rule out most serious medical conditions.

Toxicologic assessment

These distinctions can become even more difficult when dealing with chemical and biological weapon exposures that mimic psychiatric stress responses. Acute mental distress is known to manifest as somatic complaints and this effect is magnified when a disaster involves hazardous substances, even in unexposed individuals [19–21]. Confusion and disorientation are known symptoms of the cholinergic toxidrome seen after exposure to organophosphates/nerve agents such as VX or Sarin gas [17]. The antidote for organophosphate poisoning is atropine, which in excess causes an anticholinergic toxidrome that involves delirium [22]. Contact with vesicant/blister agents such as mustard gas can induce delirium through intense pain [17]. Biological weapons also have the potential to produce altered mental status through meningitis (anthrax) and viral encephalitis [22].

Psychiatric risk assessment

After ruling out any serious medical issues which require stabilization, the focus should shift to assessing the degree of traumatic exposure and individual risk factors for adverse psychiatric outcomes. Each patient will have a unique survivor experience and needs to be given an opportunity to tell their story, if desired [23]. Disasters are often multifaceted events with a cascade of maladies following the initial occurrence that can impact everyone in the surrounding area [24]. An example is a tornado which causes destruction and loss of life but also interrupts power, disrupts vital community services (fire, EMS, police), and promotes looting. A victim of these secondary effects is just as vulnerable to psychiatric distress as someone directly involved with the inciting incident.

There is a well-defined relationship between the type of event and resulting psychopathology [2]. The wide ranges of reported post-disaster PTSD rates, depending on incident type and specific details, highlight this important concept. The baseline incidence of PTSD in the U.S. is approximately 3% [14]. Natural disaster victims have been reported to have average PTSD rates of 5% [25], in contrast to 30% of mass shooting victims [26]. Due to the intimate nature of personal trauma, human-related disasters generally result in much higher rates of psychopathology [25]. The severity of the known acute and chronic psychiatric complications of disasters (such as acute stress disorder (ASD), PTSD, major depression, and anxiety disorders) also depends in large part on the individual victim's duration and intensity of exposure [25,27,28]. The mass destruction and death witnessed on 9/11 seemed to be particularly traumatizing to those in close proximity [28,29].

In obtaining the history, important aspects to cover include witnessed events, any personal loss, and injuries suffered. It is recommended to allow the victim to discuss their experience without pushing for a level of detail that could cause further traumatization [15]. Critical Incident Stress Debriefing (CISD), a detailed and formal review of the disaster experience, used to be encouraged for all survivors. However, current research indicates it does not prevent PTSD and may actually trigger distressing symptoms in survivors [6,30]. Any personal loss, especially the sudden death of a loved one or loss of home, during the event predicts an elevated risk for subsequent pathology [12,13,25]. Physically injured patients have also been identified as a high-risk group and should undergo comprehensive screening once stabilized. The EP should also inquire about any history of substance abuse or psychiatric illness, especially PTSD, as these patients are high risk for acute exacerbations of chronic disorders and the development of new psychopathology. Children, mothers with small children, pregnant women, and the elderly are other groups who appear particularly vulnerable to the traumatic effects of disaster. As secondary victims, first responders are often exposed to grotesque scenes and tremendous human suffering and are also categorized as a high-risk group [16].

Although many initial stress responses may seem extreme, for the most part they are appropriate reactions to grave circumstances and transient in nature [25]. The exceptions to the rule are severe forms of stress responses that can be categorized as pathologic and require immediate intervention [31,32]. As with routine care for patients suffering from a psychiatric crisis, screening for thoughts of harming self/others and acute psychosis must be done before discharge. Disasters can reveal maladaptive tendencies that victims are unaware of and can result in significant dysfunction. Everyone has a unique threshold of stress tolerance which is determined, in part, by past experiences, genetics, physical health, belief system, and support network. When pushed beyond the "breaking point," coping mechanisms fail and behavior may deteriorate into immobilization or fulminant psychosis. Symptoms indicating an impending collapse include agitation/rage, misdirected aggression, rambling speech, erratic behavior, loud wailing, extreme dissociation, and catatonia [4,32]. Disabling stress reactions need to be rapidly identified and treated as they can be psychologically contagious and destabilize the milieu of a disaster scene or the ED [7]. Although they are conceptually distinct processes, the psychiatric assessment and treatment of disaster victims typically occurs simultaneously.

Provision of psychological first aid

The concept of acute psychiatric care for victims of trauma is derived from the experience of military psychiatrists in handling traumatized soldiers [24]. Brief crisis interventions in the immediate post-trauma period were found to restore function, reduce the incidence of subsequent PTSD, and allow soldiers to return to battle at much higher rates [4]. This approach has been studied and refined in developing the current approach to disaster victims' care termed *psychological first aid* (PFA) [16]. As first responders, EPs should have mastery of these techniques to effectively manage the large number of victims that might present after a disaster.

Sequester

Despite the very real risk of psychiatric pathology in disaster victims, the most common response among survivors is resilience [25]; with many going on to experience post-traumatic personal growth [33,34]. All immediate interventions are designed to facilitate resilience through prompt restoration of safety, physiologic/psychological homeostasis, support networks, and coping skills. The first and most important step in PFA is to remove the victim from the disaster scene [7]. The objective is to encourage a feeling of safety and minimize any chance of repeat trauma or exposure to reminders of the event (e.g., TV coverage). It is also prudent to protect victims from media scrutiny [18]. When dealing with victims whose sense of trust in others is acutely disrupted, it is important to clearly identify yourself as the treating physician and "look the part" by wearing your white coat and a clearly visible ID badge. All interactions should be conducted with a core focus on a calm, sympathetic, and non-judgmental attitude.

Treat physical pain

When the patient arrives in a safe therapeutic environment, like the ED or a field hospital, prompt treatment and stabilization of any physical injuries and medical conditions should occur. For disaster victims, medical care has an important role in psychiatric care [35]. This principle is reinforced by research demonstrating that the early use of morphine in seriously injured soldiers resulted in significantly reduced rates of PTSD [36].

Treatment and referral

Once victims are medically stable, the EP should implement simple comfort measures, assess basic needs, and reassure the patient. Do not assume that every victim is suffering from psychiatric trauma or will want to discuss these issues. Acting in a calm, empathetic, and respectful manner will facilitate victim engagement and enhance coping [23]. Providing a quiet environment, food/drink, warm blankets, access to phones, and other practical assistance (e.g., transportation home, locating relatives, arranging shelter) is considered an important foundation for post-traumatic mental health recovery [16,37,38]. Provider flexibility during the encounter and in handling victim requests helps to reestablish locus of control and counteract feelings of helplessness [22]. When discussing the event, the EP should focus on the positive aspects of how the victim is handling the stress [16]. These efforts should help down-regulate the "fight or flight" response to stress and restore a pre-trauma state [7]. Depending on their level of distress, coping skills and support system, any individual found to meet the previously mentioned high-risk criteria for post-disaster psychopathology should have an ED psychiatric consult or urgent outpatient follow-up [23]. Those individuals demonstrating pathologic stress reactions require emergency psychiatric consultation and stabilization. This may include sedation with a benzodiazepine or antipsychotic agent to protect the milieu and prevent harm to self and others.

Pharmacologic agents also have a role in managing less severe symptoms such as anxiety or insomnia. Short-term courses of antihistamines and benzodiazepines (less than 2-week duration) can alleviate these symptoms but there is no known therapeutic agent capable of preventing the development of PTSD [39]. In victims with prominent physiologic symptoms, such as tachycardia and tremors, a short course of propranolol may be beneficial [6]. Various clinical trials have examined the role of propranolol in traumatic memory consolidation and as a potential agent for PTSD prevention in traumatized ED patients. However, propranolol is not currently recommended for PTSD prevention in disaster victims due to conflicting and inconclusive data [40,41].

Disposition

Victims with intact coping mechanisms should be discharged after instructions about what symptoms they can expect in the days to come as part of a normal stress response. This intervention should include a discussion about signs of ASD/PTSD and where to find help if they develop. A document addressing these issues should be developed as part of the preparedness plan and readily available should a disaster occur [16]. A clear list of available resources, including faith-based organizations, social services, disaster response agencies, and mental health services, should also be provided. Victims should be encouraged to engage in activities that reinforce positive coping skills, such as social gatherings, memorial services, hobbies, and getting back to work [6,23]. One of the great lessons from the aftermath of 9–11 is the critical nature of early access to mental health treatment for disaster survivors [39]. Disaster preparedness should include collaboration with our psychiatric colleagues, as a large-scale event will likely overwhelm local resources if there is no predetermined plan to scale up care and defer any non-emergent outpatient visits.

Conclusion

The increasing frequency and impact of natural disasters combined with the ever-present threat of terrorism make the management of disaster victims an essential skill for the EP. Although the primary focus is on life-threatening medical conditions, the psychiatric casualties of disasters far outnumber those who are physically injured. As a front-line physician during any disaster response, the EP can play a critical role in reducing subsequent psychiatric pathology in victims. To do so, one must understand the unique implications of these events and follow the principles outlined in PFA.

References

1. Ripley A. *Why Disasters Are Getting Worse*. Time USA. September 3, 2008. Available at: http://www.time.com/time/nation/article/0,8599,1838400,00.html (Accessed September 25, 2011).

2. World Health Organization. *Psychosocial Consequences of Disaster: Prevention and Management*. Geneva: World Health Organization. 1992. Available at: http://whqlibdoc.who.int/hq/1991/WHO_MNH_PSF_91.3_REV.1.pdf (Accessed September 23, 2011).

3. Okumura T, Takasu N, Ishimatsu S, et al. Report on 640 victims of the Tokyo subway sarin attack. *Ann Emerg Med* 1996;**28**:129–35.

4. Sadock BJ, Sadock VA. *Kaplan & Sadock's Comprehensive Textbook of Psychiatry*, (8th Edition). Philadelphia: Lippincott Williams and Wilkins; 2005. Chapter 28.9, Military and Disaster Psychiatry. Available at: Rittenhouse Digital Library. (Accessed September 25, 2011).

5. Stout CE, Weine SM. Cities of fear, cities of hope: Public mental health in the age of terrorism. In: Kimmel P, Stout CE, (Eds.). *Collateral Damage: the Psychological Consequences of America's War on Terrorism*. New York: Praeger Publishers; 2006; 189–204.

6. American Psychiatric Association. Committee on Psychiatric Dimensions of Disaster. *Disaster Psychiatry Handbook*. 2004. Available at: http://www.psych.org/Resources/DisasterPsychiatry/APADisasterPsychiatryResources/DisasterPsychiatryHandbook.aspx (Accessed September 23, 2011)

7. U.S. Department of Veterans Affairs. *VA/DoD Clinical Practice Guidelines-Management of Traumatic Stress Disorder and Acute Stress Reaction*. 2010. Available at: http://www.healthquality.va.gov/PTSD-FULL-2010c.pdf (Accessed September 26, 2011).

8. Ursano RJ, Fullerton CS, Weisaeth L, Raphael B, (Eds.). *Textbook of Disaster Psychiatry*. New York: Cambridge University Press; 2007.

9. Stoddard FJ, Pandya A, Katz CL, (Eds.). *Disaster Psychiatry: Readiness, Evaluation, and Treatment*. New York: American Psychiatric Publishing; 2011.

10. Bolz FJ, Dudonis KJ, Schulz DP. *The Counter-terrorism Handbook: Tactics, Procedures and Techniques*, (1st Edition). New York: CRC-Press; 1998.

11. Everly GS, Mitchell JT. America under attack: the "10 commandments" of responding to mass terrorist attacks. *Int J Emerg Ment Health* 2001;**3**:133–5.

12. Stellman JM, Smith RP, Katz CL, et al. Enduring mental health morbidity and social function impairment in World Trade Center rescue, recovery, and cleanup workers: the psychological dimension of an environmental health disaster. *Environ Health Perspect* 2008;**116**:1248–53.

13. Brackbill RM, Hadler JL, DiGrande L, et al. Asthma and posttraumatic stress symptoms 5 to 6 years following exposure to the World Trade Center terrorist attack. *JAMA* 2009;**302**:502–16.

14. Schlenger WE, Caddell JM, Ebert L, et al. Psychological reactions to terrorist attacks: findings from the National Study of Americans' Reactions to September 11. *JAMA* 2002;**288**:581–8.

15. NSW Institute of Psychiatry and Centre for Mental Health. *Disaster Mental Health Response Handbook*. North Sydney: NSW Health; 2000.

16. National Child Traumatic Stress Network and National Center for PTSD. *Psychological First Aid: Field Operations Guide*, (2nd Edition). National Center for PTSD. 2006. Available at: http://www.ptsd.va.gov/professional/manuals/manual-pdf/pfa/PFA_V2.pdf (Accessed September 28, 2011).

17. Fetter JC. Psychosocial response to mass casualty terrorism: guidelines for physicians. *Prim Care Companion J Clin Psychiatry* 2005;**7**:49–52.

18. Cloak NL, Edwards P. Psychological first aid: emergency care for terrorism and disaster survivors. *Curr Psychiatry* 2004;**3**:12–23.

19. Herman JL. *Trauma and Recovery*. New York: Basic Books; 1997.

20. Woodall JW. Tokyo subway gas attack. *Lancet* 1997;**350**:296.

21. Yehuda R. Post-traumatic stress disorder. *N Engl J Med* 2002;**346**:108–14.

22. DiGiovanni C. Domestic terrorism with chemical or biological agents: psychiatric aspects. *Am J Psychiatry* 1999;**156**:1500–5.

23. Watson PJ. Early intervention for problems following mass trauma. In: Ursano RJ, Fullerton CS, Weisaeth L,

Raphael B, (Eds.). *Textbook of Disaster Psychiatry*. New York: Cambridge University Press; 2007.

24. Ng AT. *Disaster Mental Health*. MIWatch.org. September 13, 2007. Available at: http://www.miwatch.org/2007/09/disaster_mental_health_1.html (Accessed September 25, 2011).

25. U.S. Department of Veterans Affairs National Center for PTSD. *Effects of Traumatic Stress after Mass Violence, Terror, or Disaster*. January 1, 2007. [updated October 6, 2010]; Available at: http://www.ptsd.va.gov/professional/pages/stress-mv-t-dhtml.asp (Accessed September 26, 2011).

26. Bryant RA. Acute stress disorder. *PTSD Res Qu* 2000;**11**:1–7.

27. Kessler RC, Galea S, Gruber MJ, et al. Trends in mental illness and suicidality after Hurricane Katrina. *Mol Psychiatry* 2008;**13**:374–84.

28. Galea S, Ahern J, Resnick H, et al. Psychological sequelae of the September 11 terrorist attacks in New York City. *N Engl J Med* 2002;**346**:982–7.

29. Bonanno GA, Galea S, Bucciarelli A, Vlahov D. Psychological resilience after disaster. New York City in the aftermath of the September 11th terrorist attack. *Psychol Sci* 2006;**17**:181–6.

30. Rose SC, Bisson J, Churchill R, Wessely S. Psychological debriefing for preventing post traumatic stress disorder (PTSD). *Cochrane Database Syst Rev* 2002;(**2**):CD000560.

31. North CS, Nixon SJ, Shariat S, et al. Psychiatric disorders among survivors of the Oklahoma City bombing. *JAMA* 1999;**282**:755–62.

32. U.S. Department of Veterans Affairs National Center for PTSD. *Early Mental Health Intervention for Disasters*. July 5, 2007. [updated March 15, 2011]. Available at: http://www.ptsd.va.gov/professional/pages/early-intervention-disasters.asp (Accessed September 26, 2011).

33. Quarantelli EL. *Organization Behavior in Disasters and Implications for Disaster Planning, Report Series 18*. Newark: Disaster Research Center, University of Delaware; 1985.

34. Calhoun LG, Cann A, Tedeschi RG, McMillan J. A correlational test of the relationship between posttraumatic growth, religion, and cognitive processing. *J Traumatic Stress* 2000;**13**:521–7.

35. Miller L. Psychological interventions for terroristic trauma: symptoms, syndromes, and treatment strategies. *Psychotherapy: Theory/Research/Practice/Training* 2002;**39**:283–96.

36. Holbrook TL, Galarneau MR, Dye JL, Quinn K, Dougherty AL. Morphine use after combat injury in Iraq and post-traumatic stress disorder. *N Engl J Med* 2010;**362**:110–17.

37. Gray MJ, Maguen S, Litz BT. Acute psychological impact of disaster and large-scale trauma: limitations of traditional interventions and future practice recommendations. *Prehosp Disaster Med* 2004;**19**:64–72.

38. Shalev AY. Treating survivors in the immediate aftermath of traumatic events. In: Yehuda R, (Ed.). *Treating Trauma Survivors with PTSD: Bridging the Gap Between Intervention Research and Practice*. Washington, DC: American Psychiatric Press; 2002.

39. Clayton NM, Nash WP. Medication management of combat and operational stress injuries in active duty service members. In: Figley CR, Nash WP, (Eds.). *Combat Stress Injury*. New York: Routledge; 2007: 219–45.

40. Pitman RK, Sanders KM, Zusman RM, et al. Pilot study of secondary prevention of posttraumatic stress disorder with propranolol. *Biol Psychiatry* 2002;**15**:189–92.

41. Nugent NR. The efficacy of early propranolol administration at preventing/reducing PTSD symptoms in child trauma victims: Pilot. *Diss Abstr Int* 2007;**68**(4-B):2665.

Trauma and loss in the emergency setting

Janet S. Richmond

Introduction

Psychological trauma involves loss, whether it is the traumatic death of a loved one, a loss of a sense of safety and security, or the shattering of one's "worldview." Trauma takes away our sense of a "just world." Bio-rhythms, belief systems, family structure, and interpersonal interactions at home or work can all be disrupted. Personal integrity can be challenged, even threatened.

Because trauma and loss are inextricably connected, this chapter focuses on both issues. Because so much loss and trauma is sudden and unexpected, it routinely presents in the emergency setting. This chapter will focus on the acutely traumatized person presenting to the emergency department (ED) and will address grief and bereavement along with the vicissitudes, various sub-types of response: acute, "impacted," delayed, traumatic, and chronic. This chapter will address how the emergency physician can best recognize and manage acute trauma and grief, and identify other presentations that may be indirect expressions of bereavement or trauma.

Because the emergency department physician and staff are frequent bearers of "bad news," discussion on how to "deliver" bad news without precipitating iatrogenic trauma will be addressed.

Overexposure to emotional trauma and loss is an occupational hazard for even the hardiest person. This chapter will examine how providers can recognize the signs of their own secondary or "vicarious traumatization" and identify strategies to prevent or remedy them.

Definitions

Psychological trauma can be defined as a witnessed or experienced event involving actual or threatened death or serious injury, or a threat to the physical integrity of self or others. Threat responses include fear, helplessness, and horror [1]. The person may become "speechless" or alexithymic, feeling absolutely alone even when others are experiencing the same event at the very same time [2–4].

Spectrum of traumatic events

A traumatic event may be variously conceptualized or categorized as *interpersonal* (rape, domestic violence, childhood neglect and abuse), or *disaster-related* (tornados, tsunamis), or *social* (terrorism). Events may be experienced *individually* (accidental injury) or *within a group* framework (wounded soldiers). Motor vehicle accidents are a common example of a traumatic event encountered in emergency department patients and in 1999 were considered to be the highest cause of post-traumatic stress disorder (PTSD) since the Vietnam War [5]. A traumatic event may be a *singular* insult or an *on-going* process, as in the case of child or domestic abuse [2,3]. It is the belief of this author that humiliation may also be a traumatic event, because it threatens the integrity of the person, is akin to "murder" of a person's reputation, and derails a person's sense of integrity and very self [6]. Various examples of traumatic events are detailed in Table 32.1. Of recognized categories, it is believed that interpersonal trauma, particularly in early childhood, leads to the development of PTSD more frequently than other traumas [2,3], because trust in others – often the very person who one needs to trust (a parent, spouse) is thwarted, resulting in the victim's perception of the world as a very dangerous place. It is generally understood that while (repeated) trauma can "erode" the adult personality, it can alter, interfere with and even "deform" normal psychological development of the child and adolescent [2,3]. In general, repetitive events and the younger a person's age at the time of traumatic events are both associated with a higher incidence and severity of PTSD [2,3,7].

Learning of a serious medical diagnosis and experiencing illness itself can be traumatic, as can be the prescribed treatment [8]. Awakening during surgery qualifies as a traumatic event because the patient is alert but unable to move or speak, completely helpless and vulnerable and potentially in pain [9]. Indeed, any physician may be perceived as perpetrator by virtue of the association with painful or difficult treatment, making subsequent ED visits re-traumatizing [2,6]. When conceptualizing humiliation as a traumatic event, the medical encounter itself can be fraught with potentially humiliating events such as disrobing or being subjected to invasive examination and procedures [6]. A routine medical encounter may trigger specific memories of previous trauma, such as rape or other physical insult. Additionally, emergency medicine physicians routinely

Behavioral Emergencies for the Emergency Physician, ed. Leslie S. Zun, Lara G. Chepenik, and Mary Nan S. Mallory. Published by Cambridge University Press. © Cambridge University Press 2013.

Table 32.1. Examples of traumatic events

Motor vehicle accidents	Childhood sexual, physical, or verbal abuse or neglect[a]
Sudden death or injury of close friend	Domestic or interpersonal violence[a]
New diagnoses of serious medical illnesses	Awaking from anesthesia during surgery[a]
Experiencing physical illness; invasive procedures	
Traumatic loss	Humiliation[a]
Abortion, miscarriage	
Directly witnessing loved one hurt or humiliated	Rape[a]
Indirect-media exposure of violence	
Vicarious/secondary traumatization	Death or serious injury notification of a loved one[a]
Media accounts of traumatic events	
Recurrent occupational exposure to others' trauma	
Terrorist attacks	War-time imprisonment (POW)[a]
Being a civilian in a war zone	
Combat exposure	
Natural disasters (tsunamis, hurricanes, earthquakes)	Emergency evacuation or re-location[a]

[a] Denotes an interpersonal traumatic event.

Table 32.2. Potential consequences of a traumatic experience

Aggression
Anger and irritability
Decreased intimacy and interpersonal relationships
Depression
Difficulty trusting others
Medical illnesses
Nonadherence to medical treatments
Personality/attachment disorders (if trauma was in childhood)
Phobias
Sense of foreshortened life or future
Shortened lifespan
Social isolation
Somatization
Substance abuse
Suicide
Work or school impairment

deliver unexpected, "bad" news, i.e., a serious diagnosis, a poor prognosis, the notification of death. Such news can indeed be traumatic for not only the patient and family, but also for care providers, specifically the physician.

Consequences of traumatic events

The consequences of trauma can affect all spheres of a person's life including impaired work and social functioning, with "sub-threshold" symptoms such as discreet startle responses or phobias [10]. Anxiety, depression, or substance abuse may develop as well. PTSD symptoms may be delayed until years after the traumatic event, often triggered by a life-cycle event (birth of a child, retirement) or the onset of a medical illness [11,12]. It has been demonstrated that patients with PTSD have a higher risk of medical comorbidities such as cardiovascular/arterial disease, lower gastrointestinal, dermatological, and muscular skeletal disorders [13]. A more complete listing of consequences is detailed in Table 32.2.

Survivors of trauma are more likely to suffer from multiple medical problems, higher morbidity, and higher mortality [2,14]. Prisoners of war in particular have been noted to have a shortened lifespan [14].

PTSD symptoms and exposure to traumatic events have been associated with greater use of medical services [13] and treatment nonadherence [2,15]. Somatization syndrome without known pathophysiology can also be a feature of PTSD (Herman [3, pp. 59–72;16]).

Epidemiology of disorders associated with acute trauma and loss

Individuals who develop some symptoms of acute stress disorder (ASD) (symptoms of PTSD that remit within 4 weeks of the traumatic event [1]) do not necessarily develop full-blown PTSD, and of those ASD patients who do go on to develop symptoms of PTSD, they are often more resilient and eventually experience some "post-traumatic growth" once their symptoms resolve [17]. Others, who never developed full-blown PTSD, may have "sub-threshold" symptoms as noted above [10].

A traumatic event does not automatically lead to the development of post-traumatic stress disorder. In fact, 85% of adults exposed to a traumatic event do not go on to develop PTSD [2]. Risk factors for the development of PTSD include past history of psychiatric disorder, particularly depression or anxiety, or a family history of psychiatric illness [17]. School-age children and adults between the ages 40 and 60 are considered at higher risk [17–19,21,23]. Female gender increases the risk, as does the association with lower socioeconomic status, lower intelligence, and less education [17,20]. Non-Caucasians are more likely to develop PTSD [19], as are those engaged in litigation or seeking disability compensation [5,17,20]. The severity of the trauma (torture, rape, assault, combat, being physically incapacitated) are highly associated [21–24]. The duration and intensity of the traumatic event(s), i.e., the longer the exposure and the higher the perceived threat to life, the higher the risk for developing PTSD [2,5,22–24]. Horrific and intrusive memories immediately following the traumatic event [5,17,22–24], the inability to make meaning out of the trauma, and feelings of shame or humiliation related to the trauma are also risk factors [3]. Peri-traumatic psychic numbing, dissociative states [27], and hyper-arousal [4,16,25], including elevated heart rate [16,25], may all be risk factors for the development of PTSD.

Protective factors include a relatively small traumatic event, flexibility, "hardiness," and resiliency (the ability to feel the emotions but to continue functioning without impairment, to "bounce back" to one's usual state of being and the ability to self-regulate emotions and physiological reactions [2]); strong social supports, food, shelter, clothing, and ability to maintain one's independence; the ability to return to one's usual routine quickly [2], good coping skills, optimism including the ability for hope in the future; self-confidence, religious connectivity, the belief that for the most part life is predictable and safe, that the traumatic incident was not routine; and the ability to avoid giving excessive meaning to the traumatic event [2, 26].

Also protective is the extent to which a person can use his or her own skills to repair or recover from the trauma (e.g., the ability to physically or monetarily help re-build a school that was damaged in a fire), particularly in the context of a community that comes together for the same cause.

Response to acute trauma

Emotional shock, a "detached calm" [2], feeling "frozen" in fear [16], dissociation, anxiety, and hyper-arousal are immediate psychological responses to acute trauma. Physiologic responses vary. Vasoconstriction can cause the victim to feel physically cold; a vasovagal response may induce fainting [16]. There is speculation that increased heart rate may be a key risk factor for the development of PTSD [12,24]. Van der kolk [4] suggests that an overall state of hyper-arousal immediately following a traumatic event is the major risk factor for developing PTSD. Other studies indicate that dissociation at the time of the traumatic event is the primary risk factor [27]. Alexithymia, as described by Sifneos [28], is one form of dissociation [1,2] as are "fugue" states, partial amnesia, and flashbacks.

During the traumatic event, time may become distorted and seconds may seem as though they are minutes or hours. If the event registers as a sensation rather than a thought, "re-living" the event might be experienced somatically rather than recalled as a verbal memory. Memories of the event may be incomplete, inaccurate, or manifest with partial amnesia, "fugue" states, or "flashbacks." Patients may report the inability to "forget" the trauma, and suffer intrusive thoughts of the event [2,3]. Dissociative experiences may be recalled. For example, Herman [3] describes a patient who at the time of a rape dissociated and found herself "looking from the side of the bed" at herself being raped, and all recollections of the rape were from the "side of the bed" rather than from the perspective of the actual experience on the bed.

The neurophysiology of trauma

Acutely, traumatic events result in increases of both catecholamine release and adrenergic activity [4,29]. Specifically, circulating norepinephrine release is coupled with the enhanced reactivity of alpha 2 adrenergic receptors [29–31]. Remotely, persistent autonomic reactivity in the amygdala can occur even years following direct exposure to a trauma (terrorism) and even in emotionally resilient, asymptomatic individuals [32].

A recent study by Murrough et al. [33] noted a marked reduction in a specific serotonin ligand, [11C]P943 BPND, in the caudate, the amygdala, and the anterior cingulate cortex [33]. Participant age at first trauma exposure was strongly associated with low [11C]P943 BPND.

The amygdala and the hippocampus are the main neuro-anatomical areas affected by acute trauma [4,31]. The amygdala is involved with the fear response, while the hippocampus is involved with the storage of memory (the verbal/cognitive content of the memory). At the time of the traumatic event, the amygdala is hyper-aroused and memories of the event imprint onto it, rather than upon the hippocampus. Thus, the memory is that of sensation, rather than the story of the trauma. Even the slightest reminder of the traumatic event can trigger marked autonomic responses rather than a verbal memory. The patient experiences the memory as a physiologic sensation – as though they were back in time, re-experiencing the trauma.

The amygdala also activates during flashbacks [31]. Anatomically, there is decreased hippocampal volume in patients with PTSD, and such changes may well be permanent [4].

The anterior cingulate is involved with memory, emotion, and selective attention. PTSD patients show under-activation in the anterior cingulate. It is hypothesized that the decreased activity results in failure of the cortex to modulate the responses of the amygdala and diminishes cognitive control in these patients [4,31].

Biochemical changes in trauma

To date, there are no clear biochemical markers to predict ASD or PTSD. Dysregulation of cortisol, serotonin, and the hypothalamic–pituitary axis (HPA axis) occur during the hyper-aroused state of trauma [29,31,33]. Low serum levels of gamma-aminobutyric acid (GABA) [27,38] also appear to be associated with a greater risk for PTSD [27,38]. These changes can be permanent, even in asymptomatic individuals [32].

Van der Kolk postulates that an overall state of hyper-arousal in the immediate aftermath of experiencing a trauma is the major risk factor for developing PTSD, and that all interventions should be aimed at reducing this hyper-aroused state [4].

The concept of resilience

The nature of resilience has become a focus of attention in the literature, both psychologically and at the neurophysiologic and anatomical level [18,34–37]. Impacted as any trauma victim, resilient people do experience acute symptoms of stress, but they are able to move on and re-establish their pre-trauma baseline faster [2]. However, with sufficient exposure, even the most resilient people may develop PTSD [2].

MRI studies have found different changes in the pre-frontal cortex of resilient trauma survivors in contrast to those who have PTSD, suggesting the possibility of a biological predisposition toward resiliency [35]. Specifically, the subgenual prefrontal cortex and nucleus accumbens area may be involved in resilience [36]. In fact, elevated cortisol levels, increased thyrotropin and decreased testosterone, total and free T4, and total and free T3 were found in a group of Special Forces subjects, chosen specifically because of their known resiliency [36].

Management of acute trauma

In the case of rape, there are prescribed workups and teams that care for the victim [38]. For other traumas, there are no such organized protocols. In general, asking the victim to describe the trauma is acceptable if he or she wants to discuss it, but debriefing by pressing the victim to describe the event in detail is contraindicated [38].

People tend to bond during traumas [2]. Thus, emergency departments should allow relatives, friends, and other victims to be together. Because of vasoconstriction, traumatized persons often feel physically cold [16], thus warm blankets and hot drinks should be provided. Chaplains and clinical social workers can assist with comfort measures and communication. A rapid return to a routine schedule is one of the main protective factors in the prevention of PTSD development and should be encouraged [2].

No particular pharmacologic intervention is known to prevent acute stress disorder or its counterpart, PTSD. Intense debriefing is not recommended but listening to volunteered information may be helpful [38,39]. Current thinking is to help the victim physiologically down-regulate. A pilot study by Pitman et al. [40] found a lower incidence of PTSD when propranolol was given to acutely traumatized persons in the ED, but further studies have not been conclusive, precluding the recommendation for routine use of propranolol. Studies of soldiers and children who received morphine for surgical pain and burns found that acute treatment with morphine prevented or reduced the risk of developing PTSD by inhibiting the consolidation of (traumatic) memories [42,43]. However, the absence of larger studies as well as ethical and medico-legal concerns precludes a recommendation for the routine use of morphine as a preventative agent at this time.

Currently in clinical trials, the neurosteroid and anticonvulsant, ganaxolone [44,45], may be a promising treatment for PTSD [45]. Another small study using methlylenedioxymethamphetamine (MDMA), otherwise known as "ecstasy," in combination with intensive psychotherapy, demonstrated improvement in treatment-resistant PTSD without side effects [46]. The proposed indication is being studied in patients with an established PTSD diagnosis, and therefore, would have no place in the ED treatment of de novo psychological trauma. There is no "morning after pill" for trauma victims, nor are there any screening scales to predict who may or may not develop PTSD [47]. For acute sleeping difficulties, anecdotal experience suggests that a few nights of a sleep compound may be of help. A referral for psychiatric care and psychotherapy is indicated for those with persistent sleep difficulty, and for those with impaired functioning due to symptoms of ASD/PTSD or comorbidites of anxiety, depression, and suicidal thoughts [12].

Delivering bad news

It has been said, "If done well, delivering difficult news will always be remembered by the patient and family. Conversely, if not done well, it also will always be remembered by the patient and family" [48–50].

Emergency departments are in themselves traumatic places where people receive unexpected "bad news" – a serious diagnosis, the need for emergency, life-threatening surgery, the loss of a loved one's life. Delivering such news can be traumatic for the physician as well as for the family and patient. It is estimated that the lifetime prevalence of PTSD diagnosis in survivors who were exposed to the news of sudden death is approximately 20% [48]. Much has been written on how to deliver "bad" news, and the reader is referred to these excellent references [48,49,51–55].

Experts agree that clear, concise wording is best – using the word "dead" is preferable to "passed on" or "gone." The physician may have to repeat that the loved one has "died" several times before it starts to "sink in." Sit, don't stand, when telling this news, and make eye contact. Prepare the family for the news, setting the stage: "I have some difficult news to give you, please sit down." Stay with the family for a few minutes after delivering the news and express your sympathy for their loss. Guide the family through the deceased's clinical course from the ambulance to the ED, what interventions were done, and, if known, the likely reasons they did not work. Any remark, which could "lay blame," such as "his lungs were in bad shape because of his smoking," should be avoided. Query the family for their understanding and entertain their questions before leaving the room. Having a nurse or carer in attendance may provide additional support and ongoing family interface. Ask the family if they wish to view the body as this may also help the family who is in shock and cannot believe that their loved one, alive and vibrant one minute and gone the next, is truly dead. [48–54]. Ask if a hospital chaplain would be helpful. The entire process takes no more than 10 or 15 minutes and has the power to help a family deal with their traumatic loss through the ministering of a caring physician and staff [46].

Bereavement and traumatic bereavement

Aside from death, the loss of a body part, of physical function and independence, loss of a pet, a miscarriage or stillbirth, or loss of an ideal can set in motion an emotional crisis and shatter one's worldview. Resolutions of grief may either lead to the deterioration of the person's psychological baseline or promote psychic growth [56].

Bereavement is a normal response to loss, and the general principle is to allow it to occur and not treat it as a medical condition [57]. The acutely bereaved patient may look shocked or startled, or may be crying or sobbing. The bereaved person may be angry or hostile, especially if he or she believes that negligent medical care contributed to the death of their loved one [12]. Cultural differences in the expression and management of bereavement do exist and, although beyond this chapter's scope, they are important for physicians to acknowledge.

Nonwithstanding, there is no way to go through bereavement without painful, anguishing emotions. Henry James tells us that bereavement "comes in waves,. . . . and leaves us on the spot [50]." CS Lewis calls loss from death "an amputation" [58]. Bereavement has its natural history. Clinical experience finds that, just when the acutely bereaved person believes that he can take no more, the acute wave of anguish stops, only to repeat itself later in another spasm of intensely gripping emotional pain. Some people describe somatic symptoms such as stomach aches, choking sensation, or nausea [59]. Hallucinations of "seeing" or "hearing" the deceased may be reported and inexplicably "seeing" the person walking down a street or at random can occur. Such phenomena are normal, and are referred to as "searching behavior." These experiences, coupled with the extremes in mood variation throughout the day, may lead a bereaved person to believe that he is "losing his mind." Reassurance that such reactions are a part of the normal grieving process can bring relief to the bereaved, who are generally unfamiliar with sudden and intense shifts in emotional states and false perceptions [12,57,59].

It is best to let people know that there is no prescribed way to grieve, and that honoring one's dead does not mean stopping one's own life. The bereaved person may feel detached from the world, confused, and angry. Their world has stopped and irrevocably changed, but the rest of the world does not. Day to day activities continue indifferently, while the bereaved person stands stuck in time, pining for the deceased [12]. To properly honor the deceased, some survivors believe a perpetual state of mourning is necessary. Alternatively, others believe that they are not grieving "properly" if they begin to enjoy a piece of music or theater, resume their usual routine, or laugh at a joke. Transient thoughts of suicide in order to join the deceased or guilt over some part of the relationship or death (e.g., "if only I had come home in time I might have witnessed the heart attack") may transiently occur.

As Zisook and Shear eloquently state, the "work of bereavement is best left to the person and his resources; bereavement is a normal part of life, and medical intervention is unnecessary and actually gets in the way of grieving" [57]. Yet, grief is not only about pain. In an uncomplicated grief process, painful experiences are intermingled with emerging positive feelings, such as relief, joy, peace, and happiness. Frequently, these positive feelings elicit negative emotions of disloyalty and guilt in the bereaved [56].

Uncomplicated grief

There is no firm time-line for grieving. The author's clinical experience indicates that 6–12 months tends to be the usual time frame, with the more acute symptoms of bereavement generally lasting 6–12 weeks [12,59]. It was once believed that keeping the deceased belongings indicated a pathological attachment to the deceased, but this is no longer considered pathological [12]. By the end of the first year, there is usually an integration of the loss; the deceased is remembered, and the importance of the lost relationship is not diminished, but has changed. Thus, there remains a "place in one's heart" [60] for the deceased, but that affection does not interfere with forming new relationships [61]. The ability to grieve, yet continue to function in one's life beyond the initial phase of bereavement (1–3 weeks), is key [12,59]. Not all emergency department deaths are unexpected. In fact, the first evidence-based study of uncomplicated bereavement was done in 2007. Acceptance, rather than denial, was the first response to hearing of the *expected* death of a loved-one [59].

Complicated grief

Symptoms of complicated grief resemble that of ASD or PTSD. Complicated, prolonged, delayed, and traumatic grieving are conceptual variations now being studied [12,56,57,62–65]. Prolonged pining or longing, continued emotional lability or dysregulation, an inability to return to usual work and social involvement, the development of major depression, and painful, intrusive, non-comforting thoughts of the deceased are the main features of a difficult grieving process. Continued disbelief or anger, survivor guilt, functional impairments including substance abuse and somatic symptoms are also features. Impaired grieving is, however, distinctly different from clinical depression; the bereaved self-esteem remains intact, guilty ruminations and even suicidal thinking are specific to the deceased. In distinguishing normal from traumatic grief, a bereaved person can talk about the loss and the deceased; the person with complicated or traumatic grief often cannot without great difficulty and may even refuse to speak about the death. The predominant affect with uncomplicated grief is sadness; in complicated grief it is prolonged pining, and in traumatic grief it is often terror or fear. Nightmares and painful or horrific visual images are noted in traumatic grief. Intrusive thoughts of the deceased are painful and do not bring comfort [2,12,62,65], whereas, the mourner with uncomplicated grief welcomes dreams of the deceased, and generally finds them comforting [2]. As with the patient with PTSD, the person suffering from traumatic grief may have a sense of foreshortened future and meaninglessness [2].

Chronic or prolonged bereavement is noted by an inability to move on – a death occurring years ago may still be as acutely painful and fresh as it was initially. If the mourner has been dependent upon the deceased, the potential for complicated bereavement increases. In some cases, where family members stay home, give up jobs, or move to care for an ill loved-one, once the death of that person occurs, the mourner's sense of meaning and purpose may be shattered. In other words, the mourner became "dependent" on the deceased to provide them with a sense of meaning and purpose, and now they must re-define their role and sense of meaning [12].

A higher risk of mortality exists among those with compli-cated grief; thus, attention must be paid to the physical health of the patient [48,51,56,62]. Somatization has been reported in persons who suffer from pathological grief and may present as stomachaches, chest pain, gastrointestinal complaints, and headaches [59,62]. Some mourners will report insomnia, and while medication is contraindicated for acute grief, some [66] medication for sleep may be in order to allow the person to continue to function during the day [12,60].

Traumatic grief

Traumatic grief occurs when there is a sudden, unplanned, particularly grotesque or stigmatized death [2,12,62,65]. The death of a small child's parent is very traumatic, as is the loss of a child. The first study of bereavement was done by Lindemann in 1944 [67]. Given the nature of his subjects' losses (a sudden, traumatic fire which took the lives of many and nearly the lives of many others, including some of the bereaved persons), it is fair to speculate that what Lindemann described was actually "traumatic," rather than uncomplicated bereavement [12]. The symptoms of traumatic grief vary from those of typical bereave-ment and are outlined in Table 32.3.

Traumatic grief is a risk factor for mental and physical morbidity [62], including an increased incidence of suicide within the first 2 years of bereavement [65]. The emergency clinician must be watchful for exacerbations of underlying psychiatric illnesses and comorbidities such as clinical depression, psychoses, and substance abuse. There is a higher incidence of cardiac illness, hypertension, and cancer in trau-matically bereaved persons [62]. Thus, for patients who present to the ED with unexplainable physical complaints and new or worsening psychiatric symptoms, an inquiry into recent loss or trauma is indicated. An evaluation of suicidal thinking should also be included [62].

Vicarious traumatization

Emergency medicine is as difficult as it is rewarding. Compassion fatigue, burnout, and vicarious traumatization are terms often used interchangeably. However, vicarious trau-matization (also named secondary traumatization or compas-sion fatigue) is a specific condition; a result of overexposure to trauma, is unrelated to "burnout," and can occur quite fre-quently in skilled and seasoned clinicians because of their capacity for empathy and years of exposure to trauma.

Table 32.3. Symptom comparison between bereavement and traumatic grief

Activity	Symptom response	
	Bereavement	Traumatic grief
Thinking or talking about the deceased	Comforting recollections, encourages conversation about deceased	Painful, wrenching sadness
		Intrusive, unwanted thoughts
		Horror, terror, fear, anger
		Potential for aggression avoidant thinking
Mood	Temporary feelings of sadness and/or anger	Chronic sadness and anger, clinical depression
Social functioning	Not impaired	Chronically impaired in several spheres
		Social isolation
		Poor concentration at work
Sleep	Transient impairment, replaced often by pleasant dreams of reuniting	Grotesque, terrifying nightmares
Sense of future	Future oriented	Sense of foreshortened life and no future
Relationship with deceased	Integrating the loss enduring, but different attachment to deceased making new relationships	"Stuck" in the loss of the relationship

Warning signs of vicarious traumatization include distancing, psychic numbing, somatization, "shutting down," loss of empa-thy, excessive or punitive limit setting, or alternatively, over-identification with the patient [2,68].

Risk factors for the development of secondary traumatiza-tion include both the intensity and frequency of exposure to others' traumatic losses, exposure to children's trauma, and the lack of variation in clinical practice beyond treating trauma patients and survivors. Clinicians with a past history of personal trauma, those who minimize their own personal or family's needs, and those "addicted" to the adrenalin rush are specifically at risk. New clinicians and those without awareness of the possibility of vicarious traumatization are also at risk. Proper supervision and administrative oversight is essential to prevent work over-load. However, with the cumu-lative exposure to the traumatic events and stories of their patients even emotionally healthy, senior clinicians may develop secondary traumatization and develop full-blown symptoms of PTSD [2].

Preventative strategies are key [2]. Varying the patient panel and practicing self-awareness of personal emotions and reactions to work events are important. Social interaction, healthy nutrition, sleep maintenance, and regular exercise are recognized habits for wellness maintenance. Planned breaks away from clinical practice and vacationing are recommended. Some hospitals and clinics provide support groups, yoga, meditation, and other activities to assist their staff in taking care of themselves. Some clinicians will require professional care, and may need referral to mental health professionals with care and sensitivity [69].

References

1. American Psychiatric Association. *Diagnostic and Statistical Manual of Mental Disorders: DSM-IV-TR.* (4th Edition). Text revision. Washington, DC: American Psychiatric Association; 2000.

2. Israel Center for the Treatment of Psychotrauma; Rothburg International School of the Hebrew University of Jerusalem. *International Course. Trauma & Resilience: Theory & Practice from the Israeli Experience.* Jerusalem: Israel Center for the Treatment of Psychotrauma; 2010.

3. Herman J. *Trauma and Recovery.* New York: Basic Books; 1997.

4. van der Kolk BA. The complexity of adaptation to trauma. In: Van der Kolk BA, McFarlane MD, Weisaeth L, (Eds.). *Traumatic Stress: the Effects of Overwhelming Experiences on Mind, Body, and Society.* New York: Guilford; 1996: 183–205.

5. Butler DJ, Moffic S, Turkal NW. Post-traumatic stress reactions following motor vehicle accidents. *Am Fam Physician* 1999;**60**:524–31.

6. Lazare A. Shame and humiliation in the medical encounter. *Arch Intern Med* 1987;**147**:1653–8.

7. Dannlowski U, Stuhrmann A, Beutelmann V, Zwanzger P. Limbic scars: long-term consequences of childhood maltreatment revealed by functional and structural magnetic resonance imaging. *Biol Psychiatry* 2012;**71**:286–93.

8. Doerfler LA, Pbert L, DeCosimo D. Symptoms of posttraumatic stress disorder following myocardial infarction and coronary artery bypass surgery. *Gen Hosp Psychiatry* 1994;**16**:193–9.

9. Osterman JE, Hooper J, Heran WJ, Keane TM, van der Kolk BA. Awareness under anesthesia and the development of posttraumatic stress disorder. *Gen Hosp Psychiatry* 2001;**23**:198–204.

10. Marshall RD, Olfson M, Hellman F, et al. Comorbidity, impairment, and suicidality in subthreshold PTSD. *Am J Psychiatry* 2001;**158**:1467–73.

11. Richmond JS, Beck J. Posttraumatic stress disorder in a World War II veteran. *Am J Psychiatry* 1986;**143**:1485–6.

12. Richmond JS. Trauma and loss. In: Glick RL, Berlin JS, Fishkind A, Zeller SL, (Eds.). *Emergency Psychiatry: Principles and Practice.* Philadelphia: Lippincott William & Wilkins; 2008: 255–64.

13. Stein MB, MQuaid JR, Pedrelli P, Lenox R, McCahill ME. Posttraumatic stress disorder in the primary care medical setting. *Gen Hosp Psychiatry* 2000;**22**:261–9.

14. Boscarino JA. Prospective study of PTSD and early-age heart disease mortality among Vietnam veterans: implications for surveillance and prevention. *Psychosom Med* 2008;**70**:668–76.

15. Shemesh E, Rudnick A, Kaluski E, et al. A prospective study of posttraumatic stress symptoms and nonadherence in survivors of a myocardial infarction (MI). *Gen Hosp Psychiatry* 2001;**23**:215–22.

16. Bracha HS. Freeze, flight, fight, fright, faint: adaptationist perspectives on the acute stress response spectrum. *CNS Spectr* 2004;**9**:679–85.

17. Price JL. *Findings from the National Vietnam Veterans' Readjustment Study –* National Center for PTSD United States Department of Veterans Affairs; September 21, 2011. Available at: http://www.ptsd.va.gov/professional/pages/vietnam-vets-study.asp (Accessed January 4, 2012).

18. Chalsa ML. *PTSD Among Ethnic Minority Veterans.* United States Department of Veterans Affairs; 2012. Available at: http://www.ptsd.va.gov/professional/pages/ptsd-minority-vets.asp (Accessed January 4, 2012).

19. Foa EB D Davidson RT, Frances A. The expert consensus guidelines series: treatment of traumatic stress disorder. *J Clin Psychiatry* 1999;**60**:1–79.

20. Breslau N, Lucia VC, Alvarado G. Intelligence and other predisposing factors in exposure to trauma and post traumatic stress disorder. *Arch Gen Psychiatry* 2006;**63**:1238–45.

21. Kennedy R. *PTSD: The Trauma After the Trauma.* 2002. Available at: http://www.medscape.com/viewarticle/441133 (Accessed August 10, 2012).

22. Yehuda R, McFarlane AC, Shalev AY. Predicting the development of posttraumatic stress disorder from the acute response to a traumatic event. *Biol Psychiatry* 1998;**15**:1305–13.

23. Bryant RA, Marosszeky JE, Crooks J, Gurka JA. Elevated resting heart rate as a predictor of posttraumatic stress disorder after severe traumatic brain injury. *Psychosom Med* 2004;**66**:760–1.

24. Shalev AY, Sahar T, Freedman S, et al. A prospective study of heart rate responses following trauma and the subsequent development of posttraumatic stress disorder. *Arch Gen Psychiatry* 1998;**55**:553–9.

25. Wild ND, Paivio SC. Psychological adjustment, coping, and emotional regulation as predictors of posttraumatic growth. *J Aggress Maltreat Trauma* 2003;**18**:97–122.

26. Foa EB, Davidson RT, Frances A. The expert consensus guidelines series: treatment of traumatic stress disorder. *J Clin Psychiatry* 1999;**60**:1–79.

27. Feeny NC, Zoellner LA, Fitzgibbons LA, Foa EB. Exploring the roles of emotional numbing, depression, and dissociation in PTSD. *J Trauma Stress* 2000;**13**:489–98.

28. Sifneos PE. Alexithymia: past and present. *Am J Psychiatry* 1996;**153** (Suppl):137–42.

29. Clayton NM, Nash WP. Medication management of combat and operational stress injuries in active duty service members. In: Figley CR, Nash WP, (Eds.). *Combat Stress Injury.* New York: Routledge; 2007: 219–45.

30. Yehuda R. Post-traumatic stress disorder. *N Engl J Med* 2002;**346**:43–9.

31. Nash WP, Baker DG. Competing and complementary models of combat stress

Injury. In: Figley CR, Nash WP, (Eds.). *Combat Stress Injury.* New York: Routledge; 2007: 65–94.

32. Tucker PM, Pfefferbaum B, North CS, et al. Physiologic reactivity despite emotional resilience several years after direct exposure to terrorism. *Am J Psychiatry* 2007;**164**:230–5.

33. Murrough JW, Czermak C, Henry S, et al. The effect of early trauma exposure on serotonin type 1B receptor expression revealed by reduced selective radioligand binding. *Arch Gen Psychiatry* 2011;**68**:892–900.

34. Brom D, Path-Horenczyk RJD, Ford JD. Resilience and the capacity to process traumatic experiences. In: Brom D, Path-Horenczyk RJD, Ford J, (Eds.). *Treating Traumatized Children: Risk, Resilience and Recovery.* London: Routledge;

35. New AS, Fan J, Murrough JW, et al. A functional magnetic resonance imaging study of deliberate emotion regulation in resilience and posttraumatic stress disorder. *Biol Psychiatry* 2009;**66**:656–64.

36. Vythilingam M, Nelson EE, Scaramozza M, et al. Reward circuitry in resilience to severe trauma: an fMRI investigation of resilient special forces soldiers. *Psychiatry Res* 2009;**172**:75–7.

37. Morgan CA III, Wang S, Mason J, et al. Hormone profiles in humans experiencing military survival training. *Biol Psychiatry* 2000;**47**:891–901.

38. Linden JA. Care of the adult patient after sexual assault. *N Engl J Med* 2011;**365**:834–41.

39. Gray M, Litz B, Papa T. Crisis debriefing: what helps, and what may not? *Curr Psychiatry* 2006;**5**:17–29.

40. Pitman RK, Sanders KM, Zusman RM, et al. Pilot study of secondary prevention of posttraumatic stress disorder with propranolol. *Biol Psychiatry* 2002;**15**:189–92.

41. Hoge EA, Worthington JJ, Nagurney JT, et al. Effect of acute posttrauma propranolol on PTSD outcome and physiological responses during script-driven imagery. *CNS Neurosci Ther* 2012;**18**:21–7.

42. Holbrook TL, Galarneau MR, Dye JL, Quinn K, Dougherty AL. Morphine use after combat injury in Iraq and post-traumatic stress disorder. *N Engl J Med* 2010;**362**:110–17.

43. Saxe G, Stoddard F, Courtney D. Relationship between acute morphine and the course of PTSD in children with burns. *J Am Acad Child Adolesc Psychiatry* 2001;**40**:915–21.

44. United States National Institutes of Health (NIH). *Post-traumatic Stress Disorder – Traumatic Brain Injury Clinical Consortium.* 2012. Available at: http://clinicaltrials.gov/ct2/show/NCT01339689; clinical trials.gov (Accessed January 12, 2012).

45. Marx CRA. *A Proof-of-concept, Double-blind, Randomized, Placebo-controlled Study of Ganaxolone in Posttraumatic Stress Disorder.* 2012. [Clinical trial of ganaxolone in patient with PTSD]. Available at: http://intrust.sdsc.edu/ganaxolone.html (Accessed January 12, 2012).

46. Mithoefer MC, Wagner MT, Mithoefer AT, Jerome L, Doblin R. The safety and efficacy of {+/-}3,4-methylenedioxymethamphetamine-assisted psychotherapy in subjects with chronic, treatment-resistant posttraumatic stress disorder: the first randomized controlled pilot study. *J Psychopharmacol* 2011;**25**:439–52.

47. Friedman MJ. Prevention of psychiatric problems among military personnel and their spouses. *N Engl J Med* 2010;**362**:168–70.

48. Hobgood C. Grief, death and dying, DNR/DNI orders: delivering effective death notifications in the emergency department. In: Tintinalli JE, Stapczynski J, Cline DM, Ma OJ, Cydulka RK, Meckler GD, (Eds.). *Tintinalli's Emergency Medicine: A Comprehensive Study Guide,* (7th Edition). New York: McGraw-Hill; 2011: 297.

49. Radziewicz R, Baile W. Communication skills: breaking bad news in the clinical setting. *Oncol Nurs Forum* 2001;**28**:1–3.

50. Applewhite A, Evans T. *And I Quote: The Definitive Collection of Quotes, Sayings, and Jokes for the Contemporary Speechmaker,* (Revised Edition). New York: Thomas Dunne Books; 2003: 129.

51. Gaehde S. *Delivering Bad News.* Boston MA: Boston VA Medical Center.

52. *Delivering Bad News.* Available at: www4.uwm.edu/libraries/ereserve/kako/csbbns.pdf (Accessed September 19, 2011).

53. Miranda J Brody RV. Communicating bad news (Commentary). *West J Med* 1992;**156**:83–5.

54. Buckman R. Breaking bad news: why is it still difficult? *Br Med J (Clin Res Ed)* 1984;**288**:1597–9.

55. Rabow MW, McPhee SJ. Beyond breaking bad news: how to help patients who suffer. *West J Med* 1999;**17**:260–3.

56. Raphael B. *The Anatomy of Bereavement.* New York: Basic Books; 1983.

57. Zisook S, Shear K. Grief and bereavement: what psychiatrists need to know. *World Psychiatry* 2009;**8**:67–74.

58. Lewis CS. *A Grief Observed.* New York: Harper Collins; 1961.

59. Maciejewski PK, Zhang B, Block SD, et al. An empirical examination of the stage theory of grief. *JAMA* 2007;**297**:716–23.

60. Shader RI. Bereavement reactions and grief. In: Shader RI, (Ed.). *Manual of Psychiatric Therapeutics,* (3rd Edition). Philadelphia: Lippincott Williams & Wilkins; 2003.

61. Zerbe KJ, Steinberg DL. Coming to terms with grief and loss: can skills for dealing with bereavement be learned? *Postgrad Med* 2000;**108**:97–8, 101–4, 6.

62. Prigerson HG, Bierhals AJ, Kasl SV, et al. Traumatic grief as a risk factor for mental and physical morbidity *Am J Psychiatry* 1997;**154**:616–23.

63. Prigerson HG, Shear MK, Frank E, et al. Traumatic grief: a case of loss-induced trauma. *Am J Psychiatry* 1997;**1**:1003–9.

64. Zisook S, Simon NM, Reynolds CF III, et al. Bereavement, complicated grief, and DSM, part 2: complicated grief. *J Clin Psychiatry* 2010;**71**:1097–8.

65. Boelen PA, Van den Bout J, De Keijser J. Traumatic grief as a disorder distinct from bereavement-related depression and anxiety: a replication study with bereaved mental health care patients. *Am J Psychiatry* 2003;**160**:1339–41.

66. Piper WE, Ogrodniczuk JS, Joyce AS, et al. Ambivalence and other relationship

predictors of grief in psychiatric outpatients. *J Nerv Ment Dis* 2001;**189**:781–7.

67. Lindemann E. Symptomatology and management of acute grief. *Am J Psychiatry* 1944;**101**:141–8.

68. Figley CR. Compassion fatigue psychotherapists' chronic lack of self care. *J Clin Psychol* 2002;**58**:1433–41.

69. *Mental Health Effects Following Disaster: Risk and Resilience Factors:* Professional Pages National Center for PTSD, U.S. Department of Veterans' Affairs http://www.ptsd.va. gov/professional/pages/effects-disasters-mental-health.asp. (Accessed February 27, 2012).

Chapter 33

Management of homeless and disadvantaged persons in the emergency department

Louis Scrattish and Valerie Carroll

Introduction

Homeless persons with mental illness frequent emergency rooms at a disproportionately higher rate than other populations due to myriad factors [1–3]. Providing optimum care for these patients requires that emergency healthcare workers understand their circumstances and unique needs. This chapter begins by describing the epidemiology of homelessness and mental illness in the United States, and by exploring some of the unique factors faced by this population. The chapter concludes by discussing the process of assessing and providing care for these patients while reflecting on systemic challenges for improving emergency care for patients with homelessness and mental illness.

Homelessness in the United States

It is estimated that 2.5 to 3.5 million people currently experience homelessness in the United States each year [1]. Approximately 100 million persons worldwide experience homelessness [2]. U.S. Department of Health and Urban Development found that 643,000 persons in the United States were homeless on an average night in 2009 [3]. A study from 2,988 U.S. counties and 1,056 U.S. cities found that 1.56 million people spent at least one night in a shelter that year [3]. The total number of persons who experienced homelessness as individuals decreased by 5%, and the number of homeless families increased for the second year in a row [4]. Nearly half of the homeless population is families with children, making it the fastest growing segment of the homeless population [1].

The homeless population in the United States is comprised of single men (44%), single women (13%), families with children (36%), and unaccompanied minors (7%) [5]. The 2008 U.S. Conference of Mayors estimated the composition of the homeless to be 42% African-American, 39% Caucasian, 13% Hispanic, 4% Native American and 2% Asian. However, these percentages vary widely, depending on the part of the country assessed [6]. Between one fourth and one third of homeless persons have a serious mental illness, 13% of homeless individuals are physically disabled, 19% are victims of domestic

violence, 13% are veterans [2], and 19% of homeless people are employed [2,6,7].

Recent demographic trends demonstrate that the number of chronically homeless persons on a single night in January 2009 dropped more than 10% from 2008 and nearly 30% from levels reported in 2006 to 111,000 [3]. Additionally, a study of adolescents found a 7.6% rate of at least 1 night of homelessness within a year [8]. However, the number of sheltered homeless persons in families increased by almost 19,000 people or 3.6% [3]. The majority of homeless individuals are currently middle-aged men of minority background, and 38% of them have some sort of disability [3].

Medical problems affecting the homeless population

The average homeless person in the United States has eight to nine medical conditions [9]. Studies have reported high rates of skin and foot disease, chronic obstructive pulmonary disease, peripheral vascular disease, arthritis and other musculoskeletal disorders, nutritional deficiencies, sexually transmitted infections (STIs) including HIV and hepatitis, alcoholism and other substance abuse, and mental disorders [10]. Traumas, particularly falls and motor vehicle accidents, are leading causes of morbidity and mortality in the homeless [11]. Respiratory infections and poor dentition are common [12]. Frostbite and hypothermia affect the homeless in the winter, while severe sunburns and heat strokes occur in the summer [13]. Chronic medical conditions including diabetes and hypertension often go undetected or untreated for long periods of time [14]. Poor nutrition can complicate chronic medical conditions. Homeless persons have decreased access to health services and increased rates of noncompliance [7]. Basic needs such as food and shelter often take priority over mental health care [7]. Lack of housing and a place to store medications while avoiding theft further complicate compliance for homeless patients.

Infectious diseases are more prevalent in homeless populations than the general population. Studies of homeless populations have reported 6.2–35% rates of HIV, 17–30% rates

Behavioral Emergencies for the Emergency Physician, ed. Leslie S. Zun, Lara G. Chepenik, and Mary Nan S. Mallory. Published by Cambridge University Press. © Cambridge University Press 2013.

of hepatitis B, 12–30% rates of hepatitis C, 1.2–6.8% rates of active tuberculosis, 3.8–56% rates of scabies, and 2–30% rates of *Bartonella quintana* infection transmitted from body lice [2]. Gonorrhea and chlamydia are also more prevalent in the homeless [15]. Risk factors prevalent in the homeless include intravenous drug use, prostitution, multiple sexual partners, and inconsistent use of condoms [15]. A study of Boston homeless found AIDS to be the leading cause of mortality in homeless persons age 25–44 [16].

Mortality in the homeless is significantly higher than the general population. Studies in the United States and Canada reported an approximately 4-fold, age-adjusted increased death rate in the homeless [11,17,18]. A study of 17,292 homeless adults in Boston found the following to be the leading causes of death in 3 different age groups: homicide in men ages 18–24, AIDS in men and women ages 25–44, and cancer and heart disease in persons 45–64 (16). The average life expectancy in the homeless population is between 42–52 years of age compared to 78 for the general population [19].

Mental illness in the homeless

Psychiatric illness, particularly schizophrenia, bipolar disorder, and major depression, have a high prevalence in the homeless population [6,7]. It is estimated that between one fourth and one third of homeless persons have a major psychiatric illness such as schizophrenia or bipolar disorder [7]. The number of homeless persons with mental illness in the United States began increasing in the mid-1950s with the de-institutionalization of the mentally ill [20]. In 1963, the Community Mental Health Centers Act was passed to shift resources for the mentally ill from inpatient hospitals to outpatient community centers [21]. Over the past 50 years, the number of occupied state hospital beds has decreased from 339 to 29 per 100,000 persons [22]. At the same time, resources such as housing, food, and treatment centers have failed to keep pace, contributing to high numbers of persons with mental illness becoming homeless [22].

Studies have found that the homeless mentally ill are only marginally served by community mental health centers [23]. In the 1980s, federal spending cuts reduced low income housing availability, further reducing basic resources for this population. From 1970 to 1985, low-cost rental units were cut from 6.5 million to 5.6 million while the number of low-income renter households had grown from 6.2 million to 8.9 million [24]. Studies show that the homeless constitute 15–18% of psychiatric admissions [7]. Homeless patients receive more care for mental health issues in hospitals than in outpatient clinics, compared to their domiciled peers [7].

Homeless persons tend to have a high risk of current or past physical and sexual abuse [25,26]. Homeless youths often have a history of extensive familial abuse, poor parental supervision, and parental substance abuse [25]. Abuse and neglect increase the propensity for mental illness, including depression, anxiety, and PTSD. Physical or sexual

abuse can be the sentinel event inciting development of PTSD [25].

Substance abuse

High rates of alcohol and substance abuse in the homeless population compound the psychiatric and medical problems [10]. A review of epidemiologic studies found alcohol abuse affects 30–40% and drug abuse 10–15% of homeless persons [27]. One study of homeless patients found 72% experienced drug abuse or addiction and 51% experienced alcohol abuse or dependence [28]. Approximately 10–20% of homeless patients have a dual diagnosis of mental illness and substance use disorders [29]. Homeless patients have higher rates of psychiatric admissions and higher mental health treatment costs when compared with domiciled patients [7].

Homeless patients in the emergency department

Homeless persons use the emergency department (ED) at a higher rate than non-homeless. In a survey of 117 million ED visits in 2007, 542,000 visits were for homeless patients, a rate twice that of their domiciled counterparts (71.8 compared with 35.9 visits per 100 persons) [30]. In San Francisco, a study found housed patients averaged 1.6 visits to the ED each year, whereas their homeless counterparts averaged 2.5 visits yearly [31]. Another study reported similar results in Boston [32].

According to a study of 1260 homeless adults in New York City in the ED, a large proportion of these visits were for trauma and victimization, with resulting limb fractures, concussions, burns, and skull fractures [33]. These types of injuries were seen 30 times more frequently when compared to the general population. Despite high rates of psychiatric illness and substance abuse in the homeless, these were not the chief reasons patients visited EDs in that particular study. However, untreated mental illness and substance abuse are risk factors for injuries [33].

Hospital assessment and interventions

In general, the assessment of homeless patients with psychiatric complaints follows a process similar to domiciled persons. However, there are several areas in which the patient's homeless status should be given special consideration. The following section will discuss these considerations and further illustrate them using case studies. We will begin this section by giving several illustrations of the circumstances leading to an ED visit by a patient who is homeless.

Case example: Phil

Phil is a 41-year-old male with a documented history of bipolar disorder and alcohol dependence. He was diagnosed with bipolar disorder at the age of 21 and became homeless at approximately the same age. He travels in and out of homeless shelters, especially during the winter months. He has had multiple ED visits for violent behavior and has been admitted to the state psychiatric facility many times. Social workers state that he is often quite quiet and calm right after leaving psychiatric facilities, but then describe that he later becomes more aggressive, loud, and sometimes violent. They believe this is because he frequently quits taking his medications once back on the streets.

Phil has currently been out of the hospital for approximately 1 month, and workers at the local homeless shelter have noticed an increase in Phil's aggressive behavior (yelling at colleagues, talking back to staff) in the last few days. Today Phil threatened a worker.

Case example: Kim

Kim is a 19-year-old mother of two young children. She left her mom's house 2 months ago for the third time after her mom's boyfriend physically assaulted her. She has been staying in different shelters around the city since then. In the past, she has taken sertraline and alprazolam for depression and anxiety. Kim was brought to the ED by paramedics when she had a panic attack after being threatened by her children's father. She complains of feeling increasingly depressed, but denies current or past suicidal or homicidal ideation. She has been obtaining food and clothing for herself and her children from shelters and volunteer centers. She has had multiple panic attacks in the past several months without going to the emergency room, but has been to three different ERs recently for trauma. She has been focusing her energy and resources on getting her children to and from school and looking for work, so she has been unable to address her deteriorating mental health.

Case example: George

George is a 52-year-old man with schizophrenia who has been homeless and in and out of psychiatric hospitals his entire adult life. He has been obtaining treatment at a community health center where he is briefly assessed, receives haloperinol decanoate injections every 2–3 weeks and counseling when necessary. He missed his last injection 2 weeks ago because he was unable to afford the bus fare. He presented to the clinic earlier today, but it was closed. He is experiencing auditory hallucinations of friends who have passed away, but denies suicidal or homicidal ideation. He presents to the ED today for a prescription refill.

Mode of arrival

Homeless patients with psychiatric complaints tend to arrive in EDs by means of emergency medical services (EMS) and police at a disproportionally higher rate than domiciled patients. Additionally, they tend to arrive more often alone: without family, friends, or caregivers [34]. This makes obtaining a

detailed description especially challenging, prompting the following considerations:

- Why were police or EMS originally called? For example, was the patient found in a situation that could cause immediate danger to herself or others? Conversely were authorities alerted because the patient was found in a park after hours or loitering in a public place?
- Who originally called EMS or police? This could give the ED caregiver contacts that would aid in further data gathering. For example, if the original EMS call came from a worker at a homeless shelter, it may be possible to obtain more detailed information regarding the patient's actions, the trajectory of symptoms, and whether or not similar episodes have occurred in the past.
- Is the patient known to the transferring providers? In some cases, certain individuals may be known to police, helping to assess whether the current presentation is similar to past occurrences, or seems distinctly different.

This process of gathering information from people other than the patient is known as gathering collateral history, and is of added importance in the care of homeless patients [34]. Finally, it is highly recommended to have the transferring personnel fill out a description of what occurred, preferably in a petition. This is especially important if the ED provider believes the patient may be in need of involuntary emergency psychiatric admission. As a legal document, it is more compelling when the people who may have actually witnessed dangerous or self-harming acts give a written account of what happened.

Case example: Phil, continued

In Phil's case, EMS brought Phil in to the ED and left before the ED providers spoke to them. Phil denies any pain or concerns and the ambulance run sheet is unclear, stating the patient was brought in for agitation. The EMS team is called to come back to ER, where they provide the additional history obtained from workers at the homeless shelter. They then fill out a petition detailing Phil's actions at the shelter. The ED and psychiatry staff then decide to involuntarily admit Phil to the psychiatry service as they deem him to be an acute danger to others.

Evaluation of medical stability

With all ED patients, the ED caregiver's primary role is to rapidly assess any patient for signs of medical instability. This is done by assessing vital signs and conducting a rapid primary survey to evaluate signs of serious medical conditions that may be mimicking a psychiatric condition. Treatment of the homeless patient is no exception: the initial evaluation is particularly important because it has been shown that homeless persons have higher rates of untreated medical conditions such as uncontrolled diabetes, trauma, and hypothermia that should be ruled out before psychiatric evaluation [10].

Chief complaint and history of present illness

This part of the ED evaluation is quite uniform whether or not the patient happens to be homeless. However, more research may be needed when the patient is homeless since she or he often arrives without family, friends, or other caregivers. Patients who are psychotic or lack insight regarding the nature of their illness are often limited historians. In these cases, obtaining information regarding the chief complaint and history of present illness from EMS, witnesses, or other community members can be helpful. Patients in this situation may also present multiple times for multiple different complaints, so a thorough review of past visits may provide clues as to why the patient came to the ED.

Past medical history

As homeless patients are known to have a higher prevalence of many comorbid conditions [16], it is critical to determine this history. This again may require gathering of collateral history and possibly review of charts from previous visits. As homeless patients also have higher rates of drug noncompliance [35], it is especially important to inquire about whether or when medications have been taken.

Past psychiatric history

As stated in previous chapters, it is critical to ask any psychiatric patient about known diagnoses, past hospitalizations, suicide attempts, and violent outbursts. It is especially critical to ask the homeless patient about past or current treatment relationships, as they are known to have less access to outpatient care [34]. Specifically, what is the nature of the psychiatric care being rendered, how often has this care been given, and have medications been recently prescribed or administered?

Psychosocial history

It is especially important to ask a homeless psychiatric patient about her or his psychosocial history and present circumstances because it may affect the patient's ultimate disposition. Specific questions may be aimed at evaluating a patient's childhood, social network, educational history, employment or other monetary sources, and past incarceration. Additional questions aimed at past or ongoing physical, emotional, and/or sexual abuse may give clues to experiences which may have triggered psychiatric conditions such as antisocial behavior or PTSD. For example, it has been shown that homeless patients have higher rates of incarceration [36] and physical and sexual trauma [37]. The clinician should also assess the patient's cognitive functioning and ability to care for self. The patient's current circumstances, such as present sleeping location, access to community behavior health sources, and reliable food sources may help to elucidate why the patient's condition has deteriorated to the point of an ED visit.

Case example: Kim, continued

With no source of income, Kim is struggling to keep two children fed, clothed, and in school. She has been physically and sexually abused by her mom's boyfriends throughout her life as well as by the father of her children. She has also suffered from depression since adolescence. She is currently depressed and anxious, but not suicidal or homicidal. Her laboratory results are unremarkable and her symptoms improve with lorazepam. The crisis worker meets with her and arranges for an appointment with a psychiatrist and a therapist. The social worker also meets with her and refers her to the public aid office and employment assistance resources.

History of chemical use

As stated previously in this chapter, homeless patients have higher rates of alcohol and drug use compared to the domiciled population [10]. History of prior use can increase risk for comorbid medical problems including malnutrition, hepatitis, and other communicable diseases. Current drug use may also sway the decision of the ED medical provider in terms of disposition. For example, a patient with current alcohol abuse may be at increased risk of hypothermia or exposure compared to domiciled patients.

Assessment and disposition

The assessment of the homeless psychiatric patient, for the most part, will follow the assessment of any other patient with psychiatric complaints, which is detailed in previous chapters. However, there are aspects of this population that warrant special consideration.

In assessing a homeless psychiatric patient, the ED provider must take into account the fact that access to outpatient care is often more difficult. These patients often lack the resources to locate clinics or mental health centers which provide affordable or free health care. They may not have a cell phone or access to a phone to schedule an appointment. Clinicians may not be able to contact the patient, making follow-up challenging. Reliable transportation can be more difficult for low-income and homeless patients to access. In addition, lack of consistent housing makes it difficult to safely store medications and medical supplies, especially if refrigeration is required.

In terms of patient disposition, there is broad agreement that any patient who is in imminent danger of killing themselves or others likely requires admission, involuntarily if necessary. It is much less clear when to admit a patient, especially against her or his will, when the main concern is "grave disability." In other words, when does a patient's inability to consistently care for her or himself become serious enough to warrant taking away her- or his free will? While this difficult question comes into play regardless of housing status, it becomes more pronounced in the homeless population as the lack of consistent housing can exacerbate the risk of being unable to care for oneself. Below are several examples in which homelessness may put a psychiatric patient at increased risk of unintended physical harm:

- The inability to ward off hypothermia or hyperthermia. While most cities do have increased shelter capacity during inclement weather, these underfunded facilities still face considerable bed shortages during weather emergencies.
- A decreased ability to safely store medications, as described above.
- An increased risk of assault or battery [33].
- A decreased ability to store and prepare foods. This is especially important when dealing with food items that may be a part of a specific medical diet. For example, plenty of fresh, low-sodium vegetables as advised by a primary healthcare provider for someone with diabetes and hypertension.
- Inconsistent access to means of communication. Patients with lack of housing may lack a private land-line through which to communicate with medical providers. They also may lack the ability to pay for cellular phone services, and most likely will have a harder time keeping these devices from being stolen or damaged. Homeless patients may also have a more difficult time receiving mail in a timely manner. Finally, while there are places in which a homeless patient can access the Internet (public libraries), this is often not feasible.
- Inconsistent access to transportation. While technically some homeless patients may own their own vehicles, this is not the case for the majority of individuals, especially in large urban centers. Additionally, public transportation may be inconsistent, unaffordable, have limited hours of operation, and be difficult to use in inclement weather.

Treatment

For patients with acute and severe psychosis, the ED provider will frequently administer anti-anxiety and/or antipsychotic medications to stabilize the patient's psychiatric state. Once the patient is calmer, the ED provider will be able to interact with her or him, and thus better determine an appropriate disposition.

If a patient remains psychotic and/or a risk to her- or himself or others, emergent hospitalization will most likely be necessary. Conversely, if a patient comes into the ED with psychosis which responds successfully to antipsychotic medications, the provider may consider discharging the patient in consultation with the patient's psychiatrist or other outpatient mental healthcare provider. During the consultation, changes in medications may be discussed and/or implemented. In this case, an admission may be avoided. However, this approach may be much more difficult in a patient who is homeless for the many reasons described previously.

Noncompliance issues such as inability to afford prescriptions or safely store them can interfere with effective treatment for the homeless population. Psychiatric patients may not understand their diagnosis or treatment, or may no longer comply with treatment if their symptoms have resolved. High rates of alcohol and drug abuse also decrease compliance. For these reasons alone, ED providers might admit homeless patients more readily.

One possible tool to improve compliance is the use of injectable antipsychotic medications such as haloperidol decanoate. As described in previous chapters, the route of drug administration allows for ideal absorption and medication activity for 2–4 weeks. This type of medication may be considered in a patient without signs of acute, severe psychosis and who has a history of noncompliance with oral medications. However, it is vital that a patient given this medication has good communication with a current mental health provider who can coordinate her or his care.

Case example: George, continued

George has schizophrenia and is hallucinating, but he is alert and oriented and acting appropriately. He is not agitated or uncooperative and is not threatening to harm anyone, including himself. He has adequate outpatient care, which he was unable to access due to transportation issues. He has a shelter at which to stay tonight. He is treated in the ED with an injection of haloperidol decanoate and discharged with a bus pass.

Systems issues affecting homeless psychiatric patients

Obtaining vital emergency psychiatric care is often difficult regardless of one's housing status. For the myriad reasons previously described, this process is usually much more arduous for a homeless patient. While many of these issues stem from individual limitations (lack of money, personal transportation), many limitations to obtaining care are, at least partially, due to systematic issues within American society and within our healthcare system.

Compared to Western Europe, the United States has higher levels of homelessness than the majority of Western European countries [38]. Additionally, the United States has higher income inequality and less generous social welfare systems than countries in Western Europe [39,40]. Also, the U.S. welfare system tends to be less centralized, as there is more emphasis on state and local programs when compared to much of Europe. This tends to cause a higher degree of variation in the types of support offered, the quality of care, and the availability of certain services depending on where a patient may live. Together, these realities of American society make it easier to become homeless and harder to find reliable housing.

In contrast to the majority of the industrialized world, we have a decidedly noncentralized healthcare system. Indeed, the latest statistics from the U.S. Census bureau demonstrate that 49.9 million people (16.2%) in this country currently do not have health insurance [41]. It is also estimated that at least 70% of all homeless patients do not currently have health insurance [32]. Lack of health insurance limits a patient's ability to seek timely primary care – both medical and psychiatric [42]. This not only adversely affects a patient's care, but also may become more expensive as the ED becomes the patient's primary source of health care.

In the United States, the Health Care for the Homeless (HCH) is currently the only federal program aimed at primarily serving the healthcare needs of the homeless [32]. HCH projects provide primary health care, substance abuse services, emergency care, dental care, mental health treatment, supportive housing, and other services. It is estimated that in 2008, HCH programs served more than 740,000 homeless people. While this program undoubtedly helps many undomiciled patients, homeless advocacy groups maintain that this level of care is insufficient [32]. Indeed this seems to be reasonable conclusion when it is noted that between 2.5 and 3.5 million people are homeless during any 1 year in the United States [1].

Overall, the combination of high rates of homelessness, a noncentralized healthcare system, and inadequate healthcare funding for the homeless, leads to an overall healthcare delivery system that fails to deliver adequate, efficient care to the homeless population. Some argue that this system actually costs more money in the long-run due to the lack of quality preventative care, and thus the overuse of EDs [32].

Compounding these systematic issues, a homeless patient often finds that the resources available to them often do not interact efficiently. Although some argue that the ultimate solution to this problem is the implementation of a centralized healthcare delivery system with more robust federal care for the homeless [32], there are also strategies aimed at connecting resources delivered on a much smaller level. An example of this is the Comprehensive Psychiatric Emergency Program (CPEP) at Columbia Presbyterian Medical Center in New York City [34]. Here emergency psychiatric service providers meet daily with Homeless Outreach Program employees and workers from local homeless shelters. In these meetings, psychiatric attendings, residents, social workers, substance abuse counselors, and others meet to discuss the progress of each client. In this setting clinical interventions can be made at the shelter or in the ED, if necessary. In the ED there is a designated "medical/psychiatric district," which is staffed by medical attendings in close consultation with psychiatric attendings. Additionally, this specialized ED is able to hold patients for up to 72 hours to give emergency providers a more robust observation period in which to create a treatment plan and ultimately decide upon the most appropriate disposition. While this multi-disciplinary program seems promising, there is a paucity of data regarding the effectiveness of this type of organization from both a medical and cost-savings viewpoint.

Conclusion

Undomiciled patients with psychiatric conditions face many hardships caring for mental health problems that are either unique to their situation, or greatly exacerbated by a lack of stable housing. Examples include a lack of caregivers, inconsistent transportation, inability to safely store medications and supplies, and difficulty efficiently communicating with mental health providers. The treatment of a homeless patient with a psychiatric complaint follows much of the same guidelines as that of a domiciled patient; however, there are aspects of such a patient's treatment in which special consideration should be given. Specifically, homeless patients have a higher rate of comorbid medical conditions, substance abuse, and often do not have a consistent relationship with a mental health provider. Providers of emergency psychiatric services may improve the short- and long-term care for a homeless patient by recognizing the unique circumstances surrounding the patient's living situation and working to link fragmented care systems to provide a homeless patient with proper outpatient psychiatric treatment.

We thank David Walker and Sharon Scrattish for their significant assistance in editing this chapter.

References

1. Levy BD, Oconnell JJ. Health care for homeless persons. *N Engl J Med* 2004;**350**:2329–32.

2. Badiaga S, Raoult D, Brouqui P. Preventing and controlling emerging and reemerging transmissible diseases in the homeless. *Emerg Infect Dis* 2008;**14**:1353–9.

3. Sullivan B. *HUD Issues 2009 Annual Homeless Assessment Report to Congress.* Washington, DC: Department of Housing and Urban Development; 2010.

4. Kautz E, Villaraigosa AR, Nutter MA, et al. *Hunger and Homelessness Survery.* Washington, DC: The United States Conference of Mayors; 2010.

5. Lowe E. *Hunger and Homelessness Report.* Washington, DC: The United States Conference of Mayors; 2000.

6. Diaz M, Nickels G, Kautz E, et al. *Status Report on Hunger and Homelessness.* Washington, DC: The United States Conference of Mayors; 2008.

7. Folsom DP, Hawthorne W, Lindamer L, et al. Prevalence and risk factors for homelessness and utilization of mental health services among 10,340 patients with serious mental illness in a large public mental health system. *Am J Psychiatry* 2005;**162**:370–6.

8. Ringwalt CL, Greene JM, Robertson M, McPheeters M. The prevalence of homelessness among adolescents in the United States. *Am J Public Health* 1998;**88**:1325–9.

9. Donohoe M. Homelessness in the United States: history, epidemiology, health Issues, women, and public policy. *Medscape Ob Gyn Womens Health* 2004;**9**.

10. Breakey WR, Fischer PJ, Kramer M, et al. Health and mental health problems

of homeless men and women in Baltimore. *JAMA* 1989;**262**:1352–7.

11. Hwang SW. Mortality among men using homeless shelters in Toronto, Ontario. *JAMA* 2000;**283**:2152–7.

12. Pizem P, Massicaote P, Vicent JR, The state of oral and dental health of the homeless and vagrant population of Montreal. *J Can Dent Assoc* 1994;**60**:1061–5.

13. Hwang SW. Homelessness and health. *CMAJ* 2001;**164**:229–33.

14. Gelberg L, Linn LS. Assessing the physical health of homeless adults. *JAMA* 1997;**262**:1973–9.

15. Radford JL, King AJC, Warren WK. *Street Youth and AIDS*. Ottawa: Health and Welfare, Canada; 1989.

16. Hwang SW, Orav EJ, O'Connell JJ, Lebow JM, Brennan TA. Causes of death in homeless adults in Boston. *Ann Intern Med* 1997;**136**:625–8.

17. Hibbs JR, Benner L Klugman L, et al. Mortality in a cohort of homeless adults in Philadelphia. *N Engl J Med* 1994;**331**:304–9.

18. Barrow SM, Herman DB, Cordova P, Struening EL. Mortality among homeless shelter residents in New York City. *Am J Public Health* 1999;**89**:529–34.

19. O'Connell JJ. *Utilization & Costs of Medical Services by Homeless Persons: A Review of the Literature & Implications for the Future*. [Monograph on the Internet]. 1999 Apr. National Health Care for the Homeless Council. Available at: http://www.nhchc.org/ Publications/utilization.html (Accessed August 22, 2011).

20. Scherl DJ, Macht LB. Deinstitutionalization in the absence of consensus. *Hosp Community Psychiatry* 1979;**30**:599–604.

21. Rochefort DA. Origins of the "Third psychiatric revolution": the Community Mental Health Centers Act of 1963. *J Health Polit Policy Law* 1984;**9**:1–30.

22. Lamb HR. Deinstitutionalization at the beginning of the new millennium. *Harv Rev Psychiatry* 1998;**6**:1–10.

23. Roth D, Bean GJ, Hyde PS. Homelessness and mental health policy: developing an appropriate role for the 1980s. *Community Ment Health J* 1986;**2**:203–14.

24. Dreier P. *Reagan's Legacy: Homelessness in America 2004 National Housing Institute*. [Monograph on the Internet]. Montclair, NJ: National Housing Institute; 2004 May/June. Available at: http://www.nhi.org/online/issues/135/ reagan.html (Accessed August 25, 2011).

25. Hyde J. From home to street: understanding young people's transitions into homelessness. *J Adolesc* 2005;**28**:171–83.

26. Kipke M, Palmer R, LaFrance S, O'Conner S. Homeless youths' descriptions of their parents' child-rearing practices. *Youth Soc* 1997;**28**:415–31.

27. McCarty D, Argeriou M, Huebner RB, Lubran B. Alcoholism, drug abuse, and the homeless. *Am Psychol* 1991;**46**:1139–48.

28. G Haugland, Siegel C, Hopper K, Alexander MJ. Mental illness among homeless individuals in a suburban county. *Psychiat Serv* 1997;**48**:504–9.

29. Drake RE, Wallach MA. Dual diagnosis: 15 years of progress. *Psychiatr Serv* 2000;**51**:1126–9.

30. Niska R, Bguiya F, Xu J. *National Hospital Ambulatory Medical Care Survey: 2007 Emergency Department Summary*. Division of Health Care Statistics: National Health Statistics Reports Number 26. August 6, 2010. Available at: www.cdc.gov/nchs/data/ nhsr/nhsr026.pdf (Accessed September 6, 2011).

31. Braun R, Hahn JA, Gottlieb SL, Moss AR, Zolopa AR. Utilization of emergency medical services by homeless adults in San Francisco: effects of social demographic factors. *AHSR & FHRS Annual Meeting Abstract Book* 2005;**12**:114.

32. National Coalition for the Homeless. [homepage on the internet]. Washington DC: National Coalition for the homeless; c2009. *Health Care for the Homeless*. Available at: http://www. nationalhomeless.org/factsheets/health. html (Accessed September 10, 2011).

33. Padgett DK, Struening EL, Andrews H, et al. Predictors of emergency room use by homeless adults in New York City: the influence of predisposing, enabling, and need factors. *Soc Sci Med* 1995;**41**:547–56.

34. McQuistin HL, Almeida C, Nossel I. Emergency psychiatric services for people who are homeless: intervention, linkage, and recovery. In: Glick RL, Berlin JS, Fishkind A, (Eds.). *Emergency Psychiatry: Principles and Practice*, (1st Edition). New York: Lippincott Williams and Wilkins; 2008: 357–69.

35. Kushel MB, Vittenghoff E, Haas JS. Factors associated with the health care utilization of homeless persons. *JAMA* 2001;**285**:200–6.

36. Burt M, Aron L, Douglas T, et al. *Homelessness: Programs and the People They Serve: Technical Report: Findings of the National Survey of Homeless Assistance Providers and Clients*. Washington, DC: Interagency Council on the Homeless; 1999.

37. Christensen RC, Hodgkins CC, Garces LK, et al. Homeless, mentally ill and addicted: the need for abuse and trauma services. *J Health Care Poor Underserved* 2005;**16**:615–22.

38. Shinn M. Homelessness, poverty and social exclusion in the United States and Europe. *Eur J Homelessness* 2010;**4**:19–44.

39. Alesina A, Glaeser EL. *Fighting Poverty in the U.S. and Europe: A World of Difference*. Oxford: Oxford University Press; 2004.

40. Smeeding T. Public policy, economic inequality and poverty: the United States in comparative perspective. *Soc Sci Q* 2005;**86**(Suppl):955–83.

41. DeNavas-Walt C, Proctor BD, Smith JC. *Income, Poverty, and Health Insurance Coverage in the United States: 2009*. Washington, DC: U.S. Department of Commerce; 2010 Sept. Available at: www.census.gov/prod/2011pubs/p60-239.pdf (Accessed August 6, 2012).

42. Schwartz K, Artiga S. *Health Insurance Coverage and Access to Care for Low-income Non-citizen Adults* [monograph on the internet]. Washington, DC: Kaiser Commission on Medicaid and the Uninsured; 2007. Available at: http://www.kff.org/uninsured/7651.cfm (Accessed September 3, 2011).

Chapter 34

Management of neurobehavioral sequelae of traumatic brain injury in the emergency department

Andy Jagoda and Silvana Riggio

Introduction

Concussion occurs when the brain is subjected to an acceleration/deceleration force or, as in the case of blast injury, to a pressure wave sufficient to disrupt brain function [1]. The term concussion and mild traumatic brain injury (mTBI) are used interchangeably in much of the literature and will be used so in this chapter. There is considerable controversy surrounding the diagnostic criteria needed to validate that a brain injury has occurred, and there is no agreed marker of injury that provides a gold standard [2]. There are several neurobehavioral sequelae, also referred to as postconcussive symptoms, that have been associated with a concussion. These symptoms encompass a spectrum of somatic and neuropsychiatric symptoms, see Table 34.1. The neuropsychiatric symptoms are subdivided into cognitive and behavioral categories. The development, severity, and duration of neurobehavioral sequelae vary; the literature is unclear on the impact of external stressors and conditions on the development and duration of these sequelae but there is no question that the expression of these symptoms is multifactorial, see Figure 34.1.

The Diagnostic and Statistical Manual of Mental Disorders, 4th Edition, Text Revision (DSM-IV-TR) proposes criteria for diagnosing "post-concussional disorder" which include physical fatigue, disordered sleep, headaches, or vertigo/dizzinesss [3]. The International Statistical Classification of Disease and Related Health Problems, 10th Revision (ICD-10) uses six diagnostic criteria to make the diagnosis of postconcussive syndrome: fatigue, dizziness, poor concentration, memory

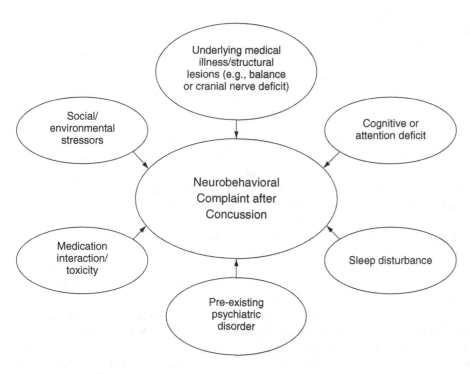

Figure 34.1. This figure demonstrates the number of factors which must be assessed and collated in the evaluation of a patient presenting with a neurobehavioral complaint after a concussion. For example, in a patient who complains of difficulty concentrating after a TBI, the clinician must consider the role of a primary injury impacting executive function plus impact from change in sleep pattern, new medications, e.g., a sedative-hypnotic for sleep, plus new social stressors since the accident.

Behavioral Emergencies for the Emergency Physician, ed. Leslie S. Zun, Lara G. Chepenik, and Mary Nan S. Mallory. Published by Cambridge University Press. © Cambridge University Press 2013.

Table 34.1. Neurobehavioral sequelae from concussion

- Neuropsychiatric

    Cognitive: e.g., deficits in attention, memory, executive function

    Behavioral:

    Primary Psychiatric disorder: e.g., mood disorder, anxiety

    Personality Disorder

    Other

- Somatic: e.g., sleep disturbance, fatigue, dizziness, vertigo, headaches, visual disturbances, nausea, sensitivity to light and sound, hearing loss, seizures

Table 34.2. Behavioral presentation correlated to anatomic brain injury to the frontal lobe or temporal lobe area (the most vulnerable areas in post-traumatic injury)

- *Dorsolateral frontal region*: Injury may be expressed as difficulties in switching parameters, planning, a certain mental inflexibility can be noted which can ultimately result in irritability, slowness in performance and/or low frustration tolerance with potential social and performance repercussion.

- *Orbito-frontal region*: Injury can manifest clinically with agitation, disinhibition and/or poor impulse control.

- *Medial frontal region*: Injury can manifest itself with apathy which can be misdiagnosed with major depression.

- *Temporal region*: Injury may cause memory disturbance and/or emotional lability problems.

- *Basal ganglia (or dorsolateral frontal region)*: Injury may result in mood symptoms, e.g., depression; resting tremor, cogwheeling, bradykinesia

- *Right hemispheric limbic area*: Injury may result in mania. Lesions to the right and left hemisphere can manifest as psychotic symptoms.

problems, headache, and irritability [4]. Few of these criteria are unique to brain trauma thus making their diagnostic and prognostic significance of questionable value [5]. That said, these neurobehavioral sequelae are reported in the literature and an awareness of them is important in evaluating, treating, and counseling patients who have sustained a concussion. Recognizing the ambiguity of current definitions for concussion and its clinical manifestations, the Department of Defense in collaboration with the Center for Disease Control and the Brain Trauma Foundation is funding a multidisciplinary task force to develop an evidence-based definition for concussion; this definition will be used to develop diagnostic criteria and to promote future research (personal communication, Dr. Jamshid Ghajar, Brain Trauma Foundation).

Identifying clear criteria that define sequelae from a brain injury is encumbered by the lack of a standardized definition of what constitutes an mTBI/concussion. Many studies use the Glasgow Coma Scale (GCS) score for identifying the study population. The GCS was developed to facilitate communication between clinicians caring for patients with severe TBI. It categorizes patients into three groups: coma, lethargic, and awake. The scale was developed before the widespread availability of computed tomography, and its use was never intended to supplant a careful neurologic and neurocognitive evaluation. The GCS score is limited in its ability to provide prognosis related to postconcussive symptoms after an mTBI. Likewise, neither computed tomography (CT) nor magnetic resonance imaging (MRI) is sufficiently sensitive to diagnose the type of injuries that predispose patients to neurobehavioral sequelae. Brain biomarkers and functional MRI (fMRI) hold promise but are still research tools without validated clinical utility. Finally, neurocognitive testing holds promise as a diagnostic criterion to demonstrate injury but unfortunately, these tests are also limited in their prognostic utility [6].

Not all mTBI is the same and sequelae that develop are most likely related to the localization and lateralization of the injury, to the medical and psychiatric comorbidities, and the pre- and post-psychosocial factors. Neurocognitive testing supports the hypothesis that some types of concussion result in impairment in brain connectivity specifically as it relates to attention. It is the impairment in attention that can then lead to difficulty with concentration, visual tracking, and task performance; impairment in these activities contributes to headaches, difficulty focusing on tasks, and difficulty with sleep, all of which are common complaints in patients after even an mTBI. The multiple factors that contribute to behavioral complaints after a concussion require that the clinician ascertains pre-morbid medical, neurological, and psychiatric conditions; obtains a history of drugs and medications; establishes baseline occupational and social function; identifies psychological and social stressors.

Pathophysiology and chronic traumatic encephalopathy

Sudden deceleration or rotational acceleration injury may generate sufficient shearing forces to result in axonal injury and edema which has been implicated as a contributing factor to the development of some postconcussive symptoms [7]. Concussion was once graded according to the presence or absence of post-traumatic amnesia (PTA) and/or loss of consciousness (LOC); however, studies have failed to demonstrate a correlation between LOC and PTA on neurocognitive performance testing after injury [8,9].

Cortical contusion can result in a loss of function served by a given brain area. White matter lesions can result in interruption of information being transmitted between cortical areas within the brain. Diffuse axonal injuries can result in slowed and inefficient information processing. There is also the possibility that head trauma causes traumatic tearing of neuronal connections impairing cortical and thalamic circuitry contributing to cognitive impairment [10]. The impact of injury on neurotransmitter function is poorly defined but clearly could provide a biological explanation for some of the behavioral changes seen after TBI. Table 34.2 presents behavioral presentations that have been associated with injury to various parts of the brain.

Chronic traumatic encephalopathy (CTE) associated with sports has gained attention in recent years. It appears that axonal and cytoskeleton alternations from repeat concussion lead to accumulations of abnormal protein aggregates expressed in neurofibrillary tangles termed tauopathy. These proteins include synuclien, ubiquitin, proganulin, TAR, DNA-binding protein 43, amyloid precursor protein and its metabolite $A\beta$ [11]. Of interest, the dementia of CTE is associated with neurofibrillary tangles and neurophil threads that are distributed in patches throughout the neocortex but spares the mesiotemporal region which is generally affected in Alzheimer's disease. In addition, the neuropathology seen in CTE tauopathy does not have the amyloid plaques seen in Alzheimer's disease.

Chronic traumatic encephalopathy has been associated with both repeat concussion and with genetic predisposition. In boxers the development of CTE has been correlated associated with the number of years of boxing and the presence of the ApoE4 allele [12]. Male boxers with more than twelve professional bouts with the ApoE4 allele have twice the risk of CTE than matched controls without the allele [13].

Epidemiology

The true incidence of concussion is unknown because the majority of these patients do not enter into any specific database. It is estimated that up to 4 million Americans sustain a recreation- and sport-related concussion annually; approximately 1.5 million Americans are evaluated annually in emergency departments for mTBI [14]. Post-deployment studies of soldiers fighting in Afghanistan and Iraq report that up to 25% of soldiers sustain a TBI, the majority of which are classified as "mild" [15]. The sports medicine literature estimates that concussion represents 9% of all high school athletic injuries; the sports with the highest risk of concussion, in descending order of prevalence, are football, girls' soccer, boys' lacrosse, boys' soccer, girls' basketball, wrestling, and girls' lacrosse [16].

Up to 80% of patients with a concussion experience at least one neurobehavioral symptoms for up to 3 months after the injury, most commonly headache [17]. Up to 45% of mTBI patients meet ICD-10 criteria for the postconcussive syndrome at 5 days post-injury [5]. Use of different study populations and varying definitions contribute to the difference in reported incidence of symptoms. Some of the risk factors which have been identified for the development of postconcussive symptoms include female gender, advanced age, pain, and prior affective or anxiety diagnoses [18].

In approximately 15% of mild TBI patients, neurobehavioral sequelae persist beyond 3 months and may contribute to long-term social and occupational difficulties [19,20]. Cognitive dysfunction in the form of impaired attention, memory, and executive function have a predominant role in patients who experience persistent symptoms [21]. A meta-analysis of neuropsychologic outcomes after mTBI reported that the majority of patients are back to baseline by three months; however, participants in litigation were reported to have longer lasting cognitive sequelae and was associated with stable or worsening of cognitive functioning over time [22].

The sports literature supports the finding that the majority of adult athletes who sustain an mTBI return to baseline by 10 days [9]. Children appear to return to baseline at a slower rate with 40% in one study not at baseline after 2 weeks and 10% still not at baseline at 6 weeks [8]. Studies have tried to identify risk factors that lead to delayed recovery, however, thus far no clinical factors, i.e., length of loss of consciousness or posttraumatic amnesia, have been found to predict which patients will have delayed recovery [23].

Patient evaluation

Before focusing on the neurobehavioral complaints of the patient who has sustained a concussion, a comprehensive history and physical exam is required. The history focuses on the events preceding and succeeding the concussion. Although LOC and PTA are important to identify, neither are prognostic in isolation. A careful neurologic exam is indicated to identify subtle deficits that may put the patient at risk for developing postconcussive symptoms or at risk for sustaining another injury. In particular, subtle cranial nerve IV and VI injuries may cause headaches due to the visual disturbances, while postural instability identified on balance testing may result in falls. Deficits identified on attention testing, see neurocognition section below, may put the patient at risk for headaches, or accidents while driving. The sports community has developed several tools that assist in acute evaluations including the Standardized Assessment of Concussion (SAC), the Balance Error Scoring System (BESS), or the Sport Concussion Assessment Tool 2 (SCAT2) [24].

The American College of Emergency Physicians in partnership with the Centers for Disease Control have developed guidelines identifying which patients with a concussion require a head CT [25]. Those guidelines do not provide insight into which patients are at risk for developing neurobehavioral sequelae. MRI is more sensitive than CT for identifying contusions, petechial hemorrhage, and white matter injury; however, there are no clear guidelines on which patients require imaging, the timing, nor the prognostic value [26]. Functional imaging, e.g., fMRI, positron emission tomography (PET), single photon emission computed tomography (SPECT) looks at metabolic and blood flow changes in the brain, and there is emerging evidence that it may assist in documenting brain dysfunction after an injury, but at this time, functional imaging remains a research tool [26].

Diffusion tensor imaging (DTI) is used to study the structural images of white matter tracts in the brain. Studies show that in mTBI structural integrity of axons within the genu of the corpus callosum is affected resulting in misalignment of fibers, edema, and axonal degeneration; this has been correlated with delays in reaction times [6]. At the current time, DTI is a research tool but holds the potential to be a diagnostic tool for concussion in the future.

Postconcussive cognitive disorders and the role of neuropsychologic testing

Cognitive dysfunction after a concussion plays a role in many of the symptoms expressed after injury. Cognitive impairment includes problems with information processing, decision making, motor function, reaction time, and memory. As a consequence of these deficits, patients may become irritable, anxious, apathetic, or depressed. Clinical expression may be misinterpreted as secondary to a primary affective disorder and lead to unnecessary pharmacologic interventions.

The use of neurocognitive testing in athletes before and after injury has contributed to our understanding of postconcussive cognitive performance. The literature is not conclusive on which neurocognitive battery best assesses postconcussive performance; Table 34.3 lists the domains that are tested. Limiting much of the literature on cognitive testing is the absence of preinjury performance, and the absence of reliable matched control data.

Historically, cognitive function has been assessed using paper and pencil tests such as Digit Symbol Substitution Test and Trail Making Tests. More recently, computerized test platforms e.g., ImPACT™ have gained acceptance [24]. It specifically assesses verbal memory, visual memory, processing speed, and reaction time. A recent study examining the construct validity of ImPACT™ with traditional neuropsychological measures suggests that ImPACT™ is a good screening tool but one that must be used carefully with an understanding of its limitations, in particular it is of more limited value if the premorbid baseline is not known [27].

An evaluation of post-TBI cognitive function is essential with a focus on assessing attention versus memory. If attention is impaired, there will be difficulty to retain information with obvious impact on memory and thus performance. If the patient has an underlying affective disorder, attention can also be impaired due to lack of interest and/or distractibility. Therefore, the assessment of memory must be placed in context of attention and a detailed psychiatric history is warranted to exclude other disorders that may interfere with performance.

Cognitive deficits after a sports-related concussion generally resolve within 10 days [28,29]. It is unclear if this pattern of

Table 34.3. Domains that can be evaluated in postconcussive cognitive testing

Verbal memory
Visual memory
Reaction time
Visual motor speed / processing speed
Impulse control
Fine motor speed
Working memory
Attention

recovery is followed in other populations such as the elderly or patients with socioeconomic stressors. Resolving this time course is made more difficult because most patients do not have an established cognitive baseline. Neither LOC nor PTA predict which patients are at risk for cognitive deficits after an mTBI: McCrea et al. performed a prospective study of cognitive functioning using pre-TBI assessments of 91 high school and college football players and compared them to performance after a mild TBI during the season [29]. The authors reported cognitive impairment relative to the athletes' own and matched control baselines immediately after TBI, even in the absence of LOC or PTA.

Performance on neurocognitive testing compared to preinjury baseline in combination with findings on symptom inventories has been reported to improve the prognostic ability of either alone; however, the sensitivity of the combined findings in predicting protracted recovery was only 65% and the specificity 80% [30]. In an emergency department-based study using ImPACT™, 25 mTBI patients were compared to 38 controls [31]. The authors reported subtle deficit in visual motor speed and reaction time; the verbal and visual memory score did not reflect a deficit. Long-term deficits were not assessed thus the study is limited in its ability to offer prognostic information. However, the study does demonstrate that computer-based neurocognitive testing can be performed in the ED and may provide a baseline that is helpful in discharge planning, i.e., return to work, and follow-up, i.e., need to see a TBI specialist.

Postconcussive behavioral disorders

Behavioral manifestations after a concussion may be due to the injury or may be due to underlying psychopathologies or medical conditions. Symptoms may also be due to an emotional response to the injury, its physical limitations, or fear of the impact on function.

Personality changes: Affective and behavioral disturbances after TBI may be expressed as personality changes appreciated by the patients or their family/caregiver. Personality changes may include aggression, impulsivity, irritability, emotional lability, or apathy [32]. Impulsivity and irritability may lead to verbal and physical inappropriateness expressed as verbal outbursts or combativeness. It may be due to impaired judgment secondary to an underlying structural lesion or the exacerbation of an underlying psychiatric disorder, or to an emotional response to trauma. Aggression is a commonly reported behavioral symptom of TBI but is reported more frequently after moderate or severe TBI. Risk factors for aggression after TBI include frontal lobe injury, premorbid affective disorder, personality disorder, or alcohol or substance abuse.

Major depression: Major depression has been reported as a sequela of concussion both acutely but also long term; the actual prevalence is unknown [33]. The degree to which a premorbid psychiatric disorder increases the risk for postconcussive major depression is unclear, but studies indicate a positive correlation especially in the more severe category of

TBI. Risk factors for developing major depression after TBI fall into two categories: premorbid psychiatric pathology and low socioeconomic status. The relationship between rates of depression and the severity of TBI is unclear.

Studies have found a link between TBI and suicidality, as well as between psychiatric comorbidity in the setting of TBI and suicidality [34]. In a retrospective study of 5034 patients, Silver et al. reported that a history of TBI with LOC posed a four times greater likelihood of attempted suicide than those without TBI; 8.1% versus 1.9% [35]. This risk of suicide attempt remained even after controlling for demographics, quality-of-life variables, alcohol abuse, and any comorbid psychiatric disorders.

Post-traumatic stress disorder (PTSD) and anxiety: Some studies report an increased risk of developing a new anxiety disorder after an mTBI [36]; other studies have demonstrated a similar incidence of anxiety disorders in mTBI patients and non–head-injured trauma patients suggesting that the brain injury per se is not responsible for the development of the new behavior disorder [5,37]. Increased age, a history of PTSD, and an avoidant coping style increases risk of acute stress symptoms after TBI [37]. In turn, a diagnosis of acute stress disorder is a risk factor for the development of PTSD after TBI. In a study of 79 patients with mild TBI, Bryant and Harvey diagnosed 14% of the patients with acute stress disorder at 1 month, and 24% were diagnosed with PTSD at 6 months post-injury; 82% of the patients diagnosed with acute stress disorder had developed PTSD by 6 months [38].

Qureshi et al. performed a systematic review of the literature looking at memory and cognitive function in PTSD patients vs. those patients exposed to trauma but without PTSD [39]. The authors reported that there exists a relationship between cognitive impairment in PTSD that is not seen in trauma patients who do not have PTSD. However, the authors emphasize that premorbid conditions and associated socioeconomic factors impact cognitive performance and that more study is required.

A growing literature is beginning to address the issue of overlap between PTSD and mTBI. Hoge et al. surveyed over 2700 U.S. Army infantry soldiers from two brigades, 3 to 4 months after returning from a 1-year deployment in Iraq [40]. Fifteen percent of the soldiers report having sustained a TBI, all but 4 of the 384 TBIs reported were mTBIs. In soldiers who reported an mTBI complaints of headache, poor memory, and concentration were frequent suggesting that a persistent postconcussive syndrome was present. Of those reporting TBI with LOC, 44% met criteria for PTSD, while PTSD was present in 27% of those reporting altered mental status without LOC. In addition, major depression was present in 23% and 8%, respectively. This high coincidence of PTSD and depression led the authors to perform a covariate analysis for the two disorders and interestingly, after adjusting for the coexistence of PTSD and depression, an mTBI history was no longer significantly associated with adverse physical health outcomes or symptoms, except for headache.

The relationship between TBI and PTSD remains controversial. There is the possibility that the two conditions are not coincidental but rather that TBI may increase the risk of developing PTSD following a psychological trauma [41]. Physical injury of any type, even if not involving the brain, has been reported to increase the risk of developing PTSD [42]. It remains unknown if a neural insult might alter reactions to psychological stressors and increase the likelihood that PTSD will develop. Current biological models of PTSD postulate that key frontal and limbic structures, including the prefrontal cortex, amygdala, and hippocampus, are involved in the development of PTSD [43].

Substance use disorders: A review of the literature by van Reekum et al. reported a 22% prevalence of substance abuse in TBI patients versus a 15% lifetime prevalence in the general population [33]. A review of subsequent studies by Rogers and Read in 2007 showed a prevalence of 12% [44]. Premorbid substance use has been found to be strongly associated with post-TBI drug use, and multiple studies have cited substance abuse as a risk factor for TBI rather than the other way around. A 30-year longitudinal study by Koponen et al. showed that 71% of TBI patients who were using drugs currently also did so pre-TBI [45].

Postconcussive somatic symptoms

Headache: The prevalence of postconcussive headache varies greatly by study, ranging from 25% to 90% of patients making it the most common postconcussive symptom [46]. Postconcussive headaches are classified as acute or chronic. According to the International Headache Society, acute post-traumatic headaches begin within 2 weeks of the injury and resolve within 2 months; chronic post-traumatic headaches begin within 2 weeks and persist for more than 8 weeks [47]. Headache often presents concommitently with other postconcussive symptoms. One study reported that 53% of patients with a postconcussive headache had at least one other somatic complaint (fatigability, sleep disturbance, dizziness, or alcohol intolerance); 49% had at least one cognitive complaint (memory dysfunction or impaired concentration/attention); and 26% had at least one psychiatric complaint (irritability, aggressiveness, anxiety, depression, or emotional lability); 17% had all three types of complaints and 17% had none [48].

A history of headache before the TBI increases the risk of post-traumatic headaches, although in the majority of these case, the headaches resolve within 3 to 6 months [48]. The presence of post-traumatic headache has not been consistently correlated with the severity of the injury; in fact, some authors have reported that mild TBI patients have higher rates of headache during the initial post-traumatic phase than patients with more severe injury [49].

Dizziness/nausea: Dizziness is the second most commonly reported somatic symptom after a concussion [50]. Most studies do not differentiate post-traumatic dizziness from vertigo, although the pathophysiology may be greatly different. Vertigo, characterized by the appearance of movement of the environment around oneself, may be peripheral or central in etiology. Peripheral etiologies include cupulolithiasis, perilymphatic fistula, post-traumatic Meniere's disease, damage to the vestibular nerve, and use of ototoxic medications. Central etiologies include damage to the brainstem involving the vestibular nucleus. Dizziness or vertigo is reported in 24–78% of mild TBI patients acutely, significantly higher than the prevalence in non-TBI patients in the community [50].

Fatigue: Fatigue is a commonly reported, potentially debilitating sequelae after concussion [51]. The presence of fatigue is associated with poorer social integration, decreased level of productive activities, and decreased overall quality of life [50]. When fatigue persists, it may present a barrier to recovery [52]. Severity of TBI and age have not been found to be predictors of severity of fatigue. Post-TBI fatigue is most likely the result of a combination of etiologies. Studies have shown that fatigue can be associated with several other postconcussive symptoms [53]. Hypopituitarism, with resultant neuroendocrine abnormalities such as growth hormone deficiency and cortisol deficiency, may also be associated with post-TBI fatigue [54]. Other possible contributing factors to fatigue include vertigo, diplopia, insomnia, and iatrogenic causes, such as psychotropic or analgesic medications.

Sleep disturbance: Sleep disturbances include difficulties in initiating sleep, maintaining sleep, or attaining restful sleep, as well as excessive daytime somnolence, and less commonly parasomnias. It is reported in up to 73% of post-TBI patients which is greater than the 32–35% prevalence reported in the general population [55]. Sleep disturbance has not been clearly linked to severity of TBI [56]. Abnormalities on polysomnography in mild TBI patients with chronic sleep disturbance have been shown, and, as with all the other somatic symptoms, the etiology is complex and therefore takes more than a prescription to solve.

Seizures: A convulsion immediately after a concussion can occur and the best available evidence suggests that these convulsions are benign and not associated with any adverse clinical, cognitive, nor neuroimaging outcomes [57]. Post-traumatic seizures developing in the days to years after a concussion are relatively rare but can occur and can present as focal or generalized, motor or nonmotor (e.g., complex partial). Complex partial seizures and other nonmotor convulsions present with a spectrum of behavioral changes ranging from inattention to psychosis. These events generally have a sudden onset and relatively sudden change back to baseline behavior with or without a significant postictal period: for the clinician, non-convulsive seizures is in the differential of a patient with atypical changes in behavior that cannot be explained; a past history of brain injury, even mTBI, may be the key to pursing the diagnosis.

Balance: Of all the physical findings after a concussion, balance has emerged as the most sensitive and specific in the identification that an injury has occurred. The Balance Error Scoring System (BESS) is the most frequently used tool in sports and tests a combination of three stances on various footing surfaces: each stance is observed with eyes closed and hands on hip and error points given for various responses e.g., opening eyes or lifting hands off the hips [6]. Studies in college football players report that 36% of concussed players have an impaired BESS score compared to 5% in controls; 24% of those impaired remained impaired at 2 days, and 9% at 7 days.

Postconcussive symptoms in nonconcussed patients

In a provocative study, Iverson and McCracken studied the prevalence of post-TBI symptoms in patients with non-TBI chronic medical conditions: They reported that 94% of these patients met criteria for commonly ascribed postconcussive symptoms [58]. They reported disturbed sleep, fatigue, and/or irritability in 81% of patients; and one or more cognitive problem in 42% of patients. Other authors have reported similar findings [59,60]. Meares et al. performed a prospective study at a level 1 trauma center; 90 patients with mild TBI were compared to 85 with non–brain-injury trauma: both groups had the same incidence of symptoms with the strongest predictor of symptoms in either group being a previous affective disorder [5]. Although this study questions the existence of a unique neurobehavioral sequelae of mTBI, a limitation of its design assigned MVA patients with non-LOC or PTA to the control group, while indeed by mechanism alone they would have been subject to a cranial acceleration/deceleration injury.

A correlation between pain and postconcussive symptoms has been reported, and pain has been associated with the persistence of symptoms [60]. Hart et al. reported that pain after TBI was associated with cognitive impairment, including deficits in attention, memory, processing speed, and reaction time. Occurrence of cognitive complaints in non-TBI chronic pain patients has been demonstrated, once again questioning the relationship between TBI per se and NBS [59].

Discharge planning and return to full activities

The key in the diagnosis and management of post-TBI complaints is to avoid premature closure on a diagnosis, to coordinate care through a multi-disciplinary team, and to involve the patient and their family in decision making. There is evidence to support the benefit of education and reassurance after TBI on outcome. Ponsford et al. studied 202 mTBI patients and reported that patients given an information booklet on mTBI and coping strategies for symptoms were significantly less symptomatic at 3 months than those who were not provided with education [19]. An extensive review of articles on early intervention after mild TBI by Borg et al. showed that early educational information reduce long-term complaints [61].

Cognitive and physical rest are key components to recovery. The American Academy of Pediatrics recommends that children who have sustained a concussion be provided with an

Table 34.4. Components of the concussion symptom inventory (modified from Randolph et al. [62])

Headache
Nausea
Balance problems / dizziness
Fatigue
Drowsiness
Feeling like "in a fog"
Difficulty concentrating
Difficulty remembering
Sensitivity to light
Sensitivity to noise
Blurred vision
Feeling slowed down

environment conducive to recovery which may include temporary leave of absence from school, shortened school day, reduction in work, longer time to complete tasks and exams [24]. In general, it is recommended that physical exertion be minimized initially and then gradually increased as tolerated. A return of symptoms with physical or mental stress is an indication that recovery is not complete and that more time is needed. Alcohol is contraindicated during the recovery phase.

In sports, Randolph et al. have developed the Concussion Symptom Inventory (CSI), which may be useful in monitoring recovery and determining return to play [62]. This inventory was derived from 27 symptom variables and the final 12 symptoms that comprise the inventory are listed in Table 34.4. At a minimum, the CSI provides a framework for clinicians to use following patients after a concussion. The scale is not validated nor has it been correlated with long-term prognosis.

Recognizing the possibility of an mTBI patient developing neurobehavioral sequelae, education is a key component of the discharge process. The CDC has collaborated with the American College of Emergency Physicians (ACEP) and developed sample discharge instructions that inform patients when to return to the ED, versus when to seek follow-up with a clinician experienced in sequelae of TBI [63]. A key component of those discharge instructions include information about post-concussive symptoms and recommendations on when to return to work, school, and sports.

Conclusions

Neurobehavioral sequelae after concussion may have both somatic and neuropsychiatric components. The neuropsychiatric symptoms are divided into cognitive and behavioral. Expression of the sequelae is multifactorial and there is evidence of a genetic contribution. The clinical presentations must be placed in the context of the patient's pre-morbid state. The evaluation consists of a history, physical, neurologic, and psychiatric examination. A careful assessment of attention and cognition, and of cranial nerves and balance may identify subtle indicators that an injury has occurred. The role of neuroimaging is of limited value in the evaluation of a patient who has sustained a concussion; functional imaging and serum biomarkers may have a future role. Management strategies are based on placing the findings on exam in context of the patient's pre-morbid state and social context. An education intervention is an important part of the patient's care plan, allowing the patient and family to understand the course of recovery. Minimizing physical and mental stress immediately after injury and then allowing for a gradual return to full activity may maximize outcomes. Caution against driving and using alcohol until symptoms resolve is advised; pharmacotherapy in general is not indicated. Referral to a specialist with expertise in traumatic brain injury should be provided for those cases in which symptoms have not resolved completely within 2 weeks post-injury.

References

1. Elder G, Mitsis E, Ahlers S, Cristian A. Blast-induced mild traumatic brain injury. *Psychiatr Clin North Am* 2010;**33**:757–81.

2. Ruff R, Iverson G, Barth J, et al. Recommendations for diagnosing a mild traumatic brain injury: a National Academy of Neuropsychology education paper. *Arch Clin Neuropsychol* 2009;**24**:3–10.

3. American Psychiatric Association. *Diagnostic and Statistical Manual of Mental Disorders (4th edition, Text Revision)*. Washington, DC: American Psychiatric Association; 2000.

4. World Health Organization. *The ICD-10 Classification of Mental and Behavioral Disorders: Clinical Descriptions and Diagnostic Guidelines*. Geneva: World Health Organization; 1992.

5. Meares S, Shores EA, Taylor AJ, et al. Mild traumatic brain injury does not predict acute postconcussion syndrome. *J Neurol Neurosurg Psychiatry* 2008;**79**:300–6.

6. Davis G, Iverson G, Guskiewicz K, et al. Contributions of neuroimaging, balance testing, electrophysiology, and blood markers to the assessment of sport related concussion. *Br J Sports Med* 2009;**43**:36–45.

7. Zink B, Szmydynger-Chodobska J, Chodobski A. Emerging concepts in the pathophysiology of traumatic brain injury. *Psychiatr Clin North Am* 2010;**33**:741–56.

8. Thomas D, Collins M, Saladino R, et al. Identifying neurocognitive deficits in adolescents following concussion. *Acad Emerg Med* 2011;**18**:246–54.

9. McCrory P, Meeuwisse W, Johnston K, et al. Consensus statement on concussion in sport – the third International Conference on concussion in sport held in Zurich, November 2008. *Phys Sportsmed* 2009;**37**:141–59.

10. DeKosky S, Ikonomovic M, Ganday S. Traumatic brain injury–football, warfare, and long term effects. *N Engl J Med* 2010;**363**:1293–6.

11. McKee AC, Cantu RC, Nowinski CJ, et al. Chronic traumatic encephalopathy in athletes: progressive tauopathy after repetitive head injury. *J Neuropathol Exp Neurol* 2009;**68**:709–35.

12. McCrory P. Sports concussion and the risk of chronic neurological impairment. *Clin J Sport Med* 2011;**21**:6–12.

13. Jordan B, Reikin N Ravdin L, et al. Apolipoprotein E episolon4 associated with traumatic brain injury in boxing. *JAMA* 2007;**278**:136–40.

14. Division of Injury and Disability Outcomes and Programs, National Center for Injury Prevention and Control, Centers for Disease Control and Prevention, Department of Health and Human Services. *Traumatic Brain Injury in the United States: Emergency Department Visits, Hospitalizations, and Deaths, October 2004*. Available at: http://www.cdc.gov/ncipc/pub-res/TBI_in_US_04/TBI_ED.htm (Accessed August 10, 2012).

15. Terrio H, Brenner L, Ivins B, et al. Traumatic brain injury screening: preliminary findings in a US Army brigade combat team. *J Head Trauma Rehabil* 2009;**24**:14–23.

16. Lincoln A, Caswell S, Almquist J, et al. Trends in concussion incidence in high school sports: a prospective 11 year study. *Am J Sports Med* 2011;**20**:1–6.

17. Lundin A, de Boussard C, Edman G, et al. Symptoms and disability until 3 months after mild TBI. *Brain Inj* 2006;**20**:799–806.

18. Baguley I, Chapman J, Gurka J, et al. The prospective course of postconcussion syndrome: the role of mild traumatic brain injury. *Neuropsychology* 2011;**25**:454–65.

19. Ponsford J, Willmott C, Rothwell A. Impact of early intervention on outcome following mild head injury in adults. *J Neurol Neurosurg Psychiatry* 2002;**73**:330–2.

20. Ruff RM, Camenzuli L, Mueller J. Miserable minority: emotional risk factors that influence the outcome of a mild traumatic brain injury. *Brain Inj* 1996;**8**:61–5.

21. Broglio S, Eckner J, Paulson H, Kutcher J. Cognitive decline and aging: the role of concussive and subconcussive impacts. *Exerc Sport Sci Rev* 2012;**40**:138–44.

22. Belanger H, Curtiss G, Demery J, et al. Factors moderating neuropsychological outcomes following mild traumatic brain injury: a meta analysis. *J Int Neuropsychol Soc* 2005;**11**:215–27.

23. Makdissi M. Is the simple vs complex classification of concussion a valid and useful differentiation? *Br J Sports Med* 2009;**43**(Suppl 1):i23–7.

24. Halstead M, Walter K. Clinical report – Sport related concussion in children and adolescents. *Pediatrics* 2010;**126**:597–615.

25. Jagoda A, Bazarian J, Bruns J, et al. Clinical policy: neuroimaging and decision-making in adult mild traumatic brain injury in the acute setting. *Clin Ann Emerg Med* 2008;**52**:714–48.

26. Jantzen K, Anderson B, Steinberg F, Kelso J. A prospective functional MRE imaging study of mild traumatic brain injury in college football players. *AJNR Am J Neuroradiol* 2004;**25**:738–45.

27. Maerlender A, Flashman L, Kessler A, et al. Examination of the construct validity of ImPACT computerized test, traditional, and experimental neuropsychological measures. *Clin Neuropsychol* 2010;**24**:1309–25.

28. Bleiberg J, Cernich AN, Cameron K, et al. Duration of cognitive impairment after sports concussion. *Neurosurgery* 2004;**54**:1073–80.

29. McCrea M, Guskiewicz KM, Marshall SW, et al. Acute effects and recovery time following concussion in collegiate football players: the NCAA concussion study. *JAMA* 2003;**290**:2556–63.

30. Lau B, Collins M, Lovell M. Sensitivity and specificity of subacute computerized neurocognitive testing and symptom evaluation in predicating outcomes after sports related concussion. *Am J Sports Med* 2011;**20**:1–8.

31. Peterson S, Stull M, Collins M, Wang H. Neurocognitive function of emergency department patients with mild traumatic brain injury. *Ann Emerg Med* 2009;**53**:796–803.

32. Tateno A, Jorge RE, Robinson RG. Clinical correlates of aggressive behavior after traumatic brain injury. *J Neuropsychiatry Clin Neurosci* 2003;**15**:155–60.

33. van Reekum R, Cohen T, Wong J. Can traumatic brain injury cause psychiatric disorders? *J Neuropsychiatry Clin Neurosci* 2000;**12**:316–27.

34. Simpson G, Tate R. Suicidality in people surviving a traumatic brain injury: prevalence, risk factors and implications for clinical management. *Brain Inj* 2007;**21**:1335–51.

35. Silver JM, Kramer R, Greenwald S, et al. The association between head injuries and psychiatric disorders: findings from the New Haven NIMH Epidemiologic Catchment Area Study. *Brain Inj* 2001;**15**:935–45.

36. Mooney G, Speed J. The association between mild traumatic brain injury and psychiatric conditions. *Brain Inj* 2001;**15**:865–77.

37. Bryant RA. Posttraumatic stress disorder and traumatic brain injury: can they co-exist? *Clin Psychol Rev* 2001;**21**:931–48.

38. Bryant RA, Harvey AG. Relationship between acute stress disorder and posttraumatic stress disorder following mild traumatic brain injury. *Am J Psychiatry* 1998;**155**:625–9.

39. Qureshi S, Long M, Bradshow M, et al. Does PTSD impair cognition beyond the effect of trauma. *J Neurospychiatry Clin Neurosci* 2011;**23**:16–28.

40. Hoge CW, McGurk D, Thomas JL, et al. Mild traumatic brain injury in U.S. soldiers returning from Iraq. *N Engl J Med* 2008;**358**:453–63.

41. Gil S, Caspi Y, Ben-Ari IZ, et al. Does memory of a traumatic event increase the risk of posttraumatic stress disorder in patients with traumatic brain injury? A prospective study. *Am J Psychiatry* 2005;**162**:963–9.

42. Koren D, Norman D, Cohen A, et al. Increased PTSD risk with combat-related injury: a matched comparison study of injured and uninjured soldiers experiencing the same combat events. *Am J Psychiatry* 2005;**162**:276–82.

43. Liberzon I, Sripada CS. The functional neuroanatomy of PTSD: a critical review. *Prog Brain Res* 2008;**167**:151–69.

44. Rogers J, Read C. Psychiatric co-morbidity following traumatic brain injury. *Brain Inj* 2007;**21**:1321–33.

45. Koponen S, Taiminen T, Portin A. Axis I and II psychiatric disorders after traumatic brain injury: a 30 year follow up study. *Am J Psychiatry* 2002;**159**:1315–21.

46. Uomoto JM, Esselman PC. Traumatic brain injury and chronic pain: differential types and rates by head injury severity. *Arch Phys Med Rehab* 1993;**74**:61–4.

47. Baandrup L, Jensen R. Chronic post-traumatic headache – a clinical analysis in relation to the International Headache Classification 2nd Edition. *Cephalgia* 2005;**25**:132–8.

48. Packard RC. Epidemiology and pathogenesis of posttraumatic headache. *J Head Trauma Rehabil* 1999;**14**:9–21.

49. Couch JR, Bears C. Chronic daily headache in the posttrauma syndrome: relation to the extent of head injury. *Headache* 2001;**41**:559.

50. Chamelian L, Feinstein A. Outcome after mild to moderate traumatic brain injury: the role of dizziness. *Arch Phys Med Rehabil* 2004;**85**:1662–6.

51. Anstey KJ, Butterworth P, Jorm AF, et al. A population survey found an association between self-reports of traumatic brain injury and increased psychiatric symptoms. *J Clin Epidemiol* 2004;**57**:1202–9.

52. Cantor JB, Ashman T, Gordon W, et al. Fatigue after traumatic brain injury and its impact on participation and quality of life. *J Head Trauma Rehabil* 2008;**23**:41–51.

53. Ashman TA, Cantor JB, Gordon WA, et al. Objective measurement of fatigue following traumatic brain injury. *J Head Trauma Rehabil* 2008;**23**:33–40.

54. Popovic V. GH deficiency as the most common pituitary defect after TBI: clinical implications. *Pituitary* 2005;**8**:239–43.

55. Rao V, Rollings P. Sleep disturbances following traumatic brain injury. *Curr Treat Options Neurol* 2002;**4**:77–87.

56. Clinchot DM, Bogner J, Mysiw WJ, et al. Defining sleep disturbance after brain injury. *Am J Phys Med Rehabil* 1998;**77**:291–5.

57. McCrory P, Bladn P, Berkovic S. Retrospective study of concussive convulsions in elite Australian rules and rugby league footballers: phenomenology, aetiology, and outcome. *BMJ* 1997;**314**:171–4.

58. Iverson GL, McCracken LM. 'Postconcussive' symptoms in persons with chronic pain. *Brain Inj* 1997;**11**:783–90.

59. Hart RP, Martelli MF, Zasler ND. Chronic pain and neuropsychological functioning. *Neuropsychol Rev* 2000;**10**:131–49.

60. McCracken LM, Iverson GL. Predicting complaints of impaired cognitive functioning in patients with chronic pain. *J Pain Symptom Manage* 2001;**21**:392–6.

61. Borg J, Holm L, Peloso PM, et al. Non-surgical intervention and cost for mild traumatic brain injury: results of the WHO Collaborating Centre Task Force on Mild Traumatic Brain Injury. *J Rehabil Med* 2004;**43**(Suppl):76–83.

62. Randolph C, Millis S, Barr W, et al. Concussion symptom inventory: an empirically derived scale for monitoring resolution of symptoms following sport related concussion. *Arch Clin Neuropsychol* 2009;**24**:219–29.

63. Center for Disease Control. *What to Expect After a Concussion*. Available at: www.acep.org/WorkArea/DownloadAsset.aspx?id=48493 (Accessed August 10, 2012).

Chapter 35

Management of psychiatric illness in pregnancy in the emergency department

Eric L. Anderson

Introduction

For many psychiatric illnesses, the onset of symptoms begins during the late teens to the early thirties [1]. This is especially concerning in women as it coincides with the childbearing years. Pregnancy was once thought to be protective from psychiatric illness. However, as the recent explosion of literature addressing the safety of psychotropic agents in pregnancy illustrates, the puerperal period is not exempt from mental illness [2–4]. The presence of mental illness in pregnancy is associated with poor compliance with prenatal care; increased tobacco, alcohol, and illicit substance use; inadequate maternal nutrition; poor mother–infant bonding; and disruption of the home environment [5].

While the diagnostic criteria are the same as in non-pregnant patients, many symptoms common in mental illness, such as fatigue, low energy, and disrupted sleep, are also normal for pregnancy [6]. Medication treatment is a controversial issue: in the case of the pregnant patient, there are at least two (or more!) patients, mother and unborn child, and many of the treatments available to address mental illness can potentially harm the fetus [3].

This chapter will present the major mental health topics of concern in pregnant patients and offer guidelines in the management of these patients in the emergency setting.

Self-injurious behavior, suicide, and violence

Perhaps most concerning is the patient with suicidal or violent ideations. These thoughts may lead to violent actions against one's self, unborn child, or another. In the emergency setting, it is imperative to assess for the safety of the pregnant patient by inquiring about these thoughts. Suicidal, homicidal, and violent ideations are the presence of a desire to end one's life, the life of another person, or to do harm to another, respectively. "Passive death wishes" differ from suicidal intent in that the person longs for death, but not at her own hands. Regardless, they too are a worrisome symptom.

The risk of suicide during pregnancy is lower than in the general United States population, with a 2% completion rate in pregnant patients versus a completion rate of 5% in all females

of childbearing age [7,8]. The rate rises in the postpartum period, with up to 20% of female deaths attributable to suicide [9]. Discontinuation of psychotropic medications potentially contributes to this increase as discontinuation before or during pregnancy is associated with a high rate of symptoms relapse [2,7,10]. Unfortunately, the recommendation to discontinue psychotropic medication is usually made before an adequate risk–benefit analysis has been conducted [9].

Suicidal and violent symptoms should be assessed in any patient presenting with emotional, psychological, or social stress. This evaluation is sometimes referred to as the "risk assessment." Direct, non-judgmental questions are advised: "Do you have any thoughts of wanting to kill yourself? Do you have any thoughts of wanting to hurt someone else, including your baby?" Contrary to popular belief, asking about these symptoms does not increase the likelihood they will occur. To the contrary, the risk often decreases [7]. Any affirmative answer necessitates further exploration: Is there a plan? Is there intent? Is there access to lethal means? Who is the intended target?

If the patient expresses a desire to harm another person, the clinician may be required to warn the intended victim. The duty to warn stems, at least in part, from the now-famous Tarasoff case. In the event there is a duty to warn, reasonable effort must be made to contact the intended victim. Barring that, law enforcement can be contacted.

Safety is paramount, both for the patient and her unborn child. The patient may be initially monitored in a safe environment in the emergency room, evaluated by a mental health clinician, and sometimes admitted to an inpatient psychiatric unit, depending on acuity. Further management and disposition of these patients does not differ significantly from non-pregnant patients.

Management of the agitated patient

The management of agitation in pregnant patients is similar to non-pregnant patients. Once the etiology is found and addressed, agitation usually resolves. However, there may be instances where either the etiology remains unknown or the agitation persists despite management of the presumed

---

Behavioral Emergencies for the Emergency Physician, ed. Leslie S. Zun, Lara G. Chepenik, and Mary Nan S. Mallory. Published by Cambridge University Press. © Cambridge University Press 2013.

etiology. Additional management strategies come in two major forms: medication and nonmedication.

Nonmedication strategies include brief, focused counseling interventions. Emergency department-based clinicians may be reluctant to use these techniques, believing it will take too much time or that they have too limited skill in counseling. However, evidence shows that these interventions do not require a great deal of time and can ultimately save time in the patient's acute management. Additionally, the ability to establish a trusting relationship between clinician and patient matters more than the specific technique used in the emergent setting [11]. Another critical step to this strategy involves discovering the patient's motivation(s). Many times agitation can be quelled simply by making the effort to meet a patient's perceived need [7].

Despite best efforts, clinicians may find more intensive management is required to keep the patient and her baby safe. Unfortunately, no specific research-based guidelines exist for the pharmacologic management of agitation in pregnancy. The American College of Obstetricians and Gynecologists (ACOG) recommends that single agents, at higher doses, be used over multiple medications [5]. Current guidelines recommend the use of oral medications, if possible, before intramuscular (IM) forms are used [12]. The Best Practices in Evaluation and Treatment of Agitation project has also presented guidelines for the management of acute agitation [13]. A collation of these recommendations is presented in Table 35.1.

On rare occasions, it may be necessary to physically restrain a pregnant patient. Special precautions are necessary for pregnant patients after the first trimester; patients should be placed in the left lateral decubitus position to prevent vena cava

Table 35.1. Treatment of agitation [12,13]

Medical condition (such as delirium)
Haloperidol 2.5–10 mg (liquid, PO, IM) + lorazepam 2 mg (PO, IM)
Risperidone 2 mg (liquid, PO, ODT) +/− lorazepam 2 mg (PO, IM)
Olanzapine 5–10 mg (PO, ODT)[a]
Intoxication and/or withdrawal
Lorazepam 1–2 mg (PO, IM, IV)
Diazepam 5–10 mg (PO)[a]
Primary psychiatric disturbance (such as psychosis)
Ziprasidone 10–20 mg (PO, IM) +/− lorazepam 2 mg (PO, IM)
Risperidone 2 mg (liquid, PO, ODT) +/− lorazepam 2 mg (PO, IM)
Haloperidol 2.5–10 mg (PO, IM) + lorazepam 2 mg (PO, IM)
Olanzapine 5–10 mg (PO, ODT, IM)[a]
Unknown etiology
Lorazepam 1–2 mg (PO, IM)

[a] Second-line options.
IM, intramuscular; PO, by mouth; IV, intravenously; ODT, orally disintegrating tablets.

syndrome [14]. Monitoring should be frequent and include regular monitoring of fetal heart tones and fetal movement [7].

Mood disorders

Unipolar disorders, such as major depression, and bipolar disorders comprise the mood disorders. They tend to have an age of onset that coincides with the peak years of childbearing. For many women, psychotherapy is insufficient to control their symptoms, making medication management necessary to function. The risk of suicide (2%) is lower than in non-pregnant women in the same age group (5%), but this risk rises dramatically in the postpartum period, especially in patients who have discontinued their medications (up to 20%)[7–9]. Infanticide rates up to 4% have also been reported in symptomatic postpartum patients [14].

Depressive disorders

The prevalence of depression varies from 12–25% in women. Depression is as common in pregnancy as it is in the non-pregnant state. It is estimated that roughly 10–16% of all pregnant women suffer from clinical depression [15–17]. In a study by Flynn et al., 31% of pregnant women screened demonstrated evidence of depressive symptoms, but only 22% of them received treatment [18]. One of the reasons cited for low treatment rates is depressive symptoms are often similar to the symptoms of normal pregnancy, including sleep problems, appetite changes, low energy, and problems with concentration [14].

Risk factors for depression include a personal or family history of depression, limited social support, history of abuse (especially sexual or physical), environmental stressors (financial, occupational, relationship, health), living alone, and the presence of substance use [15]. The presence of depression during pregnancy is associated with poor outcomes such as miscarriage, inadequate maternal weight gain, underutilized prenatal care, marital discord, inability to care for other children in the home, low birth weight, preterm delivery, neonates that are small for gestational age, and developmental delay, and suicide [14,16,18,19].

Screening is similar as in non-pregnant patients. Several tools exist, including the three-item RAND screening instrument [20], Edinburgh scale [21], and the U.S. Preventative Services Task Force rapid screen [18].

The management of depression in pregnancy depends upon the severity and course of illness, presence of depression before pregnancy, treatment before or during pregnancy, available resources, and the patient's level of support. Treatment options include psychotherapy, medications, partial or full hospitalization, electroconvulsive therapy (ECT), and repetitive transcranial magnetic stimulation (rTMS).

For patients with mild depression, referral for psychotherapy such as cognitive behavioral or interpersonal therapy may suffice [1]. A list of referral resources should be kept in the emergency department for such purposes. Emergency department personnel may find it useful to establish a working relationship with local mental health clinicians to expedite the referral process. In moderate to severe depression, medications, hospitalization, TMS, or ECT may be required.

The use of medications in pregnancy is a source of debate, but there is a high risk of symptom recurrence if antidepressant medications are discontinued [1,2,6]. Sixty-eight percent of patients who discontinue their medications relapse. This compares to a relapse rate of 26% in those who continued their medications. Half of patients relapsing did so within the first trimester, and over 90% relapsed by the end of the second trimester [15].

Despite the potential risk of relapse and subsequent complications of continued depressive symptoms for both mother and infant, medication use is not a straightforward decision. Antidepressant medications usually take several weeks to become effective. They must be monitored for side effects.

Medication use carries at least four types of potential risk that must be addressed when used in pregnancy: pregnancy loss, organ malformation, neonatal adaptability, and long-term neurodevelopmental sequelae.

The evidence regarding antidepressant use and spontaneous loss of pregnancy is conflicting as some recent studies implicate antidepressants as a general class [6,15], while other studies do not support such claims [2,22]. Furthermore, stress and depression themselves are risk factors for premature delivery and spontaneous abortion [19].

The data for organ malformation is also conflicting. Overall, there is not a statistically significantly increased risk of organ malformation when antidepressants as a class are considered [6,23]. Specific medications have been implicated in increased relative risk. Tricyclic antidepressants (TCAs), such as amitriptyline, clomipramine, and nortriptyline, are associated with an increased risk of cardiac defects, but no specific pattern has emerged [17]. Diav-Citrin el al. found an increased rate of cardiovascular abnormalities in selective serotonin reuptake inhibitors (SSRIs) exposed infants, although causation could not be determined [24]. Louik et al. found no increased risk of craniosynostosis, omphalocele, or heart defects with SSRI exposure overall. But the authors did find an increased relative risk of septal defects in neonates exposed to sertraline, with an odds ratio (OR) of 2.0 based upon 13 exposed patients [25]. In a retrospective cohort study, Malm et al. found that fluoxetine was associated with an isolated relative risk of ventricular septal defects (OR 2.03), paroxetine was associated with a relative risk of right ventricular outflow tract defects (OR 4.68), and citalopram was associated with neural tube defects (OR 2.46). While the absolute risk of these defects was small, the authors recommended against paroxetine and fluoxetine as first-line options [23]. These studies contrast with other authors who have found paroxetine [17] and fluoxetine to be relatively safe in pregnancy [1,6,14,17]. As a class, SSRIs are felt to be safe in pregnancy, with neonatal complications and rates of congenital anomalies falling within the general population rate of 1–3% [17,19,26]. Data is lacking for other antidepressants, such as venlafaxine, duloxetine, mirtazapine, and trazodone, but no significant

associations with malformations have been reported [2,3,17]. Buproprion is not associated with an increased risk of fetal malformations. It is the only antidepressant to date that has a Pregnancy Category B rating [2,27].

Late pregnancy exposure to SSRIs has been associated with an increase in premature delivery, low birth weight, and lower Apgar scores [3]. Poor neonatal adaptability (PNA) has been reported in up to 30% of newborns exposed to SSRIs [28]. PNA symptoms include irritability, abnormal crying, tremor, respiratory distress, jitteriness, lethargy, poor tone, tachypnea, and possibly persistent pulmonary hypertension of the newborn (PPHN) [27,29]. While paroxetine appears to be the SSRI most associated with these symptoms [30], a study by Lorenzo et al. found the absolute risk of PPHN in SSRI-exposed neonates was less than 1%. The major associative factor was the mode of delivery [17]. Seizures in the newborn have also been noted with exposure to TCAs such as clomipramine [6].

Croen et al. found that prenatal exposure to SSRIs was associated with a modest increase in autism spectrum disorders (ASDs). However, the authors concluded that SSRI exposure is very unlikely to be a major risk factor for ASD [31]. Most studies find no adverse neurodevelopmental issues up to the age of two for children exposed to SSRIs in utero and no significant cognitive or behavioral issues [2,22]. Remission of a mother's depression may have a positive impact on childhood development and behavior [32].

Inpatient treatment may be required for patients with severe depression, especially if psychotic or suicidal features are present. Psychoses and suicidal thoughts are psychiatric emergencies, whether or not a patient is pregnant. Inpatient psychiatric treatment seeks to ensure the safety of the patient and her unborn child.

In some cases, especially where medications may not be desired or appropriate, brain stimulation treatment may be used. The two most commonly used forms are ECT and rTMS. rTMS has not been systematically studied in pregnancy but has been found to be helpful in the treatment of depression [33]. It requires no anesthesia, has no cognitive side effects, and can be conducted on an outpatient basis. ECT is an effective treatment for severe depressive symptoms, but it requires anesthesia and the delivery of a seizure inducing electric stimulus. Cognitive impairments are common but typically limited to the actual treatment course. In a review of the literature, ECT was found to be safe and effective for the treatment of depression in pregnancy [34].

The choice of antidepressant treatment is dependent upon the patient's symptoms and preferences, a thorough risk–benefit analysis, and the ability to monitor and adjust the medications and clinical course. An algorithm for decision-making is presented in Figure 35.1 to aid in this decision process.

Bipolar disorders

The prevalence of bipolar disorders, sometimes referred to as bipolar affective disorders (BPADs), in the United States is 3.9–6.4%. Men and women are equally affected [5]. Treatments for

Figure 35.1

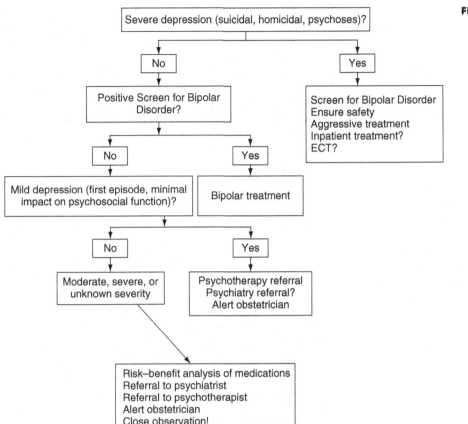

BPAD consist of the traditional mood stabilizers, such as lithium, valproic acid, lamotrigine, carbamazepine, and oxcarbazepine; and the second-generation antipsychotic (SGA) medications. First-generation antipsychotics (FGAs) and benzodiazepines are also used, but usually as an adjunct to a traditional mood stabilizer or SGA (see Table 35.2). Patients with BPAD run the risk of symptom exacerbation in the pre- and postpartum periods [35]. Relapse rates up to 71% have been reported if medications have been discontinued [36]. Nearly half of all relapses occur during the first trimester [37].

Most pregnant patients who present acutely manic or hypomanic have a prior history of BPAD. In any pregnant patient presenting with depressive symptoms, screening for BPAD should be conducted. The diagnosis does not differ from non-pregnant states. However, pregnant patients in a manic, hypomanic, or mixed episode should be considered a psychiatric and obstetric emergency due to the risk to both mother and child [2,37]. Inpatient hospitalization to stabilize the patient's mood is often required. Symptoms of a manic, hypomanic, or mixed episode include poor sleep, abnormally increased energy, agitation, irritability, euphoria, impulsivity, and flights of ideas.

Any pregnant patient with the diagnosis of BPAD should be considered a high-risk pregnancy [38]. Treatment depends upon the severity of illness but usually consists of a mood stabilizer of some kind [38]. Most mood stabilizers carry a teratogenic risk, especially if used in the first trimester [35].

Lithium is the mood stabilizer of choice in pregnancy [14]. Relative to the other traditional mood stabilizers, it is the least problematic. However, lithium's use is associated with Ebstein's anomaly, a downward displacement of the tricuspid valve, in 1:2000 live births [2,5]. For patients receiving lithium, a high-resolution ultrasound and fetal echocardiogram at 16–18 weeks is advised to assess for cardiac issues [5,35]. During the last month of pregnancy, lithium levels should be monitored on a weekly basis [3]. Lithium is not associated with intrauterine growth retardation (IUGR) or PNA, although it has been implicated in floppy baby syndrome. Floppy baby syndrome is self-limited; infants present with cyanosis and hypotonia immediately postpartum. Conservative management and monitoring is usually all that is required [35]. Some authors advocate decreasing the dose of lithium by 25% or stopping it altogether 2–3 days before delivery to prevent neonatal toxicity [3].

Other traditional mood stabilizers, such as valproic acid, lamotrigine, carbamazepine, and oxcarbazepine, are antiepileptic agents. They carry significant teratogenic risk. Folate (4–5 mg administered daily) is recommended for all pregnant patients taking one of these agents [39,40].

Valproic acid (VPA) is associated with a neural tube defect rate of 5–9% (10–20 times greater than the general population), possible IUGR, craniofacial anomalies, limb abnormalities, and withdrawal symptoms consisting of jitteriness, irritability,

Table 35.2. Bipolar and anxiety medications [5][14][39][40]

Medication	FDA classification	Selective reported adverse events [and time of risk conveyance/incidence, if known]
Lithium	D	Floppy baby syndrome (hypotonia, lethargy)[PP], thyroid abnormalities, cardiac anomalies (Ebstein's anomaly)[1]
Valproic acid	D	NTD (spina bifida)[1], cardiovascular defects [1], IUGR [1,2,3], fetal anticonvulsant syndrome [1], coagulopathy, developmental delay [NN], risk for neonatal withdrawal [PP]
Carbamazepine	D	NTD (spina bifida)[1], fetal anticonvulsant syndrome, developmental delay [NN], coagulopathy, craniofacial defects [1], risk for neonatal withdrawal [PP]
Lamotrigine	C	Nonspecific congenital malformations reported at 1–2.5% [1]
FGA	C	Nonspecific congenital malformations reported [1], risk for neonatal neuroleptic malignant syndrome [PP]
SGA	C	Nonspecific congenital malformations reported [1], risk for (except clozapine) neonatal neuroleptic malignant syndrome [PP]
Clozapine	B	Nonspecific congenital malformations reported [1], risk for neonatal neuroleptic malignant syndrome [PP]
Alprazolam, Chlordiazepoxide, Clonazepam, Diazepam, Oxazepam, Lorazepam	D	Cleft/facial defects [1], risk for neonatal withdrawal (hypotonia, respiratory problems, seizures) [PP]

feeding difficulties, and poor tone [2,3,35]. The risk of teratogenic effects increases if VPA is used in combination with other medications, or is at a dose greater than 1,000 mg daily [41]. Given these risks, ACOG recommends against VPA use in pregnancy, especially in the first trimester [5]. If VPA is deemed necessary, a first-trimester ultrasound to evaluate for neural tube defects is recommended. Other recommendations include serial ultrasounds to assess for IUGR, a fetal echocardiogram to assess for cardiac anomalies, alpha-fetoprotein at 16–18 weeks, and a late pregnancy ultrasound [40,41]. Postpartum, vitamin K (1 mg IM) should be given to the neonate to prevent valproic-acid-induced coagulopathies [40].

Carbamazepine is associated with craniofacial defects, fingernail hypoplasia, developmental delay, neural tube defects, cardiovascular abnormalities, and vitamin K deficiency [2,3,35]. Concurrent use of valproic acid increases its teratogenic potential. ACOG advises against its use, and it is therefore reserved for use only if other options are lacking. Its use should be avoided in the first trimester [5,40].

No clear guidelines exist for lamotrigine and oxcarbazepine. Lamotrigine has been associated with an increased risk of cleft palate [2,35] but the Lamotrigine Pregnancy Registry reports a less than 2% risk of fetal malformations with first-trimester exposure [3].

Antipsychotic medications are frequently used as solo or adjunct treatments for mood disorders, whether or not psychotic features are present. Unlike many traditional mood stabilizers, antipsychotics have a rapid onset of action that may begin to work in days or even hours [42]. Antipsychotic medications are broadly divided into first-generation antipsychotics (FGAs) and second-generation antipsychotics (SGAs). The FGAs are commonly used for treatment of acute mania and are felt to be relatively safe in pregnancy [6,35]. FGAs are associated with neonatal extrapyramidal side effects that can persist for several months. High-potency FGAs, such as haloperidol, are preferred because low-potency FGAs, such as chlorpromazine, have been associated with nonspecific teratogenic effects when used in the first trimester [3].

There are limited data on the safety of SGAs in pregnancy [6,35], but they do not appear to be associated with an increased risk of major malformations [3]. The major concern with SGA use in pregnancy is the propensity of this class of medications to cause maternal hyperglycemia and excessive weight gain. These agents are associated with gestational diabetes, insulin resistance, and pre-eclampsia [35].

Benzodiazepines are sometimes used in the treatment of acute mania, especially when agitation is present. Concerns for midline defects such as cleft palate exist, but it is unlikely that limited exposure to benzodiazepines carries appreciable risk to the developing child. Neonatal withdrawal symptoms are possible, especially if benzodiazepines are administered close to delivery [3,35].

Anxiety disorders

Like the mood disorders, anxiety disorders remain problematic during pregnancy; pregnancy is not protective against these symptoms. These disorders encompass a broad range of diagnoses such as social phobia, generalized anxiety disorder, panic disorder (with and without agoraphobia), obsessive-compulsive disorder (OCD), post-traumatic stress disorder, and simple phobias.

Unfortunately, there are limited data on the incidence and prevalence of anxiety disorders during pregnancy. Some disorders, such as panic disorder, have a variable course. Others, such as OCD may be exacerbated by pregnancy [36]. Anxiety disorders appear to have an adverse impact upon the developing fetus. For example, panic disorder in the mother is associated with lower neonatal Apgar scores and increased rates of maternal preterm labor and placental abruption [6]. Anxiety in general is associated with an increased incidence of delivery by forceps, prolonged labor, fetal distress, preterm delivery, and decreased neonatal adaptability [5].

One of the most effective forms of treatment for anxiety is cognitive behavioral therapy (CBT), a structured, duration-limited psychotherapy [43]. While this form of therapy may not be practical in the emergency setting, aspects of CBT may be used effectively to alleviate the patient's suffering. For example, skills such as deep breathing, guided imagery, and progressive muscle relaxation can be quickly taught to patients, allowing immediate use to combat anxiety symptoms.

Medication management of anxiety symptoms in pregnancy is controversial. Traditional antidepressants, such as the SSRIs, serotonin-norepinephrine reuptake inhibitors (SNRIs), and tricyclic antidepressants (TCAs) are also used to treat anxiety disorders. However, these medications have drawbacks, as illustrated earlier.

Benzodiazepines, such as lorazepam, are the medication class of choice for acute anxiety symptoms. While some studies demonstrate no association between extended benzodiazepine use and major malformations, other data suggest a small increase in relative risk (0.6%) for malformations such as oral cleft [44]. The use of benzodiazepines near or at delivery may result in floppy infant syndrome: hypotonia, apnea, temperature instability, and neonatal withdrawal symptoms [5,6,14].

Psychotic disorders

The psychotic disorders include psychotic disorder not otherwise specified, schizophrenia, brief psychotic disorder, and schizoaffective disorder. The general population prevalence of schizophrenia is roughly 1%. Males and females are equally affected. Recent evidence indicates a prodromal period that may be present as early as late childhood, but for most women, the peak onset of symptoms occurs between the ages of 25–35 [45]. Psychotic symptoms may be found in the presence of severe mood disorders, such as manic episodes or severe depression. The course of psychotic disorders and psychosis in pregnancy is not well understood, and the literature is sparse and contradictory [10].

A psychotic, pregnant patient is an obstetric and psychiatric emergency. Psychoses during pregnancy may interfere with a patient's ability to obtain and participate in appropriate antenatal care. The presence of psychotic symptoms may lead to a lack of cooperation at delivery [6]. Psychotic disorders are associated with a higher use of tobacco products and alcohol, lower socioeconomic status, more unplanned pregnancies, low

birth weight, preterm labor, placental abnormalities, and poor neonatal health, including postnatal death [5,10,45].

FGAs (such as haloperidol, fluphenazine, chlorpromazine, and perphenazine) and SGAs (such as quetiapine, olanzapine, risperidone, aripiprazole, ziprasidone, lurasidone, asenapine, iloperidone, and paliperidone) are the mainstay of treatment in psychotic disorders. High-potency FGAs such as haloperidol have a greater risk for acute dystonic reactions, akathisia, extrapyramidal symptoms (EPS), and tardive dyskinesia (TD) than do low-potency FGAs. However, low-potency FGAs such as chlorpromazine have a greater risk of sedation, weight gain, and seizures. With the advent of the SGAs, the risks of EPS and TD are lower, but still present to a degree. SGAs have the potential to cause metabolic disturbances, such as weight gain, hyperlipidemia, and hyperglycemia [3,45]. Hyperlipidemia is concerning as it may lead to gestational diabetes [10].

Few data exist to guide the clinician with respect to antipsychotic use in pregnancy. Some authors advise the use of high-potency FGAs over low-potency FGAs and SGAs [1]. There appears to be an increased risk of teratogenic effects, specifically congenital malformations, with the use of low-potency FGAs [10,14]. SGAs such as quetiapine and olanzapine can lead to significant weight gain, but there appears to be minimal risk for major fetal malformations [45]. For patients receiving clozapine, white blood cell counts (WBC) must be obtained every 2 weeks. A screening WBC for the neonate is also advised [40].

The choice of antipsychotic treatment for the long term is problematic, but in the emergency setting the same guidelines for acute agitation may be followed (see Table 35.1). Haloperidol is preferred especially during labor due to its potency, low sedative properties, and intravenous or intramuscular mode of delivery [6].

Substance abuse disorders

Substance abuse disorders are common in the United States, and unfortunately pregnancy is no exception. It is estimated that 4.5–10.3% of pregnant women drink alcohol to excess, 12.6–22.1% smoke nicotine, and 5.1% use illicit substances such as cocaine, marijuana, or opioids [46]. Substance use is associated with preterm delivery, low birth weight, smaller fetal head circumference, miscarriage, and fetal central nervous system damage [14].

Screening for substance use in the emergency setting should be simple, direct, and nonjudgmental. Some pregnant patients may be hesitant to disclose their substance use for fear of judgment or losing their baby to state custody. Reassuring patients that the focus of the screens is treatment, not punishment, may be necessary to obtain honest answers. Several rapid screening tests are available to assess for alcohol use. These include the T-ACE, CAGE, and TWEAK screens [47].

Management of the intoxicated patient depends upon the substance(s) ingested. Alcohol withdrawal poses a medical and obstetric emergency due to the risk of withdrawal seizures.

Prolonged seizures, especially status epilepticus, can be fatal to the fetus. Benzodiazepines are the preferred treatment. Dosing should proceed as with the non-pregnant patient.

Opioid intoxication and withdrawal may lead to fetal demise. While detoxification can be attempted, maintenance treatment with either methadone or buprenorphine is preferred to prevent withdrawal and relapse of opioid use [14]. Treatment of withdrawal from other substances such as cocaine, marijuana, and phencyclidine tends to be supportive only: provide a calm, quiet setting, with frequent monitoring of both the patient and her baby.

Some states require reporting of pregnant patients with concurrent substance use. State regulations vary from state-to-state, so emergency room clinicians are advised to know the regulations and laws for their state.

Eating disorders

Eating disorders (EDs), such as anorexia nervosa and bulimia nervosa, have a prevalence rate of roughly 4% [48]. EDs usually manifest by the patient's late teens, during the beginning and peak years of a woman's reproductive age. They are associated with a high risk of miscarriage, congenital malformations, smaller fetal head circumference, premature delivery, low birth weight, and delivery by means of cesarean section [49]. There is a greater risk of postpartum depression in women who have an eating disorder during pregnancy [50]. Pregnant patients with a concurrent eating disorder are considered high risk. Close observation throughout pregnancy is warranted to ensure proper weight gain.

Screening for eating disorders is reasonable in any pregnant patient who appears to be underweight. Questions should be direct, simple, and nonjudgmental: "Do you have any struggles with eating? Are you afraid of getting fat? Do you ever force yourself to throw up? Do you exercise several hours or more a day?" For patients demonstrating poor weight gain, an admission to an eating disorders unit may be necessary. At the very least, the patient should be referred to a therapist skilled at treating eating disorders. The National Eating Disorders Association (www.edap.org) maintains a referral hotline: 1-800-931-2237.

Domestic violence

In the United States, over 2 million women are assaulted annually, 50 million over the course of their lifetime [51]. Pregnancy fails to protect against domestic violence, although evidence suggests that pregnancy itself does not increase the rate of violence [51]. A male partner usually perpetrates the domestic violence. Its most common forms include physical abuse, sexual abuse, verbal threats, isolation, and economic abuse, such as withholding of financial resources [52]. Data are limited, but prevalence rates of violence in pregnancy are estimated at 1 to 20.6% [14,52]. This wide range is likely the result of many factors, such as the method used to screen, the population sampled, and whether or not emotional abuse was counted in the data.

Risk factors for pregnancy-related violence include low socio-economic status, low levels of social support, no prior parenting experience, unwanted or unexpected pregnancy, extremes of age, single marital status, higher parity, and substance use [51,53]. Consequences of violence include late entry into prenatal care, depression, anxiety, low maternal weight gain, emotional distress, infection, anemia, short inter-pregnancy interval, bleeding, low birth weight, uterine rupture, fetal injuries (such as fractures), and maternal or fetal death [51,52].

Warning signs of domestic violence include repeated visits, recurrent headaches, recurrent vaginitis, irritable bowel syndrome, substance use, a history of depression or anxiety, suicide attempts, a personal history of abuse or assault, and repeated visits for injuries [53]. The patient may demonstrate fright, startle responses, over-compliance, excessive distrust, flat affect, anxiety or depression symptoms, psychic numbing, and dissociation. Warning signs in the partner's behavior may include solicitousness, refusal to leave the patient, monitoring of the patient's responses, answering for the patient, hostility, and excessive demands [53].

Screening questions should be asked in private, away from the patient's partner, family, and friends. Patents should be reminded about confidentiality. The most effective means of screening is done personally in a nonjudgmental, brief, direct manner. For example: "Many women experience violence. Because it can have a negative impact on health and wellness, I ask all my patients about it." [53]

Patients with a positive domestic violence screen should be referred for treatment. Treatment varies from formal domestic violence consultations to safe havens. Accurate medical documentation is important for any future legal cases [14]. In many states clinicians are required to report acts of domestic violence (whether or not the patient is pregnant) [52,53]. It is important to know the state and local (if applicable) mandatory reporting regulations. Many clinicians feel powerless and helpless in these situations because they cannot convince the patient to leave her abusive situation. While the emergency clinician's role is to keep the patient and her baby safe as mentioned above, ultimately the woman must make the decision to end the relationship for herself [52].

Postpartum mood and anxiety disorders

The immediate period following labor and delivery is a time of significant physical adjustment for most mothers. Emotional and mental adjustments also occur and many of these changes are well within the spectrum of normal experience. Some women experience mood or anxiety symptoms in the postpartum period significant enough to warrant further management, especially if the patient has a history of a psychiatric disorder and her medications were discontinued during or before pregnancy.

Postpartum "blues" (PPB) are common, occurring in up to 75% of women postpartum. Patients with PPB feel irritable, demonstrate mood lability, and emotional sensitivity. Symptoms usually begin within one week of delivery and resolve within 1 month. The symptoms typically do not impair the patient. Supportive care is the most appropriate treatment option [4].

Postpartum depression (PPD) presents in a manner similar to MDD. The same risk factors for MDD also exist for PPD. Prevalence of PPD is 10–15%, presenting most frequently within the first 2–3 months following delivery [2]. Unfortunately, many of the symptoms of PPB overlap with PPD, making it difficult to distinguish the two. However, if there is a prior history of depression, PPD should be suspected because roughly half of all women who stop their antidepressant medications develop recurrence of their depressive symptoms within 6 months of delivery [36]. In patients with a prior history of MDD or PPD, rates of subsequent PPD are 25% and 50–62%, respectively [1,14].

Screening tools such as the Edinburgh Scale may help to differentiate PPB from PPD [21]. Untreated PPD can have a negative impact on child well-being and development, so prompt recognition and treatment is critical [2]. For mild to moderate PPD, the use of CBT and/or IPT has been studied and found to be effective [2]. In cases of more severe depression, treatment with medications, in addition to therapy, may be warranted [1].

The SSRI's are considered first-line treatment due to their low side-effect profile and tolerability, followed by bupropion and the tricyclic antidepressants [2]. Fluoxetine and its active metabolite are excreted into breast milk [22]. They have a possible association with colic, poor feeding, constant crying, seizure-like episodes, and irritability. Paroxetine is excreted in breast milk but no adverse impacts have been reported in nursing infants [22]. The lowest exposure to nursing infants appears to be with sertraline, the highest with citalopram and fluoxetine [22]. rTMS is an option for patients wishing to avoid medications. In severe cases of depression, especially if psychotic symptoms are present, inpatient psychiatric treatment with or without ECT may be necessary to stabilize the patient's symptoms.

The prevalence of manic symptoms following pregnancy is unknown. Untreated BPAD has a high rate of recurrence if it remains untreated in the early postpartum period [4], with rates reported as high as 60%. Symptoms often present less than a week following delivery [14]. BPAD should be considered in any new-onset PPD.

Symptoms of postpartum mania include precipitous deterioration, insomnia/poor sleep, labile affect, and unhealthy or paranoid preoccupation with the baby's well-being. There is a 5% suicide rate and 4% infanticide rate for untreated patients with BPAD [14]. Rapid stabilization includes a mood stabilizer and timely referral to a psychiatrist [14]. There should be a low threshold for inpatient hospitalization.

Choice of a mood stabilizer involves a risk–benefit analysis, especially for breast-feeding mothers. The American Academy of Pediatrics (AAP) advises caution in patients who are breast-feeding if they are concurrently taking lithium, with special attention being paid to potential toxicity in the

infant [35]. Lithium is readily excreted into breast milk. Toxic lithium levels in infants manifests as lethargy, cyanosis, hypotonia, and hypothermia. If possible, its use should be postponed until the infant is 5 months old, when infant renal clearance is less of an issue [40]. If its use cannot be avoided, infants should be monitored both clinically and with serum blood counts and lithium levels.

The American Academy of Neurology (AAN) and AAP both endorse the use of valproic acid and carbamazepine in breast-feeding mothers [35]. The AAP advises the monitoring of hepatic function in breast-feeding infants whose mothers take either of these two medications [6,40]. The additional benefit of valproic acid, especially in the emergency setting, is that it may be loaded as a single dose at 15–25 mg/kg. Subsequent daily dosing is adjusted to 10–15 mg/kg/day. A serum level is checked in 4–5 days so further adjustments can be made.

Data for lamotrigine are limited. The risk of serious side effects such as Stevens-Johnson syndrome is present for both mother and breast-feeding infant; close monitoring is warranted [40]. Data regarding the use of oxcarbazepine in nursing infants are lacking.

FGAs and SGAs can be used in the emergent treatment of postpartum mania, with the same guidelines as in non-pregnant patients. Data are limited for breast-feeding patients; to date no serious adverse events have been reported in nursing infants [40].

Data on postpartum anxiety disorders are sparse. Patients presenting with acute anxiety in the postpartum period may be treated using the same treatment guidelines as non-pregnant patients. In patients who are breast-feeding and receiving benzodiazepines, infants should be monitored for clinical signs of intoxication or toxicity, to include hypotonia, poor feeding, thermoregulation problems, seizures, lethargy, and irritability [3,5].

Postpartum psychotic disorders

The prevalence of new-onset psychosis in the postpartum period is not known, but estimates have placed the incidence as high as 1–2 in 1000 live births [54]. There usually is a prior history of a psychotic or mood disorder [6]. Risk factors for postpartum psychosis include a history of psychotic symptoms (especially in pregnancy), multiple hospitalizations for psychosis, and antipsychotic discontinuation or noncompliance [54].

Postpartum psychotic symptoms start rapidly after delivery, usually within 3 weeks. Some patients may demonstrate signs as early as 72 hours [2]. Symptoms include sleep disruption, paranoia, restlessness, agitation, disorganized thinking, impulsivity, risky or reckless behavior, and labile affect [4].

Postpartum psychosis is a psychiatric emergency due to the risk to both mother and child. Emergency treatment follows the same guidelines as for acute agitation (see Table 35.1). Inpatient psychiatric hospitalization may be required. ECT may be necessary to stabilize the patient's condition [2,4,14].

Conclusion

Pregnancy does not convey protection against mental illness. Pregnant patients with comorbid psychiatric problems are a special challenge to emergency department personnel. From a diagnostic standpoint, pregnant patients differ little from non-pregnant ones. However, acute management differs because one must also take the developing child's safety and well-being into consideration. The information and guidelines presented in this chapter will aid the emergency department clinician in evaluating and treating this special population of psychiatric patients.

References

1. Altshuler LL, Cohen LS, Moline ML, et al. Treatment of depression in women: a summary of the expert consensus guidelines. *J Psychiatr Pract* 2001;**7**:185–208.

2. Cohen LS, Wang B, Nonacs R, et al. Treatment of mood disorders during pregnancy and postpartum. *Psychiatr Clin North Am* 2010;**33**:273–93.

3. Jain AE, Lacy TL. Psychotropic drugs in pregnancy and lactation. *J Psychiatr Pract* 2005;**11**:177–91.

4. Chaudron LH. Critical issues in perinatal psychiatric emergency care. *Psychiatric Times* 2006;**23**:36–8.

5. ACOG Practice Bulletin. Use of psychiatric medications during pregnancy and lactation. *Obstet Gynecol* 2008;**111**:1001–20.

6. Cohen LS, Nonacs R, Viguera AC. The pregnant patient. In: Stern TA, Fricchione GL, Cassem NH et al. (Eds.). *Massachusetts General Hospital Handbook of General Hospital Psychiatry*, (5th Edition). Philadelphia: Mosby; 2004;593–611.

7. Mills MD, Berkowitz P. Psychiatric emergencies in pregnancy. In: Foley MR, Strong TH, Garite TJ, (Eds.). *Obstetric Intensive Care Manual*, (3rd Edition). New York: McGraw-Hill Inc; 2011.

8. Marzuk PM, Tardiff K, Leon AC, et al. Lower risk of suicide during pregnancy. *Am J Psychiatry* 1997;**154**:122–3.

9. Dell DL, O'Brien BW. Suicide in pregnancy. *Obstet Gynecol* 2003;**102**:1306–9.

10. Patton SW, Misri S, Corral MR, Perry KF, Kuan AJ. Antipsychotic medication during pregnancy and lactation in women with schizophrenia: evaluating the risk. *Can J Psychiatry* 2002;**47**:959–65.

11. Horvath AO, Symonds BD. Relation between a working alliance and outcome in psychotherapy: a meta-analysis. *J Couns Psychol* 1991;**38**:139–49.

12. Ladavac AS, Dubin WR, Ning A, et al. Emergency management of agitation in pregnancy. *Gen Hosp Psychiatry* 2007;**29**:39–41.

13. Holloman GH Jr, Zeller SL. Overview of Project BETA: best practices in evaluation and treatment of agitation. *West J Emerg Med* 2012;**13**:1–2.

14. Henshaw E, Marcus S. Psychiatric emergencies during pregnancy and postpartum and review of gender issues in psychiatric emergency medicine. In: Glick RL, Berlin JS, Fishkind AB, Zeller SL, (Eds.). *Emergency Psychiatry: Principles and Practice*. Philadelphia: Lippincott Williams & Wilkins; 2008;317–43.

15. Muzik M, Marcus SM, Heringhausen JE, et al. When depression complicates childbearing: guidelines for screening and treatment during antenatal and postpartum obstetric care. *Obstet Gynecol Clin North Am* 2009;**36**:771–88.

16. Yonkers KA, Wisner KL, Stewart DE, et al. The management of depression during pregnancy: a report from the American Psychiatric Association and the American College of Obstetricians and Gynecologists. *Gen Hosp Psychiatry* 2009;**31**:403–13.

17. Lorenzo L, Byers B, Einarson A. Antidepressant use in pregnancy. *Expert Opin Drug Saf* 2011;**10**:883–9.

18. Flynn HA, Davis M, Marcus SM, et al. Rates of maternal depression in pediatric emergency department and relationship to child service utilization. *Gen Hosp Psychiatry* 2004;**26**:316–22.

19. Gelenberg AJ, Freeman MP, Markowitz JC, et al. (Work Group on Major Depressive Disorder). *APA Practice Guideline for the Treatment of Patients with Major Depressive Disorder*, (3rd Edition). Washington, DC: APA; 2010. Available at: http://www.psychiatryonline.com/pracGuide/pracGuideTopic_7.aspx (Accessed June 13, 2011).

20. Kemper KJ, Babonis TR. Screening for maternal depression in pediatric clinics. *Am J Dis Child* 1992;**146**:876–8.

21. Cox JL, Holden JM, Sagovsky R. Detection of postnatal depression: development of the 10-item Edinburgh Postnatal Depression Scale. *Br J Psychiatry* 1987;**150**:782–6.

22. Hallberg P, Sjoblom V. The use of selective serotonin reuptake inhibitors during pregnancy and breast-feeding: a review and clinical aspects. *J Clin Psychopharmacol* 2005;**25**:59–73.

23. Malm H, Artama M, Gissler M, et al. Selective serotonin reuptake inhibitors and risk for major congenital anomalies. *Obstet Gynecol* 2011;**118**:111–20.

24. Diav-Citrin O, Shechtman S, Weinbaum D, et al. Paroxetine and fluoxetine in pregnancy: a prospective, multicentre, controlled, observational study. *Br J Clin Pharmacol* 2008;**66**:695–705.

25. Louik C, Lin AE, Werler MM, et al. First-trimester use of selective serotonin-reuptake inhibitors and the risk of birth defects. *N Engl J Med* 2007;**356**:2675–83.

26. Hendrick V, Smith LM, Suri R, et al. Birth outcomes after prenatal exposure to antidepressant medication. *Am J Obstet Gynecol* 2003;**188**:812–15.

27. Food and Drug Administration. *Federal Register* 1980;**44**:37, 434–67.

28. Koren G, Matsui D, Einarson A, et al. Is maternal use of selective serotonin reuptake inhibitors in the third trimester of pregnancy harmful to neonates? *CMAJ* 2005;**172**:1457–9.

29. Chambers CD, Hernandez-Diaz S, VanMarter LJ, et al. Selective serotonin-reuptake inhibitors and risk of persistent pulmonary hypertension of the newborn. *N Engl J Med* 2006;**354**:579–87.

30. Sanz EJ, De-las-Cuevas C, Kiuru A, et al. Selective serotonin reuptake inhibitors in pregnant women and neonatal

withdrawal syndrome: a database analysis. *Lancet* 2005;**365**:482–7.

31. Croen LA, Grether JK, Yoshida CK, Odouli R, Hendrick V. Antidepressant use during pregnancy and childhood autism spectrum disorders. *Arch Gen Psychiatry* 2011;**68**:1104–12.

32. Wickramaratne P, Gameroff MJ, Pilowsky DJ, et al. Children of depressed mothers 1 year after remission of maternal depression: findings from the STAR*D-Child study. *Am J Psychiatry* 2011;**168**:593–602.

33. George MS, Lisanby SH, Avery D, et al. Daily left prefrontal transcranial magnetic stimulation therapy for major depressive disorder. A sham-controlled randomized trial. *Arch Gen Psychiatry* 2010;**67**:507–16.

34. Anderson EL, Reti IM. ECT in pregnancy: a review of the literature from 1941 to 2007. *Psychosom Med* 2009;**71**:235–42.

35. Yonkers KA, Wisner KL, Stowe Z, et al. Management of bipolar disorder during pregnancy and the postpartum period. *Am J Psychiatry* 2004;**161**:608–20.

36. Altshuler LL, Hendrick V, Cohen LS. An update on mood and anxiety disorders during pregnancy and the postpartum period. *Prim Care Companion J Clin Psychiatry* 2000;**2**:217–22.

37. Viguera AC, Whitfield T, Baldessarini RJ, et al. Risk of recurrence in women with bipolar disorder during pregnancy: prospective study of mood stabilizer discontinuation. *Am J Psychiatry* 2007;**164**:1817–24.

38. Viguera AC, Cohen LS, Baldessarini RJ, et al. Managing bipolar disorder in pregnancy: weighing the risks and benefits. *Can J Psychiatry* 2002;**47**:426–36.

39. Marcus SM, Barry KL, Flynn HA, et al. Treatment guidelines for depression in pregnancy. *Int J Gynaecol Obstet* 2001;**72**:61–70.

40. Ernst CL, Goldberg JF. The reproductive safety profile of mood stabilizers, atypical antipsychotics, and broad-spectrum psychotropics. *J Clin Psychiatry* 2002;**63**:s42–55.

41. Diav-Citrin O, Shechtman S, Bar-Oz B, et al. Pregnancy outcome after in utero exposure to valproate. *CNS Drugs* 2008;**22**:325–34.

42. Goodwin GM, Consensus Group of the British Association for Psychopharmacology. Evidence-based guidelines for the treatment of bipolar disorder: revised second edition – recommendations from the British Association for Psychopharmacology. *J Psychopharmacol* 2009;**23**:346–88.

43. Otto MW, Smits JA, Reese HE. Cognitive-behavioral therapy for the treatment of anxiety disorders. *J Clin Psychiatry* 2004;**65**:S34–41.

44. Dolovich LR, Addis A, Régis-Vaillancourt JM, et al. Benzodiazepine use in pregnancy and major malformations or oral cleft: meta-analysis of cohort and case-control studies. *BMJ* 1998;**317**:839–43.

45. McKenna K, Koren G, Tetelbaum M, et al. Pregnancy outcome of women using atypical antipsychotic drugs: a prospective comparative study. *J Clin Psychiatry* 2005;**66**:444–9.

46. SAMHSA, Office of Applied Studies. *National Survey on Drug Use and Health*. Available at: http://www.oas.samhsa.gov/nsduh/2k8nsduh/2k8Results.pdf 2005, 2006, 2007, 2008. (Accessed October 17, 2011).

47. Russell M. New assessment tools for drinking during pregnancy, T-ACE, TWEAK, and others. *Alcohol Health Res World* 1994;**18**:55–61.

48. National Institute of Mental Health. *Statistics*. Available at: http://www.nimh.nih.gov/statistics/index.shtml (Accessed October 20, 2011).

49. Kouba S, Hallstrom T, Lindholm C, et al. Pregnancy and neonatal outcomes in women with eating disorders. *Obstet Gynecol* 2005;**105**:255–60.

50. Franko DL, Blais MA, Becker AE, et al. Pregnancy complications and neonatal outcomes in women with eating disorders. *Am J Psychiatry* 2001;**158**:1461–6.

51. Jasinski JL. Pregnancy and domestic violence: a review of the literature. *Trauma Violence Abuse* 2004;**5**:47–64.

52. Espinosa L, Osborne K. Domestic violence during pregnancy: implications for practice. *J Midwifery Womens Health* 2002;**47**:305–17.

53. U.S. Department of Health and Human Services Centers for Disease Control and Prevention. *Intimate Partner Violence During Pregnancy: A Guide for Clinicians.* 2011. http://www.cdc.gov/reproductivehealth/violence/intimatepartnerviolence/sld021.htm (Accessed October 20, 2011).

54. Harlow BL, Vitonis AF, Sparen P, et al. Incidence of hospitalization for postpartum psychotic and bipolar episodes in women with and without prior prepregnancy or prenatal psychiatric hospitalizations. *Arch Gen Psychiatry* 2007;**64**:42–8.

Chapter 36

Cultural concerns and issues in emergency psychiatry

Suzie Bruch

Introduction

The increasing diversification of the population has placed increased demands on the healthcare system to treat patients of different cultural backgrounds. In the field of emergency psychiatry, a person's ethnic background, race, religion, values, beliefs, customs, and language can affect the symptoms with which a psychiatric illness may present. Culture in the United States has been heavily influenced by Euro-American Protestant values including independence, autonomy, and self-sufficiency [1]. However, the complexion of the population in this country has changed dramatically over the past several decades. Between 1980 and 2010, the population of Asians in the United States increased by 319%, Hispanics by 246%, American Indians by 106%, and African Americans by 47%, in comparison to a 9% increase in the non-Hispanic white population [2].

Culture, cultural competence, and cultural formulation

The Department of Health and Human Services has defined culture as a common heritage or set of beliefs, norms, and values [3]. Culture encompasses race, ethnic background, spirituality, gender, age, sexual orientation, marital status, socioeconomic status, and education. Cultural competence refers to the set of skills and practices necessary to provide culturally appropriate care, which respects the patient's ethnocultural beliefs, values, attitudes, and conventions [4]. The notion of cultural competence aligns with the trend toward evidence-based medicine in that both represent a focus on providing effective treatment for each individual patient. Unfortunately, scientific evidence to guide treatment of patients belonging to a culture other than the majority is limited.

The charge to provide culturally competent care in the United States is rooted in the civil rights movement of the 1960s and reflects an interpretation of the Declaration of Independence to extend basic civil rights to all citizens and to outlaw discrimination [5]. Title VI of the 1964 Civil Rights Act mandated that service providers receiving federal financial assistance provide meaningful and equal access to services for people with limited

English proficiency. Transcultural psychiatry was recognized by the American Psychiatric Association as a specialty in 1969 [6]. In the 1980s, the biopsychosocial model of case formulation took hold in psychiatry. By the 1990s, states including California and New York enacted legislation to ensure provision of culturally and linguistically appropriate health care. At the same time, the American Psychiatric Association included an outline for cultural formulation in the *The Diagnostic and Statistical Manual of Mental Disorders Fourth Edition* and reference to cultural factors in its published practice guidelines for adults, providing a framework for culturally competent evaluations of psychiatric patients.

Despite the government mandate for equal access to health care and the increased focus on cultural competency, the Surgeon General's Report on Mental Health, Culture, Race and Ethnicity and the Institute of Medicine's report "Unequal Treatment" concluded that ethnic minority patients have less access to services, are less likely to receive mental health treatment, receive a lower quality of care both in terms of medical and psychiatric treatment, and are underrepresented in mental health research [3,5,6]. Yet migrant populations exhibit a higher incidence of mental illness compared with native populations, and ethnic minorities experience a greater disability burden from mental illness than do non-Hispanic whites [7,8]. While one in five Americans experiences mental illness, the majority of people with diagnosable disorders do not receive treatment, regardless of race or ethnicity [3]. As a result of his report, the Surgeon General declared that cultural competence should be a core component of any service [5]. Unfortunately, 80% of psychiatric staff feel that their professional training prepares them "very little" or "not at all" for cross-cultural clinical work [7].

A culturally competent evaluation of the psychiatric patient includes assessment of the cultural identity of the individual, the role of culture in the expression and evaluation of psychiatric symptoms, and the effect of cultural differences on the relationship between patient and clinician. In assessing a patient's cultural identity, it is helpful to assess the degree of involvement with both the culture of origin and the host culture and to note language ability and preference. This assessment may identify areas of cultural conflict pertinent to the patient's presentation. Attention to cultural relevance of stressors and

Behavioral Emergencies for the Emergency Physician, ed. Leslie S. Zun, Lara G. Chepenik, and Mary Nan S. Mallory. Published by Cambridge University Press. © Cambridge University Press 2013.

supports may help with both understanding of illness and formulation of treatment plan. The clinician needs to understand the meaning of a patient's symptoms within his culture. For example, African patients reporting crawling, burning, and itching sensations in their heads are typically not seen by members of their culture as having lost contact with reality [9]. Goals of cultural formulation include increased understanding of patients' perceptions of illness, more accurate diagnosis, more appropriate treatment, and improved access to care.

Explanatory models of illness

A patient's explanatory model of illness reflects his own cultural background. Each culture regulates its own patterns of emotional expression, determining which are socially acceptable and which are deviant. Culture influences the sources of distress, the illness experience, the symptomatology and interpretation of these symptoms, coping mechanisms and help-seeking behaviors, family and community supports, as well as the social response to distress and disability [3,10]. The cultures of the clinician and system of care influence diagnosis, treatment, and delivery of care. The stigma associated with mental illness appears to be universal cross-culturally, and alternative conceptualizations of illness may mitigate this stigma [11].

In many cultures, mood and anxiety disorders may be viewed as moral or social defect rather than illness. The United States is unique in the open expression of interpersonal conflict. Many other cultures value the suppression of both internal and interpersonal conflict, prioritizing non-confrontational interaction and social harmony. Kleinman recommended a mini-ethnographic approach to evaluating individuals from different cultures, eliciting such concerns as "Why me?" "Why now?" "What is wrong?" "How long will it last?" "How serious is it?" "Who can intervene or treat the condition?" [12]. Understanding the patient's own view of illness promotes collaboration between clinician and patient, enabling the clinician to more successfully develop and implement a viable treatment plan and leading to improved outcomes and greater patient satisfaction. When the clinician shares the patient's model of understanding distress and treatment, patient satisfaction is greatest [12]. Conflicting explanatory models may result in poor rapport, non-adherence to treatment, and dropout of treatment. The clinician should attempt to implement an evidence-based treatment which does not conflict with the patient's cultural beliefs. Conflict between patient and family explanatory models leads to family discord, shame, and impaired support system. When the patient's explanatory model differs from that of his community, he may suffer social isolation and stigmatization [1].

Language

Thirty-one million patients in the USA speak primary languages which differ from those of their healthcare providers [13]. The National Healthcare Disparities Report found that 47% of patients with limited English proficiency do not have a usual source of care and that 6% have a usual source of care which does not provide language assistance [14]. Patients with limited English proficiency are less likely to have regular health providers or to receive routine preventive treatment [15]. They experience increased frequency of medication complications and are less satisfied with clinician communication and overall health care [15].

Language barriers prove particularly problematic for patients presenting with psychiatric symptoms. Patients experiencing acute psychiatric illness may lose their ability to communicate freely in an acquired language. Whether more psychopathology is evident when a patient is interviewed in his native tongue or a second language is debated in the literature. While Marcos et al. showed that Spanish-American patients with schizophrenia displayed more psychopathology when interviewed in English than Spanish [16], Del Castillo showed that patients interviewed in their native languages displayed more psychotic symptoms [17]. The former postulate that patients with schizophrenia have difficulty expressing their experiences in general, that they may be tense when speaking English, and that they may give up, appearing emotionally withdrawn or uncooperative [16]. Del Castillo hypothesizes that the effort of communicating in a second language results in an unconscious vigilance over emotions and that patients speaking in their native languages will be more apt to freely associate, allowing their thoughts to be dominated by their unconscious minds [17]. He posits that the sheer nature of having to think in another language provides a reality check for the patient [17].

Studies assessing language in patients with depression have shown increased duration of articulations and increased pause times [16]. These same speech patterns may be present when a person is speaking in a second language and may contribute to a clinician performing an erroneous assessment [16]. Speech disturbances have also been identified as verbal indicators of anxiety, and these same traits have been observed in Spanish-American patients speaking English [16].

Interpreters, translation, and communication

Interpretation is of critical importance in the evaluation of behavioral emergencies as the mental status exam is more subjective than the physical exam and any distortion may lead to misdiagnosis or misunderstanding of treatment. In emergency situations, healthcare providers are forced to complete an evaluation in a limited period of time. Yet, it is important that sufficient time be devoted to the interview to allow the patient to present his own narrative describing symptoms and illness. This can be particularly challenging when interpretation is required.

In addition to the notion of cultural competence, we must also consider the concept of communication competency in medical interviews [18]. A translator provides a more literal interpretation of a patient's report while an interpreter provides a cultural context. When using interpreters, healthcare professionals must work to maintain basic principles of medical ethics, including patient rights, patient autonomy, patient confidentiality, and informed consent. Upholding these principles can be particularly difficult when the healthcare provider is dependant on an informal interpreter. Usage of a layperson as interpreter provides for potential distortions based on the interpreter's attitudes toward both patient and clinician. Untrained interpreters may feel uncomfortable with the personal nature of the clinician's questions or overwhelmed by the responsibility of this task. Family and friends interpreting is problematic due to their lack of objectivity and tendency to respond to clinicians' questions without input from the patient. An interpreter's inadequate understanding of the patient's culture can adversely impact the interview. Language competency, interpretative skills, and cultural knowledge are critical components in the successful evaluation of a patient presenting with a behavioral emergency.

The psychiatric interview is highly dependent on the interpreter, who has the power to control the information being exchanged. Accuracy of meaning may be diminished when an unskilled interpreter simply translates. The effectiveness of communication essential for an accurate psychiatric diagnosis and treatment plan may be altered by the dynamic of using an interpreter. In addition to the clinician–patient relationship, there now also exist relationships between patient and interpreter and between clinician and interpreter. Anxious or paranoid patients may find the presence of the interpreter problematic. Table 36.1 illustrates common errors of interpretation [7]. In addition to those errors noted, studies have shown cases of interpreters dissuading patients from disclosing information deemed stigmatizing in their culture [7]. Psychiatric evaluation is further hindered by interpretation as speech content is temporally separated from facial expression and psychomotor activity. The interpreter may focus on what the patient is saying rather than how he is saying it. Yet meanings of both verbal and nonverbal expressions are integral components of the psychiatric exam. Affect, thought process, and ambivalence can be particularly subject to distortion, in part due to difficulty in conveying the meaning of paralinguistic cues [19].

During a psychiatric interview, many questions could be considered presumptuous and adversely affect rapport if asked without appropriately empathic expression. Looking at the patient and addressing the patient directly rather than addressing the interpreter will facilitate better rapport. To prevent misunderstandings and misinterpretation, the clinician is advised to speak in short, clear sentences, avoiding slang and medical jargon, and to pause frequently to check on the patient's level of understanding.

While time is limited in the emergency setting, meetings between clinician and interpreter both before and after interviewing the patient have proven effective in minimizing distortions [7,19]. A pre-interview meeting allows the clinician to discuss the goals of the interview, including specific areas of focus and any potentially sensitive topics, and allows the

Table 36.1. Common errors of interpretation[a]

Omission	Information is partially or completely deleted by the interpreter. More likely when discussing sensitive personal issues, such as substance use or sex, or when the interpreter has a personal conflict of interest, e.g., when a family member is acting as an informal interpreter.
Addition	The interpreter includes information not expressed by the patient.
Condensation	A long or complicated response is simplified. Particularly problematic in the psychiatric evaluation of a patient with disorganized or incoherent responses or when a response is shortened such that critical information is deleted.
Substitution	The interpreter rewords the question in a manner which changes the concept.
Role exchange	The interpreter takes over the interview, replacing the interviewer's questions with his own.
Closed/Open	The interpreter alters the way the question was asked. The interpreter may elaborate with his own series of questions, delivering results of this exchange rather than an accurate response to the original question.
Normalization	The interpreter attempts to make sense of the patient's response. Particularly problematic in evaluating a behavioral emergency.

[a] Adapted from Farooq S, Fear C. [7].

clinician to assess the interpreter's attitude toward both patient and subject matter. Interpreters should be encouraged to ask both clinician and patient for clarification when needed and should be counseled not to attempt to make sense of the patient's statements. The clinician should request a verbatim translation if the response is still unclear. A post-interview meeting provides the opportunity for clarification of both interview content and dynamics of the interaction, including discussion of paralinguistic cues. The interpreter may also benefit from the opportunity to discuss and process his or her own feelings and reaction to the interview.

Interpreter services improve healthcare experiences and outcomes [15]. Despite the use of interpreters, patients with limited English proficiency are less likely to express concerns or ask questions. High-quality healthcare for patients with limited English proficiency depends on high-quality interpreter services when language concordant clinicians are not available, as patients who rate their interpreter highly are more apt to rate the healthcare received highly [15]. Patient satisfaction depends on the ability of the patient to convey information to the healthcare provider, the expertise of the physician, and the emotional tone of the encounter [18]. Enhanced communication leads to a stronger doctor–patient relationship and increased patient autonomy, allowing the patient to more effectively participate in treatment planning and make informed decisions. Therapeutic alliance is a positive prognostic indicator of treatment [20].

Language barriers influence the authenticity of the informed consent process. A patient's understanding of both illness and proposed treatment and ability to voluntarily make treatment decisions form the basis for informed consent. The clinician must attend to the patient's perspective, attempt to understand it, avoid declarations, and recognize the social context within this exchange [21]. He has the responsibility of ensuring that the patient has an accurate understanding of the totality of information required to make the decision. Recognition of an individual's autonomy, avoidance of coercion, and voluntary patient participation are essential elements of the informed consent process.

Minority populations

Increasing awareness and understanding of different cultures will aid in more accurate assessment and diagnosis. At present, patients with psychiatric illnesses are diagnosed according to the Diagnostic and Statistical Manual of Mental Disorders, 4th Edition, Text Revision (DSM-IV-TR). However, this classification system is based on Western concepts of mental health and illness and can potentially lead to patients from minority populations being misunderstood and misdiagnosed. To that end, increasing understanding of specific populations may prove useful for clinicians, particularly when evaluating for potential underlying psychiatric illness in an emergency setting.

Ethnic and racial minorities in the United States experience an environment of social and economic inequality plagued by greater exposure to racism, discrimination, poverty, and violence. People in the lowest socioeconomic strata are two to three times more likely to suffer mental illness than those in the highest strata [3]. Racism and discrimination adversely affect mental health and place minorities at increased risk of such illnesses as depression and anxiety. Mistrust of mental health services deters minorities from seeking treatment and is reinforced by clinician bias and stereotyping. Providing evidence-based treatment for minority populations is challenged by the tendency of conventional psychiatric research to reduce the complexity of illness narratives to a checklist of symptoms [10].

Education about other cultures and belief systems is an important starting point in the provision of culturally competent care. Overall, Euro-Americans align with professional disease-oriented perspectives on mental illness, seeking treatment when needed and viewing psychotropic medication as a necessary component of treatment [11]. In contrast, psychiatric patients of non-Western origin abandon treatment against medical advice far more often [9]. While the following discussion is neither complete nor exhaustive, it does provide a basic framework for understanding other cultures. Each patient must still be evaluated individually as these generalizations are not meant to invoke stereotypes or dismiss pathology as a cultural phenomenon. Even clinicians of the same ethnicity as the patient must be careful to consider each patient individually to avoid over-identification and assumptions.

According to federal classification, the four most recognized racial and ethnic minority groups in the United States are Hispanic Americans/Latinos, African Americans/Blacks, Asian Americans and Pacific Islanders, and American Indians and Alaska Natives.

Hispanic Americans

Hispanics are the largest ethnic minority population in the United States, and this population is rapidly growing with a 43% increase between 2000 and 2010 [2]. Their ancestry may trace to Africa, Asia, Europe, the Middle East, the Caribbean, or the Americas [3,20]. Latino groups experience high levels of stress and distress, which can exacerbate pre-existing conditions or increase the risk of developing substance use and psychiatric disorders [20]. Their resilience and coping skills promote mental health. Hispanic American youth experience higher rates of depression, anxiety, suicidal ideation, and suicide attempts as compared to white youth [3]. Interestingly, rates of mental illness are lower for Mexican-Americans than other Hispanics.

Limited availability of ethnically or linguistically compatible providers and lack of health insurance have limited access to psychiatric services such that Hispanic Americans are less likely than white Americans to receive needed psychiatric services [3,11]. Contributing factors include stigma associated with mental health services, cultural and linguistic barriers, poverty, discrimination, and lack of empirically based treatments [20]. Lack of culturally appropriate care contributes to premature dropout from treatment [20]. Limited outcome data suggests that Hispanic Americans are less likely to receive treatment in accordance with evidence-based guidelines [3].

Cultural factors including language, family, and beliefs about health can impact the assessment and treatment of Hispanic patients presenting with behavioral emergencies. Latinos tend to use non-biomedical interpretations of emotional, cognitive, and behavioral problems [11]. They tend to downplay their symptoms and normalize their illness experience [11]. Hispanics are less accepting of mental illness and view depression as a sign of weakness or madness. While there is limited stigma associated with the cultural syndrome of *nervios*, psychiatric labels have the potential to be socially damaging in this population [11]. Hispanics may somatize their symptoms and may prefer alternative treatment options, such as spiritual healers. Increased frequency of somatic complaints have been noted in Mexican-American and Puerto Rican patients [16]. When depressed, Hispanics are more likely to endorse appetite or weight disturbances [22]. Hispanic patients may present with atypical psychotic symptoms, including auditory and visual hallucinations, but have an otherwise unremarkable mental status exam. Hispanics tend to believe in predetermination and that a higher power is in control. Typical gender roles dictate that men are strong, loving providers for their families and that women are spiritually superior, deferring their own needs for children and family.

Deviation from these roles may lead to depression [23]. As family provides primary social support, involving relatives in treatment can be beneficial.

Incorporating cultural constructs can increase the effectiveness of service delivery to Hispanic patients. *Familismo* (family orientation) emphasizes the importance of family, loyalty, and solidarity, as well as the focus on the greater good of the family over individual needs, and it highlights the importance of family involvement in treatment [20]. *Personalismo* (personal relationship) highlights the importance of relating on a personal level and the value placed on harmonious interpersonal relationships. Getting to know clinicians on a personal level helps patients develop rapport and establish trust. Otherwise, the clinician may be perceived as cold or unpleasant, which can adversely affect treatment compliance [20]. *Respeto* (respect, mutual and reciprocal deference) refers to the adherence to hierarchical structure, in which individuals defer to those with more seniority or higher status. The patient should be addressed formally, e.g., with the use of *usted* in place of *tu*, until given permission to do otherwise, as disrespect or offensive gestures could adversely affect treatment outcomes [20]. Even though the clinician may be viewed as an authority, he must work to maintain a collaborative relationship with the patient to engage the patient in formulating a treatment plan amenable to the patient. *Confianza* (trust and intimacy in a relationship) is an essential component in establishing a therapeutic treatment alliance and typically develops in relationships based on *personalismo* and *respeto* [20]. *Dichos* are analogies, proverbs, or popular sayings commonly used in Hispanic populations, which can be used to establish rapport [20]. *Fatalismo* (fatalism) encompasses the belief that outcomes may not be entirely under one's control and that fate, luck, or a higher power may play a role [20]. Patients may refer to *Dios Quire* (God's will) or *el destino* (destiny). Exploring a patient's contributions to the achievement of his goals may be an effective means of empowering the patient and strengthening the therapeutic alliance without questioning the patient's religious or spiritual beliefs. *Contralarse* (self-containment or conscious control of negative affect) and *aguantarse* (ability to withstand stressful situations, particularly during difficult times) reflect inner strength in times of adversity [20]. *Sobreponerse* (self-suppression) refers to a particular mindset needed to overcome challenges, although the clinician must not appear to be minimizing or dismissive of the presenting issues [20]. Incorporating these cultural constructs during assessment and treatment of Hispanic patients may enhance therapeutic alliance and improve treatment outcomes.

Once respect and trust have been established in a treatment relationship, Hispanic patients prefer a more familiar tone. Latinos are generally amenable to treatment with psychotropic medication, but tend to use psychosocial interventions less frequently [11]. Latino men tend to view clinicians as a means to obtaining medication, whereas women are more likely to use psychosocial interventions such as groups and therapy [11].

African Americans

While the majority of African Americans trace their ancestry to slaves brought from Africa, this population is diversifying with the influx of immigrants and refugees from African nations and the Caribbean. The legacy of slavery, racism, and discrimination continues to affect this population. Nearly a quarter of African Americans suffer from poverty. Mortality rates are disproportionately high. Resilience is a strength of this population. Prevalence rates of mental illness for African Americans are similar to those for non-Hispanic whites [3]. Yet, African-Americans are less likely to use and receive mental health care and they are overrepresented in high need populations, including the homeless, the incarcerated, and children in foster care [3,11]. Availability of services is limited due to reliance on safety net providers and lack of African-American clinicians specializing in mental health. Access to treatment and usage of services are limited by lack of insurance and less inclination to take advantage of available services. African Americans are more likely to delay treatment until their symptoms are severe and to receive psychiatric treatment in emergency rooms and psychiatric hospitals [3]. Errors in diagnosis are more common for African Americans than whites, and African Americans are less likely to receive care directed by evidence-based treatment guidelines. When treated appropriately, African Americans respond as favorably as whites [3].

African Americans are more likely to use non-biomedical interpretations of behavioral, emotional, or cognitive problems [11]. They may attribute symptoms to supernatural or demonological forces or they may formulate characterological explanations [11]. African Americans with mental illness tend to downplay their symptoms and normalize their illness experience [11]. Those with depression are more likely to present with somatic and neurovegetative symptoms than with mood or cognitive disturbances, and they are more likely to endorse appetite or weight disturbances [22]. African Americans find mental illness stigmatizing and consider it private, family business. Diagnostic labels may have damaging social consequences, including ridicule, disparagement, and retaliation [11]. The perception that individuals with mental illness are dangerous persists in this population [11].

From a treatment perspective, African Americans are more critical of mental health services and of psychotropic medication, sensing that medication compliance is the clinician's primary concern [11]. They may become frustrated with dosing changes, feeling that they are being experimented on [11]. They tend to feel that treatment providers don't listen, don't care, and don't help solve problems [11]. They may feel treatment providers are trying to control them [11]. Difficulty communicating with clinicians constitutes a significant barrier to seeking services and engaging in treatment [11].

Asian Americans and Pacific Islanders

Over seventeen million Asians reside in the United States, and this population is rapidly growing with a 43% increase between

2000 and 2010 [2]. This minority population is remarkably diverse, accounting for 43 ethnic groups speaking over 100 different languages and dialects and representing a range of educational and socioeconomic backgrounds [3]. Given this diversity, it is not surprising that expectations may vary concerning when to seek medical treatment, the role of the physician, the roles of the patient and family, and privacy issues, including disclosure to patient and family.

Asian Americans use fewer mental health services than any other minority group, tending to access services only in crisis and to drop out prematurely [24]. Availability of services is limited due to the limited English proficiency of nearly half this population and lack of providers with compatible language skills [3]. Lack of health insurance limits access to care. Stigma and shame associated with mental illness further limit usage of services. Asians may experience trepidation when navigating an unfamiliar healthcare system, frustration when unable to effectively communicate their symptoms, and anger when feeling they are being viewed with mistrust or suspicion by hospital staff. Of those who use available services, severity of presentation is high, suggesting that Asians delay treatment until the condition is serious.

In general, strengths of the Asian population include family cohesion and motivation for upward mobility and educational achievement. In contrast to the Western focus on patient as individual, Asian culture emphasizes family, and understanding religious and social support systems may prove invaluable in formulating diagnosis and treatment plan. Family structure is patriarchal and hierarchical. Japanese Americans, in general, are highly successful, attaining high rates of educational achievement and income, and low rates of mental illness, alcoholism, and juvenile delinquency. One theory is that the highly structured role relationships in the family with their stability and predictability protect family members from outside stressors and form the basis for an individual's ability to adapt and adjust [8].

In Asian culture, there is a belief that avoiding bad thoughts can lead to mental health. Expression of feelings, particularly negative ones, and emotional distress are taboo, disgracing individual and family. Suppression of negative affect is valued. Mental illness may be indicative of character weakness or lack of self-control and can shame the family. Family members may fear they are at risk for genetic inheritance of these traits. Self-control, desire to save face, need to protect family, lack of available language to describe symptoms, and stigma associated with mental illness have led to somatization of psychiatric symptoms, which is both culturally acceptable and less stigmatizing [25]. The Asian conceptualization of mind and body as a whole has also contributed to the somatization of mental illness. In fact, somatic presentations of mental illness are seen in most patients from non-Western cultures [23]. An Asian person with depression may present to the emergency room with a chief complaint of headache, backache, muscle pain, stomachache, dizziness, low energy, or insomnia. He may be inclined to deny depressed mood to preserve his own self-image and avoid

negative reflection on his family. Asian patients tend to minimize symptoms and under-report suicidal ideation and suicide attempts, although one study did find Asian Americans more likely to endorse suicidal ideation when depressed [22,23]. Careful history taking may identify a trauma or loss precipitating onset of physical symptoms.

Treatment interventions should be problem-focused and include psychotropic medication, supportive, cognitive, or behavioral therapy, and family therapy, particularly with inclusion or support of the identified family leader. Instillation of hope is important. Patients from Asian cultures traditionally show tremendous respect toward clinicians and expect this person to be authoritative and directive once rapport has been established. Failure to provide instructions to the patient could lead the patient to conclude that the clinician is uncaring or incompetent. Traditionally recommended treatments for substance use disorders, including group therapeutic interventions such as Alcoholics Anonymous, can prove problematic due to the cultural taboo associated with public expression of emotions and group confrontation.

Cultural differences manifest in ways which may surprise even the astute clinician. A recent immigrant from southeast Asia may struggle with orientation questions on mental status exam as he may be accustomed to a lunar calendar. He may shudder at the number four, which is considered a bad omen suggestive of death. Asians with psychotic disorders are more likely to experience visual, olfactory, or tactile hallucinations than the auditory hallucinations typically experienced by Western patients [25]. Misdiagnosis of mental illness is common in this patient population with atypical nature of presenting symptoms, language barriers, lack of knowledge of Asian cultures, and lack of cultural sensitivity contributing [25].

In evaluating patients from Southeast Asia, the clinician must be cognizant of the following cultural beliefs: preference for group interest over individual interest; harmonious family relationships; respect for elders; control of emotions, including those which may be undesirable; confrontation avoidance [30]. Relevant history may include migration history and refugee status, which may provide an opening for discussion of possible past trauma. Southeast Asian refugees are at increased risk of post-traumatic stress disorder related to pre-immigration trauma. Southeast Asians may use moral, religious, magical, or medical models to explain illness. The moral model links medical or psychiatric condition to such negative traits as laziness, selfishness, and low morality and posits that correction of such behaviors is necessary for symptom resolution. Supernatural factors underlying mental illness is the central tenet of the religious model, and appeasing God or angered spirits is an essential treatment component. In the medical model, traditional Eastern therapies, including local healers, acupuncture, meditation, herbs, yoga, and dietary modification, may be preferred to Western medicine. An Asian typically turns to family for support before seeking treatment outside the home. Families may try to protect those with psychotic symptoms to save face and avoid stigma and shame [25]. Often symptoms are quite severe by the time a patient presents for treatment. Mistrust of the mental health system, conflicting Eastern and Western values, discomfort with Western treatment methods, and medication side effects impede engagement in psychiatric treatment and lead to early dropout [25].

Filipino Americans are the second fastest growing Asian immigrant group in the United States behind the Chinese [24]. They believe happiness and health result from balance and that rapid temperature changes can cause illness [24]. They have a fatalistic and passive attitude and underutilize existing mental health services, which are culturally, socially, and linguistically incompatible [23,24]. Stigma and preference for traditional healing methods, such as faith healers, inhibit Filipinos from seeking treatment. Depression may manifest with classical symptoms, somatization, or the incongruous smiling depression [24]. Suicide rates are lower, likely reflecting the influence of Catholicism as well as extended family and social support systems [24]. Some Filipinos believe that persons with mental illness are dangerously unpredictable [24]. Filipino women are at increased risk of physical and mental health problems as they are expected to work outside the home while maintaining primary responsibility for childcare and domestic duties [24]. Filipinos will express their feelings toward healthcare providers who are respectful, approachable, and accommodating, but will otherwise interact in a formal, superficial, and reticent manner, concealing emotion [24]. Affect and psychomotor behavior may be misleading. Filipino patients may look down to convey respect, smile inappropriately, or wag their heads. Respect or embarrassment may prevent the asking of questions due to desire to save face and mask any lack of understanding. Filipinos often attempt to gain familiarity with the treatment provider and are often more comfortable in the presence of family. They typically accept medications as a means of treatment.

Japanese refer to doctors using the title *sensei*, which means "master," "teacher," or "doctor" and which is shared by other professionals deemed to be morally and socially responsible public figures [13]. Doctors with greater expertise and those physicians seen as saving lives are held in higher regard. Japanese patients typically comply with their physicians' treatment recommendations. It is important to them that their physicians convey respect. Regardless of religious affiliation, there are three types of Japanese religious practices which may affect treatment [13]. The first emphasizes wish fulfillment through the power of prayer and may place greater emphasis on religious and magical prayers than on medical treatments [13]. As this practice has led to treatment refusal, Japanese doctors often do not allow it to be practiced in the hospital setting. The second religious practice is akin to determinism and emphasizes self-control [13]. Followers seek to live their lives in accordance with the will of God, gods, or spiritual principles and accept their illnesses as unavoidable fate, living their lives within these constraints [13]. The third religious practice involves the cultivation of mind through universal truth [13]. For example, Buddhism teaches patients to recognize the state of their illness in an objective manner as part of a natural reality and to seek new paths to fulfillment by transcending states of suffering [13]. Japanese avoid conversations with direct eye contact. Given that suppressing feelings of anger and sadness is considered a virtue, Japanese patients often do not want to hear the name of their illness directly from their doctor, but rather they wish to be informed indirectly so that they can be prepared [13]. Japanese patients typically present for treatment with family members. Because of stigma and potential embarrassment, Japanese patients have difficulty openly discussing mental illness. A clinician inquiring directly about personal information deemed irrelevant to the presenting illness would be considered rude and inappropriate. Japanese are frustrated by inability to adequately explain symptoms in English, and this tenet holds true even when the individual appears to have very good command of the English language [13].

Most Koreans will not seek medical treatment unless seriously ill, and even then they are apt to first consult with a physician in the family or close social circle or with a pharmacist [13]. Koreans view doctors as masters accorded absolute authority, holding specialists in higher regard [13]. They feel large hospitals have greater credibility than individual doctors [13]. Koreans trust their doctors regarding treatment choice. When illness is severe, family members will accompany the patient. Koreans may experience tension between respect for modern medicine and fundamentalist tendencies to eschew medical treatment. While Korean Protestantism emphasizes the healing power of the Holy Spirit, religious leaders do typically encourage medical attention [13]. Only the most conservative branches preach reliance on the healing power of God. Shamanism is also practiced in Korea, and shahman-nesses are thought to have magical and miraculous healing abilities. Koreans tend to view their constitution as unique and question whether Western medicine is able to effectively treat their illnesses [13]. If conventional medical treatments fail, Koreans may devote themselves to prayer [13]. Regardless of religion, Koreans believe in destiny according to cosmic providence [13].

Indians tend to use both traditional and Western approaches to medicine. Indians trust their primary care physicians and typically consult them first rather than go directly to a hospital or specialist [13]. They are accustomed to having significant personal interaction with their physicians and expect to be able to spend time with them [13]. Indians are highly respectful of physicians, particularly specialists, and tend to comply with proposed treatment [13]. Wealthier members of Indian society go to the doctor with even minor complaints, whereas poorer Indians are more apt to attempt a home remedy and go to the doctor only if it fails [13]. Ayurvedic practice is also popular. Indians may practice Hinduism, Christianity, Islam, or other religions, but religion plays a less prominent role in healthcare ideology [13]. Family members typically accompany patients to medical visits and are privy to the patient's medical information. Indians want to feel that clinicians are trying to understand them and their culture and that their lifestyle choices are respected, as this personal interest contributes to a sense of belonging [13]. Indian women tend to be shy in front of male doctors and may prefer female doctors or the presence of female nursing staff [13]. Suicide is the leading cause of death for Indians aged 15 to 24 years old [25].

American Indian and Alaska Natives

Five hundred and sixty one tribes are represented by the Bureau of Indian Affairs [3]. This minority group is the most impoverished with over one quarter living in poverty [3]. Availability of mental health services is limited by geographic location due to distance from treatment centers and lack of available specialists [3]. Lack of health insurance limits access [3]. Usage of mental health services, appropriateness of treatment, and outcomes are not well understood due to lack of research.

Prevalence rates of mental illness for American Indians and Alaska Natives are higher than the general population with individuals reporting higher rates of frequent distress [3,8]. While some tribes, including the Navajo, abstain from alcohol use, alcoholism is such a major issue that American Indians and Alaska Natives are five times more likely to die of alcohol-related causes than whites [3,8]. Both youth and adults experience increased mental illness, and the suicide rate is 50% higher than the national rate [3]. Suicide is the second leading cause of death among American Indians and Alaska Natives aged 10 to 34 years old [26]. Concern about suicide clusters necessitates a community-based, culturally competent response strategy [26].

Establishing trust with patients from American Indian and Alaskan Native communities may prove difficult as many tribal communities were destroyed by the introduction of European infectious diseases and many treaties established by the U.S. government with tribal nations were broken [26]. Casual conversation may aid the development of rapport. Showing respect is important, in part by allowing time for patients to express their opinions without interruption. Admitting limited knowledge of the patient's culture is acceptable, particularly while inviting the patient and his family or friends to educate you about specific cultural protocols in their community. Most American Indians and Alaska Natives have learned to "walk in two worlds," observing the cultural practices of the setting they are in at the time [26]. Many practice organized religion and have strong faith-based communities. They have a holistic worldview centered on the balance between mind, body, spirit, and environment. Social and health problems are often seen as spiritually based, and most use traditional and spiritual healing practices to complement Western medicine [26]. Recognizing and identifying strengths in the patient's community can provide insight for developing culturally appropriate treatment interventions. Examples of such strengths include extended family, shared sense of collective community responsibility, physical resources, survival skills and resiliency when encountering challenges, and ability to adapt to fit in with both one's traditional culture and the dominant culture [26].

American Indians and Alaska Natives communicate meaningfully using non-verbal gestures, requiring careful observation on the part of the clinician to avoid miscommunication [26]. Like Asians, they may look down as an act of deference to show respect. They may ignore someone to express disagreement or displeasure [26]. They tend to use humor when discussing difficult subjects, and smiles and jokes may mask pain [26]. American Indians are likely to endorse somatic symptoms when depressed [22]. Consultation with local cultural advisers should be considered for questions about symptomology and treatment options.

Immigration, acculturation, and mental illness

Acculturation is a process which reflects a balance of stress and resilience, and mental health reflects a complex interplay of racism, adaptation strategies, and cultural resources. Learning a new language, reconciling cultural conflicts, formation of identity, alienation from culture or family, and loss of resources are potentially stressful events associated with immigration. Overcoming these obstacles and adapting require resilience. Processes of adaptation, adjustment, and incorporation into society are not uniform, and different immigrant groups face different challenges in negotiating acculturation [27]. Some immigrants experience better mental health than individuals born in the United States, but as they become more integrated with American culture, values, and lifestyles, their mental health worsens and becomes more comparable to that of those born in the United States [27].

Acculturation in Asian Americans is inversely related to prevalence rates of mental illness and to reported symptoms, and Asian American immigrants who moved to the United States at an earlier age experience few difficulties adjusting [8]. In contrast, prevalence rates of mental illness in Mexican-Americans are directly related to level of acculturation and increase with length of time in the United States [8]. Mexican-Americans born in the United States experience higher rates of mental illness than those born in Mexico, and place of birth appears to be a more important variable in determining mental illness than age gender, or social class [8,28]. One possible explanation is erosion of family networks, which provide support and resources, exerting a protective or preventive effect. Alternatively, expectations may differ depending on place of birth such that Mexican-Americans born in the U.S. may have higher expectations for educational attainment and wealth and may feel more demoralized when they fail to achieve these goals [8].

Association between immigrant status and suicidality is unclear. Lack of social integration, low assimilation, and the high stress accompanying the immigrant experience may contribute to increased suicide risk [29]. Immigrants leave behind customs, norms, and relationships in their home country only to experience pressure to integrate and assimilate culturally, socially, linguistically, and economically with the dominant population, often at a rapid pace and with limited emotional and economic support. On the other hand, the "healthy immigrant thesis" postulates that immigrants have above average physical and mental health and are thus at lower risk for suicide [29].

Religion

Patients of different spiritual backgrounds may have different conceptualizations of their illnesses and treatment needs. Clinicians responsible for evaluating behavioral emergencies in the United States are typically trained to view religion as a protective factor in terms of suicide risk; however, this is a Western notion rooted in Christianity. It is important for the clinician to determine whether a patient's religious beliefs provide for coping skills which are positive or negative.

Hinduism

According to Ayurvedic beliefs, mental health depends on the actions, air, and personal nature of the individual. Hindus believe that mental illness may result from disrespect toward the creator, the Brahmins, and teachers. They believe that neglecting duty to God, cruelty to others, and such vices as lust and extortion lead to possession by spirits and that such fate can be avoided by keeping themselves clean, observing social obligations, and giving to charity [30].

Buddhism

Buddhism teaches that nothing is permanent and that everything is interdependent. Buddhists believe that mental health results from knowing and following the Four Noble Truths and the Eightfold Path while renouncing worldly attachments. Mental illness is caused by misdeeds of the patient or ancestors or may result from being overly ambitious or having too much desire. Therapeutic healing requires the following four components: the physician; the attendant(s); the patient; the drug, which must come from local herbs. Kindness and consideration are of particular import to the Buddhist patient. Buddhists believe that possessed individuals may be aided by worship or prayer, burning of specific incense, and following certain rituals and that meditation can lead to a tranquil state of mind [30]. Charity work may also provide benefit. Jodo Shinshu Buddhists are more willing to seek medical treatment as they believe that illness comes from causes and conditions and that eradication comes through medications and treatments [13].

Chinese spiritual beliefs

Chinese beliefs are heterogeneous, often reflecting a mix of principles based on Buddhism, Taoism, and ancestor worship. In general, there is a holistic view of mind and body as one with mental health dependent on physical health. Unbalanced, undisciplined, or excessive emotions form the primary basis for any kind of illness [30]. Taoists believe that mental illness results from an imbalance between Yin and Yang. Chinese

patients may believe in deities, devils, and spiritual beings and that certain rituals may relieve suffering. For example, schizophrenia may be explained as possession of one's spirit by angry ancestors and symptoms may include auditory and visual hallucinations of being tormented or raped by ghosts [25]. Animism is the belief that humans, animals, and inanimate objects have souls or spirits, and followers believe that mental illness is caused by the loss of one's soul or possession by evil or vengeful spirits. Chinese healing methods include herbal medicine, acupuncture, and qigong among many others.

Islam

Islamic faith tends to view people as being made up of body and soul and it is this unity that forms the psyche and reflects itself in one's behaviors [30]. Mental health is indicative of closeness to God and reflects ongoing purification of thought and deeds. Neglect of religious duties, failure to read the Qur'an, or deviation from inherent goodness may allow evil to take hold and may result in psychiatric symptoms. The belief in predestination may prevent patients from seeking medical or psychiatric treatment. Muslims may prefer folk and traditional practices to alleviate mental distress [30].

Culture-bound syndromes

Whereas a disease has identified biological underpinnings, a syndrome denotes a constellation of symptoms. Culture-bound syndromes refer to recurrent patterns of aberrant behavior and troubling experience limited to a specific culture or geographic region and do not have the broad applicability of those illnesses represented in the DSM-IV-TR. These clusters of symptoms reflect the interaction of cognitive schemata and bodily processes as interpreted in an ethnophysiologic and ethnopsychological context and may seem bizarre to the clinician from an outside culture. Neurasthenia is a Chinese syndrome of physical and emotional weakness attributed to anxiety or neurological weakness or exhaustion and characterized by the physical symptoms of headache, pain, fatigue, gastrointestinal symptoms, and sexual dysfunction and the psychiatric symptoms of irritability, excitability, dyssomnia, poor concentration, and memory loss.

Culture-bound syndromes in Hispanic populations include ataque de nervios (attack of nerves), nervios (nerves), and susto (fright or soul loss). Nervios is a common expression of psychosocial distress in Latinos in the United States and Latin America and represents instability of mood similar to general anxiety disorder. The term nervios may refer to a general state of vulnerability to stressful life experiences or a syndrome brought on by difficult life circumstances. Patients may present with physical and emotional symptoms, including affective instability, restlessness, inability to function, and feeling out of control. They may report headaches, gastrointestinal distress, dyssomnia, nervousness, or tearfulness. Typically this condition is chronic with fluctuating degree of disability. Ataque de nervios is primarily seen in Latinos from the Caribbean, but is recognized by many people of Latin

American and Latin Mediterranean descent. Like nervios, this syndrome is characterized by a feeling of being out of control but is more analogous to a panic attack, only without fear. Episodes are often accompanied by violent behavior and may include crying, screaming, shouting, trembling, palpitations, and seizure-like episodes. Typically they are precipitated by a specific event, often involving family. This condition is often associated with other psychiatric conditions, including depression and anxiety.

Approach to treatment

Clinicians should adopt open, interested, and respectful attitudes toward their patients and attempt to understand each individual's illness within a cultural context. Care must be taken to investigate unexplained symptoms and to perform a complete diagnostic medical workup rather than dismiss symptoms as somatization. Attention to precipitating, aggravating, and ameliorating factors should be paid. Review of systems will allow the clinician to screen for psychiatric symptoms. As the interview progresses and the patient engages, more sensitive topics may be broached, including psychiatric symptoms, personal or family problems, and trauma history. Clinicians should inquire about stressors as patients may not make the connection between stressors and physical symptoms. Inquiry about herbal medications is merited given that 42% of patients in the United States use some type of complementary or alternative medical treatment [23]. Common stressors, including failure to live up to own and familial expectations, threats to competence such as failure at work or school, familial conflict, recent immigration, and poor acculturation, may result in feelings of guilt or shame, isolation, and decreased functioning [23]. The more persistently a patient rejects any link between psychosocial factors and physical symptoms, the less likely the clinician recognizes and treats psychiatric illness [10].

Biological, psychological, and social methods can be used to overcome the stigma associated with mental illness and engage patients in treatment. Explaining illness in physiologic terms can dispel feelings of guilt and shame. Medication education with discussion of dosing, duration of treatment, and potential side effects promotes compliance. A psychological approach based on principles discussed in the DSM-IV-TR cultural formulation incorporates the patient's traditional beliefs and explanation of illness. Using the patient's own explanatory models of illness facilitates understanding and engagement. Involving family and spiritual or religious leaders in treatment can be beneficial. Family therapy using a psychoeducational approach is particularly helpful when treating patients from non-Western countries. Eliciting the patient's point of view and resistance to proposed treatment allows alternative options to be discussed and a viable treatment plan formulated. The clinician must convey hope and optimism regarding illness and recovery.

Treatment noncompliance rates are much higher in intercultural environments, reflecting inadequate communication and cultural differences in expectations [10]. Patients may be reluctant to question or disagree with clinicians due to etiquette, deference to authority, or desire to be viewed as a good patient [10]. Patients from ethnocultural populations dominated or marginalized by European or American powers or affected by racism may experience difficulty expressing their own concerns due to potential conflict. Concern about strength of prescribed treatment, side effects, and social stigma contribute to noncompliance [10].

Ethnicity and psychopharmacology

In addition to differences in beliefs and traditions, there are biological differences in ethnic populations. Polymorphic variability among ethnic groups may account for different responses to drugs. Mutations in cytochrome P450 enzymes affect metabolism of psychotropic medications, including selective serotonin reuptake inhibitors, selective norepinephrine reuptake inhibitors, tricylic antidepressants, and antipsychotics. Alcohol consumption, nicotine use, and diet may also affect metabolism.

African Americans are at risk for overtreatment both in terms of number of medications used and doses prescribed despite pharmacokinetic data that indicate that lower doses should be used [23]. African Americans receive more antipsychotic medications regardless of diagnosis, but fewer antidepressant medications, and they are often treated with older medications [23].

In general, Asians have difficulty metabolizing psychotropic medications [25]. Thus, lower doses are required to achieve therapeutic effect, and risk of side effects may be greater. Starting with half the recommended dose of antidepressant or neuroleptic medication has been recommended [23].

If a patient experiences side effects, the medication dose should be lowered and the possibility of using a medication metabolized through an alternative pathway should be considered. The lack of minority participation in research studies has complicated efforts to apply culturally appropriate evidence-based treatment algorithms to these populations.

The future

Individualized treatment is essential. The *LEARN* principle can be used as a model when training clinicians to perform a culturally appropriate assessment [23,30]. They should *Listen* to understand the patient's perception of the problem, *Explain* their perception to the patient, *Acknowledge* and discuss similarities and differences, and *Recommend* and *Negotiate* an agreed upon treatment plan [23,30]. Clinicians need to verify that patients understand the information discussed. The National Healthcare Disparities Report noted that 26% of hospitalized patients reported communication problems pertaining to medications and that 21% experienced problems with discharge information [14].

To develop evidence-based treatment guidelines that are culturally appropriate, research must include minority populations.

Since 1994, the National Institutes of Health have required inclusion of ethnic minorities in all research studies which they fund [3]. Researchers are examining how socioeconomic status, wealth, education, neighborhood, social support, religiosity, spirituality, acculturation, and perceived discrimination relate to mental illness [3]. Pharmacologic studies are needed to determine the effects of race, ethnicity, age, gender, family history, and lifestyle on response to medication. Culturally competent instrumentation and tested treatment protocols for specific minority populations are also needed. The development of culturally appropriate behavioral health interventions has the potential to reduce bias in the formulation of diagnosis and treatment plans, improve treatment compliance, and increase efficacy of treatment.

Improving geographic availability of mental health services, increasing access to mental health care and usage, and decreasing barriers to treatment are essential to prevent behavioral emergencies. Community education to increase awareness of psychiatric illness and integration of mental health services with primary care clinics will decrease stigmatization. Providing linguistically compatible care will ensure the necessary communication for evaluation of a patient presenting with behavioral emergency, accurate diagnosis, and comprehensive discussion of treatment. Promoting an environment which appreciates diverse cultures will be more attractive to patients seeking treatment. People who receive quality health care are more likely to stay in treatment and have better outcomes [3].

Clinicians evaluating patients experiencing behavioral emergencies must receive education and training to prepare them for treating specific patient populations present in their communities. Clinicians must be able to perform culturally competent interviews, identifying the patient's cultural beliefs, explanatory model of illness, and view of potential treatments, so that they may tailor treatment to an individual patient based on assimilation of this information rather than rely solely on assessments standardized to the majority population. The clinician must also be aware of his own cultural identity and how these similarities and differences may affect communication, rapport, transference, countertransference, and the overall therapeutic alliance. A primary goal of treatment should be symptom relief, not changing core beliefs.

References

1. Lim RF. *Clinical Manual of Cultural Psychiatry*. Arlington, VA: American Psychiatric Publishing;2006.

2. U.S. Census Bureau. Table 1. *United States – Race and Hispanic Origin: 1790 to 1990*. Washington, DC: U.S. Census Bureau; 2002. Available at: http://www.census.gov/population/www/documentation/twps0056/tab01.pdf (Accessed September 30, 2011). U.S. Census Bureau. *Overview of Race and Hispanic Origin: 2010*. Washington, DC: U.S. Census Bureau; 2011. Available at: http://www.census.gov/prod/cen2010/briefs/c2010br-02.pdf (Accessed September 30, 2011).

3. Department of Health and Human Services U.S. Public Health Services. *Mental Health: Culture, Race, and Ethnicity: Executive Summary: A Supplement to Mental Health: A report of the Surgeon General, 2001.* Available at: http://www.surgeongeneral.gov/library/mentalhealth/cre/execsummary-1.html (Accessed June 21, 2011).

4. Whitley RW. Cultural competence, evidence-based medicine, and evidence-based practices. *Psychiatr Serv* 2007;**58**:1588–90.

5. Lim RF, Luo JS, Suo S, et al. Diversity initiatives in academic psychiatry: applying cultural competence. *Acad Psychiatry* 2008;**32**:283–90.

6. Lim RF, Lu FG. Culture and psychiatric education. *Acad Psychiatry* 2008;**32**:269–71.

7. Farooq S, Fear C. Working through interpreters. *Adv Psychiatr Treat* 2003;**9**:104–9.

8. Sue S, Chu JY. The mental health of ethnic minority groups: challenges posed by the supplement to the Surgeon General's report on mental health. *Cult Med Psychiatry* 2003;**27**:447–63.

9. Kortmann F. Transcultural psychiatry: from practice to theory. *Transcult Psychiatry* 2010;**47**:203–23.

10. Kirmayer LJ. Cultural variations in the clinical presentation of depression and anxiety: implications for diagnosis and treatment. *J Clin Psychiatry* 2001;**62** (Suppl 13): 22–8.

11. Carpenter-Song E, Chu E, Drake RE, et al. Ethnocultural variations in the experience and meaning of mental illness and treatment: implications for access and utilization. *Transcult Psychiatry* 2010;**47**:224–51.

12. Bhui K, Bhurga D. Explanatory models for mental distress: implications for clinical practice and research. *Br J Psychiatry* 2002;**181**:6–7.

13. Andresen J. Cultural competence and health care: Japanese, Korean, and Indian patients in the United States. *J Cult Divers* 2001;**8**:109–21.

14. Agency for Healthcare Research and Quality. *Key Themes and Highlights from the National Healthcare Disparities Report*, 2006. Available at: http://www.ahrq.gov/qual/nhdr06/highlights/nhdr06high.htm (Accessed June 21, 2011).

15. Green AR, Ngo-Metzger Q, Legedza ATR, et al. Interpreter services, language concordance, and health care quality: experiences of Asian Americans with limited English proficiency. *J Gen Intern Med* 2005;**20**:1050–6.

16. Marcos LR, Alpert M, Urcuyo L, et al. The effect of interview language on the evaluation of psychopathology in Spanish-American schizophrenic patients. *Am J Psychiatry* 1973;**130**:549–53.

17. Del Castillo JC. The influence of language upon symptomatology in foreign-born patients. *Am J Psychiatry* 1970;**127**:242–4.

18. Bezuidenhout L, Borry P. Examining the role of informal interpretation in medical interviews. *J Med Ethics* 2009;**35**:159–62.

19. Marcos LR. Effects of interpreters on the evaluation of psychopathology in non-English-speaking patients. *Am J Psychiatry* 1979;**136**:171–4.

20. Anez LM, Paris M, Bedregal LE, et al. Application of cultural constructs in the care of first generation Latino clients in a community mental health setting. *J Psychiatr Pract* 2005;**11**:221–30.

21. Fulford B, Mordini E. Informed consent in psychiatry: cross-cultural and philosophical issues. *Bull Med Ethics* 1994;**103**:22–4.

22. Uebelacher LA, Strong D, Weinstck LM, et al. Use of item response theory to understand differential functioning of DSM IV major depression symptoms by race, ethnicity, and gender. *Psychol Med* 2009;**39**:591–601.

23. Lim RF, Lu F. *Clinical Aspects of Culture in the Practice of Psychiatry: Assessment and Treatment of Culturally Diverse Patients.* Medscape, 2005. Available at: http://cme.medscape.com/viewarticle/507208 (Accessed July 2011).

24. Sanchez F, Gaw A. Mental health care of Filipino Americans. *Psychiatr Serv* 2007;**58**:810–15.

25. Herrick C, Brown HN. Mental disorders and syndromes found among Asians residing in the United States. *Issues Ment Health Nurs* 1999;**20**:275–96.

26. Substance Abuse and Mental Health Services Administration. *Culture Card: A Guide to Build Cultural Awareness: American Indian and Alaska Native, 2009.* Available at: http://store.samhsa.gov/shin/content/SMA08-4354/SMA08-4354.pdf (Accessed August 2011).

27. Takeuchi DT, Alegria M, Jackson JS, et al. Immigration and mental health: diverse findings in Asian, Black, and Latino populations. *Am J Public Health* 2007;**97**:11–12.

28. Escobar JI. Immigration and mental health: why are immigrants better off? *Arch Gen Psychiatry* 1998;**55**:781–2.

29. Duldulao AA, Takeuchi DT, Hong S. Correlates of suicidal behaviors among Asian Americans. *Arch Suicide Res* 2009;**13**:277–90.

30. Haque A. Mental health concepts in southeast Asia: diagnostic consideration and treatment implications. *Psychol Health Med* 2010;**15**:127–34.

Chapter 37

Rural emergency psychiatry

Anthony T. Ng and Jonathan Busko

Introduction

The U.S. Census Department defines a rural community as any territory, population, or housing area outside of an urban population area of at least 50,000 residents [1]. Approximately 21% of the U.S. population lives in rural areas [2]. The delivery of health care, especially emergency health care, in rural communities can be challenging. Community mental health care may be limited. Geography, itself, can impact access. Remoteness, low population densities, and varying levels of community cohesiveness exist. There may be more or less homogeneity in rural communities, especially in areas where urban commuters populate, although one tends to encounter a greater percentage of individuals with low socioeconomic level and even poverty [3]. Many communities have residents who have been there for generations, with extended family and support networks present, but at the same time, privacy concerns or a negative social stigma of mental health illness may limit patient presentation.

Emergency care constitutes an important component of medical care in rural settings. And like their urban counterparts, rural emergency rooms have been become increasingly important in the care of psychiatric patients in crisis and emergencies [4–6]. Because access to primary and mental healthcare providers is limited, the safety net "touchstone" in rural health care is often expanded beyond the emergency department (ED) to the local emergency medical services (EMS) agency. Although generally not trained to address sub-acute, chronic, or non-emergent conditions, rural EMS providers are viewed by the communities at large as knowledgeable and are always available. Rural psychiatric emergencies present a challenge to not only EMS providers but all rural emergency medicine providers (physicians, physician assistants, nurse practitioners, nurses, case workers, etc). A lack of training in the identification and management of behavioral health emergencies may result in diagnostic delays and suboptimal care [7]. Psychiatric consultation and inpatient beds may be very limited. Because the EMS providers' scope of practice is limited and generally protocol-driven, most pharmacologic options for prehospital psychiatric management

are very limited, not only for the more prevalent basic emergency technician, but also for paramedics.

The delivery of emergency psychiatric care is one that is characterized with diverse challenges and opportunities. Such challenges range from unique clinical issues, various needs for medical and psychiatric provider collaborations, varying treatment paradigms, to diverse delivery system issues. In the following chapter, some challenges to rural emergency psychiatric care will be identified. While some of these challenges, both clinical and system related, may not be unique to rural emergency settings, an appreciation of these challenges will be critical to identify better clinical care. An appreciation of these challenges will help emergency medical and psychiatric providers collaboratively address them and prospectively develop effective, local paradigms of optimal emergency psychiatric care unique to their particular rural environment.

Challenges

Perception of behavioral disorders

The perception of mental illness by those in rural communities is an important clinical issue [8,9]. Due to the remoteness of most rural communities, self-reliance has historically been viewed as virtue. Self-reliance is expected. Mental health illness may be viewed as a character weakness, intellectual deficiency, or spiritual matter. Bias and negative stereotypes may delay presentations, bypassing what available outpatient mental health services that do exist. A psychiatric crisis may subsequently then be the initial entry to care by means of the emergency medical system. Even when prospectively sought out, rural patients and families disagree with health professionals about treatment of mental illness such as depression more than their urban counterparts [10].

Perceptions about substance use also vary. Chronic opioid use may be viewed as legitimate treatment in rural areas with limited specialty medical care. Substance abuse, including nonmedical drug use, represents a significant problem in rural settings [11,12]. Criminality and economic issues associated with rural narcotic abuse are beyond this chapter's scope. The

Behavioral Emergencies for the Emergency Physician, ed. Leslie S. Zun, Lara G. Chepenik, and Mary Nan S. Mallory. Published by Cambridge University Press. © Cambridge University Press 2013.

wide range of psychiatric issues associated with substance use, including psychosis, mood changes, depression, agitation, and suicidal thoughts and attempts are prevalent [13–15]. Substance abuse may mask an underlying mental health diagnosis. Cultural hopelessness and the lack of substance abuse services in rural settings may deter individuals from seeking care. At the same time, there may also be greater acceptance of excessive alcohol use, and subsequent medical and surgical consequences. Interpersonal violence has an association with substance abuse. The correlation between intoxication and accidental injury, such as motor vehicular trauma, farming injuries, and hunting mishaps may be underappreciated in rural communities.

Patient privacy concerns

Due to the closeness of many rural communities, it is not uncommon that individuals know others within their communities and within their healthcare delivery systems. Fear of illness disclosure and stigma, even incidentally, is a barrier to access. Privacy is difficult for the family and the patient when behavioral presentations involve law enforcement. Additionally, because healthcare providers often live in the communities they serve, patients may be hesitant to fully disclose all relevant clinical information for fear of embarrassment and shame. For the same reasons, privacy concerns extend to the prehospital setting as well, particularly in the case of volunteer first-responders.

Suicide and violence

Suicide rates across various demographic groups are higher in rural counties in comparison to urban counties [16,17]. There is a greater risk of violence, including domestic violence and violence involving rural youths [18,19]. In a survey of 69 EDs across the United States, the risk of violence to ED staff is also high [20]. Determining the level of suicidal or homicidal risks is an important component of any risk assessment in rural PES. Identifying factors that both increase and mitigate suicide and violence potential are equally important. For example, risk factors that may increase risk of suicides such as prior attempts, history of impulsivity, or substance abuse may be mitigated by factors such as a patient's level of treatment engagement, level of support, and future-oriented thinking. Many patients may be living in very isolated environments. They may have significant transportation difficulty because public transportation is often inadequate. As previously discussed, substance abuse is a significant issue. Lastly, the issue of firearms is an important consideration due to their wide availability in the rural setting. In one study, it was noted that 67% of 983 surveyed rural households had firearms [21]. The possession of firearms is accepted in the rural setting as both a means of personal protection in remote areas and for recreational hunting.

Inadequately treated agitation potentiates violence. The treatment of agitation presents an ongoing concern for emergency rooms and psychiatric emergency services, both urban and rural. It is estimated that as many as 1.7 million medical ED visits each year may involve agitated patients [22].

Approximately 20 to 50% of emergency psychiatry visits in the United States may involve patients who are at risk of agitation [23]. Agitation can be due to a diverse range of both psychiatric and medical issues [24]. Due to high patient volumes in the EDs [25] as well as staffing issues [26,27], management of agitated patients can be very challenging. With many rural EDs facing insufficient staff training on agitation de-escalation, limited staffing resources and consultation, or *locum tenems* nursing and physician staffing, the risk of inadequately recognized or undertreated agitation may be greater [28]. Agitated ED patients may injure family, patients and staff, not to mention the resultant decrease in productivity and morale for staff. Patients, families, and providers may be humiliated or otherwise traumatized by the experience [29].

Cross-cultural implications

There are unique cultural issues relevant to rural emergency care practices. While rural communities tend to be characterized as homogeneous, minority populations exist and have additional, unique circumstances relating to behavioral health. In one study, it was shown that there are greater mental health problems in rural racial and ethnic minorities residing in a predominantly Caucasian rural area [30]. The rates of specific psychiatric disorders vary among some cultural groups [31]. Cultural sensitivity to the behavioral health issues of seasonal or migrant workers is important. Generally, ethnic diversity in rural areas is less than that found in many urban settings, with less awareness of the unique ethnic and cultural issues by healthcare providers. Help-seeking behavioral differences between groups, as well as somatization of psychiatric symptoms, may result in challenging clinical situations for ED physicians [15,31,32]. Additionally, availability of medical translators may be limited, resulting in less-than-ideal translations from peers or families regarding interpersonal, private matters. There are also idiosyncratic cultural diversities between community groups in rural settings and regional differences in attitudes and beliefs. Cultural help-seeking and disease prevalence differences may be represented by occupational variation, such as those of farmers, ranchers, fishermen, etc. Lifestyles and daily routines, and seasonal variations may predispose some groups for behavioral health issues or preclude them from seeking care, even when in crisis.

Medical stabilization

Medical stabilization itself, let alone medical clearance for psychiatric hospitalization, can be a challenging issue in the rural setting. The purpose of medical stabilization is to provide care to the level of available resources capabilities. For patients requiring transfer to definitive care, physicians must affirm the completed process, identify and communicate with an accepting physician, and arrange safe transportation between facilities as required under the Emergency Medical Treatment and Active Labor laws (EMTALA) [33]. Specialty consultation is often limited in the rural environment, making the complete medical evaluation of comorbidities difficult if not impossible before psychiatric admission. Due to a lack of staff resources and limited medical back-up, some psychiatric facilities are reluctant to accept a psychiatric patient with any unevaluated comorbid conditions, requiring the referring emergency room to do a full non-emergent medical workup or force a medical admission, significantly prolonging the patient's and others' throughput times in rural EDs as well as delaying more expert psychiatric care. Alternatively, the lack of standardization to medical clearance of psychiatric patients by emergency providers may strain limited psychiatric resources as well as being adverse to patient care [34,35]. This is especially relevant in the rural setting where psychiatric facilities are often physically separate from the hospital.

Geographic isolation

Patients themselves who are in need of routine or emergency psychiatry services may be hindered in their efforts by travel distances. Public transportation is limited, particularly between rural and urban locales. The sheer cost of transportation may be prohibitive. With limited rural resources, psychiatric patients may be referred or transferred to psychiatry care far from home, limiting family support. Rural patients may refuse to be cared for at a facility that is far from their community. Interfacility transports may be delayed and lengthy. When great transfer distance exists between facilities, ongoing care may need to be provided by a registered nurse with physician order, and law enforcement may be necessary for involuntary patients. Adverse weather conditions, such as snowstorms or heavy rain, may delay or in some instances necessitate cancellation.

Safe patient transport

Although from time-to-time police or family play a role, EMS, with its limited resources, is likely the primary mode of transportation for someone in psychiatric crisis. Urban EMS systems have multiple ambulances available with other public safety agencies to provide back-up and additional support. This is not necessarily possible in the rural environment, where the entire EMS service in an area may consist of one ambulance and less than 10 volunteers. Some jurisdictions may have their own emergency personnel while others may require transport services from more distant units in other jurisdictions. Police response may consist of only one officer and police response time may be 1–2 hours. At times, police from multiple jurisdictions may be required to respond. The lack of sufficient personnel puts the responders at high risk for injury as it may be impossible to have sufficient personnel on scene in instances of an extremely agitated patient. In addition, conducted energy weapons such as tasers, which may hold significant potential to facilitate the rapid and safe control and restraint of patients with agitation, are often not available to rural police departments and sheriffs' offices.

While rural patients often have the need for more advanced EMS care delivered over much longer periods of time with experienced providers, there is a real paradox in rural EMS. Rural EMS providers are often volunteers and lack a diverse clinical experience, as they have less time to dedicate to training, typically hold only basic EMT licenses, and generally transport fewer patients per shift than their urban counterparts [36]. Even paramedic training is limited. While many studies estimate approximately that 10% of emergency cases are psychiatric in nature [37,38], psychiatric emergencies typically comprise less than 2 hours of training in a 1200 hour paramedic class and approximately 1% of the total pages of paramedic textbooks [39]; oftentimes there is no training at all on psychiatric emergencies for basic EMT classes. For law enforcement, many are small departments with few officers and very limited training resources especially regarding mental health issues. This lack of training may lead to escalation or mishandling of a potentially violent situation, thus resulting in injury or even discharge of firearms.

The vast distance between healthcare facilities in rural communities has three major implications for EMS. The first relates to actual distance a patient must move from their residence to the first ED for stabilization. The closest ED to the patient may be hours from that patient's home, resulting in a patient moving away from family, support systems, and in many cases, from the people who can provide the emergency psychiatry department with collateral past or present illness history. The second relates to length of time during the transport managing the patient. For patients who have attempted suicide, there may be unresolved traumatic or toxicologic emergencies requiring monitoring or treatment during transfer to a more equipped hospital or trauma center. For agitated patients, prolonged restraint time may increase risk of injuries to both patient and responders. Use of helicopter ambulance is a consideration for the most ill or injured patient to assure that they receive timely care as rapidly as possible, weighed against the risk of agitation during flight. Most medical flight crews can successfully treat agitation before transport. Paramedic and basic EMT's scope of practice does not generally include the use of psychiatric medication to treat agitation.

The third issue relates to the selection mode for inter-facility transport. Because many rural EDs do not have the capability to provide more than the initial assessment and stabilization, safe transfer to a higher level of care to an ED or psychiatric facility is common, and should be arranged "in the least restrictive manner possible." While obviously indicated for unstable patients, EMS transfer is often selected for patients who are not felt to pose a high risk of suicide or behavioral dyscontrol. Long wait times for these less-urgent transfers and concerns about cost of transport may deter the patient from accepting the transfer entirely, instead choosing to be discharged and self-referred to the psychiatric facility. Family or self-transport to an accepting psychiatric facility carries with it unanticipated safety risks as well as affording the patient an opportunity to negate a completed medical sobriety clearance when substance abuse occurs en route. Medical–legal risks should be considered when choosing mode of transport.

Lack of treatment centers

Additional noticeable system challenge is the general lack of psychiatric resources. While all communities, rural and urban, are facing a scarcity of mental health resources, this is nowhere more apparent than in rural communities. Both psychiatric outpatient and inpatient resources have dwindled in the past decade. As a result, psychiatric patients have had increasing difficulty accessing mental health services in timely manner, which often may precipitate or worsen any crisis. As such, many psychiatric patients have to resort to going to area hospitals ED to seek psychiatric care. Unlike an urban setting, there may be few hospitals to cover a large area; as such the demand for psychiatric crisis service may be higher. Additionally, not all EDs have readily accessible mental health services. Small hospitals, such as those designated as a Critical Access hospital, use crisis teams staffed by qualified mental health professionals (QMHP) who have varying levels of training. Often in such settings, assessment and treatment will be focused primarily on disposition, that is whether the patient needs hospitalization and if so, where. Emergent psychiatric treatment is limited to the expertise of the emergency room provider.

Provider shortages

Another significant challenge in rural emergency care is that there are less psychiatric providers in these communities. Recruitment of skilled mental health professionals and psychiatrists is difficult as practices in rural settings can be professionally isolating. Many mental health professionals may be working alone and have a heavy on-call burden. Professional collaboration and continuing education opportunities are limited. Rural providers need to be comfortable about working independently. Consultations from colleagues may not be available readily. Subspecialty psychiatric expertise is rare. Consultation for special populations, especially the case with the pediatric and geriatric would require travel or transfer. Rural emergency room nurses in Australia have cited a lack of confidence in working with the mentally ill [40]. As a result of the lack of psychiatric professionals, many rural communities resort to the use of locum tenems physicians and other health professionals. Typically these assignments are short-term precluding the development of professional teamwork and familiarity with the community's patient population, resources, and limitations.

Opportunities

While there are many challenges to rural emergency psychiatric care, there are also unique opportunities. The unique characteristics of rural communities such as extended social support, closeness of community, and to some degree a tradition of overcoming hardships may be important assets to help patients

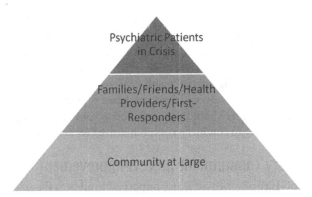

Figure 37.1. Psychiatric crisis pyramid.

cope and manage crises [3]. Like the challenges highlighted above, the opportunities are both clinical and system related. The crisis in emergency care and psychiatric emergency care is in essence a public health issue. Psychiatric crisis has a far-reaching effect. Patients' families and friends can be emotionally and financially stressed by the crisis. The community is impacted with care delays when the ED is overutilized and the EMS system resources are involved with long transports. Nonpsychiatric patients may not be seen as promptly due to lack of bed space or personnel. Safety risks exist for all groups as illustrated in Figure 37.1.

A paradigm of care should be developed and implemented in a public health approach to address rural emergency psychiatric care. In the public health model of care, there is a greater emphasis on primary prevention. Access to providers beyond emergency services is imperative. When patients are stable, they should be encouraged to discuss with their outpatient mental health provider what constitutes a crisis, and how to best access needed care.

In-home behavioral health assessment and triage

This plan can identify which crisis can be dealt with using the patient's existing resources and providers, and which crisis will warrant a higher level of care, such as an emergency room. In some instances, crisis team can be called to evaluate a patient at home, thus minimizing the potential need for transport and providing care in a less restrictive environment [41]. Additionally, after a crisis has resolved, the outpatient provider should help the patient debrief the crisis' evolution and educate the patient and their support regarding actions to take to mitigate future crises. With this emphasis on the public health paradigm, one can empower patients, families, and their treatment team to resolve crises thus potentially decreasing the burden or surge on rural emergency care.

Risk assessment education

One of the most important clinical issues in assessing behavioral health patients is the risk assessment. Covered in detail elsewhere in this book, it is important to highlight that risk assessment can be anxiety provoking for all involved parties, given what it means to the autonomy of patient as well as the medico-legal implications to providers, especially for ED providers who do not have much experience or education in acute mental health crisis [28]. Adequate risk assessment can be performed not only by mental health professionals but also by emergency room providers and primary care providers. Rural emergency providers should seek out and obtain continuing education on how to conduct a comprehensive risk assessment.

Involuntary commitment process improvement

As part of risk assessment, it is also important to address the role of involuntary commitment of patients in rural emergency psychiatric care. In many states, involuntary commitment may be initiated by a healthcare professional after determining someone to be of risk to self or others and refusing care. In the context of a busy emergency room, a provider may not have the time to explain fully the options available to the patient, thus increasing risk of the patient's refusal of treatment. As such, the provider may initiate involuntary commitment. However, involuntary commitment can lead to various short-term and long-term implications [42]. The most important short-term implication is the loss of freedom for the patient. It may increase stigma of the patient being committed. Previously committed rural patients have higher rates of recommitment [43]. Additionally, involuntary commitment may result in the loss of certain rights such as the ability to own a firearm and necessitating law enforcement transportation.

Rural health and mental health providers are assisted in their understanding on the application of the relevant involuntary commitment laws when prospective indications and processes are established. Protocols regarding the transfer of patients between institutions including the role of EMS transport and law enforcement should be clearly identified and delineated. The patient should be offered opportunities for legal counsel if they are committed. A provider should clearly communicate with the patient the reason for commitment and their treatment options. An established quality review process of the care of patients who were involuntarily committed will ensure that the commitment procedure was necessary and appropriate and education is provided for providers.

Agitation management

Despite the lack of resources in rural EDs, there is tremendous opportunity to manage agitation effectively in such environments. Importantly, prevention is paramount. The presence of family may redirect and reassure the patient during the seemingly lengthy ED evaluation and initial treatment process. Leveraging family support systems during the waiting process is important as well as using peer advocates. Drills or exercises by the unit should be conducted regularly to maintain competence in environmental and verbal de-escalation techniques. This is especially helpful in the rural environment given the potential greater use of locum tenems who are not familiar with the resources and policies and procedures of the institutions.

Pharmacologic treatment protocols can be prospectively developed with front-line clinical staff to better allow providers to manage agitation as a cohesive ED treatment team. Collaborative planning with local law enforcement and prehospital care providers will be helpful.

Psychiatric medication management

Emergency physicians have variable experience with psychiatric medication management. Patients may wish to start new psychiatric medication or re-start a noncompliant regimen due to acute distress. Patients may request existing medication regimen be changed due to ongoing distress, lack of improvement, or perceived side effects. Patients who have missed outpatient clinic appointments or who are taking more than prescribed may request a refill of their current medications. In general, medication regimen issues should be managed by the patient's primary psychiatric provider or primary care physician. The emergency room provider may not be as familiar with the patient or the medication profile. When initiating a medication, the issue of refills and adherence, as well as how to identify and manage side effects or treatment efficacy should be discussed. In an effort to lessen risks of adverse reaction, nonadherence, and pill diversion, this is especially important when a Schedule II or Schedule III drug is part of the treatment regimen. In the rural emergency room, a provider should be cautious about initiating psychiatric medication without thorough psychiatric and risk assessments, necessary medical workup, and concrete follow-up for reassessment. Continuing education for nonpsychiatric providers about commonly used psychiatric medications is easily provided. Because of the abuse and the diversion potential, the rural emergency care provider should take caution before refilling controlled medication such as opiates, benzodiazepines, or stimulants. Some state medical boards or departments of health manage prescription drug monitoring programs that can track prescribing practices. A review of this database may be helpful for the provider to determine the potential for abuse or diversion.

Establishing and monitoring expectations between providers

Medical clearance continues to be a challenging issue in rural settings. Emergency physicians are likely to interface with various psychiatric providers and facilities, often not personally knowing their colleagues. Whether or not a provider decides a patient is medically cleared may vary with experiences, requirements from receiving facility, or the workload in a busy emergency room. Joint protocols for medical clearance and transfer indications prospectively agreed upon among the providers would be both educational and establish clinical expectations. With an appreciation of the accepting psychiatric facilities' capabilities to manage urgent medical issues, such protocols should outline indicated laboratory workup, such as drug screen or alcohol levels for patients who appear intoxicated and a blood glucose determination for those with diabetes. Creating quality assurance panels to periodically review medical clearance and transfer issues would be an excellent way to monitor for improvement measures and enhance patient safety. One of the most important ways to minimize clinical friction between providers is direct consultation between the referring and the receiving providers. Professional communication can often resolve differences in medical clearance and transfer expectations.

Recruitment and retention of qualified providers

The limited access to community-based psychiatric care for rural patients can be addressed by the specific recruitment of psychiatric providers. Economic enticements, such as initial salary guarantees, may enhance recruitment efforts. Rural practice may qualify for medical school loan forgiveness programs run by state or federal government. Similarly, rural hospitals may offer such support. Although the work setting may buffer isolation associated with rural practice, transplanted practitioners' families will need community integration too. Support for continuing education should be present. Joint relationships between academic medical centers and rural hospitals and clinics provide opportunities to enhance rural job satisfaction and also increase workforce development. Rural hospital or outpatient rotations and electives during undergraduate and graduate medical education in psychiatry can provide unique opportunities for students and residents to gain exposure to rural cultures and medical practice as well as recruitment and incentive options [44]. Many rural areas also have loan forgiveness programs for postgraduate medical work and such incentives should be maximized to recruit psychiatrists. Increased role of nurse practitioners, physician assistants, and psychiatric social workers to provide psychiatric assessments and initial treatment should be promoted with similar incentives.

Telepsychiatry

Another opportunity to address the lack of psychiatric resources is the usage of telepsychiatry. Telemedicine's goal is to bring much needed specialized medical care to individuals who may otherwise be unable to access such care, usually due to distance and is being widely used in other specialties, such as trauma care [45,46]. Telepsychiatry can enhance psychiatric services, especially in rural areas, by bringing in resources from afar [47]. Telepsychiatry has been demonstrated to have broad patient and provider satisfactions with no differences in outcomes or greater risks of adverse outcomes as compared to in-person evaluation, and has been demonstrated to be cost-effective [48–51]. Telepsychiatry can provide subspeciality consultation, in particular child psychiatry [52]. Crisis intervention and treatment recommendations can be conducted by means of this modality from mental health clinics or primary care offices [53]. Lastly, telepsychiatry may be used in the rural emergency room, providing immediate psychiatric assessment to the ED patient.

To implement telepsychiatry, the participating physicians and institutions will need to implement consultation protocols, patient confidentiality protections, and develop mechanisms to streamline provider credentialing. Telepsychiatry should be culturally competent [54]. Informatics infrastructure and ongoing support is necessary. State regulations and reimbursement guidelines regarding the use of telepsychiatry should be understood, as some have a distance or needs requirement in order for reimbursement of services to occur. Specific licensing requirements from state medical boards will need to be identified. The practice guidelines and licensure requirements of some states may stipulate that patients are evaluated by a provider who is licensed in that state, regardless of the provider's physical location. Others may allow out-of-state telemedicine, but require the provider to be licensed in both the consulting and receiving locations. Quality assurance mechanisms will need to be developed to provide ongoing monitoring of any telepsychiatry service. As an extension of telepsychiatry, the greater use of hot or warm lines should be explored, permitting individuals in crisis to obtain urgent and emergent, real-time access to mental health professionals who can help rural providers assess the level of crisis and recommend temporizing interventions pending transfer or an outpatient mental health office visit [55].

EMS enhancements

Rural EMS providers have several opportunities to contribute positively to the outcomes of patients with psychiatric emergencies. These opportunities include obtaining additional training in the management of psychiatric emergencies, developing pilot projects for the EMS management of both the acute care and chronic community support of psychiatric patients, and working with the local ED to develop process for improving inter-facility transfers. Additionally, rural EMS providers can be educated to provide screening for depression [56]. There are several resources available for EMS providers to acquire continuing medical education. Physicians responsible for the oversight of EMS agencies must acknowledge the limited exposure to behavioral emergencies in EMS providers' education and work to develop educational sessions to fill this gap. The National Association of EMS Physicians' multi-text series, Emergency Medical Services: Clinical Practice and Systems Oversight provides excellent material to serve as the basis for such education [57]. Organizations such as the Continuing Education Credentialing Board for EMS (CECBEMS at http://www.cecbems.org) make distributed learning much more available to EMS providers. Many Internet-based services also exist that provide these services.

Pilot projects allow EMS agencies the opportunity to try different approaches to patient care without committing the agency to the costs of full implementation. Rural EMS agencies, particularly those operating with basic or intermediate level EMS providers, may explore expanded scope of service or expanded scope of practice care. For example, the medical director and operations director may decide to pilot a program that allows the EMT-Intermediate who is already trained to provide intramuscular epinephrine for anaphylaxis. This might further educate and allow for a similar intervention for patients with behavioral dyscontrol. Other projects could include the use of Web-based tele-consultations from the patient's home and developing alliances and crisis intervention protocols with police departments for multi-disciplinary response to behavioral emergencies.

Transfer protocols

Finally, the inter-facility transfer of a patient with a behavioral emergency typically involves EMS transport. While most EMS providers are empowered to restrain patients on the direction of a physician if necessary, it is often not feasible for EMS providers to restrain patients in the back of an ambulance. Patient should be medicated and/or restrained in the ED before the transfer. In addition, if EMS providers cannot safely meet the needs of a patient during a transfer (e.g., a depressed and suicidal patient who is also in acute alcohol withdrawal and intermittently seizing requiring a continuous benzodiazepine infusion), the transferring hospital must provide a nurse. A prospective understanding of local EMS' scope-of-practice definitions will allow for the development of a more seamless transfer process that is critical to both smooth professional interactions and patients' safety.

Short-term treatment units

A strategy to compensate for the lack of inpatient mental health treatment beds for those in crisis is the development of a designated outpatient crisis bed or area, also referred to as a crisis stabilization unit (CSU). CSUs are usually less restrictive than inpatient psychiatric units and are generally not staffed by on-site psychiatrists. They do provide a dedicated area with trained staff and ongoing assessment, supervision, and treatment for patients in behavioral crisis. CSUs focus on short-term stabilization, usually limited to a few days. Because CSUs are generally voluntary treatment settings they may not be appropriate for the more severely impaired patients.

For patients who also have co-occurring substance abuse issues, the increased availability of short-term detoxification units for acutely impaired patients, along with mental health support, may mitigate the need for inter-facility transfer once a sober assessment is accomplished. These units may be operated in collaboration between emergency medicine, medical and psychiatric specialists to provide comprehensive, but short-term assessment and intervention for dual diagnosis patients in crisis. As opposed to inpatient psychiatric treatment, substance abuse treatment may be the appropriate intervention.

Conclusion

With its unique clinical and system-based factors, behavioral emergencies pose a significant challenge to healthcare providers in rural communities. At the same time, opportunities do exist to deliver high-quality emergency psychiatric care. To do so, one must have an appreciation of the social and economic characteristics of rural communities, as well as the attendant challenges and opportunities for patients and providers.

References

1. U.S. Census Bureau Urban and Rural Classification. Available at: http://www.census.gov/geo/www/ua/urbanruralclass.html (Accessed October 25, 2011).

2. U.S. Census Bureau. *The 2010 Statistical Abstract: The National Data Book.* Available at: http://www.census.gov/compendia/statab/2012/tables/12s0029.pdf (Accessed October 25, 2011).

3. Nelson WA. The challenges of rural health care. In: Klugman CM, Dalinis PM, (Eds.). *Ethical Issues in Rural Health Care.* Baltimore: The Johns Hopkins Press; 2008; 34–59.

4. Slade EP, Dixon LB, Semmel S. Trends in the duration of emergency department visits, 2001–2006. *Psychiatr Serv* 2010;**61**:878–84;.

5. Smith RP, Larkins GL, Southwick SM. Trends in US emergency department visits for anxiety-related mental health conditions, 1992–2001. *J Clin Psychiatry* 2008;**69**:286–94.

6. Larkin GL, Claassen CA, Emond JA, et al. Trends in US emergency department visits for mental health conditions, 1992 to 2001. *Psychiatr Serv* 2005;**56**:671–7.

7. Pajonk FG, Gruenberg KAS, Moecke H, et al. Suicides and suicide attempts in emergency medicine. *Crisis* 2002;**23**:68–73.

8. Cooper AE, Corrigan PW, Watson AC. Mental illness stigma and care seeking. *J Nerv Ment Dis* 2003;**191**:339–41.

9. Wrigley S, Jackson H, Judd F, Komiti A. Role of stigma and attitudes toward help-seeking from a general practitioner for mental health problems in a rural town. *Aust N Z J Psychiatry* 2005;**39**:514–21.

10. Jones AR, Cook TM, Wang J. Rural-urban differences in stigma against depression and agreement with health professionals about treatment. *J Affect Disord* 2011;**134**:145–50.

11. Russel SF, Wang J, Carlson RG, et al. Perceived need for substance abuse treatment among illicit stimulant drug users in rural areas of Ohio, Arkansas, and Kentucky. *Drug Alcohol Depend* 2007;**91**:107–14.

12. Havens JR, Oser CB, Leukefeld CG, et al. Differences in prevalence of prescription opiate misuse among rural and urban probationers. *Am J Drug Alcohol Abuse* 2007;**33**:309–17.

13. Booth BM, Curran G, Han X, et al. Longitudinal relationship between psychological distress and multiple substance use: results from a three-year multisite natural-history study of rural stimulant users. *J Stud Alcohol Drugs* 2010;**71**:258–67.

14. Compton WM, Thomas YF, Stinson FS, et al. Prevalence, correlates, disability, comorbidity of DSM-IV drug abuse and dependence in the United States: results from the national epidemiologic survey on alcohol and related conditions. *Arch Gen Psychiatry* 2007;**64**:566–76.

15. Center for Disease Control and Prevention. *Suicide Prevention Fact Sheet.* Atlanta, GA: National Center for Injury Prevention and Control.

Available at: http://www.cdc.gov/
ViolencePrevention/pdf/
Suicide_DataSheet-a.pdf (Accessed
September 2, 2011).

16. Singh GK, Siahpush M. The increasing
rural urban gradient in US suicide
mortality, 1970–1997. *Am J Public
Health* 2003;**93**:1161–7.

17. Stark CR, Riordan V, O'Connor R.
A conceptual model of suicide in
rural areas. *Rural Remote Health*
2011;**11**:1622.

18. Krishnan SP, Hilbert JC, Pase M. An
examination of intimate partner
violence in rural communities: results
from a hospital emergency department
study from Southwest United States.
Fam Community Health 2001;**24**:1–14.

19. Kulig JC, Nahachewsky D, Hall BL,
et al. Rural youth violence: it is a public
health concern! *Can J Public Health*
2005;**96**:357–9.

20. Kansagra SM, Rao SR, Sullivan AF, et al.
A survey of workplace violence across 65
US emergency departments. *Acad
Emerg Med* 2008;**15**:1268–74.

21. Nordstrom D, Zwerling C, Stromquist
A, et al. Rural population survey of
behavioral and demographic risk
factors for loaded firearms. *Inj Prev*
2001;**7**:112–16.

22. Allen MH, Currier GW. Use of
restraints and pharmacotherapy in
academic psychiatric emergency
services. *Gen Hosp Psychiatry*
2004;**26**:42–9.

23. Marco CA, Vaughan J. Emergency
management of agitation in
schizophrenia. *Am J Emerg Med*
2005;**23**:767–76.

24. Battaglia J. Pharmacological
management of acute agitation. *Drugs*
2005;**65**:1207–22.

25. Weiss SJ, Derlet R, Arndahl J, et al.
Estimating the degree of emergency
department overcrowding in academic
medical centers: results of the National
ED Overcrowding study (NEDOCS).
Acad Emerg Med 2004;**11**:38–50.

26. Bur CW, McCaig LF. Staffing, capacity,
and ambulance diversion in emergency
departments: United States 2003–04.
Adv Data 2006;**377**:1–23.

27. Schneider SM, Gallery ME,
Schafermeyer R, Zwemer FL.
Emergency department crowding: a
point in time. *Ann Emerg Med*
2003;**42**:167–72.

28. Jelinek GA, Weiland TJ, Mackinlay C,
et al. Perceived differences in the
management of mental health patients
in remote and rural Australia and
strategies for improvement: findings
from a national qualitative study of
emergency clinicians, *Emerg Med Int*
2011;**2011**: 1–7. Available at: http://
downloads.hindawi.com/journals/emi/
2011/965027.pdf (Accessed October 30,
2011).

29. Lazare A. Shame and humiliation in the
medical encounter. *Arch Intern Med*
1987;**147**:1653–8.

30. Bonnar KK, McCarthy M. Health
related quality of life in a rural area with
low racial/ethnic density. *J Community
Health* 2012;**37**:96–104.

31. Rogers AT. Exploring health beliefs
and care-seeking behaviors of older
USA-dwelling Mexicans and Mexican-
Americans. *Ethn Health*
2010;**15**:581–99.

32. Karasz A, Dempsey K, Fallek R. Cultural
differences in the experience of everyday
symptoms: a comparative study of
South Asian and European American
women. *Cult Med Psychiatry*
2007;**31**:473–97.

33. Testa PA, Gang M. Triage, EMTALA,
consultations, and prehospital medical
control. *Emerg Med Clin North Am*
2009;**27**:627–40.

34. Szpakowicz M, Herd A. "Medically
cleared": how well are patients with
psychiatric presentations examined by
emergency physicians? *J Emerg Med*
2008;**35**:369–72.

35. Pinto T, Poynter B, Durbin J. Medical
clearance in the psychiatric emergency
setting: a call for more standardization.
Healthc Q 2010;**13**:77–82.

36. Busko JM. "Chapter 18: Rural EMS." In:
Bass RR, Brice JH, Delbridge TR,
Gunderson MR, (Eds.). *Emergency
Medical Services: Clinical Practice and
Systems Oversight, Volume 2: Medical
Oversight of EMS.* Dubuque, IA:
Kendall-Hunt; 2009:217–28.

37. König F, König E, Wolfersdorf M.
Frequency of psychiatric emergency
situations in the pre-clinical emergency
system. *Der Notarzt* 1996;**12**:12–17.

38. Pajonk FG, Bartels HH, Biberthaler P,
et al. Psychiatric emergencies in
preclinical emergency medical service:
frequency, treatment, and assessment by
emergency physicians and paramedics.
Der Nervenarzt 2001;**72**:685–92.

39. Bledsoe BE, Porter RS, Cherry RA,
(Eds.). *Essentials of Paramedic Care*,
(2nd Edition). Upper Saddle River, NJ:
Pearson Prentice Hall; 2007.

40. Kidd T, Kenny A, Meehan-Andrews T.
The experience of general nurses in rural
Australian emergency departments.
Nurse Educ Pract 2012;**12**:11–15.

41. Technical Assistance Collaborative, Inc.
2005. *A Community Based Comprehensive
Psychiatric Crisis Response Service.*
Available at: http://www.tacinc.org/
downloads/Pubs/
Crisis_Monograph_Final.pdf (Accessed
October 30, 2011).

42. Kallert TW. Coercion in psychiatry.
Curr Opin Psychiatry 2008;**21**:485–9.

43. McFarland BH, Brunette M, Steketee K,
et al. Long-term followup of rural
involuntary clients. *J Ment Health Adm*
1993;**20**:46–57.

44. Dunbain JS, McEwin K, Cameron I.
Postgraduate medical placements in
rural areas; their impact on the rural
medical workforce. *Rural Remote Health*
2006;**6**:481.

45. Duchesne JC, Kyle A, Simmons J, et al.
Impact of telemedicine upon rural
trauma care. *J Trauma* 2008;**64**:92–7.

46. Ricca MA, Caputo M, Amour J, et al.
Telemedicine reduces discrepancies in
rural trauma care. *Telemed J E Health*
2003;**9**:3–11.

47. Norman S. The use of telemedicine in
psychiatry. *J Psychiatr Ment Health Nurs*
2006;**13**:771–7.

48. Singh SP, Arya D, Peters T. Accuracy of
telepsychiatric assessment of new
routine outpatient referrals. *BMC
Psychiatry* 2007;**7**:55.

49. Hyler SE, Gangure DP, Batchelder ST.
Can telepsychiatry replace in-person
psychiatric assessments? A review and
meta-analysis of comparison studies.
CNS Spectr 2005;**10**:403–13.

50. Hilty DM, Luo JS, Morache C, et al.
Telepsychiatry: an overview for
psychiatrists. *CNS Drugs* 2002;**16**:527–48.

51. Monnier J, Knapp RG, Frueh BC. Recent
advances in telepsychiatry: an updated
review. *Psychiatr Serv* 2003;**54**:1604–9.

52. Pesämaa L, Ebeling H, Kuusimäki M,
et al. Videoconferencing in child and
adolescent telepsychiatry: a systemic
review of the literature. *J Telemed
Telecare* 2004;**10**:187–92.

53. Shore JH, Hilty DM, Yellowlees P.
Emergency management guidelines for

telepsychiatry. *Gen Hosp Psychiatry* 2007;**29**:199–206.

54. Shore JH, Savin DM, Novins D, et al. Cultural aspects of telepsychiatry. *J Telemed Telecare* 2006;**12**:116–21.

55. Joiner T, Kalafat J, Draper J, et al. Establishing standards for the assessment of suicide risk among callers to the national suicide prevention lifeline. *Suicide Life Threat Behav* 2007;**37**:353–65.

56. Shah MN, Caprio TV, Swanson P, et al. A novel emergency medical services-based program to identify and assist older patients in rural community. *J Am Geriatr Soc* 2010;**58**:2205–11.

57. Reich J. "Chapter 35: Behavioral Emergencies". In: Bass RR, Brice JH, Delbridge TR, Gunderson MR, (Eds.). *Emergency Medical Services: Clinical Practice and Systems Oversight, Volume 1: Clinical Aspects of Prehospital Medicine.* Dubuque, IA: Kendall-Hunt 2009:360–72.

Coordination of emergency department psychiatric care with psychiatry

Benjamin L. Bregman and Seth Powsner

Introduction

No one can win a relay race by him- or herself, but anyone can lose it by dropping the baton. Care of chronically ill patients, medical or psychiatric, frequently involves passing a patient from one treatment setting to the next. The complexity of caring for psychiatric patients in emergency departments (EDs) described in previous chapters suggests that a closer alignment of Psychiatric and Emergency Departments would be beneficial to both clinicians and patients. Developing and maintaining a means of coordinating care and communicating between clinicians may be unique to each practice environment. Nonetheless, the goal of this chapter is to outline general themes that arise in coordination of care between emergency and psychiatry practitioners and to articulate the non–patient-care-related benefits of having working relationships with liaison psychiatrists, including staff well-being, multidisciplinary research initiatives, joint training opportunities, quality improvement endeavors, and patient safety activities.

This chapter will address three themes relevant to the coordination of care between the emergency medicine and psychiatry clinicians: (1) who is involved in the coordination of care, (2) creating a coordination team, and (3) the benefits of nonclinical interdisciplinary collaboration. These themes were chosen to highlight differences in culture, training or approach and may provide providers with the clarity to decrease interdepartmental frustrations and improve patient outcomes.

Who is involved in the coordination of care

Coordinating care with mental health professionals suggests the challenge of understanding who's who, and who's likely to be doing what. Because there are so many kinds of mental health professionals, a list follows, arranged as an outline of organizational services.

Clinics: Mental health clinics are likely to be government operated or government funded as compared with their private or academic medical counterparts. Even though some look and run just like any medical clinic there is little tradition of around-the-clock care, and there may be no fee for service incentive. As such, their patient volume may or may not support an answering service outside of regular business hours.

Individual treaters: Often called *therapists* and *counselors* by their patients, they are often generically labeled *mental health professionals*. Individual treaters may have their own office, may share an office complex, and very frequently work in a clinic (if only to share clerical and billing overheads).

Psychiatrists: These are physicians (M.D. or D.O.) who have completed four or more years of training after medical school, training specifically focused on mental illness. They would normally be licensed by their state government as physicians able to prescribe medication, and be board eligible (completed their psychiatric training in good standing) or board certified (passed examination by the ABPN, the American Board of Psychiatry and Neurology). Although psychiatric residency training is broad in scope, and nationally regulated, individual practitioners may only accept a limited type of patient or offer only limited types of treatment (e.g., primarily medication or psychotherapy or addiction treatment or electro-convulsive therapy).

Nonpsychiatric physicians: Some internal medicine, family practice, and pediatric physicians will prescribe psychiatric medications in cooperation with non-physician mental health specialists. They may be affiliated with a mental health clinic proper, or, they may be helping one or two non-physician mental health professionals working in a traditional medical clinic. It is common in some communities to find a patient's internist or pediatrician prescribing an antidepressant on the recommendation of the patient's therapist who is a psychologist or social worker without a medical degree. Moreover, internists can now prescribe buprenorphine-naloxone, as a private practice alternative to methadone maintenance clinic treatment.

APRN, NP, PA clinicians: There are practitioners who do not have an MD or DO, but are allowed to prescribe medication, usually in collaboration with a physician. Advanced Practice Registered Nurses, Nurse Practitioners, and Physician Associates have various privileges determined by the regulatory agencies in their locale. Patients may refer to them as *doctor*, if only because they write their prescriptions. They typically graduate with less direct clinical experience than a board eligible psychiatrist, however, they can easily become seasoned clinicians as they are often 100% occupied with clinical care.

Behavioral Emergencies for the Emergency Physician, ed. Leslie S. Zun, Lara G. Chepenik, and Mary Nan S. Mallory. Published by Cambridge University Press. © Cambridge University Press 2013.

Psychologists (PhD, PsyD, MA): There are many different kinds of *psychologists*: clinical, industrial, research, and others. To further complicate matters a psychologist may or may not have doctoral-level training, and may or may not have a clinical license. If they have been licensed after receiving their doctoral degree, they have likely received more training in evaluation and psychotherapy than provided for a physician in a psychiatry residency. Psychologists usually do not prescribe medication; psychologist prescribing is only allowed in two states: New Mexico and Louisiana.

Social workers (MSW, LCSW): There are a variety of different kinds of *social workers*. They may or may not be licensed. They may or may not be specifically trained to do psychotherapy or treat psychiatric patients. And, depending on their clinical environment, they may have a variety of different assignments. Some function as a patient's regular *treater*, meeting with their patient every week or so to provide counseling and psychotherapy. Other social workers may be assigned to help patients navigate the social services system, e.g., apply for welfare benefits and Medicaid. Social workers may be designated *case managers*, implying that they keep tabs on their patients, and coordinate their overall care.

Counselors (psychological, substance abuse): *Counselors* are a very varied group. To further complicate matters, patients are not reliable about using the term *licensed professional counselor*, which suggests advanced training and licensure. Some patients use the term generically like *therapist*. In any case, the demand for lower cost mental health and addiction services has led to a growing number of clinic staff that meet routinely with patients to provide guidance, support, and therapy. It is hard to be specific about an individual *counselor's* qualifications without asking, or knowing more about their practice setting.

Outreach operations: If patients will not come to treatment, take treatment to the patients: that is the motto for outreach programs. A simple approach is to provide brief psychiatric sessions and dispense medications from a van that operates as a clinic on wheels. Unfortunately, paranoid patients may avoid even the friendliest clinic staff, and, among the severely mentally ill patients, even outreach cannot overcome their medication non-adherence.

Assertive community treatment (ACT) teams drive out to find patients, encourage them to take their medication, and help with whatever practical problems may arise, (e.g., arrange housing, welfare benefits, medical clinic visits). It turns out that a significant number of patients will accept medication and other help, when the team's persistent efforts demonstrate that someone cares. It is difficult and sometimes thankless working with a collection of these patients. Although inefficient by usual clinic metrics (visits per hour or visits per day, total number of patients carried by each clinician, etc), ACT teams can reduce hospital re-admissions and incidents in their community.

Inpatient psychiatric units: Inpatient services tackle the challenge of treating patients who are so disturbed that they could hurt themselves or someone else. Such cases can profoundly affect the operation and design of a ward: there must be staff available at all times to monitor dangerous patients, prevent any violent actions, and yet still perform routine functions of patient care (e.g., check vital signs, administer medications and conduct therapy sessions, etc.). So inpatient services are usually staffed by the same professionals that staff psychiatric clinics, but with additional nurses, aides, and security.

Inpatient services usually have ancillary support services such as physical therapy, occupational therapy, phlebotomy, and a chaplain. These staff may be shared with other wards. They are less likely to be points of contact for emergency department collaboration.

Inpatient staff frequently focus their attention on protocols, rules, and regulations governing patient admission (or discharge). Inpatient psychiatric care is subject to legal constraints and regulatory review beyond that of medical-surgical units, which generally reflect society's fears about loss of patient autonomy, risk assessments within legal protections, and perceived potential dangerousness of the mentally ill. Additionally, American inpatient psychiatric services have also been shaped by pernicious cost-cutting efforts since the late 1970s, (decades longer than other hospital services). This has led to a shortage of psychiatric beds and, consequently, it has led to a backup of psychiatric patients in general emergency departments. Admitting patients for inpatient psychiatric care is more complex than admitting medical or surgical patients.

Visiting nurses: Often called *VNA*, it is important to know that not all visiting nurses are part of a Visiting Nurse Association (which may or may not be a member of VNAA – Visiting Nurse Associations of America). In some locales there are many agencies that provide home services by registered nurses, nurse aides, and other related staff. Visiting nursing staff can provide very helpful information about a patient's baseline level of function at home, and can communicate the time course of a recent change. Occasionally, they can serve as care coordinator because they are in contact with a patient's regular prescriber. Unfortunately, newly assigned staff, or temporary covering staff, may send a patient for emergency evaluation simply because they are not familiar with poor baseline function.

Housing supervisors: Several of the seriously, persistently mentally ill (SPMI) live in settings that include some sort of *housing supervisor*. In a bordering home that accepts mentally ill, the landlord often provides supervision. Likewise, homeless shelters may employ or designate a supervisor. There are many other arrangements including rest homes and retirement homes. These *supervisors* can be very helpful, but be aware that they are unlikely to be clinically trained or selected for their clinical ability.

Low-cost housing meant for the SPMI is now more likely to include an on-site supervisor with clinical training or experience. Likewise, "crisis & respite" facilities will likely have staff on-site around the clock (temporary halfway house / group home). Although they may not be licensed clinical professionals, these staff members tend to be (self) selected for this kind of work; they can often provide information about a patient's recent behavior, and they can sometimes help assure a patient is directed to treatment.

Case managers: Outpatient case managers handle challenges much like traditional hospital social workers. They try to assure that patients are registered for care, benefits, and have housing. Unlike a medical ward social worker, they are assigned to patients for months or years, following them through emergency visits, admissions, discharges, clinical changes and alike. With phone calls and outings to transport patients to critical appointments, they can become a source of valuable patient observations. *They may also know more than any individual treater about a patient's course.* Unlike ACT Team members, they do not usually pursue patients into the community or push them into treatment.

Family and court appointed guardians/conservators: Family are often overlooked as clinical collaborators. Family can often help assure patients attend treatment, or alert 911 if there are signs of violence after skipping medication. They can often recount the time course of a patient's behavior, including stressors a patient might not report (drug use, arguments with friends, etc).

Specific information, relevant to deterioration and safety, should be elicited and factored into the evaluation. However, it is not useful to ask family if their loved one "needs to be admitted". Moreover, asking "is Mr. Jones suicidal?" may be like asking, "is Mr. Jones having a heart attack?" – most family members will translate all of these into "do you want Mr. Jones admitted today?" They may answer *yes* or *no* based on non-clinical considerations. Non-professionals are more reliable answering simple, open-ended questions, like, *what has your family member done that worries you the most?*

Legal officers: Police and parole officers are not traditionally considered collaborators. However, for some patients, only law enforcement personnel demonstrate a long-term interest. For some patients, only law enforcement agencies have any way to assure treatment. (There is no *outpatient commitment* in most locales, aka *Kendra's Law* or *Laura's Law*.)

The challenge in collaborating with law enforcement is to reasonably maintain confidentiality. Some clinicians feel this is impossible; they refuse to contact police or to even review a patient's legal record (e.g., online police blotter or court records). Other clinicians feel it is mandatory; they often cite *Tarasoff* and state laws requiring physicians to report gunshot wounds, child abuse, and such. Consultation with legal staff is recommended so that both staff and the hospital are in a defensible position.

In summary, the successful coordination of the diverse team of caretakers involved in the life of one patient could be an overwhelming task. Recognizing the training and role of each individual contributor and drawing on their strengths and abilities can create a collaborative care environment that can help patients in the short and long term. Conversely, not understanding the role of each player could contribute to frustrations and problematic communication that could ultimately worsen a patient's condition and long-term prognosis.

Creating a cohesive coordination team

In the previous section we described many of the players involved in the coordination of care for psychiatric patients. Unfortunately, as is often the case, simply having such resources doesn't mean that they work together in an efficient and frustration-free way. Creating an effective team requires additional steps, including (1) assessing the availability of willing resource-partners, (2) recognizing the abilities and liabilities of those resource-partners, and (3) designing a model for coordinating care.

The availability of psychiatric resources

Although it is more than likely that each community has many of the players listed above, whether or not they are available is a different question. The process of identifying participating partners may be as easy as transferring a patient in-house, or as difficult as "cold-calling" nearby hospitals and outpatient providers to assess whether they are currently taking patients. Local "bed-boards" offer one solution for this problem, specifically for inpatient beds. These (mostly) state-government-run services query psychiatric administrators at local hospitals daily to identify the number of psychiatric beds available, and their available services (i.e., male/female, voluntary/involuntary, substance abuse/detoxification, dual-diagnosis, adolescent, child, and full fee/Medicaid, etc). When a hospital receives a patient that they are unable to treat, they are able to call this service and quickly find whether another regional hospital is able to care for their patient, and efficiently arrange for transfer to that institution. These services offer an elegant solution to identifying the availability of psychiatric resource-partners.

Some states have a similar system to access social services. Called by a variety of names (e.g., Core Service Agency, Community Service Board), these organizations are central clearing houses for any of several services provided by the state, county or municipality for the indigent or unfortunate. Services offered by these organizations include case management, psychiatric services, substance abuse and dependence treatment, free medication services, counseling, low-income housing, food stamps/food bank/soup kitchens, homeless shelters, medical care, dental care, partial hospitals, day programs, half-way homes, and ACT teams. In addition, these organizations often have access to medical and psychiatric information on patients that can be accessed if the patient is hospitalized including diagnosis, recent hospitalizations, a recent medication list, and the phone numbers of team members associated with their care. For areas where many people access community services, having easy access to the phone number of the agency could reduce confusion over medications and time spent in the ED (i.e., the ACT team could pick the patient up), among other things.

Unfortunately, a similar system does not exist for outpatient resources for those people who do not qualify for social services. As a result, finding a psychiatrist or a therapist for a patient not requiring inpatient admission can be complex and cumbersome. This is especially true if the person requiring care does not have health insurance, has health insurance without a mental health rider, or has a language barrier. Moreover, even if a patient is able to access psychiatric care or therapy, the professional they find may not match their needs. As such, having an updated list of local resources could give patients the direction they need to access mental healthcare choices. Some recommendations for such a list include the following:

- Resident clinics at local psychiatry and psychology programs (low fee by trainees)
- Psychoanalytic institutes (low fees by trainees)
- Religious organizations (especially helpful for non-English-speaking patients)
- Veterans Administrations
- Low fee clinics (especially helpful for non-English-speaking patients)
- The mental healthcare phone number for common local insurances (e.g., BC/BS, Aetna).

If these inpatient, social services, and outpatient options do not exist a priori, it may be valuable to reach out to internal and external resources to design an ad-hoc system. In such a situation, identifying and reaching out to local hospitals and mental health professional groups such as local clinics may help to start a collaborative endeavor that could help both partners involved. Moreover, these local mental health resources may be more informed of other available mental healthcare settings, further increasing potential transfer and referral points.

Recognize each party's strengths and limitations

Beyond knowing who is available and how to access them, being aware of the strengths and limitations of each partner is vital. Certain requests for collaboration may not succeed simply because they are beyond the scope of practice for one party or the other. It is easy for each partner not to recognize critical differences between the way they and their counterpart operate. These differences do not necessarily equate to dysfunction. Indeed, as mentioned above, recognizing that a family member can recognize and report behaviors, although not necessarily symptoms, or that one type of treatment facility may be better equipped to care for one type of patient over another, may save time, frustration, money, and even prevent negative outcomes. Consequently, to create an efficient coordination effort, identify what each player can contribute and how they may be a liability if not used appropriately.

Medical and psychiatric clearance

One example of this centers on the expectation of the treatment capacities of referring and receiving facilities. For example, psychiatric inpatient facilities are much better equipped to handle medical conditions than a rest home, and probably better than a skilled nursing home. However, most psychiatric

wards will not try to maintain IV fluids, oxygen or tube feedings, and may or may not have easy access to blood testing or to an internist. No one argues that this is a good or necessary state of affairs. Although the American Psychiatric Association makes recommendations about the level of medical care a psychiatric hospital should be able to provide, implementation is variable and unreimbursed costs are a factor.

This particular limitation is best seen in the need for "medical clearance." "Medical clearance" was first addressed in Weissberg's paper [1] wherein he articulated concerns over the use and misuse of extensive pre-admission workups, identifying that they are often done for the purpose of placating a psychiatrist's feelings of inadequacy when addressing the medical care of a psychiatric patient. Since that time, other papers [2–5] have addressed the role and validity of medical clearance. Today, although the American College of Emergency Physicians (ACEP) has issued a consensus opinion that emergency physicians not perform a reflexive medical clearance on psychiatric patients [6], it is common practice for emergency departments to order laboratory and imaging studies to rule out potential medical conditions underlying psychiatric presentations.

Although not as well characterized, the converse of this limitation is true as well: medical and surgical subspecialists are often uncomfortable caring for psychiatrically ill patients without "psych clearance." This is understandable given the potential complications, financial, safety and otherwise, that accompany psychiatric patients. This limitation can be manifested as a reluctance to start a psychiatric medication on patients due to lack of familiarity with treatment indications or psychiatric medications themselves, or as an incomplete assessment for patients with substance abuse due to negative counter-transference.

In both cases, recognizing and playing to the strengths of the provider can significantly improve patient care, decrease costs to the system, and save providers from unneeded stress in providing services they feel ill-equipped to render.

Designing a coordination of care model

When a situation arises that necessitates a concerted coordinated effort of the available resource-partner, just like running a code, having a clear protocol for who does what and when before anything happens can be invaluable. Considering the unique milieu (i.e., demographic, legal, financial, academic affiliation, etc.) each institution finds itself in, it would be advantageous to have a clear picture about the extramural limitations superimposed upon one's organization. In other words, are there state-specific legal restrictions pertaining to restraints, involuntary hospitalization, isolation, involuntary administration of medications, or transfer and boarding laws that could negatively affect a well-coordinated effort between two institutions? Moreover, does the effort take into consideration the long-term needs of the patient such that the situation necessitating the coordination of care may not be necessary again in the future if particular steps are taken? In designing such a model, considerations should include:

- Which institution is responsible for arranging transportation? And who maintains the patient's safety during a transfer?
- What are the inter-state transfer laws of the jurisdiction where the patient is seen?
- What care protocols exist for patients who must wait before a psychiatric bed becomes available (i.e., visitation, in-hospital mobility, cell phone access, food)?
- Can treatment be initiated before transfer to an accepting facility?
- Can a patient be re-evaluated for admission and discharged if deemed safe?
- Is the patient admitted voluntarily or involuntary?
- Who arranges for post-discharge follow-up? What are the steps that need to be taken to ensure that a patient receives the correct referral?
- Are the financial burdens disproportionately felt by some members of the collaboration more than another?
- How does one measure and monitor the efficacy of a coordinated care program?

Taking these points into consideration, may help improve patient care in addition to reducing financial, temporal, and stress burdens on a system.

Nonclinical collaboration between the psychiatry and emergency departments

In addition to coordinating patient care, collaborations between psychiatry and emergency services can be helpful for growing departments in several ways including through education for capacity building, research initiatives, and improving well-being and morale. As Accountable Care Organizations (ACOs), interdisciplinary teams of providers who take responsibility for coordinated efforts at improving patient health, take their place in the American medical system landscape, these kinds of collaborations will become even more important.

Education

Although patients with mental illness are common visitors to acute care settings, nurses, ED techs, residents, and attending physicians may have limited training or experience in dealing with psychiatric emergencies. The reverse is also true: psychiatrists often feel unfamiliar with current treatments for common medical illnesses encountered in inpatient and outpatient settings. Engaging both Emergency Physicians and psychiatrists to provide frequent lectures and trainings can reframe care for psychiatric patients in acute care settings, improve familiarity and comfort in dealing with psychiatric patients,

and communicate the importance of attending to psychiatric issues for the ED staff. In addition, updates on nonpsychiatric medications and treatment protocols, refresher courses on medical codes, and conversations about treatment protocols for psychiatric patients in the ED can help psychiatrists feel more comfortable with patients who might have previously been subjected to unnecessary testing and consults under the care of the psychiatry team.

Educational seminars are currently being taught at the supporting institution of one of the authors (B. Bregman). Three separate seminars are provided on a weekly to monthly basis for ED staff including one for nurses and techs, one for residents, and one for medical students. In addition to going over role-specific information, and talking about the psychiatric concepts of transference and countertransference, these seminars provide the opportunity for the learners to talk about their experiences with psychiatric patients. This aspect of the seminar serves both to allow the students to learn from each other and to provide an informal "psychiatric supervision" that has been reported to be helpful in mitigating the negative feelings elicited by working with psychiatric patients.

Research

Although it is a growing area of interest, relatively little has been written on the field of emergency psychiatry. Organizations such as the American Academy of Emergency Psychiatry (AAEP) and the Society for Academic Emergency Medicine (SAEM) have spearheaded efforts to improve research in this area; however, more needs to be done to further explore this interdisciplinary intersection. In addition to examining psychopharmacological interventions, research on ultra-brief psychotherapeutic interventions, psychiatric trauma, first-break psychosis, access to care, somatization, psychiatric and medical comorbidities in the ED, and recidivism are just a few potential topics in this rich untapped research field.

Morale and well-being

Caring for patients can be physically and emotionally taxing. This is especially true for psychiatric patients, who often contribute to the overall level of tension in the ED, and perhaps generate additional stress in an already stressful work environment. In such settings, psychiatrists can play an additional role in the coordination of care, specifically that of caring for the caretakers.

A psychiatric liaison can help to prevent, reframe, and resolve the impact of negative patient interactions in several ways. First, through interactive educational modules, such as the one described above, ED staff can discuss their experiences concerning psychiatric patients thereby providing a forum for peer learning, and offering a time for "psychiatric supervision." In addition to education, these classes allow for time to deal with potentially harmful negative feelings that arise between ED providers and patients with psychiatric issues (if not complaints). Second, asking for a psychiatrist to be available to participate in debriefing of difficult cases can help to resolve frustration with other staff members and patients by shedding light on intrapsychic conflicts that patients bring to and foist upon ED staff. Clarifying these patient–system conflicts can be comforting to staff members who may be exhausted from dealing with complicated patients or traumatized from poor outcomes. Finally, having a psychiatrist on emergency department committees can provide a different and possibly beneficial perspective on an administrative level. Having a psychological perspective on potential staff and patient interpersonal dynamics may give committees information that can raise awareness of potential "flashpoints" before they become active problems. Tasks could include the creation of an interdisciplinary plan for problem patients and creating safe and effective protocols for managing agitated and aggressive patients. Including a psychiatrist in these functions can build resilience in the ED staff, improve morale, and prevent staff burnout.

Conclusion

Given the high volume of psychiatric patients seen in acute care settings, creating and sustaining a relationship between the psychiatry and emergency medicine departments can decrease patient length of stay, increase safety for patients and ED staff, increase awareness of mental illness in patients and staff, and improve patient outcomes. As there are differences in clinical training and approaches to patient care, improving communication and developing an awareness of expectations can improve overall interdepartmental coordination of patient care.

As the American medical landscape continues to adapt to new political and economic pressures, interdisciplinary collaborations will be vital to maintaining excellent, safe, and cost-effective health care. In addition, having an awareness of the mental health of one's staff and an informed approach to maintaining their morale can help maintain patient care excellence in acute care settings.

References

1. Weissberg MP. Emergency room medical clearance: an educational problem. *Am J Psychiatry* 1979;**136**:787–90.

2. Dolan JG, Mushlin AL. Routine laboratory testing for medical disorders in psychiatric patients. *Arch Intern Med* 1985;**145**:2085–8.

3. Riba M, Hale M. Medical clearance: fact or fiction in the hospital emergency room. *Psychosomatics* 1990;**31**:400–4.

4. Korn CS, Currier GW, Henderson SO. 'Medical clearance' of psychiatric patients without medical complaints in the emergency department. *J Emerg Med* 2000;**18**:173–6.

5. Pinto T, Poynter B, Durbin J. Medical clearance in the psychiatric emergency setting: a call for more standardization. *Healthcare Q* 2010;**13**:77–82.

6. Lukens TW, Wolf SJ, Edlow JA, et al. Clinical policy: critical issues in the diagnosis and management of the adult psychiatric patient in the emergency department. *Ann Emerg Med* 2006;**47**:79–99.

Chapter 39

Integration with community resources

Jennifer Peltzer-Jones

Introduction

In the United States, emergency departments (EDs) have become primary access points to obtain emergent psychiatric care. In 2007, the Agency for Healthcare Research and Quality reported 12.5% of U.S. ED visits were related to a psychiatric complaint [1]. Management of a psychiatric crisis in the ED is complicated by several factors. First, the United States lacks a standardized delivery model of emergency mental health care. Patients who present to an ED in crises may or may not speak with a mental health professional. The training of the mental health professionals who do work in the ED also varies: social workers, psychiatric residents, psychologists, or psychiatrists may conduct the ED evaluations.

Additionally, ED physicians are not universally trained during the course of their residency to manage psychiatric crises [2,3]. Variance in delivery systems and ED physician knowledge contribute to variance in disposition recommendations from one emergency department to the next [4,5]. Because ED physicians may be unaware of alternative care choices for patients, inpatient psychiatric hospitalization may be overutilized in the management of psychiatric emergencies [1,5,6]. When patients are referred to inpatient care, this contributes to a larger problem within the ED: boarding of psychiatric patients. The U.S. Department of Health and Human Services' Literature Review: Psychiatric Boarding [7] provides a comprehensive examination of the contributory factors specific to psychiatric boarding, one of which includes the decreased number of emergency psychiatric beds available across the United States. The Treatment Advocacy Center determined in 2005, there were 17 public psychiatric beds available per 100,000 people. In their estimation, this equals a national shortage of 95,820 psychiatric beds in the United States [8]. While opening more inpatient psychiatric beds is a necessary part of the solution for psychiatric patient boarding, this is not a solution an ED can control. There are some solutions for psychiatric boarding EDs could enact such as better collaboration with existent outpatient psychiatric care resources. As EDs continue to serve as de facto safety nets for psychiatric crises, ED personnel will need to increase their understanding of non–hospital-based

community alternatives to assist in safe crisis management. If EDs can enhance partnership with existent community resources to create alternative crisis pathways for patients, the number of psychiatric patients and their length of ED stay could potentially decrease without sacrificing quality of patient care. The aim of this chapter is to familiarize ED physicians with the community mental health model and to introduce non-inpatient community resources along the psychiatric crisis continuum.

Organization of mental health services

In reviewing community mental health resources, it is critical to understand the structure of the mental health system and the definition of "community". Of the patients who present to EDs in psychiatric crisis, it has been found that only one quarter of these patients have private insurance coverage; the majority of patients who come to an ED in psychiatric crises receive healthcare through public funding sources such as Medicare and Medicaid [1,9,10]. While advantageous to have private insurance coverage for medical problems, patients with private healthcare coverage can have insufficient benefit options for mental health (if their medical plan allows for any mental health benefit at all). Although government-supported community resources may exist in a community, patients with private coverage may be ineligible to use these resources. Per the Surgeon General's 1999 Report on Mental Health Care, "Health insurance, whether funded through private or public sources, is one of the most important factors influencing access to health and mental health services" [11]. In 2002, when he created the President's New Freedom Commission, President Bush emphasized how private insurance treatment limitations and a fragmented mental health system were two core obstacles for patients to obtain needed mental health care [12]. It is within this context of complicated pay structures and poorly connected private and public sectors that ED physicians are left to naively navigate appropriate resources. The disorganized structure of mental health care and the inconsistency in care delivery across states and funding streams leaves ED staff disconnected from appropriate system resources. Because the

Behavioral Emergencies for the Emergency Physician, ed. Leslie S. Zun, Lara G. Chepenik, and Mary Nan S. Mallory. Published by Cambridge University Press. © Cambridge University Press 2013.

greater percentage of patients who present in psychiatric crisis to EDs lack private coverage benefits, this chapter will primarily focus on publicly funded community resources.

Community psychiatric services

Deinstitutionalization has often been cited as the single most important factor contributing to the current mental health system crisis. In the mid-20th century, when the deinstitutionalization movement gained strength, large numbers of patients were in state institutions receiving subpar care. Deinstitutionalization proponents believed patients living in home communities would receive improved illness management and care. If needed, acute stabilization could be provided in local community hospitals for episodes of psychiatric decompensation and crises. Treatment in the community, rather than locked hospitals, continues to be a guiding principle in the structure of today's mental healthcare system: "The new priorities of psychiatric hospitalization focus on ameliorating the risk of danger to self or others ... Inpatient units are seen as short-term intensive settings to contain and resolve crises *that cannot be resolved in the community*" [11]. However, while community mental health programs have been given the burden to stabilize patients within the community, historically there has not been appropriate funding to provide for a comprehensive delivery system.

Brief history of community mental health

The National Mental Health Act of 1946 was the first major federal law supporting community-based care as the recommended treatment for mentally ill patients. Under this act, the National Institute for Mental Health was formed to help distribute grants to fund outpatient care [13]. As a result, over one thousand outpatient mental health clinics were in practice and receiving state assistance to care for patients in the community by 1955 [13]. The next important legislation in the development of community mental health in the U.S. was the Mental Health Study Act of 1955. This act called for a team of experts to perform a "comprehensive review of the mental health system in America" [14]. In the subsequent report generated in 1960, the Joint Commission on Mental Illness and Health listed three major conclusions about the mental health system: (1) there was a need for increased research about mental illness, (2) there was a need for an increased number of mental health providers, (recommending specifically one mental health clinic for every 50,000 people), and (3) "spending for public mental health services should be greatly expanded – doubled in the next 5 years, tripled in the next 10 years" [14]. Throughout the 1960s, despite the discovery of antipsychotic medication, there were still between 500,000–600,000 patients hospitalized in state institutions across the country. The estimated costs of care for these patients were around $1.8 billion [14]. It was at this time President Kennedy proposed the Community Mental Health Centers Act (CMHC), which called for an increase in funding for mental health as well as a concerted effort to decrease the

number of patients institutionalized by 50% over 1–2 decades [14]. As many programs were already in place, the President believed strong increases in funding could support the movement of patients from state hospitals to the community, and federal grants and research monies would shift from state legislatures to local hospitals and non-profit care organizations [14–16]. When the CMHC Act was passed in 1963, concerns about the funding of staff in community care programs, prompted by the American Medical Association's fears about socialized medicine, limited federal monies to the new community mental health centers' programs to $150 million [14]. This figure represented less than 10% of existent costs for treating state psychiatric patients, yet was expected to fund the transition of at least half the institutionalized population to outpatient care. These funding proposals also failed to account for people who were not institutionalized, but who still needed mental health care and had no other recourse but to go to community mental health centers [13]. With the passage of the CMHC Act, deinstitutionalization as a national agenda was born, but without the appropriate financial backing needed to fully realize a true community-based care model.

Since passage of the CMHC Act over 50 years ago, programming-funding discrepancy continues to impact care delivery as community-based programs experience continued budgetary cuts for mental health care. According to the National Alliance on Mental Illness (NAMI), states cut more than $1.6 billion in general funds from their state mental health agency budgets for mental health services from 2009 to 2011 [17].

Current structure

The Substance Abuse and Mental Health Services Administration (SAMHSA) designates State Mental Health Agencies (SMHAs) responsible for "assuring the provision of mental health services to persons with mental illnesses and emotional disturbances" within each state. The SMHA sets programmatic state goals for care, ensures quality of care, and distributes federal monies to state-based programs. In sum, SMHAs are the organizers of community mental health [18]. In the National Alliance for Mental Illness (NAMI) report, *State Mental Health Cuts: A National Crisis* [17], the expectations of state-based care is defined:

> "State general funding of mental health care is the "safety net of last resort" for children and adults living with serious mental illness. Although Medicaid is an extremely important funding source, many people with mental illness do not qualify for Medicaid, either because their income is slightly higher than the Medicaid threshold (which is well below poverty level in most states) or because they are too ill to take the steps necessary to apply and qualify for Medicaid. Additionally, Medicaid does not pay for some vital mental health services, most notably inpatient psychiatric treatment".

The number of people served in these community mental health programs has steadily risen. In 2009, 6,401,613 people received some type of service which was partially or wholly funded by a SMHA; an increase from 2007 by 300,000 patients [17]. Because such a large number of patients in need of mental health care must go through community mental health, a large number of patients seen in the ED are already or will need to be connected with their local Community Mental Health Centers (CMHCs). CMHCs are structured to provide a variety of mental health programs. They are organized under State Mental Health Agencies (SMHAs) and serve cohorts of patients in their immediate "catchment" areas. According to the Centers for Medicare and Medicaid Services, the core services a CMHC must have to qualify for Medicare reimbursement are:

- Outpatient services, including specialized outpatient services for children, the elderly, individuals who are chronically mentally ill, and residents of the CMHC's mental health service area who have been discharged from inpatient treatment at a mental health facility
- 24 hour-a-day emergency care services
- Day treatment, or other partial hospitalization services, or psychosocial rehabilitation services
- Screening for patients being considered for admission to State mental health facilities to determine the appropriateness of such admission" [19].

Additional treatment modalities offered may include: Medication Management Programs, Case Management, ACT (Assertive Community Treatment) Services, and Supported Employment Programs. CMHCs employ a variety of professionals, including psychiatrists, psychologists, nurse practitioners, registered nurses, social workers, case managers, and peer support specialists.

CMHCs can be contacted through each state's Department of Mental Health or Department of Health and Human Services, or by contacting the SMHA. CMHCs may be organized under regional authorities or may be directly managed by individual counties. Thus, given the wide range of services and the increasing population CMHCs serve, EDs *must* develop strong partnerships with their area CMHCs or SMHA to understand specific crisis services and outpatient programs available for patients.

Services along the crisis continuum

The Community Mental Health Centers Act and the deinstitutionalization movement did not seek to transfer the care of state hospitalized patients to community hospitalized patients. The basis of these movements as described above, were to create a more comprehensive care system for the mentally ill in the safety of the home community. While the comprehensive visions of the past have not been fully realized today, there are multiple examples of programs which function to meet the needs of patients in the community. Examples of the types of programs and interventions that may avert the need for inpatient care are provided below.

Mobile crisis teams

Mobile crisis teams are a type of service along the psychiatric crisis continuum which consist of trained mental health and/or law enforcement personnel organized to respond to psychiatric crisis in a variety of locations. These programs may be community based, hospital based, or clinic based. Dependent upon how the teams are structured, they may serve the dual purpose of psychiatric consult or screening agents for the counties or SMHAs [20]. There is no one agency which organizes these units across the country. Effectiveness of mobile crisis teams is subjective according to the structure goals of the program because mobile crisis teams differ in their purpose. For example, in one study, mobile crisis teams were evaluated to determine if mobile crisis team intervention strengthened outpatient follow-up for suicidal patients (they did not), while in another study, patients who were evaluated in a hospital-based setting had a 51% higher chance of psychiatric hospitalization than patients who were seen by a mobile crisis team [20,21]. While further large-scale research is needed to address what are appropriate measures of success, mobile crisis teams can still serve as an additional resource for ED physicians.

Mobile crisis teams are primarily contacted through a crisis telephone line. Depending on the type of mobile crisis team, hours may vary, and thus, some emergency lines redirect individuals to go to the nearest ED. Calls can be made to the crisis lines by anyone, including patients, families, local police departments, medical physician offices, or even EDs. Once calls are received and triaged, the clinician fielding the calls may send out a team to the site. At the site of the crisis, the mobile crisis team meets with the individual and/or family and determines if the patient can be linked to outpatient care, or, in more intense situations, assists the family members with involuntary hospitalization steps. This may then require the patient to be transferred to an ED for psychiatric medical clearance, insurance authorization, and/or bed placement. Mobile crisis teams may also offer the availability of follow-up postincident visits by the team. Because many mobile crisis teams are linked through local suicide hotlines and "warmlines" (suicide prevention resources specifically staffed by patients in mental health recovery themselves), patients form strong connections and relationships with their contacts.

CIT, or crisis intervention team, is a specific model of police response to psychiatric crisis. This model entails collaboration of mental health professionals and police officers who undergo specialized education about mental illness and crisis response. When a crisis occurs, departments with a CIT send out at least one trained officer to help problem solve the situation. In establishing a CIT response effort, local resources establish predetermined access to a variety of disposition options, including a designated single point of entry for emergency care. This type of program requires investment from both the community (mental health providers, hospitals) as well as police departments [22]. Outcomes reported from this type of collaborative partnership have included decreases in the arrests of mentally ill individuals, reduced police officer stigma toward the mentally ill, and decreased officer and patient injuries [23]. As of September 2011, only four states in the United States had not formally adopted this type of training in any of its counties.

Unfortunately, there are no current Federal Regulations mandating the use and standards of mobile crisis teams. While providing a professional and fiscally smart alternative to ED use, their services are not billable under Medicare, are not covered by many private insurance policies, and may only be reimbursed by Medicaid depending on the state in which the service is found. Because Medicaid does not fund inpatient psychiatric admissions (Medicaid saddles SMHAs with the fiscal burdens of this care), there is little incentive to reimburse mobile crisis teams. However, patients who attend EDs for psychiatric crisis will still have a Medicaid bill generated for the visit. Thus, it is fiscally wise for Medicaid agencies to invest in alternative treatment pathways for psychiatric crises. If mobile crisis teams can achieve this, Medicaid programs may want to reconsider funding. As stated earlier in the chapter, the Centers for Medicare and Medicaid Services (CMS) do require some type of 24-hour emergency coverage in CMHCs that have partial hospital programs, and some states require state funded Psychiatric Emergency Services to have a mobile crisis team. EDs should investigate their local CMHC patient care plans.

Residential services

Crisis residential services, respite services, and transitional housing programs are all community levels of care which may be available from an ED at time of discharge for patients served in the community. Crisis residential services can vary from organized, insurance reimbursed settings to consumer run levels of care. Crisis residential treatment is a voluntary level of care agreed to by the patient. Crisis residences are unlocked facilities. Like mobile crisis teams, there is not a uniform definition or standard for crisis residences. Depending on how and by whom they are run, patients may or may not need to have a primary home residence established. That is, these residences may be available for patients who have stable homes, but need the assistance of non-family members for their crises, or, they may target patients who are homeless and in psychiatric crisis to avoid the use of a shelter in the time of crisis.

The START Model, or Short Term Acute Residential Treatment Model, in San Diego has demonstrated how this type of alternative level of care can provide an improved quality of life while reducing symptom severity equal to that seen in patients hospitalized on inpatient units [24]. There were no significant differences on selected symptom measures between the groups who were in START versus the hospitalized patients at time of discharge and at 2-month follow-up, despite having almost equal number of days in each program setting. These findings, and those of similar studies [25,26], suggest patients in acute crisis can be safely and effectively managed in crisis

residential services. In the START model, the average length of stay in the program was 9 days. Patients lived in a remodeled home which housed approximately 10–12 patients. The programmatic structure included two community meetings, two group sessions, individual counseling, medication meetings with psychiatrists, recreational activities, and participation in chore and meal preparation for participating patients. There was a low patient to staffing ratio, and the staff consisted of master's and doctoral level prepared clinicians.

Day treatment programs

Day treatment programs, Partial Hospital Programs (PHPs), and Intensive Outpatient (IOP) services are intensive, full or half day (4–9 hours), personalized treatment regimens for patients. These programs target the population who may be transitioning from an inpatient psychiatric level of care, or who need intensive treatment, but not inpatient stabilization. They may or may not be used in conjunction with a crisis residential program, but if so, the program is delivered at a different location than the actual crisis residence. The general structure of a day treatment program consists of group and individual therapy under medical management delivered 1–5 days per week, and potentially includes evening or weekend hours. Patients do not live at the site of care. These programs may be offered for primary mental health or substance abuse problems, or may be offered as a way to treat co-occurring disorders. Day treatment programs may be based at the site of a hospital or in an outpatient clinic. These programs are not restricted to Medicaid patients, as both private insurance companies and Medicare typically reimburse this level of care. Several agencies set minimum standards or provide accreditation for day treatment models, including the Association for Ambulatory Behavioral Healthcare and Commission on Accreditation of Rehabilitation Facilities (CARF). Patients who present to the ED in crisis may benefit from this intense level of care. If the patient has private insurance, the behavioral health benefits would need to be verified to see if this level of care is covered. For Medicare patients, referrals for PHP would go to the local CMHC or possibly to a hospital-based program. Medicaid patients would be referred to CMHC day treatment programs.

Case management

Several agencies define the expectations of effective case management. CARF defines case management as a level of care that "provide(s) goal-oriented and individualized support focusing on improved self-sufficiency for the persons served through assessment, planning, linkage, advocacy, coordination, and monitoring activities. Successful service coordination results in community opportunities and increased independence for the persons served. Programs may provide occasional supportive counseling and crisis intervention services, when allowed by regulatory or funding authorities [27]." The National Association of State Mental Health Program Directors (NASMHPD) further state case management "is a range of services provided to assist and support patients in developing their skills to gain access to needed medical, behavioral health, housing, employment, social, educational, and other services essential to meeting basic human services; linkages and training for patient served in the use of basic community resources; and monitoring of overall service delivery" [28]. In practice, case management typically refers to a level of care in which a mental health professional, usually a clinically trained psychiatric social worker, provides individualized assistance to patients. Case managers may assist patients with clinical care as well as navigation of the complex mental health system. They may provide crisis counseling as well as assist in access to clinical and social services such as housing. Case management philosophies focus on meeting patients at their current level of function and helping them better function within their own communities.

Intense case management strategies, such as Assertive Community Treatment (ACT), also called Programs of Assertive Community Treatment (PACT), are highly standardized, intense service delivery models that target the most seriously mentally ill patients. ACT programs are deemed as evidence-based best practices according to SAMHSA as this model has repeatedly been shown to decrease both inpatient acute hospitalizations as well as incarcerations for severely mentally ill patients. Essential features of the ACT model include low patient to psychiatric staff ratios; the availability of 24-hour crisis coverage; a multidisciplinary team; and comprehensive patient-centered planning which incorporates medication management, supportive therapy, and rehabilitative support. Peer support, transportation, and community outreach to assist with the delivery of care are additional basic tenets of the model [29]. ACT teams have very distinct admission criteria for patients, but are not time limited. Despite the many studies which demonstrate the positive outcomes of an ACT model, many insurance companies are reluctant to fund this level of care, and the lack of an "end" may overshadow the long-term financial benefits to fund such a plan. Regardless, EDs may not be aware the patients they are evaluating have these services, and may not know to ask the patients who present in crisis for the name and contact information of their ACT advocate. If an ED is not aware of, and connected to, the local ACT programs in its area, opportunity to link patients with available resources may be missed. Because ACT programs are clinical services unconnected to payer services, the only way an ACT program knows a patient has presented to the ED is if the patient reports the visit to their team or if the ED makes contact with the ACT program. For patients who repeatedly present in crises and who do not know what an ACT team can provide or that ACT teams exist, the ED may serve as the referral agent. Local ACT teams are usually found through local CMHCs or can be located through the SMHA.

Summary

ED personnel are increasingly treating primary psychiatric crises, and knowledge of all available referral options may decrease unnecessary hospitalization which can result in extended boarding times for the ED. While navigating the mental healthcare system can be frustrating, EDs can connect with the community through State Mental Health Agencies and local Community Mental Health Centers. If EDs can increase their knowledge base of community resources and enhance partnerships with existent community resources, the number of psychiatric patients presenting to the ED and their length of ED stay could decrease while quality of patient care could improve.

References

1. Owens PL, Mutter R, Stocks C. *Mental Health and Substance Abuse-related Emergency Department Visits Among Adults*, 2007. HCUP Statistical Brief #92. July 2010. Agency for Healthcare Research and Quality, Rockville, MD. Available at: http://www.hcup-us.ahrq.gov/reports/statbriefs/sb92.pdf (Accessed September 19, 2011).

2. Olfson M, Marcus SC, Bridge JA. Emergency treatment of deliberate self-harm. *Arch Gen Psychiatry* 2012;**69**:80–8.

3. Baraff LJ, Janowicz N, Asarnow JR. Survey of California emergency departments about practices for management of suicidal patients and resources available for their care. *Ann Emerg Med* 2006;**48**:452–8.

4. Douglass AM, Luo J, Baraff LJ. Emergency medicine and psychiatry agreement on diagnosis and disposition of emergency department patients with behavioral emergencies. *Acad Emerg Med* 2011;**18**:368–73.

5. Alakeson V, Pande N, Ludwig M. A plan to reduce emergency room 'boarding' of psychiatric patients. *Health Aff (Millwood)* 2010;**29**:1637–42.

6. Stefan S. *Emergency Department Assessment of Psychiatric Patients: Reducing Inappropriate Inpatient Admissions*, August 2006. Available at: http://www.medscape.com/viewprogram/5768. (Accessed September 2, 2011).

7. Bender D, Pande M, Ludwig M. *A Literature Review: Psychiatric Boarding*. Washington, DC: Office of Disability, Aging and Long-Term Care Policy, Office of the Assistant Secretary for Planning and Evaluation, U.S. Department of Health and Human Services. 2008. Available at: http://aspe.hhs.gov/daltcp/reports/2008/PsyBdLR.pdf (Accessed September 19, 2011).

8. Torrey EF, Entsminger K, Geller J, Stanley J, Jaffe DJ. *The Shortage of Public Hospital Beds for Mentally Ill Persons: A Report of the Treatment Advocacy Center*. Available at: http://www.treatmentadvocacycenter.org (Accessed July 27, 2011).

9. Kaiser Commission on Medicaid and the Uninsured. *Mental Health Financing in the United States: A Primer*. Washington, DC: Henry J. Kaiser Family Foundation; April 2011.

10. Larkin GL, Claassen CA, Emond JA, Pelletier AJ, Camargo CA. Trends in U.S. emergency departments visits for mental health conditions, 1992 to 2001. *Psychiatr Serv* 2005;**56**:671–7.

11. U.S. Department of Health and Human Services. *Mental Health: A Report of the Surgeon General-Executive Summary.* Rockville, MD: U.S. Department of Health and Human Services, Substance Abuse and Mental Health Services Administration, Center for Mental Health Services, National Institutes of Health, National Institute of Mental Health; 1999.

12. President's New Freedom Commission on Mental Health. *Achieving the Promise: Transforming Mental Health Care in America.* July 22, 2003.

13. Grob GN. Mad, homeless, and unwanted: a history of the care of the chronic mentally ill in America. *Psychiatr Clin North Am* 1994;**17**:541–59.

14. Rochefort DA. Origins of the "Third psychiatric revolution": the Community Mental Health Centers Act of 1963. *J Health Polit Policy Law* 1984;**9**:1–30.

15. Prepared by C. Koyanagi from the Judge David Bazelon Center for Mental Health Law, for the Kaiser Commission on Medicaid and the Uninsured. (2007). *Learning from History: Deinstitutionalization of People with Mental Illness as Precursor to Long Term Care Reform.*

16. Klerman G. Better but not well: social and ethical issues in the deinstitutionalization of the mentally ill. *Schizophr Bull* 1977;**3**:617–31.

17. NAMI. *State Mental Health Cuts: A National Crisis.* A report by the national alliance on mental illness. Changes in Number of People Served By the State Mental Health Authority, March 2011. Available at: http://www.nami.org/ Template.cfm? Section=state_budget_cuts_report (Accessed September 19, 2011).

18. Substance Abuse and Mental Health Services Administration. *Funding and Characteristics of State Mental Health Agencies, 2009.* HHS Publication No. (SMA) 11-4655. Rockville, MD: Substance Abuse and Mental Health Services Administration; 2011.

19. Centers for Medicare & Medicaid Services. *Certification & Compliance for Community Mental Health Centers.* Available at: https://www.cms.gov/ CertificationandComplianc/ 03_CommunityHealthCenters.asp May 31 2006. (Accessed September 3, 2011).

20. Guo S, Biegel DE, Johnsen JA, Dyches H. Assessing the impact of community based mobile crisis services on preventing hospitalization. *Psychiatr Serv* 2000;**52**:223–8.

21. Currier G, Fisher S, Caine E. Mobile crisis team intervention to enhance linkage of discharged suicidal patients to outpatient psychiatric services: a randomized control trial. *Acad Emerg Med* 2010;**17**:36–43.

22. Dupont R, Cochran S, Pillsbury, S. *Crisis Intervention Team Core Elements.* 2007 Available at: http://cit.memphis.edu/ pdf/CoreElements.pdf. (Accessed September 29, 2011).

23. NAMI. *CIT Toolkit CIT Facts.* Available at: http://www.nami.org/Content/ ContentGroups/Policy/CIT/ CIT_Advocacy_Toolkit.htm (Accessed September 29, 2011).

24. Hawthorne WB, Green EE, Gilmer T, et al. A randomized trial of short term acute residential services for veterans. *Psychiatr Serv* 2005;**56**:1379–86.

25. Sledge WH, Tebes J, Rakfeldt J, et al. Day hospital/crisis respite care versus inpatient care, part 1: clinical outcomes. *Am J Psychiatry* 1996;**153**:1065–73.

26. Fenton WS, Hoch JS, Herrell JM, Mosher L, Dixon L. Cost and cost-effectiveness of hospital vs. residential crisis care for patients who have serious mental illness. *Arch Gen Psychiatry* 2002;**59**:357–64.

27. Commission on Accreditation of Rehabilitation Facilities. *Behavioral Health Programs Descriptions.* 2011. Available at: http://www.carf.org/ WorkArea/DownloadAsset.aspx? id=23988 (Accessed September 28, 2011).

28. National Association of State Mental Health Program Directors Research Intitute, Inc. *Proposed New HCPCS Procedure Codes for Mental Health Services* [definitions]. Alexandria, VA: NASMHPD; 1996.

29. NAMI. *Assertive Community Treatment: Investments Yield Outcomes.* Fact sheet. September 2007. Available at: http://www.nami.org (Accessed September 16, 2011).

The role of telepsychiatry

Avrim B. Fishkind and Robert N. Cuyler

Introduction

Telemedicine and telehealth both describe the use of medical information exchanged from one site to another by means of electronic communications. This process is described in the American Telemedicine Association's Practice Guidelines for Video-Conferencing for TeleMental Health as "electronic communication between multiple users at two or more sites which facilitates voice, video, and/or data transmission systems, and the audio, graphics, computer, and video systems required to do so" [1].

Emergency telepsychiatry involves the delivery of direct patient care or physician consultation to emergency departments (EDs) by a qualified psychiatrist over audio–visual communication systems. The discipline of emergency psychiatry dates back to the period from the mid 1950s to early 1960s; a time in which psychiatric patients were being discharged from largely rural state psychiatrist hospitals due to the availability of the first antipsychotic medication, chlorpromazine [2]. Many mental health patients gravitated toward urban environments, often without sufficient community-based care, resulting in frequent presentation to medical emergency rooms or jails in acute crisis.

Early pioneers in emergency psychiatry moved into these emergency departments to assist with such patients [3]. These early emergency psychiatrists were few in number and largely concentrated in tertiary care hospitals with affiliated medical schools and departments of psychiatry. Even in the present era, the penetration into medical emergency departments by emergency psychiatrists has remained minimal, while overcrowding and boarding by psychiatric patients in EDs has continued with few novel solutions [4].

The uneven availability of psychiatrists and the fact that psychiatrists do not typically do physical examinations helped shape pioneering efforts in telemedicine, including the first telemedicine project in the United States in 1956 [5]. In 1968, the first emergency telepsychiatry project was done by Dartmouth's Department of Psychiatry who provided simultaneous audio and video transmission to a rural affiliate hospital. Dwyer described a project in 1973 in which psychiatrists from the Massachusetts General Hospital used closed circuit television to see psychiatric emergency patients at the nearby airport [6]. This project was noteworthy for the first use of the term "telepsychiatry" and the use of remote-controlled cameras with pan, tilt, and zoom capability.

Obstacles preventing expansion of emergency telepsychiatry include limited cross-state licensure, uneven recognition and reimbursement by third-party payers, lack of efficacy studies, uneven availability of fast broadband, cost and ease of use of videoconferencing equipment, availability of technical support, and privacy requirements. It is important to note that patients have been accepting of the use of telepsychiatry, in fact more so than psychiatrists, who have often been quick to doubt that therapeutic relationships can develop by means of remote connection [7].

For the most part, these obstacles are being overcome. The most commonly asked question, whether telepsychiatry can substitute for "face-to-face" psychiatry, is gradually being answered [8–10]. The accumulating evidence for telepsychiatry suggests diagnostic accuracy and efficacy of interventions is equivalent to in-person care for most populations. In general, whether a patient can be assessed and treated by means of telepsychiatry has more to do with the idiosyncratic viewpoints of the provider and patient, rather than the use of videoconferencing or the patient's individual mental health diagnosis.

Advantages to using telepsychiatry in the emergency department

The American Hospital Association reports that 40% of American Hospitals cannot maintain adequate psychiatric coverage of their emergency departments [11]. The intermittent volume of psychiatric patients in most Emergency Departments makes full-time psychiatric coverage cost-ineffective. Hospitals are challenged to maintain sufficient call rotation among members of the psychiatric medical staff, who may feel burdened by interference with office practice hours and the need to travel to the hospital (sometimes repeatedly) on evenings and weekends. Telepsychiatrists can provide improved access to psychiatric evaluations for emergency departments. One telepsychiatrist can serve multiple emergency departments on a given shift,

Behavioral Emergencies for the Emergency Physician, ed. Leslie S. Zun, Lara G. Chepenik, and Mary Nan S. Mallory. Published by Cambridge University Press. © Cambridge University Press 2013.

without the limitations and inefficiencies of travel. The on-call psychiatrist can even take calls from a home office as long as a HIPAA-compliant environment is maintained [12]. The growth of telepsychiatry holds promise for increasing the number of psychiatrists willing to "go" into emergency departments to provide consultation and treatment.

Additionally, telepsychiatry can improve specialist response time to the ED, facilitating the care of the agitated or aggressive patient. More rapid response may also reduce ED elopements by agitated or dissatisfied patients. Telepsychiatrists are able to use several crisis intervention methods including verbal de-escalation, cognitive reframing, and the offering of oral medications for agitation just as if they were on-site [13]. Thus, rapid diagnosis and intervention can help the ED clinicians avoid more coercive interventions such as seclusion, restraint, and medication overobjection [14,15].

Emergency telepsychiatrists can provide much help in the evaluation and disposition of suicidal and homicidal patients, particularly those with personality disorders. The decision to discharge such patients is filled with real and perceived medical legal risk, and, in response, many ED physicians will board psychiatric patients until an inpatient bed is available [16–18]. The telepsychiatrist can do an evaluation to determine the safety of discharging such patients, which can lead to less boarding and more rapid throughput in the ED. As more rigorous suicide assessment standards are required by regulatory bodies such as The Joint Commission, hospitals are increasingly challenged to secure the medical expertise to evaluate and manage such emergencies [19].

The emergency psychiatrist can assist the ED with focused medical examinations, and reduce usage of low-yield or unnecessary laboratory and diagnostic tests. Other cost reductions may flow from reduced length of stay, boarding time, and one-to-one sitters. Expensive transportation costs by EMS or law enforcement personnel can be avoided either through discharge to the community, instead of to the hospital, or by clearing the patient for transportation provided by family or other responsible party. Telepsychiatry also allows emergency departments to better manage their behavioral health dollars by purchasing services only when needed. Many of these cost savings remain theoretical due to lack of economic research in emergency telepsychiatry [20].

ED clinicians may find that significant amounts of time and resources may be taken up by inappropriate, high utilizers of ED services. The patients include malingering patients, patients with substance abuse disorders, and personality disordered patients, especially borderline personality disorder. The emergency telepsychiatrist can quickly engage these patients to minimize the likelihood that they escalate in agitation or aggression, and help to develop treatment plans that decrease the likelihood of such patients returning to the ED.

Another advantage to using telepsychiatry is that consultation and education of staff can be done by means of the same teleconferencing equipment used to see patients. In this case, the telepsychiatrist meets with the ED physician, nurse, or social worker, rather than the patient. The consulting telepsychiatrist may recommend pharmacologic interventions which are less sedating to facilitate rapid discharge or transfer. The telepsychiatrist can also help in determining whether the patient is appropriate for an alternative to hospitalization including outpatient crisis counseling, crisis residential and respite units, or intensive outpatient programs, and day hospitals. Time-consuming transportation of patients in remote areas to urban EDs can be deferred through such consultation. Telepsychiatrists can do monthly or bimonthly lectures to ED staff including nurses, social workers, and techs on a variety of issues [21]. The education can include the use of ED protocols for the agitated, suicidal, or homicidal patient, as well as updates on diagnosis and treatment of less common presenting psychiatric disorders.

Review of the literature

Overall, the literature on emergency telepsychiatry is small, but steadily increasing [22]. The first review of telemedicine in emergency psychiatry was published by Meltzer in 1997 [23]. He was the first to note the high level of acceptance of telepsychiatry by patients, doctors, nurses, and other persons in the emergency department. This acceptance was very dependent on "synchronization of speech and visual images." Meltzer also noted that, even though medical examination presupposes physical contact, emergency telepsychiatry allowed for necessary physical examinations to be done by nurses and ED physicians.

The first dedicated use of telepsychiatry for emergency consultation occurred in 1996 when a telemedicine link was set up between a Scottish hospital and a general practitioner on the island of Inishmore [24]. A series of nine patients were seen in crisis over an eight-month period. The use of telepsychiatry for emergencies was noted to be "acceptable and satisfactory for patients and staff alike." Patients were followed until they could be managed in an outpatient clinic. Satisfaction was the only outcome measured. A similar study was carried out in 2002 using telepsychiatry between the Maudsley psychiatric hospital in London and an acute facility on Jersey in the Channel Islands [25]. Fourteen crisis assessments were performed with very high satisfaction levels but no other outcome measures. In 2004, Jong evaluated the management of suicidal patients in remote emergency facilities in Canada by means of telepsychiatry. He also noted high satisfaction, and in this case, highly significant cost savings as patients did not have to be transported hundreds of miles to urban treatment facilities [26].

In 2002 and 2005, Sorvaniemi and colleagues published studies from Finland looking at telepsychiatry in emergency consultations [27,28]. Sixty patients were followed subsequent to admission for acute psychiatric disorders. Mean consultation time was 37 minutes with a range of 15–120 minutes. Ninety-two percent of the patients preferred the use of videoconferencing to waiting for an outpatient appointment with a psychiatrist. The authors found that, in follow-up, "no harm that could possibly have been caused by videoconferencing was detected." Satisfaction with audio and picture quality was high.

In a study presented in 2007, the length of stay before and after telemental health screening was measured. Length of stay in the ED was reduced from an average of 4.2 days to less than one day for more than 80% of patients. ED staff felt discharges were more appropriate and occurred earlier, there were fewer inappropriate hospital admissions, and discharge planning improved [16]. Telemedicine may also decrease ED visits as one study showed that the use of telemedicine by psychiatric nurses in the outpatient setting decreased the incidence of depressed patients going to the emergency department in crisis [29]. Lyketsos showed that telepsychiatry provided at long-term care facilities could also prevent ED visits and psychiatric hospitalization for geriatric patients [30].

In an article published in 2008, Yellowlees et al. point out that emergency telepsychiatry can improve patient care and satisfaction, reduce boarding of ED psychiatric patients, improve the accuracy of psychiatric diagnoses made in the emergency department, and decrease the baseline admission rate to psychiatric hospitals [31]. The authors states, "It appears that almost all psychiatric emergencies can be managed by means of telemedicine, with the exception of patients who are actively engaged in violence or selfharm." Even in these situations, the psychiatric can provide support to the ED team working with such patients.

Promising results were noted in a presentation on a major emergency telepsychiatry initiative at the 2011 American Psychiatric Association Annual Meeting. A series of 6000 telepsychiatry encounters provided in the Emergency Departments of 25 South Carolina hospitals in a grant-funded initiative were reported. Outcomes were compared to matched controls at nonparticipating hospitals. Length of stay of telepsychiatry patients declined from an average of four days in the control group to three days in the study group. Rates of community follow-up within 30 days for patients with severe mental illness was markedly improved compared to control patients (85% and 22%, respectively). Mean charges per patient were reduced by 29% for Medicaid patients, and by 38% for commercially insured patients [32].

Emergency telepsychiatry guidelines

Due to the lack of research in emergency telepsychiatry, Shore et al. published a set of emergency management guidelines for telepsychiatry in 2007 to spur interest [33]. The authors drew from their combined clinical experience of 14 years and over 5000 telehealth sessions in six western states in the United States and Australia. Notably, the patient represented a wide cultural sample (Caucasian, African American, Hispanic, American Indian, and Australian Aboriginal) and range of diagnoses (anxiety, mood, psychotic, cognitive, and substance abuse). Several of the guidelines are more relevant to the emergency department physician.

First, per the guidelines, it is important that a telepsychiatrist perform a remote site assessment before initiating services. This visit helps the telepsychiatrist to understand the idiosyncratic hospital, city, and county regulations and resources, as well as practice patterns within the facility. Knowledge of these factors helps the telepsychiatrist more easily acculturate to the distant facility, and therefore integrate more easily with the facility staff. During the site visit, the psychiatrist can then work with the ED doctors, nurses, and other staff to create emergency protocols. The protocols should clearly define what clinical situations warrant a telepsychiatry consult, how the telepsychiatry consultant is contacted, and how the consult is initiated, including use of teleconferencing equipment. Protocols should also include local civil commitment procedures and duty to warn regulations [34]. It can be helpful to think of the protocols as layered, the first level being written protocols for the agitated or suicidal patient, then phone consultation, with the ED physician, followed by video consultation with the ED physician and/or patient.

Second, the onsite assessment should be used to help the telepsychiatrist become aware of local collaborators and service agencies [35]. This is the key to rapid assessment, treatment, and discharge. Local resources may include walk-in clinics in community mental health centers, mobile crisis outreach teams, or crisis residential units to which the ED patient may be rapidly referred [36]. Often an emergency department will have a discharge coordinator who can work with the telepsychiatrist to facilitate transfer to these community resources or a psychiatric hospital.

Third, the guidelines indicate there should be attention to certain clinical issues. Agitated patients may be able to more easily express their strong emotions by means of videoconferencing as compared to a direct conversation with the ED physician. It is the job of the telepsychiatrist to prepare that patient to "return" to the ED environment calmer and in better control, so as not to jeopardize the safety of the patient or ED staff. Procedures should define in detail what steps the ED staff should take if the patient suddenly leaves the telepsychiatry interview. Family members and significant others can be included in the telepsychiatry interview so the telepsychiatrist can obtain collateral information and prepare the family to support the patient after discharge.

Implementing telepsychiatry consultation to emergency departments

Identification and selection of qualified consulting telepsychiatrists and associated support systems are key to a successful collaboration in the ED. The consulting psychiatrists may come from a variety of sources, including private telepsychiatry groups, university medical centers, and community mental health centers. The structure of the relationship with the ED can range from equipping existing psychiatric members of the medical staff with videoconference technology to full-time coverage of the ED for psychiatric consults by a new external entity.

Table 40.1. Identification of patients for telepsychiatry consultation

1. Evaluation of a patient who is acutely agitated, and 1 of the following:

    - Not responding to conventional verbal de-escalation
    - Not responding to conventional pharmacologic intervention
    - Needing a psychiatric consultant to intervene due to the presence of complex psychological factors

2. Suicidal or homicidal ideation and 1 of the following:

    - Staff uncertainty as to the safety of discharging the patient or releasing from involuntary hold
    - Staff uncertainty as to the need for inpatient hospitalization.
    - Patient is asking for hastened death, physician-assisted suicide

3. Patient presents with a psychiatric disorder, but his/her medical condition requires medical/surgical hospitalization. The patient might benefit from the following:

    - Prompt psychiatric assessment and initiation of psychotropic medications in ED
    - Development of a treatment plan which can be implemented on the medical /surgical floor

4. Other cases presenting with the following:

    - Risk of a prolonged stay in the emergency department and psychiatric consultation can be expected to assist in shortening length of stay in the ED
    - Risk of patient or staff injury resulting from acuity of a psychiatric illness which might by reduced by prompt consultation or crisis de-escalation
    - Psychiatric intervention to address inappropriate re-admissions and over-utilization of ED resources

Issues related to fees, billing and collections, and insurance should be discussed carefully during initial meetings.

The ED and telemedicine group optimally will conduct a needs assessment to review existing resources. A determination will need to be made as to whether the telepsychiatry program will supplement an existing pool of on-call psychiatrists who already provide evening and/or weekend coverage, or will assume full responsibility for psychiatric call.

Early in the implementation process, information technology (IT) staff should be involved. Issues that need to be addressed by IT include the selection and purchase of video-conference systems, testing of video and audio quality to insure adequacy for healthcare applications, and the methods by which information will be transferred back and forth between facilities including shared electronic medical records, and secure email and faxing. IT staff should also determine how they will deliver technical support personnel to assist with telemedicine connectivity and trouble-shooting.

Clinical staff from the ED and the telepsychiatry group should develop policies and procedures detailing systems for scheduling, communication, access to medical records and collateral information. Clear delineation of the responsibilities of the consulting psychiatrist in relation to the attending ED physician should be addressed. The hospital ED formulary should be included in the procedures so the telepsychiatrist knows what is available on site, and should also address what to do if equipment fails. Credentialing and privileging of the telepsychiatrists should be started as early as possible as this process usually takes 2 to 3 months.

The final phase of implementation involves staff training. ED staff should know what the criteria are for getting a telepsychiatry consultation (see Table 40.1). ED personnel should be trained in the operation of the videoconference systems to both make and receive video calls. ED nurses should be trained in how to present information about the patient to the telepsychiatrist.

Conclusion

A convergence of factors including a shortage of psychiatrists, increasing numbers of psychiatric patients presenting to EDs, and advancements in technology and acceptance of telemedicine are shaping the growth of telepsychiatry. Emergency telepsychiatry provides a pathway for improved patient outcomes and satisfaction, rapid stabilization, and improved throughput in the ED.

References

1. Grady B, Myers K, Nelson E. *Practice Guidelines for Video-conferencing for Telemental Health.* Washington, DC: American Telemedicine Association Publication; 2009.

2. Fakhoury W, Priebea S. Deinstitutionalization and reinstitutionalization: major changes in the provision of mental healthcare. *Psychiatry* 2007;**6**:313–16.

3. Bassuk EL, Birk AW. *Emergency Psychiatry: Concepts, Methods, and Practices.* New York: Plenum Press; 1984.

4. American College of Emergency Physicians. *ACEP Psychiatric and Substance Abuse Survey 2008.* Available at: http://www.acep.org/uploadedFiles/ ACEP/Advocacy/federal_issues/ PsychiatricBoardingSummary.pdf (Accessed August 14, 2012).

5. Wittson CL, Affleck DC, Johnson V. Two-way television in group therapy. *Ment Hosp* 1961;**2**:22–3.

6. Dwyer TF. Telepsychiatry: psychiatric consultation by interactive television. *Am J Psychiatry* 1973;**130**:865–9.

7. Bishop JE, O'Reilly RL, Maddox K, Hutchinson LJ. Client satisfaction in a feasibility study comparing face-to-face interviews with telepsychiatry. *J Telemed Telecare* 2002;**8**:217–21.

8. Hilty DM, Luo JS, Morache C, Marcelo DA, Nesbitt TS. Telepsychiatry an overview for psychiatrists. *CNS Drugs* 2002;**16**:527–48.

9. Frueh BC, Deitsch SE, Santos AB, et al. Procedural and methodological issues in telepsychiatry research and program development. *Psychiatr Serv* 2000;**51**:1522–7.

10. O'Reilly R, Bishop J, Maddox K, et al. Is telepsychiatry equivalent to face-to-face psychiatry? Results from a randomized controlled equivalence trial. *Psychiatr Serv* 2007;**58**:836–43.

11. American Hospital Association. *The State of America's Hospitals – Taking the Pulse: 2007 Survey of Hospital Leaders.* Available at: http://www.aha.org/aha/%20resource-center/Statistics-and-Studies/studies.html (Accessed May 19, 2008).

12. HIPAA Security Series. *Security Standards – Implementation for the Small Provider.* Available at: http://www.hhs.gov/ocr/privacy/hipaa/administrative/securityrule/smallprovider.pdf (Accessed December 10, 2007).

13. Fishkind A. Calming agitation with words, not drugs: 10 commandments for safety. *Curr Psychiatry* 2002;**1**:32–9. Available at: http://www.currentpsychiatry.com/pdf/0104/0104_Fishkind.pdf (Accessed June 13, 2011).

14. Fishkind A. Agitation II: de-escalation of the aggressive patient and avoiding coercion. In: Glick RL, Berlin JS, Fishkind AB, Zeller SL, (Eds.). *Emergency Psychiatry: Principles and Practice.* Philadelphia, PA: Wolters Kluwer Health/Lippincott Williams & Wilkins; 2008;125–36.

15. Stefan S. *Emergency Department Treatment of the Psychiatric Patient: Policy Issues and Legal Requirements.* New York, NY: Oxford University Press; 2006.

16. Augusterfer EF, Cavanagh N. *Telemental Health in the Emergency Room.* American Telemedicine Association Annual Meeting 2007 Nashville, TN. Available at: http://www.atmeda.org/conf/2007/Presentations/Tuesday/GOVB/%201045%20Augusterfer%20Governor's%20B%20Tue/Telemental%20Health%20in%20

20the%20Emergency%20Room.ppt (Accessed May 2008).

17. Mitchell AM, Garand L, Dean D, Panzak G, Taylor M. Suicide assessment in hospital emergency departments: implications for patient satisfaction and compliance. *Emerg Med* 2005;**27**:302–12.

18. Baraff LJ, Janowicz N, Asarnow JW. Survey of California emergency departments about practices for management of suicidal patients and resources available for their care. *Ann Emerg Med* 2006;**48**; 452–8.

19. Screening for Mental Health. *A Resource Guide for Implementing the Joint Commission 2007 Patient Safety Goals on Suicide.* Available at: http://www.stopasuicide.com/downloads/sites/docs/Resource_Guide_Safety_Goals_2007.pdf (Accessed February 14, 2011).

20. Hilty DM, Bourgeois JA, Nesbitt TS, et al. Cost issues with telepsychiatry in the United States. *Int Psychiatry* 2004;**3**: 6–8.

21. Janca A, Gillam D. Development and evaluation of an ICD-10 telepsychiatry training programme in Western Australia. *J Telemed Telecare* 2002;**8**:120–2.

22. California Healthcare Foundation. *Telepsychiatry in the Emergency Department: Overview and Case Studies.* Publication of the Abaris Group for the California Healthcare Foundation. Available at: http://www.chcf.org/publications/2009/12/telepsychiatry-in-the-emergency-department-overview-and-case-studies (Accessed December 2009).

23. Meltzer B. Telemedicine in emergency psychiatry. *Psychiatr Serv* 1997;**48**:1141–2.

24. Mannion L, Fahy TJ, Duffy C, Broderick M, Gethins E. Telepsychiatry: an island pilot project. *J Telemed Telecare* 1998;**4**(Suppl 1):62–3.

25. Harley J, McLaren P, Blackwood G, Tierney K, Everett M. The use of videoconferencing to enhance tertiary mental health service

provision to the island of Jersey. *J Telemed Telecare* 2002;**8**(Suppl 2):36–8.

26. Jong M. Managing suicides via videoconferencing in a remote northern community in Canada. *Int J Circumpolar Health* 2004;**63**:422–8.

27. Sorvaniemi M, Santamaki O. Telepsychiatry in emergency consultation. *J Telemed Telecare* 2002;**8**:183–4.

28. Sorvaniemi M, Ojanen E, Santamaki O. Telepsychiatry in emergency consultations: a follow-up study of sixty patients. *Telemed J E Health* 2005;**11**:439–41.

29. Lyketsos C, Roques C, Hovanec L, Jones BN. Telemedicine use and the reduction of psychiatric admissions from a long-term care facility. *J Geriatr Psychiatry Neurol* 2001;**14**:76–9.

30. Haslam R, McLaren P. Interactive television for an urban adult mental health service: the Guy's Psychiatric Intensive Care Telepsychiatry Project. *J Telemed Telecare* 2000;**6**(Suppl 1):50–2.

31. Yellowlees P, Burke M, Marks S, Hilty D, Shore J. Emergency telepsychiatry. *J Telemed Telecare* 2008;**14**:227–81.

32. Otto MA. *ED Telepsychiatry Cuts Admissions, Saves Money at South Carolina Hospitals.* Clinical Psychiatry News, June 2011: 8.

33. Shore JH, Hilty DM, Yellowlees P. Emergency management guidelines for telepsychiatry. *Gen Hosp Psychiatry* 2007;**29**:199–206.

34. Herbert PB, Young KA. Tarasoff at twenty-five. *J Am Acad Psychiatry Law* 2002;**30**:275–81.

35. Shore JH, Manson SM. Rural telepsychiatry: a developmental model. *Psychiatr Serv* 2005;**56**:976–80.

36. Fishkind A, Berlin J. Structure and function of psychiatric emergency services. In: Glick RL, Berlin JS, Fishkind AB, Zeller SL, (Eds.). *Emergency Psychiatry: Principles and Practice.* Philadelphia, PA: Wolters Kluwer Health/Lippincott Williams & Wilkins; 2008;9–24.

Emergency medical services psychiatric issues

Joseph Weber and Eddie Markul

Introduction

As the prevalence of mental illness increases in the United States, emergency medical services' (EMS) role in the care of the psychiatric patient continues to grow. In 2004, an estimated 25% of adults in the United States reported having a mental illness in the previous year [1]. A recent study found that 15% of geriatric patients transported by EMS tested positive for moderate depression [2]. Mental illness also significantly affects and impairs the lives of 10% of all children and adolescents in the United States. The World Health Organization has estimated that by the year 2020, childhood neuropsychiatric disorders will become one of the five most common causes of morbidity, mortality, and disability among children. Studies have estimated that 2.5–10% of pediatric EMS calls were for behavioral emergencies [3].

Despite the increasing role EMS plays in the care of the psychiatric patient, there is a paucity of peer-reviewed literature addressing the care of these patients in the field. Standard EMS treatment protocols for psychiatric patients have been extrapolated from emergency departments and psychiatric centers, leaving prehospital providers and EMS Medical Directors with little evidence from prehospital-based studies. However, as EMS professionals know, the prehospital environment differs significantly from the "controlled" setting of an emergency department. In this chapter, we will address care of the psychiatric patient in the prehospital setting by focusing on issues unique to the out of hospital environment.

Scene safety

One of the most unique aspects of prehospital medical care is the uncontrolled environment. Violence against emergency medical services personnel is a daily occurrence in some systems. Although the prevalence varies from system to system, violence against EMS providers is estimated to occur in 0.8–5% of all calls [4]. Suspected psychiatric disorder calls were strongly predictive for violence against providers [4]. Restraint use, often required for behavioral emergencies, was also a significant risk factor for violence against EMS providers. In one system, providers were assaulted in 28% of cases where restraints were

applied [5]. Weapons are also regularly encountered in the uncontrolled prehospital environment. A survey of Boston and Los Angeles EMS providers, found that greater than 60% of providers have found weapons on patients [6]. This often violent environment puts additional risks on the EMS provider already at significant risk for blood and body fluid exposure. One study estimates that paramedics across the United States have close to 50,000 total exposures per year, including 10,000 needle sticks [7].

This uncontrolled and often dangerous prehospital environment requires the EMS provider to do a thorough scene assessment when caring for the patient with a potential behavioral emergency. This should begin with assessment of the scene for potential indicators of a patient with cognitive impairment. Unkempt or destroyed property, drug paraphernalia, weapons, or combative bystanders may give the first indication of an unsafe scene. When possible, the patient should be assessed from a distance to identify any behavior patterns that may indicate a potential for violence. Once the potential for violence is identified, all prehospital providers should retreat to a safe area and await the arrival of law enforcement. Prehospital providers should never knowingly enter an unsafe scene. Although, timely care of the psychiatric patient is the goal of EMS, the number one priority should be the safety of the provider. EMS systems should have a policy that addresses care of the potentially violent patient, and should work closely with local law enforcement to ensure the best outcome for both provider and patient [8]. Online medical control should be available for consultation.

Patient assessment

Once a scene is felt to be safe, EMS providers should carefully approach the patient and attempt to perform a medical assessment. The goal of the brief initial survey is to identify a potentially reversible medical cause for the patient's abnormal behavior. Although multiple organic disorders may manifest as altered behavior (Table 41.1), few are treatable in the prehospital setting. Antidotal therapy for hypoglycemia, hypoxia, opioid overdose, and seizures are usually carried by advanced life support (ALS) providers and thus assessment for these

Behavioral Emergencies for the Emergency Physician, ed. Leslie S. Zun, Lara G. Chepenik, and Mary Nan S. Mallory. Published by Cambridge University Press. © Cambridge University Press 2013.

Table 41.1. AEIOU-TIPS causes of altered mental status in the prehospital setting

A	Alcohol
E	Electrolytes, epilepsy
I	Insulin (hypo/hyperglycemia)
O	Opiates, oxygen
U	Uremia
T	Trauma, temperature (hypo/hyperthermia)
I	Infection
P	Psychiatric, poisoning
S	Shock

conditions should be carried out on all patients. If other organic causes of abnormal behavior are identified, supportive treatment and rapid transport should take place.

After the brief initial survey, a more thorough patient assessment should take place. This should be performed in a non-threatening manner. As with any scene, be aware of the exits and make sure they remain accessible at all times. Standing in front of exits can make a patient feel trapped. The home should again be assessed for signs of violence, substance abuse, or lack of basic hygiene, which may indicate that the patient is a danger to self or others. For the nonviolent, nonsuicidal patient, a complete evaluation should follow. The most common psychiatric conditions encountered in the prehospital setting include depression, schizophrenia, bipolar disorder, anxiety disorder, and substance abuse. Safety should be continually reassessed throughout the patient encounter. If the EMS provider feels threatened at any point during the patient encounter, they should leave immediately and stay away from the scene until law enforcement can arrive and secure the patient [9]. In rare circumstances, providers may be unable to avoid a physical confrontation. In those instances, the provider should use the minimal force necessary to escape from the scene, while trying to avoid harm to the patient.

The actively suicidal patient creates unique challenges for the prehospital provider; however, intervention by the EMS system may be the last opportunity to provide help and avoid a tragedy. As with any patient encounter, scene safety is a primary goal. If weapons are identified, providers should remove themselves from the scene until law enforcement arrives. Once secure, the scene should be assessed for other items with the potential for self-injury. Pill bottles, household- or automobile-related chemicals and pesticides, if present, may have been ingested by the patient. An inventory of these items should be brought with the patient to the receiving hospital. The patient should be interviewed in a non-threatening manner. These patients should be treated with the same urgency as any other critically ill patient [10]. For the stable, cooperative patient the goal is transport to a hospital for further psychiatric care. EMS systems should have a policy addressing transport of the suicidal patient. Because of the potential for self-harm, and the chaotic prehospital environment, some EMS systems require law enforcement assistance for transport of all suicidal patients.

The violent patient represents one of the most challenging encounters for the prehospital provider. The causes of violent behavior are diverse so the EMS provider must consider a broad differential diagnosis when attempting to assess and treat these patients (Table 41.1). In one metropolitan EMS system, 9% of violent patients encountered by EMS were suffering from hypoglycemia [11]. Medical stabilization of potentially reversible conditions must take priority, however, patients most likely to be violent or aggressive are the mentally ill and those intoxicated with alcohol and drugs [12]. Violent or potentially violent patients must be dealt with using extreme caution and as with all encounters, a scene safety evaluation should be performed upon arrival. Local law enforcement should be present on scene for all violent or potentially violent patients, before any assessment or treatment can take place. Risk factors for potential violence should be identified and include previous history of violence, psychiatric disorder, and drug or alcohol abuse. If a potentially violent patient is coherent, verbal de-escalation through negotiation or appeal to reason should be attempted. Research has shown that this type of interpersonal communication is effective in calming agitated patients and preventing escalation [12]. If a potentially violent patient cannot be controlled quickly, it is best to remove from the scene all people and objects that may be contributing to the patient's agitation. Sometimes a subtle show of force may be enough to keep a potentially violent patient in check, however, this can also serve to further agitate the patient. When de-escalation techniques fail, EMS should allow law enforcement to secure the scene before resuming care. Physical and/or chemical restraint by EMS in conjunction with law enforcement, may be needed. Excited delirium is one type of violent patient who deserves special mention. It is characterized by a hyperthermic patient with acute onset of bizarre, violent, delusional behavior. There are thought to be multiple causes including underlying psychiatric disorders and acute stimulant intoxication. Since EMS or police are frequently the first to encounter these patients, caution is warranted in any restraint techniques used. Sudden death has occurred in multiple cases and is thought to be related to multiple factors including restraint-related positional asphyxia, metabolic acidosis, rhabdomyolysis, and catecholamine-induced sudden death [13].

Treatment and transport

The goal of EMS systems is safe transport of the psychiatric patient to the hospital for further evaluation and care. The cooperative patient can usually be transported without physical or chemical restraint, or law enforcement assistance. The actively suicidal patient, even when cooperative, is often placed in restraints and transported with the assistance of law enforcement. EMS systems should have a clear policy defining their transport, based on local resources. Transport of the violent patient requires the assistance of law enforcement and when verbal de-escalation techniques fail, physical and possibly chemical restraint is often needed. The chosen method of restraint should be the least restrictive method that assures the safety of the patient and EMS personnel. While restraint methods are often applied in a stepwise manner, violent patients may require immediate physical restraint to assure the safety of the patient and EMS personnel.

Physical restraint is accomplished with devices and techniques that create restriction of movement of the person who is considered a danger to self or others. Devices include soft restraints (sheets, wristlets, and chest poseys) and hard restraints (plastic ties, handcuffs, and leathers). In general, EMS systems should avoid the use of hard restraints [14]. If a system uses hard restraints, all providers should be trained in their use and the restrained extremities should be frequently assessed for neurovascular compromise. Four-point restraints are preferred over two-point restraints. Tethering of the thighs may prevent kicking. A hard cervical collar may limit a patient's cervical range of motion if attempting to bite. A surgical mask may be used to prevent spitting. Ideally, a minimum of five people should be present to safely apply physical restraints, allowing for control of the head and each limb, however, this may be difficult in some EMS systems. Prone restraint position may be necessary while gaining initial control of the patient, however, supine four-point position should be achieved before transport. A hobbled or "hog-tied" position (prone with arms and legs tied together behind the back) should never be used. Once restrained, a patient should not be left unattended. Some recommend cardiac monitoring in all restrained patients when possible [15]. The known complications of physical restraints include strangulation (from vest restraint), aspiration, impaired circulation, neurovascular extremity injury, psychological injury, and sudden death [12]. The rate and type of restraint-related complications in the prehospital setting remains unclear. One study found a small rate (7%) of minor complications from restraint use in the emergency department [16]. Severe injuries and deaths related to restraints were not found. In general, for the safety of EMS personnel, physical restraints applied in the field should not be removed until the patient is evaluated in the emergency department [14].

A patient who has undergone physical restraint should not be allowed to continue to struggle against the restraints. This may lead to rhabdomyolysis, severe acidosis, and fatal arrhythmia. Often, chemical restraint is required. The goal of chemical restraint is to subdue excessive agitation and struggling against physical restraints [14]. EMS systems may use a variety of agents for chemical restraint of the agitated or combative patient. Ideally, this pharmacologic sedation will change the patient's behavior without causing altered mental status, hypotension, or respiratory depression. Prehospital studies of chemical restraint are limited. Two studies found that droperidol effectively sedated combative patients without serious adverse events [17,18]. Shortly thereafter, droperidol received a "black box" warning of potential QT prolongation and torsade de pointes related to its use. Current recommendations from the manufacturer suggest that droperidol should be used in patients who fail other treatments, and following determination of the QT interval before drug administration. Thus, droperidol has fallen out of favor as a chemical restraint. Alternative agents include haloperidol, lorazepam, and midazolam. None of these has been studied in the prehospital setting, however, an emergency department-based study compared the three for management of the violent and agitated patient. Midazolam was found to have a significantly shorter time to onset of sedation and arousal, with all having similar efficacies [19]. No adverse events occurred with midazolam. Despite the lack of prehospital data, many EMS systems currently use midazolam as part of a prehospital chemical sedation protocol for patients with violence and agitation. Midazolam has the advantage of being a single agent not requiring refrigeration that can be administered intravenously (IV), intramuscularly (IM), or intranasaly (IN). Typical doses are 1–2 mg IV and 5 mg IM or IN. Further prehospital studies are needed. Patients who have undergone physical and/or chemical restraint should be expeditiously transported to the hospital, just as any other critically ill patient.

Electronic control device exposure

In cases of the extremely violent or agitated patient in whom de-escalation techniques have proved futile, law enforcement may elect to use an electronic control device (ECD) to subdue the patient. More than 7,000 law enforcement agencies currently use ECD technology. Electronic control devices are electrical weapons designed to temporarily incapacitate a person. These devices are commonly referred to as "stun guns" or "tasers," although taser represents a specific model. These devices work by firing metal darts connected to the device by means of conducting wires into the person and delivering an electric current for approximately 5 seconds. The electric current causes involuntary muscle contraction resulting in the person falling to the ground. After incapacitation, the patient can be cautiously approached with law enforcement to attempt an assessment. After ECD exposure, there are the additional patient concerns of dart injury and injuries sustained from the fall. While the darts usually affect the trunk or back, they may impact any area of the body. Dart injuries have included eye injuries, pneumothorax, testicular injuries, and intracranial perforation. If the EMS provider can identify the location of the dart it should not be removed in the field but rather secured with tape or gauze. Trauma care including spinal immobilization should be considered for anyone who sustained a significant fall during electric current delivery. Controversy exists on ECD's role in sudden death or possible cardiac rhythm disturbances. Numerous deaths have been temporally associated with ECD use, although no direct link to fatal injury has been made. While there have been more than 850,000 ECD exposures in human volunteers without serious cardiac side effects, these results may not be applicable to the field where the majority of field ECD exposures involve alcohol intoxication, illicit drug usage, or psychiatric disease [20]. In an analysis of deaths temporally related to ECD use, patients who died within 24 hours of ECD use were more likely to be male, have significant cardiovascular disease, stimulant intoxication, and behavior consistent with excited delirium [21]. The most common causes of death as listed by the medical examiners report were stimulant intoxication (48%) and cardiac arrest/arrhythmia (32%) [21]. Thus, it is important for EMS personnel to monitor for cardiac rhythm disturbances as soon as safely possible after ECD exposure. Law enforcement should always accompany EMS personnel during transport of the ECD patient.

Refusal of care

Refusal of care in the psychiatric patient poses a challenging dilemma. The violent and agitated patient clearly lacks decision-making capacity. However, EMS providers may arrive to find a calm and cooperative person wishing to refuse care. In these cases friends and family members may have activated the EMS system because they believe the patient may cause harm to themselves or others. Transporting a patient against their will can result in accusations of battery and false imprisonment. However, allowing a truly suicidal patient to refuse care can result in their untimely death. Adding to this dilemma is the fact that "competence" is a legal determination that can only be rendered by a court. Thus EMS personnel need to determine decision making capacity in the difficult prehospital environment. EMS providers should try discerning who requested EMS and clarify their concerns regarding the patient. It is important to perform a thorough scene assessment looking for signs that the patient may lack decision-making capacity (unkempt home, signs of drug or alcohol use). EMS providers should also obtain a history of medical or mental illness, suicide attempts, recent attempts at self-harm including ingestions, and recent statements regarding self-harm. If there is concern for patient safety the EMS provider should calmly explain their concerns, reassure the patient they are there to help, and try to convince them to consent to transport to the hospital. If resistance is met the EMS provider should contact medical oversight. Allowing the patient to directly speak with a physician may facilitate their cooperation. If, despite all reasonable efforts, the patient still refuses to cooperate they will need to be transported against their will. Local law enforcement should be present for patients being transported against their will.

Patients who refuse care, but appear to have decision-making capacity, represent a more difficult situation for the EMS provider. EMS systems have responded by adopting operational policies intended to guide field personnel in the management of patient refusals. Eighty six of the largest EMS systems in the country were surveyed and 91% have a formal written refusal policy [22]. However, the content of those policies varies greatly. Three elements are most commonly recognized in the medical and legal literature as crucial to a refusal of service policy. Competence or decision-making capacity plays a central role in determining whether a refusal should be honored, however, 17% of these systems did not have assessment of competence as part of their policy [22]. Physician consultation through online medical control was only required by 22% of these policies, leaving the burden of these decisions on the shoulders of the field provider. Finally, documentation of the refusal is also found to be lacking in most policies. Minimum documentation should include general appearance, vital signs, findings on physical exam, presence of drugs or alcohol, and the nature of the treatment offered by EMS. In addition, the patient should be asked to sign an "AMA" against medical advice form. Unfortunately, only 17% of the surveyed systems require all of these minimum documentation standards in their policy [21]. Overall, only 29% of the systems surveyed used all of the recommended medico-legal criteria in their refusal of transport policy. This not only creates significant medico-legal risk for the system, but also creates risks for the patient who may not have been thoroughly assessed.

Summary

As EMS systems continue to play a larger role in the care of the patient with a potential behavioral emergency, they need to have evidence-based guidelines in place to direct the care of these patients in the field. Guidelines should dictate that provider safety is of paramount importance. Scene safety should always be assessed before and during any patient encounter. Organic causes of abnormal behavior, such as hypoglycemia, should always be considered. Assessment should always be done in a nonthreatening manner. When required, restraints should be applied with the least amount of force needed to protect the patient and provider. Chemical restraint indications and use should be clearly delineated. Because local law enforcement is required for many patients, they should be included in policy development and training. Thorough documentation of the patient encounter should be included in the EMS provider's medical record. For patients with decision-making capacity, who are not considered a danger to self or others, refusal should be carried out with the involvement of an online medical control physician.

References

1. Reeves WC, Strine TW, Pratt LA, et al. Mental illness surveillance among adults in the United States. *MMWR Surveill Summ* 2011;**60**(Suppl 3):1–29.

2. Shah MN, Jones CMC, Richardson TM, et al. Prevalence of depression and cognitive impairment in older adult emergency medical service patients. *Prehosp Emerg Care* 2011;**15**:4–11.

3. Hoyle JD, White LJ. Treatment of pediatric and adolescent mental health emergencies in the United States: current practices, models, barriers and potential solutions. *Prehosp Emerg Care* 2003;**7**:66–73.

4. Grange JT, Corbett SW. Violence against emergency medical services personnel. *Prehosp Emerg Care* 2002;**6**:186–90.

5. Cheney PR, Gossett L, Fullerton-Gleason L, et al. Relationship of restraint use, patient injury, and assaults on EMS personnel. *Prehosp Emerg Care* 2006;**10**:207–12.

6. Thomsen TW, Sayah AJ, Eckstein M, et al. Emergency medical service providers and weapons in the prehospital setting. *Prehosp Emerg Care* 2000;**4**:209–16.

7. Leiss JK, Ratcliffe JM, Lyden JT, et al. Blood exposure among paramedics: incidence rates from the national study to prevent blood exposure in paramedics. *Ann Epidemiol* 2006;**16**:720–5.

8. Jenkins WA. Scene safety: situational awareness saves lives. *J Emerg Med Serv* 2011;**36**:30–3.

9. Ahlert B, (Ed.). *Paramedic Practice Today: Above and Beyond*, (1st Edition). St. Louis, MO: Mosby JEMS; 2010.

10. Reich J. Behavioral emergencies. In: Cone DC, O'Connor RE, Fowler RL, (Eds.). *Emergency Medical Services: Clinical Practice and Systems Oversight*, (4th Edition). Dubuque, IA. Kendall-Hunt; 2009.

11. Tintinalli JE, McCoy M. Violent patients and the prehospital provider. *Ann Emerg Med* 1993;**22**:1635.

12. Brice JH, Pirallo RG, Racht E, et al. Management of the violent patient. *Prehosp Emerg Care* 2003;**7**:48–55.

13. Park KS, Korn CS, Henderson SO. Agitated delirium and sudden death: two case reports. *Prehosp Emerg Care* 2001;**5**:214–16.

14. Kupas DF, Wydro GC. Patient restraint in emergency medical services systems. *Prehosp Emerg Care* 2002;**6**:340–5.

15. Vilke GM, Chan TC, Neuman T. Patient restraint in EMS. *Prehosp Emerg Care* 2003;**7**:417–19.

16. Zun LS. A prospective study of the complication rate of use of patient restraint in the emergency department. *J Emerg Med* 2003;**24**:119–24.

17. Rosen CL, Ratliff AF, Wolfe RE. The efficacy of intravenous droperidol in the prehospital setting. *J Emerg Med* 1997;**15**:13–17.

18. Hick JL, Mahoney BD, Lappe M. Prehospital sedation with intramuscular droperidol: a one year pilot. *Prehosp Emerg Care* 2001;**5**:391–4.

19. Nobay F, Simon B, Levitt A, Dresden GM. A prospective, double blind, randomized trial of midazolam versus haloperidol versus lorazepam in the chemical restraint of violent and severely agitated patients. *Acad Emerg Med* 2004;**11**:744–9.

20. Pasquier M, Carrin PN, Vallotton L, Yersin B. Electronic control device exposure: a review of morbity and mortality. *Ann Emerg Med* 2011;**58**:178–88.

21. Strote JS, Range H. Taser use in restraint related deaths. *Prehosp Emerg Care* 2006;**10**:447–50.

22. Weaver J, Brinsfield KH, Dalphond D. Prehospital refusal-of-transport policies: adequate legal protection? *Prehosp Emerg Care* 2000;**4**:53–6.

Triage of psychiatric patients in the emergency department

Mark Newman, Margaret Judd, and Divy Ravindranath

What is triage?

Patients arrive in emergency departments (EDs) with concerns needing rapid assessment and effective clinical management. Providers in the ED have an obligation to rule out any apparent life-threatening presenting conditions. Ensuring efficiency and safety is easy when patients come to the ED one at a time. However, patients arrive in the ED at different rates and with different acuities of illness. Facilitating efficiency and safety, triage is the process by which multiple patients are rapidly assessed for risk and queued for care by the ED providers. Patients assessed to be at the highest risk for deterioration or in need of immediate intervention are seen first, while patients with less urgent concerns may be asked to wait.

The physical organization of each individual ED influences this process. Some hospitals have dedicated Psychiatric Emergency Services with an independent triage and evaluation process. More commonly, the initial triage of patients with psychiatric complaints is accomplished in the ED's triage area. Medical emergency room physicians perform the initial evaluation, and the mental health service acts as consultants to assist in assessment and disposition. Regardless of location, the staff responsible for triage should receive training in the assessment of mental health emergencies: what to determine before patient arrival, what to determine on arrival, how to manage the waiting room to keep patients safe, and what issues are specific to direct psychiatric admissions and inter-hospital ED to ED transfers. A cautionary section on patient hand-offs is also provided.

What can be determined before arrival?

Before conducting an assessment and formulating a treatment plan with psychiatric patients in the ED, clinicians are encouraged to obtain pre-arrival patient information whenever possible. Because some patients with emergent psychiatric complaints are unwilling or unable to report their medical or psychiatric histories, gathering collateral information can be extremely useful. It is particularly helpful when the patient's treatment records are not available to the ED clinician.

A variety of sources can be used to obtain pre-arrival information, such as community providers, law enforcement personnel, and family members. Each source provides a slightly different perspective and can be contacted at any point during the ED encounter to solicit information. However, the triage professional is likely to have contact with at least one of these sources before the patient arrives. In this circumstance, information needed to prepare the ED for the patient's arrival should be obtained. Contact information for the referral source and other interested parties should also be recorded to facilitate gathering additional collateral information during the patient's stay.

Community providers and crisis hotlines

Patients may already be involved with the community mental health system, substance use disorder treatment clinics, or private therapists or psychiatrists. When these providers call the ED to advise that a patient is on the way, triage staff should document the reason for ED referral, the time course for the current crisis, the patient's baseline demeanor, and whether there is suspicion of substance misuse. Information about the patient's history of suicidal ideation and suicide attempts, history of homicidal ideation and other violent or dangerous behaviors, current mental health diagnoses, and medications should also be obtained.

Law enforcement and EMS

Law enforcement agents may become involved in a patient case secondary to a 911 or suicide crisis line call by the patient, a family member or friend, or the patient's outpatient treatment provider. These agents usually bring patients to the ED and can give a brief report upon arrival. This report should include details about the reason they became involved, i.e., is the patient intoxicated, behaviorally unstable, suicidal or homicidal, how they became involved, and whether the referral source can be contacted to elicit additional information.

EMS personnel, similarly, become involved secondary to a crisis call and arrive at the ED with the patient. Beyond the reporting of vital signs and symptoms while en route, EMS

Behavioral Emergencies for the Emergency Physician, ed. Leslie S. Zun, Lara G. Chepenik, and Mary Nan S. Mallory. Published by Cambridge University Press. © Cambridge University Press 2013.

personnel can also provide important information about a patient's initial presentation, cooperativeness, and medical status. This may include details about the condition of the patient's living environment and information transmitted from witnesses or family members. Again, a way to contact the initial referral source should be sought.

Friends and family

Friends and family provide valuable information regarding the current mental status and past histories of patients. Spouses, children, and neighbors often have intimate knowledge of a patient's mental health history and baseline functioning. Determining any current psychosocial stressors such as pending legal issues, the recent death of a loved one, or the loss of a job will help the ED clinician assess the impact of situational factors on the patient's presentation.

What can be determined at arrival?

Safety assessment

Ambulatory patients with psychiatric complaints may present to triage alone or arrive with family or friends, and the degree of their cooperation can vary widely. It is advisable to have a protocol for determining the location of initial triage based on the circumstances of arrival. A patient who self-presents with a calm demeanor can fill out paperwork and sit in the waiting room until triage staff is available. On the other hand, patients who arrive in an agitated state clearly require immediate attention in a pre-designated, secure triage area. The challenging cases lay in between, i.e., a patient who was brought in against their will but has been cooperative thus far.

Initial assessment

For cooperative patients, the triage process begins with ascertaining the chief compliant, gathering of basic demographic data, and patient registration. The patient should undergo a face-to-face interview with a triage clinician as soon as possible upon arrival to the ED.

This interview represents the formal triage process. It has been defined as "a brief intervention that occurs when a patient initially presents to the ED during which the patient is interviewed to help determine the nature and severity of his or her illness" [1]. This tightly focused assessment includes a brief history of chief complaint, brief mental status exam, vital signs, and targeted medical screening. The rest of this section provides further detail about this process and its implications for subsequent evaluation.

Indications for restraint

One critical determination is the need for behavioral management. This should be evaluated immediately at presentation and periodically throughout a patient's ED visit. The fundamental consideration is the level of danger a patient poses to

themselves or others. Agitated patients create such risk through actions like intimidating or threatening speech, striking walls, attempted elopement, and physical violence toward others. They also create a distraction for staff and a disturbing environment for other patients and families. Detailed management of agitated patients is covered elsewhere in this text; the focus here is on identification and immediate management of this behavior. Policies and procedures that outline the institution's approach to behavioral management are advisable.

The safety of patients and staff is the first priority. In cases where the risk is unclear or there is limited time for assessment, clinicians should always err on the side of safety, as patients can easily be removed from secure areas of the ED and/or restraints once they are calm. Patients brought in by police or EMS, particularly if agitated in the field, should be triaged in a contained environment if possible. Patients who arrive in restraints should remain in them during the initial assessment. Patients who arrive verbally agitated should be taken to a secure area of the ED immediately. Clear behavioral indications for transfer to a secure area include throwing inanimate objects, striking the wall, or attempted elopement. Indications for restraint include repeated threatening comments or gestures, striking oneself, or lashing out at others.

Several methods exist to quantify agitation, such as the agitation subscale of the well-known Positive and Negative Syndrome Scale (PANSS). Brevity and ease of use are particularly important in fast-paced EDs, however. Schumacher et al. suggest using the Behavioral Activity Rating Scale. This is a single-item, 7-point scale initially developed to monitor behavioral activity in psychotic patients during pharmaceutical trials. It has demonstrated reliability and validity and takes minimal time to complete. In their investigation, a BARS score over 5 reliably distinguished patients who required behavioral management but was not associated with subsequent psychiatric hospitalization (Table 42.1) [2,3].

Indications for medical evaluation

Another critical function of triage is to identify patients who, although their chief complaint may be psychiatric in nature, have medical issues that must be addressed. These patients fall into two broad categories: those with an acute medical condition manifesting with psychiatric symptoms, and those with

Table 42.1. Behavioral Activity Rating Scale [3]

1 Difficult or unable to rouse
2 Asleep but responds normally to verbal or physical contact
3 Drowsy, appears sedated
4 Quiet and awake (normal level of activity)
5 Signs of overt (physical or verbal) activity, calms down with instructions
6 Extremely or continuously active, not requiring restraint
7 Violent, requires restraint

chronic but significant medical problems that are incidental to their current presentation. The high incidence of comorbid medical problems in patients with psychiatric complaints is well-established, ranging from 25–40% in studies [4]. However, the practice of requiring "medical clearance" for all patients is inefficient, expensive, and exposes patients to unnecessary risk. Thus, establishing guidelines for which patients require medical assessment is an important task. Despite the frequency with which this issue arises, there is little evidence to guide decision making.

Certain criteria should prompt immediate medical assessment and deferral of further psychiatric evaluation. Unstable vital signs are clearly a red flag, as are serious medical complaints such as chest pain, focal neurological deficits, or shortness of breath. Inebriated patients are not appropriate for psychiatric assessment, although there is no consensus on a specific blood alcohol content at which they can be interviewed [1]. In addition, new-onset of altered mental status in a patient without psychiatric history should prompt an evaluation for organic causes before being attributed to a psychotic disorder. Similarly, visual hallucinations are more characteristic of organic disorders than primary psychosis [5]. Finally, altered mental status in any elderly patient should be investigated medically due to the high incidence of delirium [6].

On the other hand, without specific medical concerns, there is no evidence to support obtaining "routine labs" such as CBCs, metabolic panels, or urine studies. These tests are typically low yield and rarely uncover medical problems that would not have been discovered by history and physical exam. In one retrospective observational analysis, 19% of patients presenting to the emergency department with psychiatric complaints had some active medical condition. History alone demonstrated 91% sensitivity for detecting these conditions. Less than 1% of patients who denied medical problems subsequently had any positive medical finding. Moreover, less than 1% of patients had a medical condition serious enough to require treatment, and all of these were also diagnosable by history, physical exam, and vital signs. Even the detection of drug use was not significantly aided by routine urine toxicology screens, as patient self-report alone had an 88% positive predictive value and 94% negative predictive value [6].

There have been efforts to address this issue with screening tools. For instance, an Illinois Department of Mental Health Task Force [1] published best practice guidelines on this subject in 2007. They recommend a checklist, developed by the authors, which includes components such as new onset of psychiatric condition, active medical illness, abnormal vital signs, abnormal physical exam, or altered level of consciousness. They suggest that patients without these findings do not benefit from further laboratory testing. Shah and colleagues later developed a similar screening tool for patients initially identified as having primary psychiatric complaints. In addition to collecting basic history, the tool attempts to detect patients with primary medical disorders underlying their psychiatric symptoms. For instance, to be deemed medically stable, patients were

required to have stable vital signs, a prior psychiatric history or age under 30, to be fully oriented, to have no evidence of acute medical problems, and to not have visual hallucinations. In their retrospective review of 500 consecutive patients presenting to an urban ED, none of the patients who were "cleared" with this tool subsequently required medical or surgical admission [7].

Urgency of psychiatric evaluation

After addressing any acute medical issues or agitation, the urgency of patients' psychiatric complaints is assessed. Patients present to emergency services for many reasons, ranging from an interest in social services without specific psychiatric complaint to severe depression with acute suicidality. Consideration should be given to a formal triage process in which urgency of need determines the timing of assessment, as is standard for patients with medical complaints. The 5-level triage systems such as the commonly used Emergency Severity Index (ESI) that is endorsed by the Emergency Nursing Association (ENA) and the American College of Emergency Physicians [8] or the Canadian ED Triage & Acuity Scale (CTAS) define acceptable durations of waiting based on severity of presenting concern, and, in the case of the ESI, availability of clinical resources. For example, a patient rated with a triage level of I in the CTAS protocol, such as an actively violent patient, should be seen immediately, whereas a patient with a level of V may be asked to wait for up to 120 minutes. Under the ESI system, a patient requiring immediate resuscitation should be in level 1, a patient with a very urgent concern should be in level 2, and other patients are assigned a level of 3, 4, or 5 based on the number of clinical resources they may need [9].

Each ED has the latitude to choose which triage protocol to use, although calls for uniformity of approach in U.S. EDs have resulted in widespread adoption of the ESI system. Unfortunately, the use of both patient characteristics and clinical resource usage results in a non-nuanced approach to mental health patients. Moreover, the ESI does not assign an acceptable duration of waiting time even for general ED patients. Alternatively, the CTAS classifies an acutely psychotic and agitated patient as Level II/Emergent and a severely depressed patient without suicidal thoughts as Level IV/Semi urgent [10]. A level II patient should be seen within 15 minutes, whereas a level IV patient can be seen within 60 minutes. Another system, the Australasian Triage Scale (ATS), has been adapted specifically for psychiatric emergencies into the Mental Health Triage Scale. It assigns patients with psychiatric complaints to four categories as described in Table 42.2 [11].

There are no quantitative criteria for assigning triage categories. However, the developers recommend consideration of factors such as manifest behavioral disturbance; presence of or threatened deliberate self-harm; perceived or objective level of suicidal ideation; patient's current level of distress; perceived level of danger to self or others; need for physical restraint; accompaniment by police; disturbances of perception; manifest

Table 42.2. Mental Health Triage Scale [11]

Category	Description	Patient characteristicsis
2	Emergency	Patient is violent, aggressive, suicidal, a danger to self/others, has/may have a police escort
3	Urgent	Patient is very distressed or psychotic, likely to become aggressive and is a danger to self and/or others, patient is experiencing a situational crisis and is very distressed
4	Semi-Urgent	Patient has a long-standing, semi-urgent mental disorder/problem. May have a supporting agent present.
5	Non-Urgent	Patient has a long-standing non-acute mental disorder. No supportive agency present.

evidence of psychosis; level of situational crisis; descriptions of behavior disturbance in the community; current level of community support; and presence of caregiver/supportive adult. Even before the most recent revisions, this assessment tool was shown to decrease mean emergency waiting times and transit times in an Australian sample [12]. It is a valid assessment with no association found between triage rating and either perceived business of the ED or perceived patient cooperation [13].

The ATS has been studied head-to-head against the CTAS protocol in an urban U.S. patient sample. This study showed correlations between the ATS score, patient level of agitation, and some self-reported symptoms. Psychiatric patients were generally deemed less urgent using the ATS in comparison to the CTAS protocol. There was no difference in terms of patient waiting time or throughput time [14].

Other scales have been used for assessment, such as the Crisis Triage Rating Scale and the Brief Psychiatric Rating Scale. However, these studies focused on association with admission rather than pure triage assessment [15,16].

Regardless of the protocol used, patients should be assigned a level of acuity, queued for care in relation to other patients in the ED, and asked to wait as appropriate for their situation. The majority of patients will have to wait for at least a short amount of time before being seen for their concern.

How can the waiting room and waiting intervals be managed?

As in any other area of medicine, continual reassessment of patient status is critical, especially as they wait for clinical care. After the initial triage and immediate management, a process must exist to monitor patients for new onset of medical issues, agitation, or self-injurious behavior. As always, safety is the primary concern in mental health emergencies. In addition, Clarke et al. noted that "an inherent mismatch exists between the needs of an individual or family experiencing a psychiatric emergency and the treatment norms in general hospital EDs" [17]. Patients without mental health concerns present to the

emergency department with a reasonably clear goal in mind. However, psychiatric illness itself may cloud the patient's understanding of the need for treatment or their willingness to participate in treatment. Thus, a patient may appear safe for the waiting area after initial triage, but become unsafe after being forced to wait, encountering another person in the waiting area, experiencing disturbing hallucinations, and so on. Moreover, a mental health patient may lack the wherewithal to report worsening of their state to staff and receive needed attention. This mismatch can be mitigated by appropriate training, proactive monitoring, and careful consideration of the process by which mental health patients are navigated through the ER.

Medical evaluation

As with any other patient, individuals with psychiatric complaints should have a periodic brief review of systems to assess patient comfort. In addition, vital signs can be checked on a regular basis. Abnormal blood pressure and heart rate may simply result from anxiety, but they may also herald the onset of alcohol or benzodiazepine withdrawal. Finally, given the long lengths of stay often associated with behavioral emergencies, staff should inquire about scheduled, prescribed medications, both psychiatric and medical. It is all too easy for the patient and staff to forget their bedtime dose of a medication, but this mistake can be easily avoided with adequate communication.

Suicidality

Suicidality is a common reason for patients to present to emergency departments. All patients endorsing suicidal thoughts should be closely monitored while they remain in the ED. There are two major concerns: potential for elopement and potential for self-harm while in the ED. Careful observation can lessen, but not eliminate, both of these risks.

All patients presenting with suicidal ideation are at elevated risk of self-harm, although their ultimate disposition will depend on full psychiatric evaluation. While this is pending, the patient should not be allowed to leave the ED. This decision must be made at the initial triage. Of course, if the patient is being hospitalized, they must remain in the ED until transferred. There are various ways to achieve direct patient supervision and safety. Some psychiatric emergency rooms have locked areas where high-risk patients are boarded. Without such facilities, one approach is to mark high-risk patients with a wristband or other identifier to indicate that they are not to leave the ED [18]. If the patient does elope, security should be immediately notified and will be able to identify the patient by this marker. When returned, these patients should be placed in a secure area of the ED.

Actual self-injurious behavior while in the ED is rare but difficult to predict. Patients with a history of such behavior, psychotic patients, and those who are visibly anxious may be at higher risk. The use of a standardized screening instrument, like the Risk of Suicide Questionnaire [19], may help identify patients who are at particularly high risk for suicide and warrant additional monitoring while waiting for definitive assessment. Patients who are unable to keep themselves safe should clearly be monitored directly. However, any patient identified as at risk for suicide should have their belongings held and their person searched for potential weapons. Increasing the level of observation throughout the ED, for instance by video monitoring, provides an additional layer of security. Finally, patients who harm themselves, or attempt to do so, should be temporarily placed under direct observation or in restraints.

Agitation and violence in the ED

Unfortunately, violence in EDs is not an uncommon phenomenon. While definitive statistics are hard to come by, several studies have revealed high lifetime prevalence of assaults toward staff. A 1999 survey of Canadian EDs found that 55% of employees, by self-report, had themselves been physically assaulted in some manner, and 86% had witnessed either a physical assault or threats of violence toward other staff [20]. Most violence occurred toward nursing and security personnel. Minimizing these incidents is imperative.

While high-quality evidence is lacking in this area, observational studies have suggested several steps to decrease the incidence of violence. The key theme is early identification and intervention. General steps include increasing staff-to-patient ratios and incorporating video surveillance, both of which have been associated with decreases in need for seclusion and restraint. There are also more targeted interventions. For instance, tools such as the Overt Agitation Severity Scale [21] and Overt Aggression Scale [22] are "designed to assist in the identification of prodromal behaviors that increase the risk of violent or aggressive behavior". Examples of prodromal signs include moaning, tapping fingers, wringing hands, and flexing or twisting a foot. These may precede more concerning behavior such as vocal perseveration, cursing, rocking back and forth, and pacing [22]. Completion of these scales does not require patient cooperation and can even be done by means of video monitoring. Periodically administering these measures to appropriate patients in the waiting area (and in the ED) can assist staff in managing potential agitation before it escalates, thus preventing assaults [23]. Interdisciplinary education in the recognition of prodromal behaviors of violence should be considered, to include security, nursing, and physician staff.

How can hand-offs be safer?

At various points in this chapter, we have discussed the movement of patients from one clinical environment to another. Each transition includes an attendant hand-off between clinical providers. For example, a patient referred from the clinic to the ED will be seen by the ED clerk and the triaging provider, then by the ED physician, the bedside nurse, and perhaps a mental health professional associated with the ED. Thus, each patient may be transitioned through four or five professionals before the appropriate disposition.

Each transition point risks loss of critical information. Patient hand-offs between providers are well-documented to be high-risk times for medical errors [24]. An available technique to reduce the risk of error in hand-off is the performance and documentation of a standardized protocol, or checklist [25].

It is also often the triaging provider's responsibility to collate information available about the patient's case, organizing it in an easily comprehensible package for use by the ED physician or mental health consultant. Opportunities abound for misplacement of information, unduly influencing the clinical decision making of the rest of the team.

Standardizing the triage process can help mitigate these risks. For example, the ED could develop a flowsheet in the patient's medical record (electronic or paper record) used for jotting notes from telephone calls about patients referred to the ED. This can include prompts covering those topics listed in the first section of this chapter. This sheet could be available at the clerk's desk when the patient arrives, at which time it would be attached to another element of the medical record prompting determination of chief complaint, vital signs, and necessary screening questions. This data can then determine whether the patient is safe to wait in the common waiting area, will need to be in a more secure space, or will need to be in restraints with immediate, brief assessment by the physician. These documents would then be available for the physician to review before formally seeing the patient.

Direct admissions and transfers from other EDs

At times, a patient will be sent to the emergency department en route to an inpatient psychiatric unit, for example, from a psychiatric clinic. These directly admitted patients have already been accepted to a psychiatric ward associated with the ED in question. However, there may be medical questions to be answered before admission. These patients may have disclosed dangerous behaviors to their outpatient clinician, and the clinic may lack the resources to ensure that the patient's medical conditions are stable enough for psychiatric admission. Thus, they are assessed in the ED before moving to the psychiatric ward. At arrival to the ED, these patients should be considered dangerous and should be afforded the same safety measures applied to any patient awaiting disposition to a mental health facility.

Because some hospital medical staff's lack the expertise or the hospital lacks the resources to formally assess the behavioral health of ED patients, an inter-hospital ED-to-ED or ED-to-Emergency Psychiatry Services transfer may be arranged. Deterioration may occur during transfer, which at times may be lengthy with either EMS or family. When possible, these patients should receive necessary medical evaluation at the transferring hospital. Despite apparent stabilization, transferred patients should be afforded the same safety measures applied to any patient at high risk of dangerousness to self or others while awaiting full assessment at the receiving hospital.

In either circumstance, it is very helpful when the referring clinician contacts the emergency department with a report about the patient, including at a minimum the patient's identifying information, the clinical concern prompting referral, and

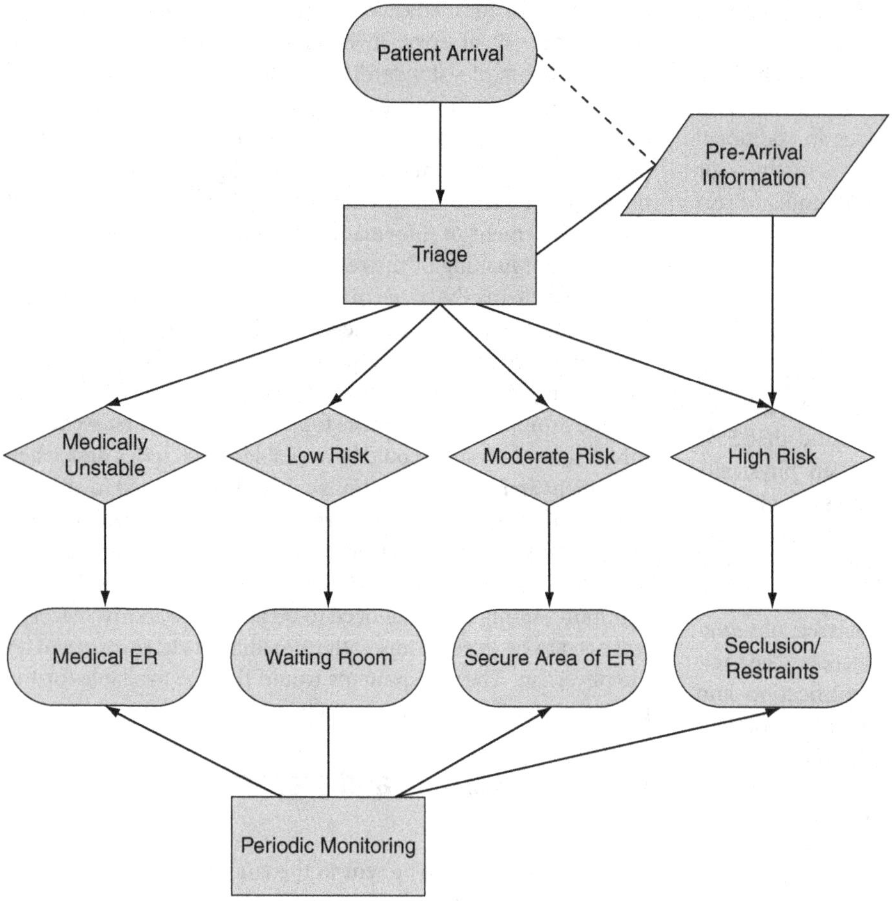

Figure 42.1. Triage flowsheet.

details of the patient evaluation up to that point. Prior acceptance by the receiving ED physician or accepting psychiatrist is mandated by statute when patients are transferred from ED-to-ED, or ED-to-inpatient bed. All emergency departments have structured procedures and documents to facilitate transfer of clinical information about patients between providers, and the mental health transfer is not exempt from these requirements.

Summary

This chapter has covered the details of mental health triage, the process by which the urgency of a patient's case is determined and cases are prioritized so as to maximize efficiency and safety. Figure 42.1 summarizes the process of information integration from various pre-arrival informants and the signs and symptoms discovered during the triage assessment. Based on this integration, the patient should be directed to the common waiting area, a more secure area of the ED with prioritized assessment by the physician, or into restraints with immediate assessment by the physician. Mental health patients may be uniquely unable to communicate deterioration to staff; therefore, each ED must have a system for periodic brief reassessment of mental health patients who are awaiting the next step in the assessment and disposition process. A standardized flowsheet documenting the development of the patient's case can minimize errors associated with patient hand-offs. Direct admissions and ED-to-ED transfers constitute special cases.

Acknowledgments

The authors thank Kathy Adamson RN for her comments during the preparation of this chapter.

References

1. Slade M, Taber D, Clarke MM, et al. Best practices for the treatment of patients with mental and substance use illnesses in the emergency department. *Dis Mon* 2007; 53:536–80.

2. Schumacher JA, Gleason SH, Holloman GH, McLeod WT. Using a single-item rating scale as a psychiatric behavioral management triage tool in the emergency department. *J Emerg Nurs* 2010;36:434–8.

3. Swift RH, Harrigan EP, Cappelleri JC, Kramer D, Chandler LP. Validation of the behavioural activity rating scale (BARS): a novel measure of activity in agitated patients. *J Psychiatr Res* 2002;36:87–95.

4. Carlson RJ, Nayar N, Sur M. Physical disorders among emergency psychiatric patients. *Can J Psychiatry* 1981;**42**:99–102.

5. Norton JW, Corbett JJ. Visual perceptual abnormalities: hallucinations and illusions. *Semin Neurol* 2000;**20**:111–21.

6. Olshaker JS, Browne B, Jerrard DA, et al. Medical clearance and screening of psychiatric patients in the emergency department. *Acad Emerg Med* 1997;**4**:124–8.

7. Shah SJ, Fiorito M, McNamara RM. A screening tool to medically clear psychiatric patients in the emergency department. *J Emerg Med* 2010 [Epub ahead of print].

8. Fernandes CMB, Tanabe P, Gilboy N, et al. Five-level triage: a report from the ACEP/ENA five-level triage task force. *J Emerg Nurs* 2005;**31**:39–50.

9. Gilboy N, Tanabe P, Travers DA, Rosenau AM, Eitel DR. *Emergency Severity Index, Version 4: Implementation Handbook*. AHRQ Publication 2005. 0046(2). Available at: http://www.ahrq.gov/research/esi/ (Accessed August 10, 2012).

10. Bullard MJ, Unger B, Spence J, Grafstein E. Revisions to the Canadian Emergency Department Triage and Acuity Scale (CTAS) adult guidelines. *CJEM* 2008;**10**:136–51.

11. Australasian College for Emergency Medicine. *G24 – Guidelines for the Implementation of the Australasian Triage Scale in Emergency Departments.* 2005. Available at: http://www.acem.org.au/media/policies_and_guidelines/G24_Implementation__ATS.pdf (Accessed August 10, 2012).

12. Smart D, Pollard C, Walpole B. Mental health triage in emergency medicine. *Aust N Z J Psychiatry* 1999;**33**:57–66.

13. Happell B, Summers M, Pinikahana J. Measuring the effectiveness of the national Mental Health Triage Scale in an emergency department. *Int J Ment Health Nurs* 2003;**12**:288–92.

14. Downey LA, Zun LS. *Comparison of Canadian Triage System to Australian Triage System for Psychiatric Patients.* San Francisco, CA: American Psychiatric Association-Institute for Psychiatric Services; October, 2011.

15. Brooker C, Ricketts T, Bennett S, Lemme F. Admission decisions following contact with an emergency mental health assessment and intervention service. *J Clin Nurs* 2007;**16**:1313–22.

16. Hooten WM, Lyketsos CG, Mollenhauer M. Use of the brief psychiatric rating scale as a predictor of psychiatric admission for non-suicidal patients. *Int J Psychiatry Med* 1998;**28**:215–20.

17. Clarke DE, Brown AM, Hughes L, Motluk L. Education to improve the triage of mental health patients in general hospital emergency departments. *Accid Emerg Nurs* 2006;**14**:210–18.

18. Macy D, Johnston M. Using electronic wristbands and a triage protocol to protect mental health patients in the emergency department. *J Nurs Care Qual* 2007;**22**:180–4.

19. Folse VN, Hahn RL. Suicide risk screening in an emergency department. *Clin Nurs Res* 2009;**18**:253–71.

20. Fernandes C, Bouthillette F, Raboud J, et al. Violence in the emergency department: a survey of health care workers. *CMAJ* 1999;**161**:1245–8.

21. Yudofsky SC, Kopecky HJ, Kunik M, Silver JM, Endicott J. The Overt Agitation Severity Scale for the objective rating of agitation. *J Neuropsychiatry Clin Neurosci* 1997;**9**:541–8.

22. Yudofsky SC, Silver JM, Jackson W, Endicott J, Williams D. The Overt Aggression Scale for the objective rating of verbal and physical aggression. *Am J Psychiatry* 1986;**143**:35–9.

23. D'Orio BM, Purselle D, Stevens D, Garlow SJ. Reduction of episodes of seclusion and restraint in a psychiatric emergency service. *Psychiatr Serv* 2004;**55**:581–3.

24. Philibert I. Use of strategies from high-reliability organizations to the patient hand-off by resident physicians: practical implications. *Qual Saf Health Care* 2009;**18**:261–6.

25. Phillips A. The effect of a standardized form in guiding communication between peers during the hand-off of patients in a hospital setting. *Stud Health Technol Inform* 2009;**146**:885.

Chapter 43

The Emergency Medical Treatment and Active Labor Act (EMTALA) and psychiatric patients in the emergency department

Derek J. Robinson

Required disclaimer

This chapter was prepared or accomplished by Dr. Derek J. Robinson in his personal capacity. The opinions expressed in this chapter are the author's own and do not reflect the view of the Centers for Medicare and Medicaid Services, the Department of Health and Human Services, or the United States government. Furthermore, this chapter was prepared as a tool to assist providers and is not intended to grant rights or impose obligations. The official Medicare Program provisions are contained in the relevant laws, regulations, and rulings, which may change over time.

Federal law has an important role in safeguarding access to emergency care at Medicare participating hospitals. The Emergency Medical Treatment and Active Labor Act (EMTALA) was enacted in 1986 as a component of the Consolidated Omnibus Budget Reconciliation Act of 1985. Congress enacted EMTALA in response to concerns that indigent and uninsured patients were refused emergency care at hospital emergency departments (EDs) or inappropriately transferred to other hospitals. It is important that physicians, hospitals, and ancillary staff members involved in the care of patients understand the requirements of this federal law to ensure compliance and avoid serious penalties.

EMTALA mandates that any individual who presents to the ED of a hospital must be provided a medical screening exam (MSE). It must be appropriate for the presenting complaint and performed within the hospital's capability and capacity [1]. There should be no disparity in the MSE based upon actual or perceived ability to pay for medical care, citizenship, race, religion, or other factors. The hospital's capability and capacity includes its ancillary services, on-call physicians, and physical resources [2]. This requirement is also applicable in instances where a medical complaint is made on the individual's behalf or is apparent to a prudent layperson. The MSE must be performed by a physician or qualified medical personnel (QMP) of the hospital, designated in its bylaws as qualified to perform the MSE [1]. While a QMP is commonly a mid-level provider, such as a physician assistant or nurse practitioner, the standard for appropriateness of the MSE is not lowered for such providers. Even among physicians, the standard required

does not differ based upon the professional's training, license, or other credentials. It is important to note that ED triage is not a MSE.

The purpose of the MSE is to determine whether the individual (patient) has an emergency medical condition (EMC), which may require the consultation and physical presence of an on-call physician, if requested by the emergency physician or QMP [4]. An EMC is defined by EMTALA as "a medical condition manifesting itself by acute symptoms of sufficient severity (including severe pain, psychiatric disturbances and/or symptoms of substance abuse) such that the absence of immediate medical attention could reasonably be expected to result in: (i) Placing the health of the individual (or, with respect to a pregnant woman, the health of the woman or her unborn child) in serious jeopardy; (ii) Serious impairment to bodily functions; or (iii) Serious dysfunction of any bodily organ or part [2]."

The emergency physician must ensure that a psychiatric presentation is not masking or coinciding with another illness, such as an occult head injury, metabolic disturbance, or toxic ingestion. A thorough history (including review of EMS records and information provided by family or police) and physical exam are imperative. Several emergency medical conditions may exist and require clinical judgment to prioritize the necessary resources for evaluation, management, and stabilization.

If an EMC is not present after an appropriate MSE has been performed, no further obligations are required under EMTALA. When a patient is determined to be a danger to self or others, such as the case of patients expressing suicidal or homicidal ideations or plans, an EMC is present; this is an important distinction to be well understood in psychiatric emergency care. Further obligations are imposed upon Medicare participating hospitals and physicians when an EMC, including a psychiatric illness, is present. Specifically, stabilizing treatment must be rendered without delay within the hospital's capability and capacity [3].

The medical community commonly uses terms such as *emergency*, *stable*, and *transfer* differently than the definitions prescribed in the regulation. Therefore, it is necessary to understand

Behavioral Emergencies for the Emergency Physician, ed. Leslie S. Zun, Lara G. Chepenik, and Mary Nan S. Mallory. Published by Cambridge University Press. © Cambridge University Press 2013.

how this federal law defines and applies these and other terms to ensure compliance. Under EMTALA, stabilized means "that no material deterioration of the condition is likely, within reasonable medical probability, to result from or occur during the transfer of the individual from a facility [2]." Furthermore, it defines *transfer* as "the movement (including the discharge) of an individual outside a hospital's facilities at the direction of any person employed by (or affiliated or associated, directly or indirectly, with) the hospital, but does not include such a movement of an individual who (i) has been declared dead, or (ii) leaves the facility without the permission of any such person [2]." After an EMC has been treated to a point where a clinician can be reasonably confident that the patient's condition will not deteriorate in the absence of further ongoing care, the EMC is likely stabilized. *Transfer* is not defined under EMTALA as the movement of a patient from one hospital to another; it is the movement of the patient from the hospital. Physicians with experience completing certification forms upon sending patients to another hospital are familiar with an area that requires the selection of *stable* or *unstable*, in reference to the EMC. This determination should not be based upon the hemodynamic status of the patient and the likelihood of survival during transport. It should be based upon the definition discussed above.

Considering the variable manner in which patients with psychiatric emergencies present to the ED, security guards and clinical staff managing the waiting room and triage areas should be aware of how the law defines transfer and the implications of their actions on the hospital's compliance with EMTALA. Some individuals with psychiatric emergencies may become unruly in the waiting room. In attempt to maintain accepted decorum, staff may violate EMTALA by directing such individuals to leave the ED or having them arrested, without meeting the MSE requirement.

The EMC can be considered stabilized when the patient no longer requires immediate psychiatric or medical care, direct observation, and is not considered a threat to self or others. In other words, when the patient is deemed safe for discharge home, the EMC may be considered stabilized. Suicidal or homicidal patients requiring further immediate care or patients requiring emergency/involuntary admission should not be considered to have a stabilized EMC. The use of chemical restraints for the safety of the patient or staff is a temporizing measure; it does not stabilize the EMC and terminate the obligations of hospitals and physicians under EMTALA. When the EMC persists despite treatment, the physician and hospital have an obligation to admit the individual for continued treatment within its capability and capacity, without regard to the patient's ability to pay. Upon a legitimate or good faith inpatient admission to the hospital, the EMTALA obligation ends [4].

The inpatient psychiatric needs of patients and the resources available to provide the appropriate level of care at hospitals may vary. If the capability and capacity needed to stabilize a patient's psychiatric emergency are unavailable, then a hospital may request the services of another hospital that has the capability and capacity to stabilize the EMC [5]. In such a circumstance, an individual with an EMC that is not stabilized can be appropriately transferred. The decision to admit an individual from the ED with an EMC to the inpatient psychiatric unit of a hospital, or effect an appropriate transfer to another hospital, should not depend upon the individual's financial status.

When arranging an *appropriate transfer* the referring physician must certify, in writing, a summary of the medical benefits of stabilizing care expected at the receiving hospital, which outweigh the risks of the transfer. The physician should take care to avoid confusing medical benefits and financial benefits during this certification process. Furthermore, the receiving hospital must accept the transfer and have the capability and capacity to stabilize the EMC. While physician-to-physician communication is a good practice during an inter-hospital transfer, it is not required; the name of the accepting physician should be documented. All available records and results pertaining to the EMC should be sent along with the individual at the time of transfer or as soon as possible following the transfer. Where applicable, the name and contact information of any on-call physician that failed to appear in a reasonable period of time or refused to render stabilizing treatment must also be provided. It is necessary to use qualified personnel and equipment during movement of the individual to another hospital [6]. The referring hospital and physician are responsible for the patient until arrival at the receiving hospital. The transfer of a patient with an EMC that has not been stabilized to an outpatient office, mental health clinic, or outpatient detoxification center is a high-risk activity that may violate EMTALA and does not represent an appropriate transfer. Such locations do not have EMTALA obligations.

There are circumstances where a patient may refuse care. A patient who has the capacity to make medical decisions can request a transfer (i.e., discharge home, transfer to another hospital) even when the capability and capacity to stabilize the EMC exists at the current facility. However, such a request may not be the result of financial coercion by the hospital or physician. The specific reason for the patient's transfer request must be documented along with acknowledgment of the hospital's obligation and willingness to provide stabilizing care, the associated risks and benefits of transfer [7].

It is commonplace for mental health screeners from the community to participate in the evaluation of patients with psychiatric emergencies and assist in locating inpatient availability when the EMC is not stabilized and inpatient care is required. The emergency physician or QMP located at the referring hospital remains ultimately responsible for the MSE, determination of the presence of an EMC, and the treatment rendered, not the mental health screener or a physician that has not evaluated the patient. Should the ED's on-call psychiatrist make a requested appearance to the ED to evaluate an individual, the psychiatrist may also participate in this decision process. Because intoxication is widely accepted as a clinical diagnosis, on-call physicians should avoid specifying a lab value as a pre-requisite for making an appearance in the ED to provide stabilizing treatment or to accept an appropriate transfer from a referring hospital.

EMTALA imposes specific responsibilities upon Medicare participating hospitals with specialized capabilities, regardless of whether such hospitals have an ED onsite. These recipient hospital responsibilities state that a hospital "that has specialized capabilities or facilities may not refuse to accept from a referring hospital, within the boundaries of the United States, an appropriate transfer of an individual who requires such specialized capabilities or facilities if the receiving hospital has the capacity to treat the individual [8]." While the on-call physician at a recipient hospital may provide some clinical input to the referring physician in the course of professional dialogue, the legal responsibility for determining the MSE, the existence of an EMC, and the care of individual being transferred from one hospital to another is that of the referring hospital and physician. Recipient hospital responsibilities under EMTALA do not apply to patients admitted at a referral hospital; however, it does apply to patients on *observation status* at a referral hospital [9] as they are technically outpatients.

The refusal of an appropriate transfer by an on-call physician at a recipient hospital does not remove the recipient hospital's obligation to accept an appropriate transfer. Because some inter-hospital transfers may not involve direct physician-to-physician communication, it is important that all staff members involved in the inter-hospital transfer process understand the law. Excessive delays in accepting an appropriate transfer, tactics such as requiring unnecessary tests or an involuntary admission certificate as a pre-requisite for acceptance, and refusing an appropriate transfer due to insurance status are examples of high-risk activities, which may violate EMTALA [10]. Both referring and receiving hospital providers should be aware of these requirements, even if local practices have historically ignored them.

Disputes may arise between the referring and receiving hospital during the arrangement of an inter-hospital transfer regarding the appropriateness of the MSE, the status of the patient's EMC, or the capability of on-call staff and bed availability at the referring or receiving hospital. If the referring hospital believes that a recipient hospital refused an appropriate transfer, it should attempt to secure stabilizing treatment for the patient at another hospital and report its suspicion to the Centers for Medicare and Medicaid Services (CMS) regional office or the respective state survey agency. It is often difficult and not the role of hospitals and physicians to determine the capability and capacity of another hospital in real time. While recipient hospitals cannot refuse an appropriate transfer from anywhere within the United States, sending hospitals must ensure their compliance with EMTALA. More specifically, the referral hospital should understand its bed capacity, resources, and on-call staff capability at the time it initiates a transfer and feel comfortable with a retrospective review of the actions taken. Any time that a recipient hospital has reason to believe that it may have received an individual with an EMC that was not stabilized, in violation of the statute, it is required under federal law report the incident to the state survey agency or CMS within 72 hours [11]. When the recipient hospital fails to report such incidents, its Medicare provider agreement may be subject to termination [12].

Many physicians and hospitals are uncertain as to how to respond when local or state laws are not consistent with EMTALA. When such concern arises, it is prudent to seek legal counsel. State and local laws may regulate areas such as the care of intoxicated individuals, the authority to involuntarily commit an individual, or which facilities can care for psychiatric patients by payer type or geographic boundaries, for example. These laws may also provide authority for a restraining order against an individual. As a federal law, EMTALA preempts conflicting state and local laws. Consequently, physicians and hospitals must remain cognizant of the federal requirements pertaining to the care of all individuals that present to the ED of a hospital, including those in police custody. Complying conflicting state or local law is not a viable defense to violating EMTALA [13]. Instances may occur where a physician or staff member of a hospital secures a restraining order against a patient. It should be clearly understood that the hospital and on-call physician's obligations under EMTALA preempt the restraining order.

Upon receiving a credible allegation of an EMTALA violation, the CMS regional office may authorize the state to perform a complaint investigation of an accredited hospital. This process may involve the review of many items such as medical records, diagnostic results, paging or call logs, transfer and acceptance logs, hospital census information, hospital video surveillance, transcripts or recordings of calls to a transfer center, ED on-call lists, and privileges of on-call physicians at the transferring and/or receiving hospital. Physicians, staff, patients, family members, EMS, police, and others may be interviewed during an investigation. Upon review of the evidence gathered, CMS will determine if a violation occurred. When necessary, a professional review from the quality improvement organization (QIO) may be obtained when a clinical issue is present [14]. However, when a MSE is not performed, the Office of the Inspector General may take the case immediately [15]. When EMTALA has been violated, CMS will initiate steps to revoke or terminate the hospital's Medicare provider agreement [16]. In hospitals with less than 100 beds, the Office of the Inspector General (OIG) may impose civil monetary penalties (CMP) of up to $25,000 per violation, whereas hospitals with 100 or more beds could face fines of up to $50,000 per violation. The OIG may also impose CMPs against physicians in an amount up to $50,000, for each negligent violation of EMTALA; repetitive or flagrant violations may lead to exclusion of a physician from participation in the Medicare and Medicaid program [17].

Failure to comply with EMTALA can lead to substantial consequences for hospitals and physicians. Emergency psychiatry involves a broad healthcare team and members vary in their level of responsibility and education. Understanding the requirements imposed by EMTALA is an essential compliance topic for each team member.

References

1. Special responsibilities of Medicare hospitals in emergency cases, 42 CFR 489.24 (a)(1)

2. Special responsibilities of Medicare hospitals in emergency cases, 42 CFR 489.24 (b)

3. Special responsibilities of Medicare hospitals in emergency cases, 42 CFR 489.24 (d)

4. Special responsibilities of Medicare hospitals in emergency cases, 42 CFR 489.24 (a)(1)(ii)

5. Special responsibilities of Medicare hospitals in emergency cases, 42 CFR 489.24 (e)

6. Special responsibilities of Medicare hospitals in emergency cases, 42 CFR 489.24 (e)(2)

7. Special responsibilities of Medicare hospitals in emergency cases, 42 CFR 489.24 (d)(3)

8. Special responsibilities of Medicare hospitals in emergency cases, 42 CFR 489.24 (f)

9. Special responsibilities of Medicare hospitals in emergency cases, 42 CFR 489.24 (d)(2)

10. Special responsibilities of Medicare hospitals in emergency cases, 42 CFR 489.24 (d)(4)

11. Special responsibilities of Medicare hospitals in emergency cases, 42 CFR 489.20(m)

12. State Operations Manual, Interpretive Guidelines for 42 CFR 489.20(m)

13. State Operations Manual (SOM), Interpretive Guidelines for 489.24(a)

14. Special responsibilities of Medicare hospitals in emergency cases, 42 CFR 489.24 (h)

15. Special responsibilities of Medicare hospitals in emergency cases, 42 CFR 489.24 (h)(3)

16. Special responsibilities of Medicare hospitals in emergency cases, 42 CFR 489.24 (g)

17. Special responsibilities of Medicare hospitals in emergency cases, 42 CFR 1003.103

Chapter

44

Assessing capacity, involuntary assessment, and leaving against medical advice

Susan Stefan

Introduction

Patients who leave the emergency department (ED) against medical advice (AMA) are at increased risk of morbidity and mortality, and are more likely than other patients to show up at the hospital again within 30 days [1]. There is little research about psychiatric patients leaving EDs AMA, but studies do show that psychiatric patients leave inpatient units AMA at a higher rate than medical patients, and that psychiatric patients who leave AMA are also more likely to be readmitted [1]. Because of the significant differences between psychiatric and medical disorders, a psychiatric patient returning to the ED after leaving AMA is not necessarily an indicator of problematic care by the ED [2]. Yet proposed new government regulations would penalize hospitals when a disproportionate number of patients are readmitted within 30 days [3].

Like medical patients, psychiatric patients have the legal right to refuse treatment, even life-saving treatment, and to leave the hospital, unless their condition renders them a danger to themselves or others or unless they are not legally competent to make treatment decisions. The language surrounding this issue is sometimes confusing: the medical profession assesses and makes determinations of a patient's "capacity," while statutes, regulations, and court decisions almost uniformly refer to "competence." In this article, I use the term "capacity" when referring to a physician's assessments and judgments, and "competence" when referring to legal standards or statutes. Both medical standards and legal standards recognize that psychiatric patients cannot be detained against their will simply because they need treatment. Involuntary detention is limited to situations where a patient meets stringent standards of dangerousness related to mental illness. In an emergency, a hospital may also involuntarily detain a patient who has been determined to lack decisional capacity to make the decision to leave while it finds someone statutorily authorized to make a decision on the patient's behalf. If a hospital attempts to restrain a patient from leaving who is later determined to be legally competent and nondangerous, it faces potential charges of false imprisonment and/or violation of constitutional rights.

Whereas federal law does require EDs to screen for life-threatening conditions, including psychiatric conditions, and to provide stabilizing treatment if an emergency condition is found to exist, it also mandates that a patient can refuse such treatment, and must be permitted to leave (unless he or she meets involuntary commitment standards). Chapter 48 discusses these legal requirements in detail. This chapter addresses the question of how emergency departments should handle the situation of a person with a psychiatric condition who wishes to leave the ED AMA, especially in situations where the patient's capacity to make the decision is in doubt.

The legal answers to these questions combine state law, which governs false imprisonment, civil commitment, and malpractice, and federal constitutional and statutory law, including Emergency Medical Treatment and Active Labor laws (EMTALA) and other requirements under the Medicare/Medicaid statute. Although each state's law is different, there are some patterns that consistently emerge from a survey of research and case law in this area.

First, judges and juries are generally unsympathetic to litigation by psychiatric patients – or even their estates – and are particularly unsympathetic to litigation seeking compensation for adverse outcomes after the patient leaves AMA. A variety of legal doctrines embody this lack of sympathy. For example, the doctrine of contributory negligence enables juries to apportion the blame for adverse outcomes between the facility and the patient. Often juries find the patient completely or mostly at fault in ignoring medical advice. In some states, if the patient's fault exceeds 50%, no finding of liability can be returned against any defendant. The unsurprising exceptions are cases where the hospital claims that the patient left AMA after suitable warnings, but the patient's chart reflects no documentation of this at all. Almost every plaintiff victory in litigation is tied in some way to incomplete or defective documentation.

The best outcome, of course, is not to win a lawsuit but to prevent one from being filed. There are practical ways to respond to situations where a psychiatric patient wishes to leave AMA. These responses feature common sense, flexibility, listening to a patient's concerns in a respectful way, and negotiation.

This chapter suggests different approaches to a patient wishing to leave AMA based on the different reasons

Behavioral Emergencies for the Emergency Physician, ed. Leslie S. Zun, Lara G. Chepenik, and Mary Nan S. Mallory. Published by Cambridge University Press. © Cambridge University Press 2013.

underlying the patient's determination to be discharged. Threats or attempts to leave AMA generally fall into four categories, each requiring different responses from ED staff.

> **Four primary categories of reasons for leaving AMA**
>
> - Dissatisfaction or frustration with delays, ED environment, proposed treatment or disposition, or with how the patient is being treated
> - Conflicting social or financial obligations
> - Presenting problem has resolved
> - Confusion associated with intoxication, organicity, or psychoses.

This chapter will begin by discussing the differences and similarities, clinically and legally, between medical patients and psychiatric patients that wish to leave AMA, the legal landscape relating to departures AMA, the essential elements of a hospital policy relating to AMA departures by psychiatric patients who arise from this landscape, and practical ways that ED staff can respond to patients with potential psychiatric presentations who wish to leave AMA.

In some situations, ED staff will have to assess the patient's competence to make informed decisions to leave or refuse treatment. Although there is no standardized instrument to measure capacity to make medical decisions in EDs, the fundamental components of an assessment will be described. Even if the patient is deemed to lack decisional capacity to make treatment decisions, generally he or she cannot be detained and treated without the consent of legally authorized surrogate decision makers unless assessment of the patient's condition reveals the likelihood of a life-threatening condition. What constitutes an "emergency" and the crucial distinction between these emergencies justifying treatment and a behavioral emergency justifying restraint or seclusion will also be detailed.

Distinctions between leaving before being seen, elopement, and leaving AMA

Patients who leave without being seen are far more common than patients who leave AMA [4]. There is some indication that leaving without being seen is more associated with ED overcrowding than is leaving AMA [4]. Leaving without being seen raises fewer liability issues, except when delay in seeing a clearly serious emergency creates an EMTALA issue [5,6].

Nor should elopement or escape be conflated with leaving AMA [7]. Although in the past elopement of psychiatric patients was often called "leaving against medical advice," elopement generally represents a different and more serious liability issue. Whereas judges and juries are generally hostile to claims brought by patients who left AMA, they tend to be more sympathetic to claims brought by patients or the estates of patients who escaped or eloped. Even in elopement cases, plaintiff victories tend to be based on extreme circumstances. For example, a psychiatric inpatient who had attempted suicide was placed on a gurney in the ED after experiencing cardiac problems. After waiting for transfer to the medical floor for 48 hours, he left the ED and hanged himself from a tree very close to its entrance. The case settled on the eve of trial for $700,000 [8].

Hospitals have tried to prevent patient elopement through a variety of policies and architectural modifications. Some of these policies – one-to-one observation of patients, or having a secure and more quiet area to evaluate people presenting with psychiatric conditions – are generally considered improvements in care. Others – requiring psychiatric patients to remove their clothing, or introducing armed security guards into the ED – may create legal issues of their own (see Chapter 48). If a psychiatric patient elopes, the ED clearly must undertake a search of the premises surrounding the ED, including the parking lot and the area immediately outside the ED, and make every effort to find the patient, as well as notifying any individual listed by the patient as a person to contact in an emergency.

Why do psychiatric patients leave AMA?

The rate of departure AMA from EDs by medical patients has increased in the past 10 years [9]. Patients who leave AMA are often dissatisfied, and they sue ED physicians and hospitals at nearly 10 times the rate of the typical ED patient [9].

Although the rates of psychiatric patients leaving EDs AMA have not been well documented, it is no secret that many patients in psychiatric crisis at an ED do want to leave. At least some psychiatric patients are brought to the ED involuntarily, so they never wanted to be at the ED in the first place. However, psychiatric patients who come to the ED voluntarily seeking help also leave, or at least try to leave. They may be more vulnerable to the stresses of waiting, or to the uncomfortable, noisy, crowded conditions of the ED, or a combination of both [10]. They may just be hungry or thirsty or want to smoke or need to take their medications. They may feel that the problem that brought them to the ED has subsided.

In addition, emotional factors that have been identified as being associated with medical patients leaving AMA–anger, anxiety, and helplessness–may be particularly pronounced in psychiatric patients. People who are psychotic may want to leave because the stimulating environment is exacerbating their condition, or because they are confused. Finally, the patient profile associated with high AMA rates in medical patients–young, male, substance- or alcohol-abusing, Medicaid or no insurance, and past history of leaving AMA [1,7] may be more common among psychiatric patients than the general medical population.

Provider variables associated with leaving AMA, e.g., the failure to establish a supportive doctor–patient relationship [7] may also be higher among psychiatric patients in the ED than medical patients. ED staff may become angry or frustrated with psychiatric patients in a general hospital ED [11]. In addition, there is evidence that patients with psychiatric diagnoses who present at the ED for medical issues are suspected of malingering or mistaking psychiatric symptoms for medical ones. While this is sometimes true, it does not make it less frustrating for patients who actually have medical conditions, many of whom try to leave when the response to their medical complaints is a psychiatric assessment.

Hospital policies and practices: responding to the request of a behavioral health patient to leave AMA

Recommended staff practices when a patient wishes to leave

If an individual arrives for help with psychiatric issues, and desires to leave before being evaluated, the ED staff to whom the request is communicated should immediately notify the nurse responsible for the patient's care. If the nurse cannot respond right away, the staff-person should engage the patient, and try to determine, in a sympathetic and respectful way, the reason that the patient wants to leave. *Do not immediately respond to a request to leave with the statement that the patient cannot leave.* Even if a person is under legal detention, a first response that the patient cannot leave is likely to create resentment or begin an escalating power struggle rather than elicit needed information and enhance communication and cooperation. Acknowledging the desire to leave, and the right that patients generally have to leave, accompanied by a concerned and respectful inquiry into the reason that the person wants to leave, is likely to assist in separating the patient into one of the four rough categories outlined in the box above. When the nurse arrives, the staff-person can attempt to summarize the patient's concerns, turning to the patient and asking if he or she is accurately characterizing the situation.

If the reason the patient wishes to leave falls into one of the first two categories, the identified problem may be addressed and resolved. The patient may be given something to eat, or drink, or to keep warm; the lights may be turned lower or dimmed; a staff-person with whom the patient is having difficulties may be replaced by another staff-person (this is often worth doing in terms of long-term outcome and creating an alliance with the patient).

If the problem is delay, sometimes it can be resolved by an apology and an honest explanation of the source of the delay [12]. Too often, ED staff feel that nothing can be done for the patient while waiting for the mental health evaluator to arrive or the lab tests to come back. In fact, this is the time when a patient is likely to be most anxious, having no information about what will happen next and when it will happen. *The fact that ED staff lack information is no reason to avoid the patient; it is during this time that efforts should be made to ensure comfort, and to reiterate the current status of the process and what will happen next.* ED staff should avoid making promises or assurances that cannot be kept, but a staff member can and should make a promise to check on sources of delay and report back to the patient within a certain amount of time.

If the patient disagrees with proposed tests or treatment, as do many patients who leave AMA [13], the physician may attempt to negotiate a course more acceptable to the patient. In the author's experience, some psychiatric patients will attempt to leave AMA upon learning that the proposed inpatient admission is to a particular hospital. One patient refused to return to a hospital where she had been sexually assaulted. If a patient is willing to be voluntarily admitted to one hospital but not another based on past experience, a genuine attempt to honor the patient's wishes may be worthwhile in terms of avoiding escalation, attempts to elope, and restraint. If it is not possible, the patient should be asked if anything can be done to reduce or alleviate their concerns about the facility. Sometimes patients are simply worried about proposed treatments and need to be reassured. Flexibility and negotiation may prevent departure AMA.

If the patient has social or financial responsibilities, these should be taken seriously and the hospital should have means to assist in addressing them. If telephone calls need to be made to arrange child care or notify employers, and the ED does not have a portable phone, the patient should be escorted to a pay phone or permitted to use a hospital phone to make these calls. If the patient is worried about insurance issues, these should be clarified by the social worker if possible.

Sometimes the problem cannot be resolved. The patient is convinced he or she doesn't need to be there and the hospital judges, based on the patient's conduct or collateral information, that a professional assessment is essential; or the patient is clearly very intoxicated or possibly incompetent. If so, a physician or other staff member with the authority to assess and either discharge the patient or sign the documents necessary for involuntary retention should be summoned *immediately*. Often, ED staff are reluctant to summon an on-call doctor who is not on-site. But a voluntary patient's explicit desire to leave AMA both converts a previously voluntary stay into an involuntary detention, and signals a conflict which may very well escalate. It must be understood by all staff, including on-call professionals, as a situation that needs attention without delay. No patient should be detained involuntarily without prompt efforts to meet the requirements of the law. The convenience and comfort of on-call specialists, while a very real concern for ED staff, is not an excuse that judges and juries will find plausible for extended delay, especially if during this delay the patient escalates and is restrained and injured, or escapes from the hospital.

While waiting for the physician to arrive, the nurse can both help the patient feel heard and assist the doctor's assessment by asking key questions to elicit both risk factors and protective factors, including support at home, presence of a weapon at home, follow-up in the community, what triggered the crisis, and how it will be avoided next time [14]. These questions can be phrased in a way that is supportive of the patient's desire to leave, while conveying that discharge cannot take place until the patient has a conversation with the doctor. The questions can include practical issues such as how the patient will be picked up from the

ED, and whether anyone is at home or available to come to the ED. If so, can the patient share contact information, if the hospital does not already have it? Can the nurse assist in making a follow-up outpatient appointment? If the ED staff has not already initiated attempts to contact collateral sources of information, this is a good time to do it, with the patient's permission.

Needless to say, all of the efforts outlined above should be documented in the patient's chart and on the AMA form, using the patient's own words. If the patient is determined to leave AMA, physicians, social workers, and other staff should make all mitigating efforts possible to reduce the risks involved in the patient's departure. Anger at patients for leaving AMA, while understandable, should not prevent scheduling outpatient appointments, making follow-up telephone calls, and writing follow-up letters.

Essential elements of written hospital policy

When a patient who has presented with a potential psychiatric emergency asks to leave, the request should trigger a set of consistent staff responses that are embodied in a hospital policy. This policy should be readily accessible to ED staff (i.e., not simply stored in an enormous plastic binder in the Human Resources office). All staff having patient contact should receive regular training about the policy and the roles of various staff in implementing it. The policy should be familiar to staff in the ED, and hospital quality assurance departments should conduct audits to ensure that it is implemented as a standard practice.

A hospital AMA policy should include the following:

- A statement of guiding principles (e.g., the presumption of a right to autonomy and informed consent, a reminder that treatment and safety is best achieved through respect and empathy rather than coercion, and a reiteration that a patient's desire to leave AMA may signal a problem with the care received that may be addressed and resolved)
- A standard AMA form, in all the languages routinely used by hospital patients
- Designation of staff authorized to discharge psychiatric patients AMA[1]
- Time frames to complete all assessments if the patient is held involuntarily
- Specific documentation requirements in the patient's chart and/or the AMA form:
  - Patient's vital signs at time of request and at discharge
  - Mental status and orientation at time of request and discharge

- Specific finding of capacity to make decision to refuse treatment and leave
- Follow-up appointments for patients
- Specific discharge instructions, including urging return to the ED if patient changes his or her mind, and any symptoms that should raise particular concern
- Community supports, including family, therapist, etc.
- Patient offered the opportunity to ask questions/what questions patient asked
- Diagnostic tests and their results
- Suicide risk assessment and results
- Any request for interpreters and implementation of that request

There should be a procedure to ensure that any test results that come in after the patient leaves are recorded and the patient is notified, especially if the results show a need for further care. In *Lyons v. Walker Regional Medical Center*, test results after the patient left showed that he was suffering from diabetic ketoacidosis, treatable but fatal if untreated. The hospital did not notify officials at the jail where the patient returned, and the prisoner died several days later. The hospital won the case, in part because the patient was found to have left AMA [15].

The court in *Lyons* was troubled, however, as to whether the patient's information had been specific enough (he was told he might die if he left, without specific information about his potential diagnosis and condition and why a patient in his specific condition was better off in the hospital). A patient leaving AMA should be informed of his or her diagnosis and condition, as well as *why* the departure is AMA, and what the patient and his or her family can do to mitigate any risks created by his or her departure. For example, the patient or family should be asked about the availability of weapons in the home, and advised to dispose of them or secure them elsewhere. In addition, the patient and family should be informed of signs to watch out for that might signal the need to return immediately. The documentation must include any collateral contacts that have been made (with the patient's permission) and the information these contacts have been given about the patient's condition and instructions for aftercare. Most of these items are, of course, routinely documented as part of patient care.

Some patients seek to leave before full medical clearance or psychiatric evaluation. While the hospital cannot legally enforce a policy prohibiting *any* patient who arrived for psychiatric reasons from leaving before being evaluated (see Chapter 48), some patients who arrive voluntarily and have not yet been professionally evaluated clearly should *not* be

---

[1] In some states, such as Massachusetts, only specifically certified physicians can sign forms to involuntarily detain an individual under the state commitment law. In these states, it may be illegal for a physician who does not have this certification to discharge a patient who has been involuntarily detained. See *Dimilla v. Fairfield et al.* Case No. CV 2005–00941, 2010 MA JAS Pub LEXIS (certified emergency physician signs involuntary detention papers and blank discharge and transfer orders for inpatient psychiatric unit; non-certified physicians discharged patient to less secure community facility without signing any discharge orders; certified physician found not liable for patient's subsequent escape and suicide; hospital found negligent through acts of non-certified physician for $521,201.00, reduced by prior stipulation to $171,201.)

permitted to leave. These include patients who are grossly psychotic, severely intoxicated patients, or who articulate imminent suicidal plans. Although clinically clear cases, the involuntary detention of these patients occupies a gray area of the law. The law permits involuntary detention only on the basis of determinations of dangerousness or lack of capacity, yet these patients have not been assessed by a professional with the legal authority to make those determinations (the law does permit a "reasonable" period of time to obtain such an assessment, see Chapter 48).

The hospital's AMA policy should clearly distinguish between psychiatric patients permitted to leave AMA and those who will not. The latter category includes anyone under a legally authorized involuntary detention order, or who is judged at triage by a trained nurse to represent a significant risk of substantial harm to themselves or others. Patients who arrived voluntarily and do not want a medical or psychiatric assessment, should be allowed to leave unless they meet the criteria outlined above. The hospital should also have clear procedures to obtain the appropriate psychiatric evaluations for patients being held involuntarily without delay.

The AMA policy and form should be prepared with the assistance of experienced legal counsel familiar with federal and state mental health law. In some states, there are restrictions on which professionals can discharge an individual involuntarily detained under the state's law. As discussed in more detail below, other states limit the time a psychiatric patient can be held involuntarily in an ED setting, and courts take these time limits seriously. If this is the case, the hospital must have procedures and personnel in place that ensure the evaluation will be conducted within that time, including any "extras" that may be reasonably anticipated, such as the need for an interpreter or for lab test results.

The policy should require data collection on the number of patients who leave AMA, as well as data collection on time frames between arrival and medical clearance, and medical clearance and mental health evaluation (some hospitals do both simultaneously, and save time), and an accountable individual with responsibility and authority to ensure that the evaluations are happening in a timely manner.

Leaving AMA and the law: exceptions to the right to leave

The basic starting point of the law is that the common law doctrine of informed consent includes the right to refuse treatment [16]. People with psychiatric conditions are not uniformly dangerous or incompetent. Therefore, a blanket hospital policy that all patients presenting for psychiatric reasons cannot leave before medical clearance or before psychiatric evaluation is not legal.

However, there are three well-known exceptions to this basic and fundamental legal principle. The first permits the involuntary detention of a person who is mentally ill and dangerous to himself or herself or others. The second allows

an ED to temporarily detain a patient determined to lack capacity to make his or her own treatment decisions while it finds a legally authorized substitute decision maker. The third involves a patient who is under arrest or is otherwise in lawful custody of police or correctional officers.

Detention pursuant to involuntary commitment statutes

A person who is mentally ill, dangerous to himself or herself or others, and who has difficulties controlling that dangerousness, may be prevented from leaving the ED AMA by certain professionals. Although many hospitals have created involuntary detention forms with a few boxes to check, and three or four lines to record the professional's observations, it is important to specifically document the basis for findings of mental illness and dangerousness. For example, rather than merely recording conclusions that the patient is "agitated" or "noncompliant," describe the behavior and/or language that forms the basis for this conclusion. These descriptive details should be included on any required form and in the patient's chart. This is true whether the patient is to be detained or discharged. Observation and specificity are key, rather than generalized conclusions. Any available information from collateral sources should also be documented. Dr. Jon Berlin and this author have prepared a guide that assists in appropriately documenting discharges [14].

It is crucial to accurately note the time of arrival, detention, and examination. Some states have time limitations on a patient's ED detention, and it is important to know when the clock starts, to note that time explicitly in the patient's record, and to adhere to those time limits. For example, in Pennsylvania, an individual brought in for psychiatric evaluation must be examined by a physician within 2 hours of arrival [17]. Although Pennsylvania law grants ED staff immunity from civil or criminal liability for ordinary negligence in the course of evaluating a person for involuntary commitment, a Pennsylvania court recently found that a complaint stated a claim for gross negligence when a woman was restrained for 4 hours and forced to use a bedpan before being seen by a physician in violation of the 2-hour limit [17]. As the court stated:

> If plaintiffs can produce evidence to support the claim that Cheryl James was left strapped to a gurney for 4 hours before being examined, they can show that the medical defendants grossly deviated from the standard of care, because the law requires a patient be seen within 2 hours [17].

The court held that plaintiff had stated a claim for punitive damages. In this case, the court also described problems with the hospital's documentation: the documentation justifying the patient's restraint stated that she had removed her clothing and attempted to escape naked from the ED, but a separate notation made 1 minute after the restraint order recorded the patient as still wearing her street clothes.

In some states, agencies external to the ED staff make the final determination about whether the patient meets commitment standards. In Washington, the statutory 6-hour time limit begins to run when ED staff conclude that a county-designated mental health professional must be notified to determine whether an individual can be held involuntarily [18]. However, the Supreme Court of Washington also held that its citizens' constitutional due process rights limit the amount of time a person can be held involuntarily between his or her arrival and the decision to notify the community-designated mental health professional, and that the burden is on the hospital to demonstrate that any delay was justified by the individual circumstances of the case. In *C.W.*, the Supreme Court affirmed a lower court holding that two of the appellants were subject to unconstitutional delay – one because of an unexplained 3.5-hour delay between medical clearance and the social worker's psychiatric evaluation, and the other because of an almost 3-hour delay in psychiatric evaluation when there were no medical clearance issues [18].

When a decision has been made to involuntarily detain a person because of dangerousness, hospital policy should require a respectful explanation to the individual, along with explanation of the process. The ED staff should emphasize that theirs is not the final determination, because the patient will be evaluated by others at whatever facility will be receiving the patient. If he or she still disagrees with the result, there is a right to a hearing and legal representation. It is helpful to have a clear page or pamphlet setting out the steps of the process and relevant contact information. Several model forms exist designed for ED patients in individual states [19,20]. Obviously, a different form would have to be prepared for each state, because state laws differ.

A determination that an individual is mentally ill, and dangerous to self or others as a result of that mental illness, does not necessarily translate into incompetence to make treatment decisions, although in some cases a patient may fall into both categories. Nor does the determination that an individual may be involuntarily detained under the state's commitment statute provide justification under federal regulations for physical, mechanical, or chemical restraint or even seclusion (see Chapter 48).

Incompetent/lacks capacity to decide to leave AMA

The issue of lack of capacity to make the decision to leave AMA is complex. As courts now recognize, competence is not an all or nothing proposition. A patient may be incompetent to make financial decisions, and competent to make treatment decisions [21,22]. Thus, the fact that a patient is under guardianship does not necessarily equate with incompetence to make treatment decisions [22]. In addition, competence is not related to the wisdom or folly of the treatment decision, but rather the ability to receive information and make and communicate a decision on the basis of that information.

Second, competence (or capacity, the term more often used by medical professionals) can fluctuate with time. This is seen most commonly in EDs in relation to people who are extremely intoxicated or high or having adverse reactions to medications such as steroids [23,24]. These individuals may regain their capacity over a period of hours.

In addition, a legal distinction that is very relevant to EDs is between the incompetence of a patient experiencing a medical emergency and one who is not. All states have an exception for medical emergencies when a person is incompetent and/or unconscious and permit a legally authorized decision maker to make those decisions. These vary from state to state, but generally begin with the person's spouse, and go on through adult children, parents, and siblings. The definition of what constitutes a medical emergency also varies tremendously from state to state, with some (e.g., Georgia and South Carolina) having quite broad definitions and others (Massachusetts and Washington) having far narrower ones. EDs may be permitted to treat a patient in a medical emergency if they cannot locate a substitute decision maker. However, reasonable efforts must be made, even in an emergency. In the case of *In v Estate of Allen*, the physician did not know whether the patient had taken a fatal overdose, and she was refusing diagnostic tests. Although the court found that she was not competent to make an informed decision, it also held that the physician should at least have made an effort to contact her sister for permission [25].

A medical emergency should be distinguished from a behavioral emergency justifying restraint and seclusion under federal standards (see Chapter 48). A patient who is violent or self-destructive and cannot be verbally de-escalated may present a behavioral emergency requiring restraint, but these restraints are not treatment, and CMS standards for restraint must be followed.

Finally, a distinction that often emerges in the practice of EDs is the one between those patients arguably lacking in capacity who assent to treatment, and those who refuse it. Assenters often receive treatment without understanding either their conditions or having provided informed consent to the treatment. Their questionable capacity is rarely documented. On the other hand, those patients of questionable capacity who refuse treatment, or want to leave, are often restrained. Obviously, the reason for the distinction is the belief by ED staff that patients incompetently assenting to medically beneficial treatment do not raise the same risk of harm as patients' potentially incompetent refusal of treatment and departure. However, failing to note capacity issues for assenters is risky, because the ED may be subject to later charges of treatment without informed consent [26]. In addition, if the person later decides to refuse treatment or to leave, courts will look askance at a hospital's apparent assumption that a patient was competent until he or she began to refuse treatment.

Standards of capacity to leave AMA

Different standards have been articulated for competence or capacity to make treatment decisions [26–28]. A person articulating a desire to leave AMA meets the broadest definition of competence in that he or she is capable of expressing and communicating a treatment decision. However, most would agree that merely expressing the desire to leave does not mean the person is competent to make the decision, because many highly intoxicated, extremely psychotic, or very demented patients express the desire to leave and are not competent do so. State statutes usually contain a definition of competence to make treatment decisions, and hospital policy should track that definition.

All state statutes begin with the presumption that adults are competent. In addition to being able to communicate a preference, an individual must generally also understand the basics of the physician's opinion of his or her condition, and the proposed treatment for it. Disagreeing with the opinion is not per se evidence of incompetence. Rejecting the treatment because of superseding values – keeping a job, religious values, hating the side effects of medication, fear of the stigma of hospitalization – is not evidence of incompetence. It is extremely important to note that intoxication, psychosis, or a diagnosis of dementia, standing alone, do not necessarily equate with incompetence [24,26,29]. Nor is a suicidal patient – or even one who attempts suicide – necessarily incompetent [27]. Of course, a person who attempts suicide can be considered dangerous to him- or herself and detained under the involuntary commitment standard. There is no hard and fast rule that any particular condition (except truly severe dementia or psychosis) automatically means a patient is incompetent. It is axiomatic that each decision must be made and documented individually.

Determining incompetence to leave AMA

Although most competence evaluations are made on the basis of subjective interviews, research has shown that unstructured clinical determinations of competence are not reliable; in one study, clinicians achieved a rate of agreement that was no better than chance [26]. It is far better for a hospital to have a policy that requires a brief structured assessment of competence [26,28]. Using a systematic set of questions for competence assessments leads to far more interrater agreement, as well as agreement with expert judgments of competence [28].

Using structured questions also ensures that the prerequisites for informed consent are met: the patient must have actually been provided with understandable information about the condition, and the decision-making must be voluntary. The Joint Commission has found that failure to provide truly informed consent is a common problem for EDs [30]. Surveys by this author of psychiatric patients in EDs across the country support this conclusion: patients routinely complained that they were given insufficient information about their diagnosis, proposed treatment, and the process being followed in the ED. In a few cases, patients stated that they were given medication without its even being identified by staff (let alone being given the opportunity for informed consent), leading in one case to serious medical complications [31].

Thus, a capacity assessment must ensure that (1) the patient receives adequate information about his or her condition and recommended and alternative treatments in an accessible language and format; (2) the patient understands that information; and (3) the patient is making his or her decision by reasoning in some way with the information provided. This does *not* mean making a decision that ED staff consider "reasonable." Competence assessment focuses on the process and not the outcome [26].

To provide information to the patient, it is axiomatic that staff must use language that is understandable to that patient– not only sign language for deaf patients or interpreters for those who do not understand English, but simple enough language for people whose fear and stress makes it hard for them to understand. This information should be given in small amounts, and may have to be repeated. After each unit of information, the patient should be given the opportunity to ask questions. This interaction, properly done, provides the staff with sufficient information to assess competence. The interaction may also take more time than ED staff are accustomed to spend performing this task, but if a potentially incompetent patient wishes to leave AMA, the time taken to provide information and seek understanding may persuade the patient to stay. Whether such a patient is permitted to leave or involuntarily detained on the basis of incompetence rather than dangerousness, a careful assessment process that is carefully documented is both good patient care and good legal insurance.

When assessing the patient's capacity, the fact that a patient's description of his or her condition or symptoms varies from the ED staff's diagnosis is not, by itself, sufficient to find incompetence, nor does a denial that the patient has the particular condition named by ED staff. For example, denying that one is depressed, or has a mental illness, but acknowledging being "very sad" or confused, does not indicate incompetence. The patient's own language to express his or her condition should be respected, particularly for patients from different cultures. However, staff should ensure that the patient does understand what he or she has been told about the ED staff's diagnosis and proposed treatment. The patient should be assured that being able to repeat this information does not mean that the staff believes that the patient agrees with it.

Specific legal issues related to leaving AMA

Leaving AMA and the minor

There are two basic issues involved in minors leaving AMA: minors who wish to leave when their parents are unavailable, and parents who wish to remove their children from medical care AMA. The latter issue is litigated far more frequently than the former. However, because presentations by minors for psychiatric reasons often raise different legal issues than presentation for medical reasons, the hospital should ensure that its policies reflect any distinctions embodied in state and/or federal law. This is particularly true in the areas of confidentiality and involuntary commitment. For example, in Massachusetts, minors 16 years of age and older have the same rights as adults, both to admit themselves conditionally for mental health treatment without their parents' knowledge or consent, and to consult with an attorney regarding their rights. Different states have varying requirements and exceptions involving the legal decision-making authority of minors beginning at age 14, and the hospital should be aware of the laws applicable in its state [32].

Although parents' decisions regarding their children must generally be respected, there is an enormous difference between the law – and especially courts' interpretation of the law – regarding an adult's right to refuse treatment on his or her own behalf, and the rights of parents to refuse treatment for their child. Because the state has a *parens patriae* obligation in the case of children that it does not have in the case of adults, hospitals and physicians who believe a parent's decisions about care may endanger the life of their child, or are likely to cause serious injury, can and should take measures to protect the child. Outraged parents may litigate, but in the overwhelming majority of cases, courts side with the hospital that treated or detained the child over the parents' objections [33,34].

Leaving AMA and the intoxicated person

One complication presented by people in psychiatric crisis seeking to leave AMA is when they appear intoxicated, and refuse blood or urine tests. An added wrinkle is the outright unwillingness of some inpatient psychiatric units to accept patients who are intoxicated, regardless of their behavior. Thus, many EDs unfortunately serve as very expensive waiting rooms for psychiatric hospitals.

Both professional standards and the courts agree that the determination of whether an intoxicated patient is competent to make medical decisions is an individualized one, and that there can be no hard and fast rule equating certain blood alcohol levels with incompetence [24,35]. In the case of a person who is intoxicated, it is particularly important to conduct and document a suicide risk assessment and to attempt to rule out medical causes for the apparent intoxication. If the individual appears to have the capacity to make the decision to leave, and is not requesting medical or psychiatric treatment, getting a friend or family member to provide transportation home is optimal; if this cannot be accomplished, a taxi voucher or bus token may be appropriate. Courts have little patience with plaintiffs who sue EDs for false imprisonment or battery due to being restrained or prevented from leaving when the plaintiffs presented with signs of intoxication, especially disruptive intoxication.

Leaving AMA and the person under guardianship

There are several important principles to bear in mind in discussing the rights of a patient under guardianship and the responsibilities of a hospital toward the patient and his or her guardian. First, not all guardianships result in the loss of an individual's right to make medical decisions. Many states provide for limited guardianship to protect a person's property or

finances, without removing the right to make treatment decisions. Thus, a hospital should not automatically assume that a patient under guardianship has lost the right to informed consent, or to make his or her own treatment decisions [21,22].

Leaving AMA: the psychiatrically disabled patient with a medical complaint

Although most ED physicians are more concerned about permitting the AMA departure of a person at the ED with a primarily psychiatric complaint, there is ample clinical research suggesting that an equal, if not greater, mortality and morbidity concern lies in underestimating the seriousness of medical complaints of people with psychiatric disabilities. People with psychiatric disabilities often have comorbid medical conditions, and sometimes the only treatment they receive for these conditions is in EDs. A recent study of unexpected deaths seven days after departure from an ED found that mental illness and substance abuse was a strong predictor of unexpected deaths from medical etiology [47] and several cases charging that ED physicians misdiagnosed a medical complaint as just another manifestation of psychiatric symptomatology confirm this finding. These issues are discussed in greater detail in Chapter 48.

Practical solutions: how to prevent departure AMA

By definition, patients who want to leave AMA are, in the clinical opinion of the medical or mental health professional who assessed them, better off staying at the hospital for observation or to receive treatment. Therefore, staff should make – and document – respectful efforts to resolve the problems leading to the patient's decision to leave AMA. There has been some suggestion that at least some overcrowded and overworked EDs may be all too eager to permit disruptive psychiatric patients to leave AMA [36].

The strategies outlined below may not only assist in reducing AMA departures, but also increase patient satisfaction, and reduce disruptiveness and staff frustration.

Address nicotine, alcohol, and drug dependence issues

Often, patient agitation or restlessness in the ED after a long wait is caused or exacerbated by hospital rules preventing smoking, as well as precluding going outside to smoke. Several attempts to elope or escape, as well as departures AMA, have been attributed to the difficulties inherent in withdrawing from nicotine, alcohol, or painkillers during an extended wait in an ED. Case law also reflects this, including one case where a man who left the ED to go home and get methadone was prevented from re-entering the same ED later that evening [37].

While most EDs have protocols for treating alcohol withdrawal, many do not attend to the difficulties for patients of going without smoking. All EDs should have nicotine gum, patches, or some similar substitute, for patients for whom this is medically appropriate.

Attend to environmental comfort issues

Many EDs provide warmed blankets, which are very helpful when the ED is perceived by patients as cold. Others have substituted more sturdy pajamas for the paper or flimsy cloth johnnies that patients are asked to wear as they wait for assessment. Because many psychiatric patients have histories of sexual abuse, and find hospital gowns exacerbate feelings of vulnerability, the clothing that is provided may make a difference between a patient's severe anxiety or refusal to change clothes and willingness to do so [31]. It is difficult enough for a person in psychiatric distress or suffering from psychosis to be in a loud and chaotic ED [11]; there should be a way to dim lights in the patient cubicles at night, as the Brackenridge Hospital Emergency Department does in Austin, Texas, while permitting sufficient lighting at nurses' stations, security guard outposts, and in the halls. At least one class action lawsuit against psychiatric EDs raised unending bright lights as an issue; dimmed lights at night was one of the provisions of the settlement (see Chapter 48).

Address nonclinical reasons for delay in mental health evaluations

ED delays are at least partially responsible for psychiatric patients wishing to leave AMA [10]. These delays have several causes, some of which can be addressed. As mentioned above, it should be clear that the on-call mental health professional is expected to come at night. Rather than wait for medical clearances before even calling a mental health professional to perform an evaluation, EDs should consider conducting the evaluations concurrently, or at least calling the psychiatric consult while the medical clearance is ongoing. The clearance need not be extensive for many patients. There are several protocols articulating streamlined medical clearances for patients with low risk factors [38,39]. Elaborate medical clearances are often done simply because psychiatric hospitals require them to agree to admit the patient. Treatment for patients with psychiatric needs is delayed to the point that some decide to leave; the inflexible insistence on medical testing by receiving hospitals frustrates the very treatment that these hospitals were designed to provide.

Peers in the ED

The single research paper that examined initiatives to reduce leaving AMA from a psychiatric inpatient unit found that the presence of a patient advocate accomplished this goal [40,41]. Some EDs, such as Maine Medical Center, Regions Hospital in Minneapolis, Kingston Hospital and King's County Hospital in New York, use "peers" – individuals with psychiatric disabilities who understand and can provide support, including help making phone calls [41,42]. While many hospitals resist the introduction of peers in the ED, the hospitals that use them have been pleased with the additional attention available to psychiatric patients, who often want to talk at greater length than is comfortable for ED staff. Reassuring patients, providing them company, and assisting with worry and stress about external obligations can reduce the likelihood of leaving AMA and increase cooperation in assessment and diagnostic procedures.

Reward staff who work well with psychiatric patients

Clinical literature on patients who leave AMA emphasize the importance of communication skills [1,40]. It is important for all ED staff (including security guards) to receive at least some training in how to interact with people who have psychiatric disabilities, and especially to understand the different approaches needed with different conditions [11]. Most EDs use at least one or two staff who are known to have particular talents or gifts at working with psychiatric patients: doctors who understand the symbolic importance of sitting down and slowing down when they speak to psychiatric patients who are dissatisfied; nurses who are flexible and kind; security guards who can persuade patients to return to their cubicles using words instead of restraints. Yet, these staff members are rarely recognized and rewarded for these exceptional skills. The author visited one psychiatric emergency service where the hospital paid for a janitor who clearly had outstanding patient skills to obtain her nursing license as an LPN. This was clearly a win–win situation for the woman, the hospital, and the patients. Rewards need not be this dramatic, but if hospital leadership takes visible steps to recognize and reward staff members with these skills, they will accomplish an informal but very effective training for all staff.

Mitigating potential harm and/or liability when a psychiatric patient leaves AMA

Sometimes, the best course of action, especially with a patient already known to ED staff, is not to engage in a conflict over whether the patient should leave, but to urge the patient to return if his or her problems are not resolved. Good patient care and reinforcement of treatment alliances should not be undermined by fear of liability over the potential consequences of permitting a psychiatric patient to depart AMA [14]. There are ways to both try to minimize the risk of potential harm to the patient who is departing AMA and to limit liability for adverse outcomes when a patient leaves AMA and comes to harm.

Minimizing the risk of potential harm to the patient

Happily, some of the techniques to minimize the risk of potential harm to the patient also assist in insulating a facility and its staff against liability. For example, documentation of competence assessment, robust and specific information at discharge, follow-up appointments (with concurrent inquiries or arrangements about transportation to ensure the patient can actually make the appointment), and follow-up with any test results that come in after the patient's discharge, is important and should be documented [15,26]. Patients should be urged to come back if they change their mind.

In addition, often a patient's presentation in psychiatric crisis to an ED reflects not simply an individual crisis, but a crisis in the patient's system of support, e.g., his or her family, landlord, group home, or school. Often these individuals are present in the ED. As Drs. Factor and Diamond suggest, they should be involved (with the patient's permission) in formulating discharge plans and constructive resolution of the problems that triggered the presentation [43]. Drs. Factor and Diamond outline specific strategies to work with all parties to resolve conflicts that brought the patient to the ED. This may prevent harm or even reduce the possibility of an immediate return to the ED, especially when the patient's presentation was instigated by family members, whose anger and frustration with having the respite they envisioned by the patient's admission may sabotage successful return to the community.

Minimizing the risk of liability for adverse outcomes

First, courts are generally hostile to litigation by patients or their estates seeking to recover from hospitals for adverse consequences resulting from a patient's departure AMA. This is true even in relatively extreme fact situations: a doctor barring the door to prevent a patient who left AMA from returning to seek care [37]; a prisoner discharged AMA when the hospital's tests showed he had diabetic ketoacidosis, a condition which predictably would (and did) prove fatal [15]; or an 80-year-old stroke victim who was allowed to leave AMA and suffered a second stroke shortly thereafter [29].

In some states, such as Alabama, a patient's leaving AMA could mean that the patient was "contributorily negligent" or "assumed the risk" for any adverse outcome associated with leaving AMA [15].

Of course, all of this assumes that the fact that the patient left AMA, rather than being discharged by a physician, is well documented. Before an ED patient with an emergency medical condition leaves AMA, EMTALA, as well as the standard of care, require the physician to inform the patient of the risks of leaving, and document that the patient was informed. Cases in which the hospital claims that the patient left AMA but cannot substantiate it with documentary evidence tend to result in plaintiff verdicts [44]; at the very least, the absence of the AMA form is a significant issue at trial [45].

Especially in the case of psychiatric patients who have been given sedating medication, a hospital has no right to hold a competent, nondangerous person who wishes to leave, but specific warnings about driving or undertaking similar tasks should be given (repeatedly) and documented [46].

In cases of doubt regarding competence to sign out AMA, it is always helpful to ask for a consultation, especially when collateral sources such as family members or an individual's therapist are advocating involuntary detention. Of course, obtaining a consultation means that the results of this consultation should be heeded; several cases premise liability on the failure to follow the recommendations generated by the consultation [23]. By the same token, consultations that support the professional's decision are protective.

Conclusion

The reasons that psychiatric patients leave AMA are important in determining whether and how to reduce them. Psychiatric patients departing AMA can simply reflect the gap between the need for treatment and the involuntary commitment standard. If no psychiatric patient is leaving AMA, the ED is probably overcommitting patients. It could be that departures AMA do not reflect anything about the ED. Psychiatric patients may simply be more difficult to persuade than medical patients that inpatient hospitalization will benefit them.

To the extent that departure AMA reflects anger and frustration at delay, the ED environment, or differential staff treatment of medical and psychiatric patients, it can be a quality control marker offering useful data about ways to improve hospital care.

There is no question that the departure of psychiatric patients AMA raises concern among ED staff about bad outcomes and potential litigation. This concern should not interfere with good clinical practice that respects the rights of competent patients to make their own treatment decisions. Courts understand that the ED is not a guarantor of good outcomes. If ED physicians and mental health professionals simply engage in thoughtful assessment, listening to the patient and treating him or her with respect and concern, paying particular attention to medical complaints of psychiatric patients, their patients will benefit.

References

1. Alfrandre DJ. "I'm going home": discharges against medical advice. *Mayo Clin Proc* 2009;**84**:255–60.

2. Stefan S. *Emergency Department Treatment of the Psychiatric Patient: Policy Issues and Legal Requirements*. New York: Oxford University Press; 2006.

3. Department of Health and Human Services, Center for Medicare and Medicaid Services. Proposed changes to the hospital inpatient prospective payment systems for acute care hospitals and the long-term care hospital prospective payment system and fiscal year 2012 rates: proposed rule. *Fed Regist* 2011;**76**:257–88.

4. Ding R, Jung JJ, Kirsch TD, et al. Uncompleted emergency department care: patients who leave against medical advice. *Acad Emerg Med* 2007;**14**:870–6.

5. Johnson v. Nacogdoches County Hospital. 2003 Tex.App.LEXIS 7230 (August 20, 2003).

6. Correa v. San Francisco Hospital. 69 F.3d 1184 (1st Cir. 1995).

7. Brook M, Hilty DM, Liu W, et al. Discharge against medical advice from inpatient psychiatric treatment: a literature review. *Psychiatr Serv* 2006;**57**:1192–8.

8. Ruiz v. XYZ Hospital. 1997 FL Jury Verdicts Review LEXIS 512 (April 1997).

9. Monico E, Schwartz I. Leaving against medical advice: facing the issue in the emergency department. *J Healthc Risk Manag* 2009;**29**:6–9, 13, 15.

10. Jayaram G, Triplett D. Quality improvement of psychiatric care: challenges of emergency psychiatry. *Am J Psychiatry* 2008;**165**:1256–60.

11. Gilbert S. Psychiatric crash cart: treatments for the emergency department. *Adv Emerg Nurs J* 2009;**31**:298–308.

12. Taylor DM, Wolfe R, Cameron PA. Complaints from emergency department patients largely result from treatment and communication problems. *Emerg Med* 2002;**14**:43–9.

13. Dubow D, Propp D, Narasinham K, Emergency department discharges against medical advice. *J Emerg Med* 1992;**10**:513–16.

14. Berlin JS, Stefan S. *Brief Documentation of Release/Mitigation of Risk.* (2011). Available from Dr. Jon Berlin, Milwaukee County Behavioral Health Division, 9455 Watertown Plank Road, Milwaukee, WI 53226.

15. Lyons v. Walker Regional Medical Center. 868 So.2d 1071 (Ala. 2003).

16. Washington v. Glucksberg. 521 U.S. 702 (1997).

17. James v. City of Wilkes-Barre. 2011 U.S. Dist.LEXIS 90575 (M.D.Pa. Aug. 15, 2011).

18. In re C.W., 105 Wn.App. 718 (2001), aff'd 147 Wn.2d 259 (2002).

19. Disability Rights Texas. *Mental Health Detention in an Emergency Room.* Available at: www.disabilityrightstx.org/ resources/healthcare (Accessed September 20, 2011).

20. Center for Public Representation. *Patients' Rights in Hospital Emergency Rooms.* Available at: www. centerforpublicrep.org/litigation-and-major-cases/emergency-rooms. (Accessed October 1, 2011).

21. Woods v. Commonwealth of Kentucky. 142 SW3d 24 (Ky.2004).

22. In re Estate of Austwick, 275 Ill.App.3d 275 (Ill.App. 1995).

23. Thomas v. Christ Hospital and Medical Center. 328 F.3d 890 (7th Cir. 2003).

24. Miller v. Rhode Island Hospital. **625** A.2d 778 (R.I.1993).

25. In re Estate of Allen, 365 Ill.App.3^d 378 (2006).

26. Appelbaum P. Assessment of patients' competence to consent to treatment. *N Engl J Med* 2007;**357**:1834–40.

27. Appelbaum P, Guttheil T. *Clinical Handbook of Psychiatry and the Law,* (4th Edition). Philadelphia: Lippincott, Williams and Wilkins; 2006.

28. Etchells E, Darzins P, Silberfeld M, et al. Assessment of patient capacity to consent to treatment. *J Gen Intern Med* 1999;**14**:27–34.

29. Cavender v. Sutter Lakeside Hospital. 2005 U.S.Dist.LEXIS 33766 (N.D.Ca. Sept. 6, 2005).

30. Joint Commission on Accreditation of Health Care Organizations. *Accreditation Issues for Emergency Departments.* Chicago: Joint Commission Press; 2003.

31. Maryland Disability Law Center and the Center for Public Representation. *Maryland Citizens in Psychiatric Crisis: Improving Emergency Department, and Community Care for People with Psychiatric Disabilities.* Baltimore: Maryland Disability Law Center; 2007.

32. Hartman RG. Coming of age: devising legislation for adolescent decision-making. *Am J Law Med* 2002;**28**:409–53.

33. In re LJMS, 844 SW2d 86 (Mo.App. 1992).

34. Miller v. HCA. 118 SW3rd 75 (Tx.2003).

35. Lukens TW, Wolf SJ, Edlow JA, et al. Clinical policy: critical issues in the diagnosis and management of adult psychiatric patients in the emergency department. *Ann Emerg Med* 2006;**47**:79–99.

36. Lincoln A. Psychiatric emergency room decision-making, social control, and the 'undeserving sick.' *Sociol Health Illn* 2006;**28**:54–75.

37. Pugh v. Doctors Medical Center. 2010 U.S.DistLEXIS 71807 (N.D.Ca. July 16, 2010).

38. Massachusetts College of Emergency Physicians. *Consensus Statement on Medical Clearance.* Available at: www. macep.org/practice_information_ medical_clearance.htm (Accessed on October 1, 2011)

39. Zun LS, Downey L. Application of a medical clearance protocol. *Prim Psychiatry* 2007;**14**:47–51.

40. Targum SD, Capodanno AE, Hoffman HA, Foudraine C. An intervention to reduce the rate of hospital discharges against medical advice. *Am J Psychiatry* 1982;**139**:657–9.

41. The Amistad Community. *Our Programs: Emergency Room at Maine Medical Center.* Available at: www. amistadinc.org/programs/php (Accessed Sept. 30, 2011).

42. MI Watch. *Peer Counselors Support Consumers in Emergency Rooms.* Available at: www.miwatch.org/2010/ 08/peer_counselors_support_con sumers_in_emergency_room.htm (Accessed September 29, 2011).

43. Factor R, Diamond R. Emergency psychiatry and conflict resolution. In: Vaccarro JV, Clark GH, (Eds.). *Practicing Psychiatry in the Community: A Manual.* Arlington: American Psychiatric Press; 1996: 51–76.

44. Parker v. Florida Emergency Physicians. Case No. CI99–3260, 2000 Medical Litig. Alert LEXIS 2100 (April 11, 2000).

45. Thomas v. Hardwick. 231 P.3d 1111 (Nev. 2010).

46. Young v. Gastro-Intestinal Center. **361** Ark. 209 (2005).

47. Sklar DP, Loeliger E, Edmunds K. Unanticipated death following discharge to home from emergency department. *Ann Emerg Med* 2007;**49**:735–45.

Chapter

45

Best practices for the evaluation and treatment of patients with mental and substance use illness in the emergency department

Maureen Slade, Deborah Taber, Jerrold B. Leikin, and MaryLynn McGuire Clarke

Required disclaimer

The information contained in this Report reflects the views of the authors of the research cited and of the members of the Illinois Hospital Association Behavioral Health Constituency Section Steering Committee and its Best Practices Task Force. The "best practices" described in this Report are offered to aid in the consideration and discussion of practices that might be appropriate for an institution, based upon the circumstances at that institution. They do not constitute either clinical or legal advice. It is also important to remember that "best practices" reflect current knowledge and practice, and necessarily evolve with time and experience. Significant portions of this chapter were published in Disease-a-Month, 2007;**53**: 536–580 under the title of "Best Practices for the Treatment of Patients with Mental and Substance Use Illnesses in the Emergency Department" authored by Illinois Hospital Association Behavioral Health Constituency Section Steering Committee and its Best Practices Task Force: Slade M, Taber D co-chairs.

Introduction

The Illinois Hospital Association (IHA) Behavioral Health Steering Committee established a Task Force on Best Practices in 2006. As its initial project, the committee chose the emergency department (ED). Its charge was to (1) examine from a clinical perspective emergency care delivered in Illinois hospital EDs to patients with mental or substance use disorders; (2) research the literature and evidence-based/best practices for emergency services, as applied to patients with these conditions; (3) identify models of care and practices used in Illinois hospitals that were viewed by the committee as being exemplary or worthy of note; and (4) keeping in mind the six aims of quality health care articulated by the Institute of Medicine, to make recommendations about practices that could be used in EDs.

This Report considered the following: the structure of EDs; common staffing, patient flow, ED settings such as the physical design and layout, including whether or not there are separate spaces designated for psychiatric patients; the literature relevant to best practices and evidence-based practices related to the treatment of patients [1–7] with mental illness and substance use

disorders in the hospital ED; survey of a representative sample of hospital EDs about systems of care, structural and operational components in their respective EDs; and made recommendations about practices and structures that benefit patients. The committee also identified areas for future research.

This chapter is a summation of the findings of the task force. It is designed to be a treatise of current practice structure and recommendations for the best practice for the care of the patient in EDs throughout the country. The chapter reviews the current process for protocols, staffing, and space and made recommendations concerning the following.

Protocols

Across the board, hospitals surveyed indicate there are no differences between the treatment protocols for general psychiatric patients and substance abuse patients, with the exception of a patient's level of intoxication requiring medical intervention. Larger urban/suburban hospitals reported a significant number of dual diagnosis patients more so than rural hospitals.

Space

In most facilities, psychiatric patients are housed in regular ED rooms or bays, either near a nursing station or with a security officer. Hospitals with a dedicated space transfer psychiatric patients to the area after medical clearance, using regular ED beds for overflow as necessary. Nearly every facility requested either a dedicated area, if they did not have one, or an expansion of existing space if they did.

Staff

In most facilities the patient receives medical care, such as medications, from the general ED nursing staff and psychiatric staff evaluate the patient's psychiatric symptoms (typically Licensed Clinical Social Workers [LCSWs]). However, only in the large facilities found in urban settings does care and monitoring after medical clearance become the responsibility of the psychiatric staff. This can be attributed to the fact that most of the smaller rural hospitals rely on Community Mental Health Centers (CMHCs) to do psychiatric evaluations and do not

Behavioral Emergencies for the Emergency Physician, ed. Leslie S. Zun, Lara G. Chepenik, and Mary Nan S. Mallory. Published by Cambridge University Press. © Cambridge University Press 2013.

have trained psychiatric personnel on staff 24 hours a day, 7 days a week (24/7).

Also evident is the fact that the smaller hospitals tend to have more entry level trained staff, if any, other than consultants. Some of the larger urban facilities are using highly skilled, advanced degree personnel such as Psychiatric Advanced Practice Nurses for the majority of their 24/7 staffing patterns; some even staff Board Certified Psychiatrists for regular hours in the ED.

Triage

Triage is a brief intervention that occurs when a patient initially presents to the ED during which the patient is interviewed to help determine the nature and severity of his or her illness. Patients with acute illnesses are admitted to the department more rapidly than those with less severe symptoms or injuries. The brief intervention should include, but is not limited to, the patient's or significant other's description of presenting symptoms or complaints, vital signs, and an assignment of disposition based on gathered information (Table 45.1).

Smart et al. developed a Mental Health Triage Scale (MHTS) which integrated psychiatric patients into the National Triage Scale (NTS) used throughout EDs in Australia (Table 45.2). The authors stated, "Motivating factors for the development of the mental health triage scale included a perceived unfairness in the way mental health presentations were integrated leading to long delays in medical assessment and long transit times."

Coupled with comprehensive training of the nurses, staff using the MHTS reported they felt well equipped and more confident, reporting a greater understanding of mental health presentations. The mean waiting time was reduced from 34.3 minutes (26.4 minutes for medical patients) to 29.1 minutes. Proper triage level also positively impacted mean time to disposition which was reduced from 149.2 minutes to 131.8 minutes. Through education and implementation of a mental health triage scale, the authors realized for their 306 patients over a 3-month period, a reduction of 88.9 patient hours (Tables 45.2 and 45.3) [12].

Table 45.1. National Triage Scale for emergency departments in Australia

National Triage Scale	Numerical code	Treatment acuity: Time to be seen by a doctor	Color code
Resuscitation	1	Immediate	Red
Emergency	2	10 Minutes	Orange
Urgent	3	30 Minutes	Green
Semi-urgent	4	60 Minutes	Blue
Non-urgent	5	2 Hours	White

Source: Smart, D., Pollard, C. & Walpole, B. (1999). Mental health triage in emergency medicine. Australian and New Zealand Journal of Psychiatry, 33:57–66. Reproduced with permission.

Recommendations for triage

The Task Force strongly recommends the use of a predetermined triage system or scale to ensure timely and appropriate evaluation and treatment of psychiatric patients.

Table 45.2. Mental Health Triage Scale[*]

Triage category	Patient description	Treatment acuity
2 "Emergency"	Patient is violent, aggressive or suicidal, or is a danger to self or others, requires police escort	Within 10 minutes
3 "Urgent"	Very distressed or acutely psychotic, likely to be aggressive, may be a danger to self or others	Within 30 minutes
4 "Semi-urgent"	Long-standing or semi-urgent mental health disorder and/or has supporting agency/escort present	Within 1 hour
5 "Non-urgent"	Patient has a long-standing or non-acute mental disorder/problem but has no supportive agency/escort – may require a referral to an appropriate community resource.	Within 2 hours

[*]It is considered advantageous to "up-triage" mental health patients with carers present because carers' assistance facilitates more rapid assessment.

Source: Smart, D., Pollard, C. & Walpole, B. (1999). Mental health triage in emergency medicine. Australian and New Zealand Journal of Psychiatry, 33:57–66. Reproduced with permission

Table 45.3. Factors considered in assigning mental health triage categories

i.	Manifest behavioral disturbance
ii.	Presence of or threatened deliberate self-harm
iii.	Perceived or objective level of suicidal ideation
iv.	Patient's current level of distress
v.	Perceived level of danger to self or others
vi.	Need for physical restraint/accompanied by police
vii.	Disturbances of perception
viii.	Manifest evidence of psychosis
ix.	Level of situational crisis
x.	Descriptions of behavior disturbance in the community
xi.	Current level of community support
xii.	Presence of carer/supportive adult

The first six factors favor triage to categories 2 or 3.

Source: Smart, D., Pollard, C. & Walpole, B. (1999). Mental health triage in emergency medicine. Australian and New Zealand Journal of Psychiatry, 33:57–66. Reproduced with permission.

Medical clearance

The term "medical screening" is frequently used interchangeably with "medical assessment." For our purposes, we will define medical screening as a determination of need for further evaluation, however, to establish the existence of an emergency medical illness or condition by a physician or, in limited cases, another qualified medical person. During the medical assessment the ED physician would conduct a history and physical examination, determine if the patient is intoxicated or under the influence of a drug, establish if the patient's symptoms are caused by or exacerbated by a medical illness, and stabilize any acute medical illness that necessitates intervention.

It is generally accepted that "medical clearance" occurs after completion of the medical assessment and any pertinent laboratory or radiological tests to conclude there is no organic etiology. The patient is considered, within reasonable medical probability, to be medically stable and to have the appropriate cognitive status to undergo psychiatric evaluation. Medical clearance does not indicate the absence of ongoing medical issues that can be easily managed and that will not interfere with psychiatric evaluation and treatment. If such conditions exist, the clearing physician should include the recommended level of medical observation and treatment.

Lukens et al., from the American College of Emergency Physicians, published a clinical policy in 2006 for the adult psychiatric patient in the ED [13]. The authors recommend using the term "focused medical assessment" as they believe the term "medical clearance" can suggest different things to psychiatrists and emergency physicians. They believe the term "focused medical assessment" better approximates the process "in which a medical etiology for the patient's symptoms is excluded and all other illness and/or injury in need of acute care is determined and treated." The authors recognized "a difficult aspect of the focused medical assessment is clearly determining when a patient is not only medically stable, but has the cognitive status suitable for the psychiatric interview."

According to Zun, the components of the medical clearance process include taking a history and conducting a physical examination, a mental status examination, testing, when appropriate, and treatment, when necessary. He notes there is no clearly accepted protocol adopted by emergency physicians as to the standard procedures to perform on psychiatric patients presenting to the ED [14].

Notwithstanding this, a decade ago a group of psychiatrists and emergency physicians in Illinois developed a mutually agreeable protocol for the medical clearance process that occurs in EDs for patients with psychiatric complaints. The group authored a paper on the process that evolved into a medical clearance checklist, this checklist may be found in Appendix A [15]. The medical clearance checklist was designed to walk the emergency physician through the process and provide the psychiatrist assurance that the patient had an adequate medical clearance process. The checklist does not require any testing, unless the patient has a new onset of psychiatric illness. The checklist has been tested in a before and after study, finding no difference compared to the emergency physician's usual assessment [16]. The usual medical clearance performed by emergency physicians and that required by psychiatrists varies from physician to physician but there is a discordance of testing between specialists [17]. Another study demonstrated that the costs were significantly reduced by using this medical clearance protocol [18].

In 2003 the Massachusetts College of Emergency Medicine, together with the Massachusetts Psychiatric Society, published a Consensus Statement on medical clearance exams that also challenges the use of the term but deemed it too "ingrained" to eradicate. Massachusetts is one of at least two states where emergency physicians and psychiatrists worked together to reach consensus on guidelines for medical clearance. The Task Force found this document useful. It is included in Appendix B in its entirety [19].

Recommendations for medical assessment/clearance

The Task Force solidly endorses the use of the term "focused medical assessment" in place of medical clearance but, like our Massachusetts Colleagues, believes that it is likely too deeply embedded in ED culture to be changed.

The Task Force also strongly endorses the Consensus Statement on Medical Clearance from the Massachusetts College of Emergency Medicine and the Massachusetts Psychiatric Society.

The Task Force endorses the protocols of the "Psychiatric Medical Clearance Checklist".

Patients with substance use disorders or co-occurring substance use and psychiatric disorders

We recognize that many patients presenting to the ED abuse drugs or alcohol, and these drugs may mask or exacerbate other psychiatric symptoms. For purposes of this paper we are defining terms and care levels for these patients as follows: Intoxication is a nervous system abnormality (usually involving the central nervous system) due to a drug. Inebriation is the inability to perform activities of daily living (ADL) due to a drug. Impairment is an increased risk for being involved in an accident [15].

Intoxication without psychiatric illness or chemical dependence: The patient is simply under the influence of a drug and intoxicated and does not require psychiatric intervention and should remain solely a patient of the medical portion of the ED.

Intoxication, primary chemical dependence diagnosis, without psychiatric illness: The patient should be maintained in the medical portion of the ED until he/she is deemed to be sober enough to undergo psychiatric assessment. In most instances this patient will require referral to an addictions treatment facility.

Intoxication with co-morbid psychiatric illness and chemical dependence: The patient should be maintained in the medical portion of the ED until he/she is deemed to be sober enough to undergo psychiatric assessment. A patient who is inebriated cannot undergo psychiatric assessment.

In the article, Clinical policy: Critical Issues in the Diagnosis and Management of the Adult Psychiatric Patient in the Emergency Department, the authors [13] consider issues surrounding testing in alert patients with normal vital signs; urine drug screens; point of time at which a psychiatric exam can be conducted in an intoxicated patient; and the most effective pharmacologic treatments for acutely agitated patients. Their recommendations are based on a thorough review of the literature and the guidance of physicians with relevant clinical experience. Their recommendations for patient management are classified according to their level of clinical certainty, which reflects the strength of the evidence of the literature: Level A is a high degree of clinical certainty, level B is a moderate degree of clinical certainty, and level C strategies are based on preliminary, inconclusive, or conflicting evidence, or committee consensus.

For purposes of this chapter, we are focusing on the recommendations of Lukens et al. related to urine drug screens and the time to conduct the psychiatric evaluation in an intoxicated patient. The specific question posed and answered is as follows: "Do the results of a urine drug screen for drugs of abuse affect management in alert, cooperative patients with normal vital signs, a noncontributory history and physical examination, and a psychiatric complaint?" Ranking this issue as Level C, they concluded that routine urine toxicologic screens do not affect ED management and need not be performed as part of the assessment. They also conclude that if these tests are performed for a receiving psychiatric facility, they should not delay patient evaluation or transfer [13]. The Massachusetts College of Emergency Medicine and the Massachusetts Psychiatric Society Joint Task Force reached a similar conclusion that drug screens of medically stable psychiatric patients should not delay transfers of patients to psychiatric facilities [19].

Regarding the initiation of a psychiatric evaluation of a cooperative patient with normal vital signs and a noncontributory history and physical examination, the authors conclude that "The patient's cognitive abilities, rather than a specific blood alcohol level, should be the basis on which clinicians begin the psychiatric assessment." They further recommend that the clinician use a "period of observation to determine if psychiatric symptoms resolve as the episode of intoxication resolves" [13]. In making this Level C recommendation, they note that there are no evidence-based data to support a specific blood alcohol concentration at which the psychiatric evaluation should begin. They further note that there are no studies that show an individual regains adequate decision-making capacity when he or she reaches the legal limit for driving. There also is no evidence in the literature to support the delay of the evaluation.

> **Recommendations related to urine toxicology screens**
>
> Routine urine toxicologic screens need not be performed as part of assessment (in medically stable patients); Drug screens should not delay patient transfers to psychiatric facilities.

> **Recommendations regarding laboratory tests**
>
> The examining physician should determine whether and what tests to order based on the patient's presentation.

> **Recommendations related to time at which to conduct**
>
> **The psychiatric assessment of an intoxicated patient**
>
> The patient's cognitive abilities, rather than a specific blood alcohol level, should be the basis upon which psychiatric assessment begins.

Medications

In response to Task Force inquiries of emergency physicians in Illinois, we found that they generally do not endorse standard medications for psychiatric patients. The American College of Emergency Physicians do make limited recommendations for agitated patients who may or may not have a psychiatric illness such as the use of benzodiazepines (lorazepam or midazolam) and/or an oral antipsychotic (risperidone) for agitated and cooperative patients [13].

> **Recommendations regarding medications**
>
> Psychiatrists on the Task Force and with substantive experience in managing the acutely decompensated psychiatric patient report using the following medications:
>
> - Acutely agitated (non-psychotic) patients – oral benzodiazepine
> - Acutely agitated (not psychotic) and uncooperative with oral medications – IM benzodiazepine
> - Acutely agitated, psychotic, cooperative – dissolving oral antipsychotic (Zyprexa Zydis or Risperdal M tabs)
> - Acutely agitated, psychotic, uncooperative – injection of Zyprexa IM or haloperidol IM
> - Psychiatric history, without agitation but with other presenting symptoms such as irritability or anxiety – benzodiapine for anxiety or antipsychotic for psychotic symptoms.
>
> Finally, the Task Force notes that the use of benztropine whenever haloperidol is given to reduce the possibility of a dystonic reaction. Although the occurrence rate is low, it can be such an unpleasant experience for the patient that it may discourage them from future medication use.

Emergency psychiatric evaluation

The American Psychiatric Association in 2006 adopted Practice Guidelines for the Psychiatric Evaluation of Adults [20] which set forth parameters of practice for several different types of psychiatric evaluations and examination, including the emergency psychiatric evaluation. The guideline notes that there are several specific approaches to the emergency psychiatric evaluation, and that they include the following:

1. Assess and enhance the safety of the patient and others.
2. Establish a provisional diagnosis (or diagnoses) of the mental disorder(s) most likely to be responsible for the current emergency, including identification of any general medical condition(s) or substance use that is causing or contributing to the patient's mental condition.
3. Identify family or other involved persons who can give information that will help the psychiatrist determine the accuracy of reported history, particularly if the patient is cognitively impaired, agitated, or psychotic and has difficulty communicating a history of events. If the patient is to be discharged back to family members or other caretaking persons, their ability to care for the patient and their understanding of the patient's needs must be addressed.
4. Identify any current treatment providers who can give information relevant to the evaluation.
5. Identify social, environmental, and cultural factors relevant to immediate treatment decisions.
6. Determine whether the patient is able and willing to form an alliance that will support further assessment and treatment, what precautions are needed if there is a substantial risk of harm to self or others, and whether involuntary treatment is necessary.
7. Develop a specific plan for follow-up, including immediate treatment and disposition; determine whether the patient requires treatment in a hospital or other supervised setting and what follow-up will be required if the patient is not placed in a supervised setting.

> **Recommendation regarding emergency psychiatric assessment**
>
> The Task Force agrees with the recommendations of APA regarding the Emergency Psychiatric Assessment.

Throughput

According to the Illinois Hospital Association's 2005 Emergency Department Utilization Survey, 59% of Illinois hospitals reported that their throughput times in the ED had increased between 2002 and 2004. The average wait time was 163 minutes with a median of 144 minutes, an average increase of 5.4%. According to the report, only 9.6% of hospitals maintain statistics specifically for behavioral health patients, but of those that did, the average turnaround time was 297 minutes. The longest throughput times take place in large urban areas. Also of note is that hospitals that provide psychiatric services reported longer throughputs in the ED than those that do not provide services. The hospitals with inpatient psychiatric services reported an increase in throughput time in the ED of 11%.

The largest reported influencing factor for increases in throughput time was difficulty in finding placement, including placement at State Operated Hospitals (SOHs). Reporting hospitals also cited increases in total patient volume and behavioral

health volume; insufficient staffing in the ED; and procedures instituted with Screening Assessment and Support Services (SASS) and Crisis and Referral Entry Services (CARES) systems, a state-mandated prescreening program for youth.

As this survey and experience would indicate, increased ED throughput time is related to both extrinsic and intrinsic factors. Many of the extrinsic factors in our environment, such as a lack of sufficient substance abuse facilities or insufficient inpatient acute psychiatric beds, confound our ability to expedite a disposition for the psychiatric patient. Yet, if we are to deliver patient-centered care that recognizes the essential connection between mental and overall health, we must address disparities between mental and physical health. Differences in throughput or wait times in the ED for psychiatric, substance abuse, and other medical patients is a disparity that is worthy of our attention and study.

> **Recommendations regarding throughput**
>
> In the interest of creating a seamless system of care for all of our patients, the Task Force recommends that hospitals measure and evaluate the variance in throughput for psychiatric and other medical patients, in order to better understand those factors contributing to longer lengths of stay in the ED and to determine ways in which throughput can be improved.

Staffing

Larger hospitals with a significant number of psychiatric presentations have dedicated psychiatric staff to assess and treat patients within the ED. The Task Force recognizes that facilities in rural areas as well as those with low psychiatric presentations, may consider alternate forms of treating the psychiatric patient who presents to the ED. Many of the facilities use non-medical staff, such as ED social workers or use a licensed mental health professional for consultation services. It is not uncommon for facilities to use a combination of approaches when caring for psychiatrically ill patients. For example, a social worker may be on duty for 16 hours per day and a consultant on call for the remaining 8 hours. Although none of the facilities the Task Force surveyed used a mobile assessment team, the concept is a viable one and is successful in other areas either in lieu of or as an adjunct to ED care or as a mechanism to prevent ED presentations by linking the patient directly from the community to the proper level of care. When considering the needs of the state of Illinois, the Task Force found the following table to be a reasonable guideline [21].

One large urban facility commented that although their bed size was over 500, their psychiatric presentations were far lower than most urban hospitals. They cautioned that percentage of psychiatric presentations should also be considered when determining the appropriate model and space for each facility. The Task Force does not consider bed numbers to be an absolute guideline. Each facility needs to factor in their unique characteristics. For example, downstate hospitals may draw from a

Table 45.4. Models of emergency psychiatric services to emergency departments

	Staffing cost	Hospital size	Mental Health take early responsibility	Acceptance by ED staff	ED staff mental health skills
Consultation model CAT or CL Service	+	<250 beds	No	+	+++
ED based mental health nurses	++	250–500 beds	No	++	++
Psychiatric Emergency Centre	+++	>500 beds	Yes	+++	+

a+, low; ++,medium; +++,high.
CAT – Crisis and Assessment Team, CL – Consultation Liaison, ED – Emergency Department
Source: Frank R, Fawcett L, Emmerson B. Development of Australia's first psychiatric emergency centre. Australasian Psychiatry. 2005;13:266–72. Reproduced with permission.

broader geographic area, that combined with a Level I or Level II trauma level designation of the facility may indicate a model that differs from what is recommended by the corresponding bed size.

> **Recommendations regarding staffing**
>
> Facilities with significant psychiatric presentations should consider dedicated, psychiatrically trained staff.

Physical space

No matter the size or location of the facility, patient safety, privacy, and comfort should be paramount in the psychiatric ED. Most EDs struggle with lack of patient privacy. Proximity of bays or rooms, overflow patients in half-beds in corridors all contribute to not only lack of privacy but an environment that exacerbates some patients' illnesses.

Some psychiatric patients are vulnerable to the environment of the waiting room. Often crowded, noisy and sometimes chaotic, the waiting room can aggravate psychiatric symptoms. Although most facilities report trying to place agitated patients into a room immediately, a quiet room or separate waiting area for psychiatric patients is ideal. In an article in the *International Journal of Mental Health Nursing*, Timothy Wand cautions that we should take care not to "generate the impression of a segregated system of healthcare that further stigmatizes mental health" by completely separating the psychiatric component from the ED [22]. However, providing "special care areas" within the ED for those in need is optimal. One hospital calls their dedicated psychiatric rooms "SNUs" – Special Needs Units, and another hospital has both a separate low stimulus waiting area available as well as a "family friendly" interview room.

With time in the ED increasing, comfort is a concern. Many facilities report throughput of well over 8 hours with the patient in a stark environment. Although most EDs are built for function and leave little room for ambiance, psychiatric rooms typically are even more austere by virtue of patient safety concerns. Most rooms contain only a bed – which often is fixed to the floor- and little else. It is important to consider what effect 8 hours in this environment will have on the patient. Some facilities report soft murals or subdued colors and decorative border trim in the rooms. One facility has an enclosed television in the room for the patient, and another has a small table and chair fixed to the floor in the corner of the room. This allows the patient an alternate to the bed/gurney to take a meal at the table or sit with staff to fill out paperwork. Any furniture that does go into the room should be stationary and not pose any type of potential physical harm to the patient.

Sometimes, it may be possible to prevent an inpatient psychiatric admission by stabilizing the patient psychiatrically. For example, there could be beds devoted to a 24–48 hour stay for crisis stabilization and linkage to appropriate level of care. It is imperative that the physical space be designed to effectively care and treat these patients while maintaining their safety; and the environment should be soothing and supportive.

Safety: Keeping a patient safe from harm is our obligation; however, doing so may require the use of restraints or seclusion when a patient is at risk of immediate physical harm to himself or to others. These devices only should be considered when all other less restrictive alternatives have been considered and applied by staff trained in their safe use, pursuant to federal and state law. It is essential that each facility have the means to safely contain an agitated patient, ideally, in a room which can function as a seclusion room, if necessary. If this physical space is not possible, a patient room/area should have a stationary or fixable bed and ensure privacy.

In addition to the staff that evaluates the patients, facilities may use security or public safety officers to monitor the safety of patients in the ED. Smaller facilities that lack sufficient security support may rely on local police to assist with violent patients. Some areas also rely on specially trained police officers (e.g., Crisis Intervention Teams) to assess disturbances in which a mentally ill individual may require evaluation. EDs should work closely with hospital security and local police to establish protocols regarding the care of psychiatric patients and to maintain the safety of staff. Psychiatric rooms and/or staff should have panic alarms to summon emergency help. To deter elopement, psychiatric rooms and patients should not be housed near entrances/exits and should be in the direct line of sight of the nursing station, if not separately staffed.

Specially trained staff and dedicated space would be the ideal for the care of the psychiatric patient in the ED. Wherever this is not achievable, at a minimum, the model should include the assurance of patient privacy, comfort, and safety; qualified staff; and space that may range from a flexible room to an area specifically designed for psychiatric patients. Bed size is a fair predictor of needs, but when considering the impact psychiatric patients presenting to the ED will have on resources, it is just as pertinent to consider the number of psychiatric admissions, what types of mental health services are provided, and the complexity of associated responsibilities.

Recommendations for physical space, patient safety, and comfort

The physical space should be soothing and supportive, promote healing and help to de-escalate agitated and psychotic patients. For circumstances in which there is a question whether the patient meets medical necessity criteria for inpatient admission, provide special areas in the ED, or in an alternative location, in which that patient can remain from 24 to 48 hours for crisis stabilization and linkage to the appropriate level of treatment.

Additional recommendations

The following are additional recommendations related to the care of the psychiatric patient in the emergency department:

Referral source guide

The Task Force recommends every hospital maintain a comprehensive Referral Source Guide which contains at a minimum:

- Other area hospitals, including levels of treatment available
- Area treatment centers (such as substance abuse, psychiatric clinics), including diagnoses and populations they serve
- Area clinicians: discipline, specialty

Community Centers

- State Operated Facilities
- Other resources: Pastoral care, self-help groups, NAMI consumer guides.

Notations for each should include details such as ages served, diagnoses served, accepted funding sources, "catchment area" or network information, etc. Although local and state agencies do publish directories, the Task Force recommends each hospital maintain this smaller, readily available resource manual that details their respective area in a quick and concise manner.

Staff qualifications

According to American Psychiatric Association standards and The Illinois Mental Health and Developmental Disabilities

Code, psychiatric evaluations must be conducted by Licensed Independent Mental Health Practitioners/"qualified examiners" [23]. The IHA Emergency Department Utilization Survey revealed that most EDs that have access to staff trained in behavioral health typically use Licensed Clinical Social Workers (82.5%). All EDs have physicians and registered nurses; however, access to 24-hour behavioral health professionals is much more limited in hospitals that do not provide inpatient psychiatric services. Less than one fifth of these providers have 24-hour access to trained mental health personnel [1]. Not surprisingly, lack of psychiatric staff can contribute significantly to overall length of stay.

Staff education

In reviewing the Graduate Medical Education Guidelines for Emergency Medicine, minimal training in psychiatry is present. Most facilities with dedicated psychiatric staff find the medical ED staff have limited interaction with psychiatric patients as there is no need to hone these skills with trained personnel immediately available.

Surveyed hospitals reported few psychiatrically focused presentations, educational sessions, or professional consultations for the ED staff. Academic medical centers reported few grand rounds on psychiatric presentations in the ED, but those that did occur were not attended by ED staff. Wright et al. found that ED staff members with more training or "a personal connection to someone with a psychiatric problem increased the staff members subjective understanding of a mental health patient's needs" [24]. One urban academic medical center uses an Advance Practice Nurse as clinical coordinator within the ED. By means of patient coordination, this position provides both formal and informal education for the ED staff as well as fostering the relationship between the medical ED staff and the dedicated psychiatric staff. Wright et al. would contend that the improved relationships would change the organizational climate, thereby enhancing the ED staff's positive perception of their working environment. The authors found that "work group cooperation and facilitation emerged as the strongest predictor of more clinical involvement" with psychiatric patients [24].

Recommendations regarding staff qualifications, education, and training

Depending upon the model of service in use, if a hospital does not have dedicated, psychiatrically trained staff, the ED physicians, medical staff, and nursing staff need substantive training regarding psychiatric patients. This may include bringing in outside consultants to provide the training and education. The Task Force also recommends on-going continuing education for all medical and nursing staff in the ED staff regarding the care of the psychiatric patient.

This chapter did not consider legal issues associated with medical screening and stabilization under Emergency Medical

Treatment and Active Labor laws (EMTALA) or Mental Health Code requirements related to such issues as involuntary treatment or admission. It also did not address issues related to financing of ED services, which are significant, given the large number of ED patients who are uninsured or whose care is covered by public payors at below the cost to deliver it.

The Task Force recommended additional work be done to address the needs of older adults, and child and adolescent patients in the ED. We also recommended that attention be given to emerging technologies that are available to improve access to care, patient throughput, staff communication about patients in the ED, medication management and patient information in general. We are experiencing the rapid adoption of information and other patient technologies that promise new efficiencies and safer, evidence-based care. Electronic message boards in the ED, for example, provide up to the minute information about a patient's status, lab tests ordered, their status, and the time in which the patient has been in the ED. The use of telemedicine can bring psychiatrists and mental health professionals with special skills to rural communities, as well as to settings in which patients do not speak English or have physical handicaps. And finally, the best practice is that which delivers safe, effective, and compassionate care [25,26].

Appendix A Psychiatric Medical Clearance Checklist

	Yes	No
1. Does the patient have a new psychiatric condition?	☐	☐
2. Any history of active medical illness needing evaluation?	☐	☐
3. Any abnormal vital signs before transfer	☐	☐

Temperature >101°F

Pulse outside of 50 to 120 beats/min

Blood pressure systolic <90 or >200; diastolic >120

Respiratory rate >24 breaths/min

(for a pediatric patient, vital signs indices outside the normal range for his/her age and sex)

4. Any abnormal physical exam (unclothed)   ☐   ☐
    a. Absence of significant part of body, eg, limb
    b. Acute and chronic trauma (including signs of victimization/abuse)
    c. Breath sounds
    d. Cardiac dysrhythmia, murmurs
    e. Skin and vascular signs: diaphoresis, pallor, cyanosis, edema
    f. Abdominal distention, bowel sounds
    g. Neurological with particular focus on:

     i. ataxia
     ii. pupil symmetry, size
     iii. nystagmus
     iv. paralysis
     v. meningeal signs
     vi. reflexes

5. Any abnormal mental status indicating medical illness such as lethargic, stuporous, comatose, spontaneously fluctuating mental status?   ☐   ☐

If no to all of the above questions, no further evaluation is necessary. Go to question #9

If yes to any of the above questions go to question #6, tests may be indicated.

6. Were any labs done?   ☐   ☐
7. What lab tests were performed? _____

   What were the results? _____

   Possibility of pregnancy?   ☐   ☐

   What were the results? _____

8. Were X-rays performed?   ☐   ☐

   What kind of X-rays were performed? _____

   What were the results? _____

9. Was there any medical treatment needed by the patient before medical clearance?   ☐   ☐

   What treatment? _____

10. Has the patient been medically cleared in the ED?   ☐   ☐

11. Any acute medical condition that was adequately treated in the emergency department that allows transfer to a state operated psychiatric facility (SOF)   ☐   ☐

   What treatment? _____

12. Current medications and last administered? _____

13. Diagnoses: Psychiatric _____

   Medical_____

   Substance abuse _____

14. Medical follow-up or treatment required on psych floor or at SOF: _____

15. I have had adequate time to evaluate the patient and the patient's medical condition is sufficiently stable that transfer to ___SOF or ___ psych floor does not pose a significant risk of deterioration.

           (check one)

         _____MD/DO

          Physician Signature

Appendix B

The Massachusetts College of Emergency Medicine and the Massachusetts Psychiatric Society in 2003 developed consensus guidelines on the components of the medical clearance exam. We present it verbatim and in its entirety:

The Medical Clearance Exam

1. There was general agreement by task force members that the term medical clearance may convey unwarranted prospective security regarding the absence of any prospective medical risks. However, given the deeply ingrained use of the term, task force members felt it would not be possible to eliminate its use or introduce an alternative term.

2. Medical clearance reflects short-term but not necessarily long-term medical stability within the context of a transfer to a location with appropriate resources to monitor and treat what has been currently diagnosed.

3. Any patient with psychiatric complaints who is examined by the emergency physician should be assessed for significant contributing medical causes of those complaints. Medical clearance of patients with psychiatric complaints in an emergency facility should indicate that:

   - within reasonable medical certainty, there is no known contributory medical cause for the patient's presenting psychiatric complaints that requires acute intervention in a medical setting;

   - within reasonable medical certainty, there is no medical emergency;

   - within reasonable medical certainty, the patient is medically stable enough for the transfer to the intended dispositional setting (e.g., a general hospital, a psychiatric hospital, an outpatient treatment setting or no follow-up treatment);

   - the emergency physician who has indicated medical clearance shall, based on his or her examination of the patient at that point in time, indicate in the patient's medical record the patient's foreseeable needs of medical supervision and treatment. This information will be used by the transferring physician who will make the eventual disposition of the patient (See item # 13).

4. Medical clearance does not indicate the absence of ongoing medical issues which may require further diagnostic assessment, monitoring and treatment. Neither does it guarantee that there are no as yet undiagnosed medical conditions.

5. Task force members agreed to make reference to and use of the EMTALA definition of the medical screening and stabilization exam. By that definition, transfer of a patient requires that the patient be medically stable for transfer or that the benefits of transfer outweigh the risks.

6. No consensus in the literature was found that delineated a proven, standardized approach to the evaluation and management of psychiatric patients requiring medical evaluation in the emergency department. There was general agreement, based on clinical experience, to establish Criteria for Psychiatric Patients with Low Medical Risk.

7. The Criteria for Psychiatric Patients with Low Medical Risk recommended by the task force included:

   - Age between 15 and 55 years old

   - No acute medical complaints

   - No new psychiatric or physical symptoms

   - No evidence of a pattern of substance (alcohol or drug) abuse

   Normal physical examination that includes, at the minimum:

   - a. normal vital signs (with oxygen saturation if available)
   - b. normal (age appropriate) assessment of gait, strength and fluency of speech
   - c. normal (age appropriate) assessment of memory and concentration

8. A typical physical examination in the emergency department is focal, driven by history, chief complaints and disposition, and is not a replacement for a general, multisystem physical examination. The extent of the physical examination performed on a psychiatric patient by the emergency physician should be documented in the patient's medical record.

9. It was agreed and recommended that routine diagnostic screening and application of medical technology for the patient who meets the above low medical risk criteria is of very low yield and therefore not recommended.

10. Patients who do not meet the low medical risk criteria are not automatically at high medical risk. For patients who do not meet the low medical risk criteria, selective diagnostic testing and application of medical technology should be guided by the patient's clinical presentation and physical findings.

11. Once a patient has been medically cleared and accepted by the receiving facility, the receiving facilities may nevertheless request that the emergency department initiate laboratory tests (e.g., drug levels, renal function etc.) only if such tests will facilitate the patient's immediate care at the receiving facility. However, awaiting the results of these lab tests should not delay the transfer process.

12. It was agreed that during a psychiatric patient's medical assessment, the decision of when to begin the patient's psychiatric evaluation should be a clinical judgment. The psychiatric component of a patient's emergency department evaluation should not be delayed solely because of the absence of abnormality of laboratory data.

13. When crisis or inpatient psychiatric treatment is recommended for a patient who has been cleared by an emergency physician, the transferring physician should consider:

   - a. the patient's anticipated needs for medical supervision and treatment as outlined in the medical record by the examining emergency physician and

   - b. the medical resources available at an intended receiving psychiatric facility. The receiving facility's medical resources should be accurately represented to the transferring physician by a qualified professional of the receiving facility.

14. To facilitate the transferring physician's choice of an appropriate inpatient psychiatric facility, the task force recommends the development of a list of New England psychiatric units indicating the respective availability of concurrent medical care, nighttime and weekend medical coverage, locked and unlocked beds and separate and concurrent substance abuse treatment.

15. In the event that transfer to a crisis or inpatient psychiatric facility is recommended, it is often desirable to have direct communication between the transferring physician and the psychiatrist accepting the transfer at the receiving facility.

    · a. Before having accepted a medically cleared patient for transfer, a potential receiving facility's request for additional diagnostic testing of the patient should be guided by that individual patient's clinical presentation and physical findings and should not be based on a receiving facility's screening protocol.(See paragraphs 6–10)

    · b. After having accepted a medially cleared patient for transfer, a receiving facility may request that the emergency department initiate laboratory tests (e.g., drug levels, renal function etc.) only if such tests will facilitate the immediate care at the receiving facility. Awaiting the results of these laboratory tests should not delay the transfer process.

16. Task force members felt that direct physician to physician communication was required to resolve concerns arising between the transferring physician and the receiving facility regarding:

    · a. the need for an inpatient psychiatric hospitalization;
    · b. the appropriateness of one facility versus another;
    · c. a request for certain diagnostic testing;
    · d. any general clinical disagreement;
    · e. significant ongoing medical issues or treatment recommendations.

17. In view of the focal nature of the emergency physician's medical assessment and clearance, task force members strongly recommend that all psychiatric patients transferred to an inpatient facility be considered for a timely, comprehensive medical evaluation during the course of their hospitalization.

Massachusetts College of Emergency Medicine and Massachusetts Psychiatric Society Consensus Statement, 2003

Appendix C

The Six Aims of Quality Health care [25]

The Institute of Medicine has identified six aims for improvement in quality of healthcare delivery:

Safe – avoiding injuries to patients from the care that is intended to help them

Effective – providing services based on scientific knowledge

Patient-centered – providing care that is responsive to individual patient preferences, needs and values, assuring that patient values guide all clinical decisions.

Timely – reducing wait and sometimes harmful delays for both those who receive care and those who give care

Efficient– avoiding waste, including waste of equipment, supplies, ideas and energy

Equitable – providing care that does not vary in quality because of personal characteristics such as gender, ethnicity, geographic location or socio-economic status

The Quality Chasm's Ten Rules to Guide the Redesign of Health Care [26]

1. Care based on continuous health relationships. Patients should receive care whenever they need it and in many forms, not just face-to-face visits. This rule suggests that the healthcare system should be responsive at all times (24 hours a day, every day) and that access to care should be provided over the Internet, by telephone, and by other means in addition to face-to-face visits.

2. Customization based on patient needs and values. The system of care should be designed to meet the most common types of needs but have the capability to respond to individual patient choices and preferences.

3. The patient as the source of control. Patients should be given the necessary information and the opportunity to exercise the degree of control they choose over healthcare decisions that affect them. The health system should be able to accommodate differences in patient preferences and encourage shared decision making.

4. Shared knowledge and the free flow of information. Patients should have unfettered access to their own medical information and to clinical knowledge. Clinicians and patients should communicate effectively and share information.

5. Evidence-based decision making. Patients should receive care based on the best available scientific knowledge. Care should not vary illogically from clinician to clinician or from place to place.

6. Safety as a system property. Patients should be safe from injury caused by the care system. Reducing risk and ensuring safety require greater attention to systems that help prevent and mitigate errors.

7. The need for transparency. The healthcare system should make information available to patients and their families that allows them to make informed decisions when selecting a health plan, hospital, or clinical practice, or choosing among alternative treatments. This should include information describing the system's performance on safety, evidence-based practice, and patient satisfaction.

8. Anticipation of needs. The health system should anticipate patient needs, rather than simply reacting to events.

9. Continuous decrease in waste. The health system should not waste resources or patient time.

10. Cooperation among clinicians. Clinicians and institutions should actively collaborate and communicate to ensure an appropriate exchange of information and coordination of care.

Appendix D

The following statistics were considered during discussions and writing. They are excerpts from NAMI Fact Sheet "Mental Health: An Important Public Health Issue – Know the Facts" revised January 2006.

National Statistics

- 62.5 million Americans (22.2%) experience some form of mental disorder each year
- 8.76% of the U.S. population have a severe mental illness
- More than 50% of adults and 70–80% of children are not receiving any treatment for their mental illness
- Between 85 and 90% of adults with severe mental illness end up unemployed
- Mental illness accounts for more than 15% of the overall burden of disease from all causes (slightly more than that of cancer)
- By the year 2020, depression alone will be the third leading cause of disability worldwide
- Nationally, the direct treatment costs in 1997 were estimated at 150 billion, the estimate for 2005 is 200 billion
- The average annual growth for national healthcare expenditures from 1986–1996 was 8.3%, for mental health 7.2%
- The cost of treating serious mental illness is comparable to the cost of treating many other chronic medical conditions
- For every $1 spent on mental health services, $5 is saved in overall healthcare costs.

References

1. Illinois Hospital Association. *2005 Emergency Department Utilization Survey*. Naperville, IL: The Illinois Hospital Association; 2006.

2. American College of Emergency Physicians. *Emergency Departments see Dramatic Increase in People with Mental Illness*. Washington, DC: American College of Emergency Physicians; 2004.

3. The Lewin Group. *Emergency Departments – An Essential Access Point to Care*. AHA Trend Watch, 3, 1. March, 2001. Available at: http://www.aha.org/aha/trendwatch/2001/twmarch2001.pdf (Accessed August 13, 2012).

4. Institute of Medicine. *Hospital-based Emergency Care: At the Breaking Point*. Committee on the Future of Emergency Care in the U.S. Health System. Washington, DC: National Academy Press; 2006.

5. Illinois Hospital Association. *Memorandum: Psychiatric Bed Data*. Naperville, IL: Illinois Hospital Association; 2004.

6. Larkin GL, Claassen A, Emond JA. Trends in U.S. emergency department visits for mental health conditions, 1992 to 2001. *Psychiatr Serv* 2005;**56**:671–7.

7. Haugh R. Stressed out. *Hosp Health Netw* 2006;**80**:50–2.

8. Substance Abuse and Mental Health Services Administration. *Blueprint for Change: Ending Chronic Homelessness for Persons with Serious Mental Illnesses and Co-occurring Substance Use Disorders*. DHHS Pub. No. SMA-04–3870, Rockville, MD: Center for Mental Health Services, Substance Abuse and Mental Health Services Administration; 2003.

9. The Kaiser Commission. *Medicaid and the Uninsured. The Uninsured: A Primer*. October 2006.

10. Substance Abuse and Mental Health Services Administration. *Drug Abuse Warning Network, 2005: National Estimates of Drug-Related Emergency Department Visits*. March, 2007. SAMHSA's Office of Applied Studies. Available at: http://oas.samhsa.gov/DAWN/2k5ed.cfm (Accessed August 13, 2012).

11. Brauser D. *Psychiatric Patients Often Warehoused in Eemergency Departments for a Week or More*. January 24, 2011. Medscape Medical News. Available at: http://www.medscape.com/viewarticle/736187_print (Accessed December 8, 2011).

12. Smart D, Pollard C, Walpole B. Mental health triage in emergency medicine. *Aust N Z J Psychiatry* 1999;**33**:57–66.

13. Lukens TW, Wolf SJ, Edlow JA, et al. Clinical policy: critical issues in the diagnosis and management of the adult psychiatric patient in the emergency department. *Ann Emerg Med* 2006;**47**:79–99.

14. Zun LS. Evidence-based evaluation of psychiatric patients. *J Emerg Med* 2004;**28**:35–9.

15. Zun LS, Leikin JB, Stotland NL, Blade L, Marks RC. A tool for the emergency medicine evaluation of psychiatric patients. *Am J Emerg Med* 1996;**14**:329–33.

16. Zun L, Leikin J, Downey L. Prospective medical clearance of psychiatric patient. Submitted for publication.

17. Zun LS, Hernandez R, Thompson R, Downey L. Comparison of EPs' and psychiatrists' laboratory assessment of psychiatric patients. *Am J Emerg Med* 2004;**22**:175–80.

18. Zun L, Downey L. Application of a medical clearance protocol. Submitted for publication.

19. Pearlmutter MD, Summergard P. *Consensus Statement on Medical Clearance and Toxicology Screening*. 2012. Available at: www.macep.org/index (Accessed August 13, 2012).

20. American Psychiatric Association. *Practice Guideline for the Psychiatric Evaluation of Adults*, (2nd Edition). 2006. Available at: www.psych.org/practice/clinical-practice-guidelines (Accessed August 13, 2012).

21. Frank R, Fawcett L, Emmerson B. Development of Australia's first psychiatric emergency centre. *Australas Psychiatry* 2005;**13**:266–72.

22. Wand T. Psychiatric emergency centres, reinforcing the separation of mind and body. *Int J Ment Health Nurs* 2005;**14**:218–19.

23. Illinois Mental Health and Developmental Disabilities Code. 405. ILCS. 5/1–122.

24. Wright ER, Linde B, Rau NL, Gayman M, Viggiano T. The effect of organizational climate on the clinical care of patients with mental health problems. *J Emerg Nurs* 2003;**29**:314–21.

25. Kohen T, Corrigan JM, Donaldson MS, (Eds.). *To Err is Human: Building a Safer Health System.* Washington, DC: National Academy Press; 2000.

26. Institute of Medicine. Improving the quality of healthcare for mental and substance-use conditions. In: Daniels A, England MJ, Page A, Corrigan JM, (Eds.). *Crossing the Quality Charm: Adaptation for Mental Health and Addictive Disorders.* Washington, DC: National Academy Press; 2006.

Chapter 46

Improving emergency department process and flow

Peter Brown, Stuart Buttlaire, and Larry Phillips

Introduction

The demands placed on emergency departments (EDs) today make it essential that every possible avenue be explored to improve flow and outcome of care. No consumer wants to spend many hours waiting for care or for placement in the appropriate service. Staff members find the delay in serving behavioral health clients especially frustrating, and delaying care can often lead to an exacerbation of symptoms, complicating treatment and disposition. Average length of stay in EDs across the nation has risen to more than 6 hours, but for behavioral health clients, it is all too often measured in days. This can create trauma for clients, major issues for ED staff, lost revenue for hospitals, and many wasted resources at a time of decreasing funding.

This chapter will address the basic problem of improving ED flow and reducing trauma and dissatisfaction for consumers and staff alike. Unlike other chapters which address an extensive variety of important aspects of treatment, this chapter looks at the ED as an overall system. It is dedicated to giving you ways to change your operation so you have a better, more therapeutic and less expensive system of care. It will also give you some examples of successful efforts to make this type of improvement in ED operations. If you master the process described in this chapter and apply it effectively, your ED and your hospital will be able to serve more consumers at no increased cost and with an overall improvement in the public reputation of your hospital and its financial success. Later in this chapter, we will describe the changes that hospitals who participated in a learning collaborative made which gives credence to this promise of improvement.

The ED is sometimes viewed as the "early warning" system for healthcare system stress or failure, and the last resort for care in a general and behavioral healthcare system, which is often challenged to meet client needs. Across the United States, State Mental Health Programs were reduced by 4% in 2009, 5% in 2010, and were estimated to be cut by more than 8% in 2011 (Stateline.org). Approximately four million people seek care for behavioral health problems each year in hospital EDs compared to less than three million in 1999. Visits per 1000 have increased from 17.1 to 23.6 over the past 10 years [1]. In 2007, 12 million

visits were for behavioral health care. Of that number, 66% were for mental health (MH), 25% for substance use (SU) and the rest for both MH/SU. Some 41% of those 12 million visits resulted in admission to the hospital, which is 2.5 times the rate for other conditions. This higher admission rate is not surprising in a setting often overburdened and under-resourced. This can lead to inadequate care and poorer outcomes, negative patient experience, and staff dissatisfaction.

Systems improvement background

In order to make what is known as "breakthrough improvement," which means really dramatic improvement, the ED has to be viewed as a system and as part of a larger system. By considering this or any other process or organization as a system, we remove the personal connection and look at the overall operation. We also look at all aspects: the things which go into the creation and operation of that entity; the processes which are used; and the results achieved.

Any system is an organized structure for achieving a specific outcome, product, or objective. The system itself is the sum of the inputs, such as materials and labor, brought to address a specific issue or product; the process used in utilizing those resources; and the end sum of these processes is the product achieved from applying the resources. Each aspect of the system needs to be evaluated to create improvement.

In every case, the ability to improve a result requires the participation of the people responsible for the product creation. Don Berwick, MD, is often quoted as saying "Every system is perfectly designed to achieve the results it gets" [2]. By this he means: if you want better results: change the system, don't just try to get people to work harder, they are already working as hard as you can expect them to work. However, any chance of success for change must include the people who actually provide the labor which drives the system or it will be extremely difficult, if not impossible, to make a new system work effectively. A number of techniques and methods have been developed to redesign systems and achieve improved results, and are well documented. These methods include in part: ISO 9000 Quality Management, Quality Circles, Total Quality Management [3], Zero Defects, Kaizen, Lean, Six Sigma, Model for Improvement, and IDEO

Behavioral Emergencies for the Emergency Physician, ed. Leslie S. Zun, Lara G. Chepenik, and Mary Nan S. Mallory. Published by Cambridge University Press. © Cambridge University Press 2013.

Deep Dive, which has been used extensively to completely redesign both products and processes.

Theories of systems change

Walter Shewhart and W. Edwards Deming originated the 20th century development of quality improvement. Shewhart held a doctorate in Physics from University of California at Berkley when he went to work for Bell Labs in 1924 and met Deming there, a PhD from Yale. One of the more recent and extensively used quality improvement methodologies is Six Sigma [4]. Shewhart set as the level of quality desired a limit of three standard deviations, or Three Sigma, for reduction of errors from the desired results. The standard deviation can be calculated based on actual results, but in general a Three Sigma deviation would mean an error in the normal process less than 1% of the time. A Six Sigma level of defect control would mean no more than 3.4 errors per million opportunities or products. The Six Sigma system was developed at Motorola and later adopted and aggressively utilized by General Electric and other corporations. If this level of perfection were achieved in an ED, death of a patient due to errors would be an extremely rare occurrence.

The Six Sigma system of improvement utilizes experts in the quality improvement process. The process begins with Executive Management commitment to the process and establishment of the organization's goals. They select a Senior Champion to assure organizational support and resolution of road blocks and problems. There are Deployment Champions responsible for general implementation, Project Champions who drive specific projects, Master Black Belts who are the most highly trained in the techniques of systems analysis and improvement and are full-time improvement specialists, Green Belts who are trained in the improvement process but work part-time on specific projects, and Team Members who have basic training in the improvement process and work on specific projects part-time under direction of Black Belts. Projects typically begin with identification of a problem or failure in the current product or outcome. The team is assembled under the Black Belt with a few Green Belts and Team Members who review the current system and map the process in use. They identify the failure points and devise changes to address the specific failures in the process leading to the poor results. Finally, they supervise the implementation of the changes they have developed for the system. This system works well for many corporations especially those with specific production processes and industrial technology.

Another quality improvement methodology is Lean or Lean Production developed by Toyota in the 1980s. Lean is dedicated to eliminating waste of any kind from a process, whether manufacturing or service based. There is a long history to waste control and many specific strands to the overall development of Lean. Some of this success is credited to Deming. While Deming began his work in the United States and was later recognized as a giant in the field, he spent some particularly important time in Japan with the occupation after World War II when he was asked by the Army to help organize the Japanese census effort. During that time, he was invited to speak to the Japanese Union of Scientists and Engineers. The Japanese took his message to heart much more aggressively than had US manufacturers of the time. Toyota's adoption of the Lean Production system was most likely heavily influenced by Deming's models.

The Lean quality improvement system uses the concepts of *Continuous Improvement* and *Respect for People*. It breaks Continuous Improvement into three basic principles: *Challenge*, or having a long-term vision of the challenges one needs to face. Principle two is *Kaizen*: There is never a perfect process or it is never *Good Enough*. The third principle is *Genchi Genbutsu*: going to the source to see the facts for oneself, and making the right decisions, creating consensus, and making sure that the goals are attained at the best possible speed. There are no Black or Green Belts but there are experts, team members who are selected and contribute to the establishment of goals with senior management assurance of support and direction.

More recently the two concepts, Lean and Six Sigma, have been combined into a single concept of developing a dedicated team for improvement and having them work directly with production members to address significant issues in process management. Lean and Six Sigma together help to create a major system for restructuring processes and improving outcomes in many organizations. This system still establishes teams of experts and provides dedicated support from the Executive level. It works on specific aspects of a production system to eliminate waste as a key ingredient of failure but also works on assuring a high level of reliability.

Each of these improvement methods have been tried and used with some success in health care. These methods have been used most successfully with processes that have a specific function, such as a call center or production operation. They also have their critics. Critics complain the process is time consuming and expensive with an overemphasis on training Black and Green Belts. In addition, the dependence on a team of experts has the tendency to cut out of the process the workers most affected by change. In any major change process, it is crucial to have the support of the workers. Furthermore, when empowered, line workers are usually the best source of new ideas for improving results. These systems tend to implement new processes all at once and lose the opportunity to bring the whole workforce into the implementation process.

The breakthrough collaborative (BC) constitutes an especially successful method of quality improvement specifically aimed at improving healthcare outcomes. The Institute for Healthcare Improvement has been a particularly strong proponent of using a breakthrough collaborative as one of the best models for change [5]. The BC process includes a number of aspects of Lean/Six Sigma and other quality improvement methods, but is not so heavily directed toward cost reduction or establishment of costly full-time experts in improvement.

Instead it involves the people who are regularly involved in working within the process, ward, or service.

A breakthrough series collaborative is a short-term (6- to 15-month) learning system that brings together a large number of teams from hospitals or clinics to seek improvement in a focused topic area to help make "breakthrough" improvements in quality while reducing costs. Participating organizations learn both specific methods of improvement and general methods for trying new approaches. They learn from experts and especially from each other. The BC requires upfront overt support and establishment of a champion from the executive level. This method then calls for creation of a team of key people from the area of the project. For a hospital-based project, this team should include at least one physician as champion for the project. It should also have the key decision makers from the specific service. Typically, this includes a senior member of the nursing personnel, a chief of service, a manager and at least one person at the primary working level, such as a floor nurse. The team can be as large as the group wants to make it and should include at least one representative of everyone who has a role in the operation of the service.

A key ingredient of the Breakthrough Collaborative is the use of the Plan Do Study Act (PDSA) process of testing and implementing improvements. In this process, the team will select a change they feel will make a difference in the success of a specific activity. Success may be measured as reducing morbidity or other unwanted results or it may be improving a benchmark such as shortening the length of stay or even reducing overall mortality. The team then selects a place to test the new technique or modification, identifies a person and time to carry out the test and a specific outcome measure. The test is performed for only a limited time, usually no more than one day or less. The results are collected and the team reviews the results. If the trial is successful the change is tried on a larger sample or for a longer period of time. If it was not successful the change is either discarded or modified for a second trial using the same process. Only after a series of successful trials of the change done over larger groups and for longer duration, is it determined to be ready for implementation.

Staff involvement with the change leads to a greater likelihood of implementation. Typically, change occurs when it is easier to change than it is to continue to perform old negative behavior. Payment to change can be a major inducement, however in most cases this is not a feasible approach. Change required as a result of some other adverse outcome, such as being fired, is also a major inducement. However, this approach can create animosity, and implementation is likely to be grudging and less effective. If staff are offered more education in how to be more effective with fewer negative results it can be a powerful inducement to make change.

The importance of culture

A lot of work has been done on the significance of culture and its relation to outcome. Ted Sperof et al. said "Organizational cultures that emphasize teamwork and innovation have been found in alignment with quality improvement, whereas bureaucratic, hierarchical cultures, which inherently promote stability and resist change, are less suited for quality improvement" [6].

Langley et al in The Improvement Guide (1996) pointed out that people have to be willing to look critically at current practices and recognize their failings to develop new approaches to care [7]. Don Berwick has repeatedly pointed out that if the culture of a hospital does not encourage teamwork and innovation it will be difficult to develop a process which will engage in self-evaluation and be open to the significant restructuring usually needed to make major improvements in outcomes. Bureaucratic organizations have difficulty accepting the possibility of finding better methods of operation. To determine the culture of any hospital, The Agency for Healthcare Reach and Quality (AHRQ) has provided on its website an instrument, Hospital Survey on Patient Safety Culture: Items and Dimensions. This free instrument and related scoring document provide a good method for evaluating the culture of the hospital [8]. For any organization scoring high in bureaucracy, their first step is to recognize that this is a problem and to begin a conversation with senior management underlining how their organizational structure will interface with the improvement process and desired change. The next step is to select candidates for a redesign team, to examine potential solutions. There are many resources which can be employed in helping to reshape the culture of the hospital. A crucial first step is to identify the problem and obtain strong senior executive commitment to changing the culture.

Quality improvement for emergency departments

With increasing wait times, overcrowding, and concerns about results, EDs have become a major focus of concern and have caused hospitals and others to direct attention at changing the method of operation. In one of the earlier efforts at improvement Harvard University-affiliated hospitals agreed to a project to evaluate and improve ED care in 1993 [9]. An on-site questionnaire asked patients about socio-demographic characteristics and utilization of primary care services, emergency department, hospital services in the previous year, and other health-related issues [10]. The follow-up telephone interview assessed patient satisfaction with ED care, self-reported problems with the process of care, and discharge instructions. After reviewing the data on results and satisfaction each hospital was allowed to organize its own quality improvement project. Following the improvement projects a representative sample of patients was again interviewed and researchers found a five to ten percent improvement in satisfaction. Clearly an improvement though modest had been achieved.

A number of efforts have since been mounted to change ED systems of care. One of the largest and most successful was the Institute for Healthcare Improvements Learning and Innovation Community on Operational and Clinical Improvement in the ED, which ran for several years between 2005 and 2009 and involved over 200 EDs. IHI adopted objectives of the Collaborative: Reduce Total Length of Stay, Length of Stay for Admitted Patients, Length of Stay for ED Patients, Length of Stay for Fast Track, Walk-always (patients who left the ED before or after the Medical Screening Exam and who leave Against Medical Advice) and ED Diversions (the number of hours per month the ED is closed to ambulance admissions). The IHI Collaborative required about a year and involved three face-to-face meetings plus extensive consultation with faculty and with the other hospitals participating in the program [11].

IHI relies on many aspects of the Lean and Six Sigma process but does not require heavy investment in establishing change managers. The IHI approach focuses on training key workers from the area involved, in this case the ED, to lead and to create innovative new methods. Each collaborative is provided what is known as a Change Package. These are the "good ideas" for which there is some body of evidence they produce improved results. The participating hospitals are encouraged to adopt some of these ideas but to create their own process for implementing them. All participants are trained in the rapid tests of change. These are small experiments that provide continues feedback and gather evidence of successful change as the trials proceed. All participants share their data on results and on changes attempted with all other participants, allowing everyone to learn from each other. This process has produced successful results and led to significant improvement in patient satisfaction [12].

Patient satisfaction

Many studies have evaluated patient satisfaction with EDs. Although we have not found one that specifically identifies the satisfaction of behavioral health patients apart from the general ED population, we believe that the same concerns and findings identified in previous studies including Beaudraux and O'Hea (2004), Press Ganey (2005), and The Gallup Poll in its annual satisfaction of patients in EDs (2007) apply to behavioral health clients as well. The key drivers of satisfaction include the patient and MD and nurse interaction and the patient feeling listened to, cared for, being treated courteously, and their concerns taken seriously. The other important factor is wait time in the ED, the longer the wait the less satisfied the patient. However, patients who experience longer waits can be highly satisfied if kept informed about delays and receive information and explanation about the delays. The issue of wait times is particularly problematic for Behavioral Health clients as shown by the American College of Emergency Physician (ACEP) survey of EDs that found longer wait times for Behavioral Health Clients in EDs. The ACEP survey found 79% of the hospitals said psychiatric patients are boarded in their ED while 60% of psychiatric patients needing admission stay in ED over 4 hours. This is not likely to produce satisfied consumers or staff (American College of Emergency Physicians, "Psychiatric and Substance Abuse Survey 2008" [13].

Improving care for behavioral health clients

Much remains to be done in improving ED operations for patients, but even more improvement is needed in emergency care for behavioral health clients. In Australia there have been several attempts to develop improved emergency care for behavioral health clients. A Monash University School of Nursing research team in Victoria, Australia, chose a participatory action research strategy. Jointly executed with staff from the Peninsula Health Care Network, the research process brought together the multiple disciplines involved in the care and management of behavioral health patients for a number of meetings.

In the United States, there have been a number of projects to evaluate various aspects of emergency care. Some examples include: A systematic intervention to improve patient information routines and satisfaction in a psychiatric emergency unit [14]; Quality assurance for psychiatric emergencies. An analysis of assessment and feedback methodologies [15]; Measuring quality of care in psychiatric emergencies: construction and evaluation of a Bayesian index [16]; and A survey of emergency department psychiatric services [17]. Unfortunately, these efforts in most cases did not go beyond the research level and have only slowly found their way into any aspect of practice.

Nearly two decades ago there began a development of specialized Psychiatric Emergency Services and Comprehensive Psychiatric Emergency Programs (CPEPs) to improve emergency care for behavioral health clients. The PES units provide more specialized care in psychiatric emergency centers separate from the general care provided in the EDs of larger hospitals. CPEPs offer short-term Crisis Intervention beds in the ED for 72 or more hours. CPEPs also coordinate outpatient follow-up services to continue the stabilization of the crisis and to help the patient return to a precrisis state. These outpatient services are usually independent of the hospital and are usually not run by the hospital and typically have not reported outcomes and are not subject to any regulatory reporting requirements such as the Joint Commission or the National Commission on Quality Assurance. Without reporting requirements the outpatient program outcomes remain unknown as well as not easily lending themselves to process improvement.

Improving the system of care in EDs

The atmosphere and culture in many EDs can actually, and inadvertently, encourage destabilization in people who appear with behavioral health problems. ED staff are trained to be professional, efficient, effective, and calm in their approach. In many cases, this can be interpreted by the patient and family as uncaring, distant, and brusque. ED staff members, from physicians to aides, can see behavioral health clients as requiring a significant investment of time and resources that could be better invested in patients with "true" medical or surgical emergencies. Behavioral health issues are complex yet somehow not viewed as "real" emergencies. While a diabetic reaction brought on by excess sugar consumption is an emergency, a wish to rid one's head of voices demanding anti-social actions may be perceived as just a waste of time. Behavioral health problems can be as life threatening and debilitating as many more traditional general health issues. All these mental health conditions can be life threatening conditions just as heart disease or carcinoma can be life-threatening. Suicide is the 10th leading cause of death in the United States, ahead of colorectal cancer, breast cancer, and prostate cancer [18].

ED staffs may be without behavioral health resources entirely or inadequately staffed with individuals with behavioral health expertise. Inadequate resources, negative previous experiences, and perhaps unrealistic expectations may lead ED staff to try to maintain a distance both physically and emotionally from such people. For clients suffering behavioral health issues serious enough to arrive at the ED, this combination of distance, intrapsychic emotional pain, and inadvertent neglect are likely to exacerbate an already difficult existence. Common negative experiences are poignantly described in Susan Stefan's book; Emergency Treatment of the Psychiatric Patient [19]. Even in specialty psychiatric emergency units specifically designed for the behavioral health clients, there can be a tendency for staff to fall victim to insensitivity and negativity. None of us appreciate treatment we feel is depersonalizing, and people with behavioral health problems, as described in Susan Stefan's work, are especially likely to react negatively to what they see as insensitive treatment.

Several successful improvement efforts have started with keeping the patient's experience of the ED in mind. In addition, every initiative to improve a system of care should involve the local consumer in the process in order to obtain invaluable feedback. Contra Costa Regional Medical Center took this approach and significantly improved ED care as well as outcomes and financial results [20].

The breakthrough collaborative to improve EDs care for people with behavioral health problems

The Institute for Behavioral Healthcare Improvement (IBHI) is a not-for-profit organization (501c3) formed in 2006 dedicated to improving the quality and outcome of behavioral health care [21]. In response to the many problems of caring for behavioral health clients in EDs, IBHI led a Breakthrough Collaborative to improve care for people with behavioral health problems in EDs in 2008. The aim of this Collaborative was to:

- Reduce the suffering of clients
- Improve knowledge for better care of persons with behavioral healthcare needs in EDs
- Improve hospital functioning and effectiveness as measured by
  · Reduced overall time for care
  · Reduction of use of, and time in, restraint

- Improved patient and staff satisfaction
- Reduced congestion and conflict in EDs
- Establish subsequent collaborative efforts nationally.

When IBHI began work on the Collaborative, IHI had been offering The Breakthrough Series methodology in its collaborative for hospitals on Improving Flow in EDs but had excluded the behavioral health component and clientele. IBHI began developing the Collaborative by hosting an expert panel to identify the best available practices. This was the beginning of development of a Change Package and also helped develop faculty. The domains identified for the Change Package that would be the core of the improvement efforts were: Clinical Outcomes, Operations, and Patient and Staff Satisfaction.

The pioneering IBHI Collaborative began in January of 2008 with six active participating hospital emergency departments. A report from one of them is included below.

Formation and operation of the Collaborative

The Collaborative included participant hospitals from Colorado, Louisiana, Minnesota, New York, Oklahoma, and the State of Washington. They all agreed to collect and share data on their results, committed to the improvement process for a 10-month active phase, and to share data for an additional 6 months. A pre-work assignment provided a reference for organizational readiness, baseline data, and reporting of patient experience. It required the hospitals to:

- Obtain clear and firm support from the senior administration of the hospital
- Form a team of people from both general and behavioral health who would organize and develop the change process at the hospital;
- Have one of the members of the team go through the process of becoming a client of the ED
- Interview two to four former patients who were recently served in the ED who had needed behavioral health care.

IBHI faculty provided a model for improvement, the rapid tests of change process and the change package, which made good ideas readily available to the teams. This included measuring results, crucial to making improvement in a Breakthrough Collaborative. The Collaborators mutually agreed to collect the following set of measures of success:

- Overall length of stay in the ED
- Length of time from door to behavioral health provider who can evaluate the consumers' condition
- Number and percent of total consumers presenting who must be placed in restraints
- Average amount of time consumers are in restraints
- Consumer satisfaction as measured by the portion of consumers who are highly satisfied or would be willing to recommend the service to others.

The Change Package

The Change Package is a collection of specific practices for which there is evidence of effectiveness. If there is not a sufficient array of specific recognized evidence-based practices the next best choice is a set of practices with a significant body of favorable expert opinion behind them. To overcome the evidence gap IBHI created the expert panel who met for a full day developing specific recommendations.

The Change Package contained specific concepts to improve outcomes in each of the following areas:

- Increase client/patient collaboration with assessment and treatment
- Simplify and expedite assessment and disposition processes
- Make treatment effective at reducing stay and return
- Address the boarding burden
- Improve patient and family satisfaction
- Improve staff satisfaction.

The Change Ideas for increasing client collaboration with assessment and treatment:

- Train all staff in de-escalation techniques at least yearly (e.g., Mandt, Crisis Prevention Institute [22])
- Develop a goal of restraint *reduction* (e.g., 10–30% per year)
- Adopt a program such as the NTAC program to reduce the use of restraint [23]
- Develop skills for a step-wise approach to verbal interventions to reduce agitation
- Identify environmental and ED process "trigger points," that lead to patient agitation, and seek to modify, mitigate, or eliminate
- Get reviews by client representatives of ED receptiveness
- Train staff and security in sensitivity and non-escalation techniques – consider security part of treatment team
- Be respectful and receptive to patients' perceptions Ask: "How can we help you today?"
- Eliminate asking identical questions by multiple evaluators
- Seek and use information gathered from patients
- Create mental health liaison position for each shift to be on hand at all busy times; equip this person with cell phone or radio and give them authority and backup
- Post explanation in waiting room of ED process, including name and phone number of liaison individual(s) and hospital grievance person
- Ensure liaisons are responsive to requests for information
- Assure every psychiatric patient has ED staff face-to-face contact every hour (sitters don't count) to answer any questions, arrange for snack or water, etc.
- Ensure that patients are permitted to be accompanied if desired
- Allow patients to retain their clothing unless individualized assessment is made that retention would be dangerous and constant observation is not sufficient.

Data collection

Obtaining data, especially satisfaction data, proved most difficult due to the lack of simple stratification elements on BHC clients in existing patient satisfaction data collection surveys. All the Collaborators ultimately developed systems for collecting this information, but with some difficulty. Good data quickly collected is essential to assess change process progress and know when to modify specific processes to improve results. Without this data the Collaborative efforts will be difficult to maintain beyond the Collaborative.

Achievements

Collaborative members were presented with assault prevention models emphasizing the early warning signs of possible assault and de-escalation techniques. Patients' rights were emphasized, both the importance of respecting the individual's psychological vulnerabilities as well as identifying the trigger points which might cause behavioral escalation in the process of admitting and managing behavioral health clients. For example, the necessity of having clients disrobe as part of the admission process was questioned extensively because it was identified as a potential cause of escalation, particularly in previously sexually traumatized clients. A leader in patient advocacy described the use of well-trained Peer Counselors in EDs to help guide a patient through their emergency room experience. This can be a very cost-effective and patient-centered approach in behavioral health, which helps lessens patients' anxiety about being in the noisy fast-paced ED [24]. The group chose to adopt the specific measures cited previously.

Some specific changes hospitals have made

Participant hospitals developed and/or adapted a significant number of changes derived from other participants, faculty, the change package, and other benchmarking. In order to have sustained success each hospital must develop its own set of changes. Imposing change from the outside is rarely successful and usually leads to other problems.

The following are some examples of these changes:

- Held emergency de-escalation intervention training for all staff
- Developed a second triage area
- Developed a short stay 1–5 day psychiatric unit
- Developed behavioral early response team for BH emergencies. . . Placed a behavioral health professional in the ED waiting room as a patient "greeter" who also identified potential behavioral health clients
- Established protocols and workflow process for medicating agitated patients and brought in outside expert to discuss with MDs
- Created medication guidelines in the use of atypical antipsychotics in addition to typicals

- Developed a psychiatric transport, versus police transport of patients, that proved cost-effective
- Met with community physicians, mental health programs, agencies, and outpatient programs to develop exit resources
- Developed a geriatric community diversion program
- Psychiatric Emergency Service recidivist program– system-wide case conferences
- Developed an electronic alert system at entry
- Developed order sets for psychiatric patients
- Provided a new procedure for having patients medically cleared before transfer to Mental Health ER. Patients with high alcoholic levels, when stable are discharged from the ER vs. transferring to MHER
- Decreased number of restraints through use of de-escalation techniques, early use of anti-psychotics, time out room, diversion activities, and one-to-one observation by a psych aide
- Increased focused on community resources and discharge planning; including National Alliance on Mental Health, assertive community treatment teams and homeless shelters and provision of vouchers for transportation and medication refills

- Intensive 2-day training to teach hospital security on use of restraints
- Monthly meetings to review all seclusion/restraint
- Established a violence reduction protocol
- Focused on continuous education of staff and increased flexibility for patients, e.g. free phones, healthy snacks, grooming supplies, showering as requested
- Improved ED/BH relationships, bi-weekly workgroup meeting, monthly MD meetings
- Increased ED psychiatric bed capacity, opened short-stay unit, improved physical space to increase safety
- Increased ED Crisis Social Workers, added psychiatry with e-call rotation, moved from uniformed security guards to psychiatric aids
- Increased education and training to identify high-risk clients, teach de-escalation, use medications in earlier and standardized fashion
- Psychiatric emergency response protocols created
- Developed community round table leading to ability to divert ambulance traffic to other hospitals when needed
- Worked more with referral resources.

References

1. Larkin GL, Claassen CA, Emond JA, Pelletier AJ Carmargo CA. Trends in US emergency department visits for mental health conditions, 1992 to 2001. *Psych Serv* 2001;**56**:671.

2. Berwick DM. A primer on leading the improvement of systems. *BMJ* 1996;**312**:619–22.

3. International Standards Organization ISO 9000 Quality Improvement http://www.iso.org/iso/iso_catalogue/management_and_leadership_standards/quality_management.htm (Accessed January 27, 2012).

4. Harry M, Schroeder R. *Six Sigma, the Breakthrough Management Strategy Revolutionizing the World's Top Corporations*, Doubleday, a division of Random House; 2000.

5. *The Breakthrough Series: IHI's Collaborative Model for Achieving Breakthrough Improvement* Available at: http://www.ihi.org/knowledge/Pages/IHIWhitePapers/TheBreakthroughSeriesIHIsCollaborativeModelforAchievingBreakthroughImprovement.aspx (Accessed October 31, 2011).

6. Sperof T. *Qual Saf Health Care* 2010 **19**:592–596 doi: 10.1136/

qshc.2009.039511 http://qualitysafety.bmj.com/content/19/6/592.full.html (Accessed October 31, 2011).

7. Langley G. *The Improvement Guide*, San Francisco, CA: Jossey Bass Books; 1996.

8. *Agency for Healthcare Research and Quality*. Hospital Survey on Patient Safety. http://www.ahrq.gov/qual/patientsafetyculture/hospscanform.doc (Accessed October 31, 2011).

9. http://ww.amjmed.com/article/s0002-9343%2899%2900269-7/abstract.

10. Burstin HR, Conn A, Setnik G, et al. *Benchmarking and Quality Improvement: The Harvard Emergency Department Quality Study*. Department of Medicine, Brigham and Women's Hospital, Boston, Massachusetts 02115, USA. http://www.ncbi.nlm.nih.gov/pubmed/10569298 (Accessed October 20, 2011).

11. *Optimizing Patient Flow: Moving Patients Smoothly Through Acute Care Settings*. IHI Innovation Series white paper. Boston: Institute for Healthcare Improvement; 2003.

12. www.IHI.org (accessed October 20, 2011).

13. Heslop L. http://onlinelibrary.wiley.com/doi/10.1046/j.1365-

2648.2000.01251.x/abstract. *Improving Continuity of Care Across Psychiatric and Emergency Services: Combining Patient Data Within a Participatory Action Research Framework*. Article first published online: 9 Oct 2008 DOI: 10.1046/j.1365–2648.2000.01251.x http://onlinelibrary.wiley.com/doi/10.1046/j.1365-2648.2000.01251.x/abstract (Accessed October 20, 2011).

14. Johnsen L, Oysaed H, Børnes K, Moe TJ, Haavik J. A systematic intervention to improve patient information routines and satisfaction in a psychiatric emergency unit. Haukeland University Hospital, Division of Psychiatry, Bergen, Norway. *Nord J Psychiatry*. 2007;**61**:213–18 http://www.ncbi.nlm.nih.gov/pubmed/17523034 (Accessed October 20, 2011).

15. Sateia MJ, Gustafson DH, Johnson SW. Quality assurance for psychiatric emergencies. An analysis of assessment and feedback methodologies *Psychiatr Clin North Am*. 1990;**13**:35–48. Dartmouth Medical School, Hanover, New Hampshire. http://www.ncbi.nlm.nih.gov/pubmed/2156240 (Accessed October 20, 2011).

16. Gustafson DH, Sainfort F, Johnson SW, Sateia M. Measuring quality of care in psychiatric emergencies:

construction and evaluation of a Bayesian index. University of Wisconsin-Madison. *Health Serv Res.* 1993;**28**:131–58. http://www.ncbi.nlm. nih.gov/pubmed/8514497 (Accessed October 20, 2011).

17. Brown JF. A survey of emergency department psychiatric services. Department of Integrative Systems, School of Nursing, Virginia Commonwealth University, Richmond, VA, USA. jbrown35@vcu.edu *Gen Hosp Psychiatry.* 2007;**29**:475–80. http://www. ncbi.nlm.nih.gov/pubmed/18022039 (Accessed October 21, 2011)

18. National Institute of Mental Health. *Suicide in the U.S.: Statistics and Prevention.* http://www.nimh.nih. gov/health/publications/suicide-in-the- us-statistics-and-prevention/index. shtml (Accessed October 20 2011).

19. Stefan, S J D. *Emergency Treatment of the Psychiatric Patient,* New York Oxford University Press; 2006.

20. Kelley J. *Adapting and Implementing New Strategies for Patient Centered Care.* Mental Health/Psychiatry Contra Costa Regional Medical Center, Martinez, CA http://www.katedudding.com/ibhi/ref- lib-papers/Kelley%20slides%20April% 202011.pdf (Accessed October 21 2011).

21. Institute for Behavioral Healthcare Improvement (www.ibhi.net) (Accessed October 20, 2011).

22. The Mandt System http://www. mandtsystem.com/MH/mh.ms (Accessed October 20, 2011).

23. National Association of State Mental; Health Program Directors National Technical Assistance Center Six Core Strategies for Reducing Seclusion and Restraint Use© 2001 http://www. nasmhpd.org/nasmhpd_collections/ collection5/publications/ntac_pubs/ Debriefing%20p%20and%20p%20with %20cover%207-05.pdf (Accessed October 20, 2011).

24. Emergency Services by Projects to Empower http://www. projectstoempower.org/ (Accessed October 20, 2011).

Chapter 47

Physical plant for emergency psychiatric care

Patricia Lee and Joseph R. Check

Introduction

Emergency departments (EDs) are often crowded, noisy, and chaotic places with limited privacy. In recent years, the number of patients presenting to EDs with psychiatric complaints has been growing, in part due to funding and budget cuts which have curtailed support for outpatient treatment. Increasingly, EDs find themselves providing not only the initial acute stabilization of a psychiatric patient, but also the management of these patients, often for days, until care is transferred to an appropriate psychiatric treatment facility. It is not uncommon for patients to be stabilized and discharged from the ED before an inpatient bed becomes available. However, a typical ED lacks the ideal amount of space to effectively manage psychiatric patients, especially those requiring a quiet, nonstimulating environment [1]. As the paradigm shifts from a triage model to a treatment model, the need for an Emergency Psychiatry Service becomes more apparent.

It is estimated that 50% of all psychiatric emergencies requiring acute intervention in a hospital occurs in the ED. Although the majority of psychiatric patients are not violent, the potential for unexpected violence toward self or others is always present [2]. Since 1995, suicide has ranked in the top five most frequently reported events to the Joint Commission, who maintains a Sentinel Event Database. The database finds that 8% of all in-hospital suicides occur in the ED [2]. In addition, patients treated in a non-psychiatric hospital reporting suicidal ideation will attempt suicide earlier and with less warning than suicidal psychiatric inpatients. Two studies showed that suicide attempts within the general hospital environment were more violent (hanging, jumping, or gunshot) than those on psychiatric units [2,3,5].

The two main events that drive many of the safety-related design choices for the treatment of emergency psychiatric patients are acts of self-harm and elopement. Even though the Joint Commission requires EDs to screen all patients for suicide risk, suicide remains the second most frequently identified Joint Commission Sentinel Event [1]. A November, 2010 Joint Commission Sentinel Alert acknowledged that suicidal patients are often admitted to EDs that "are not designed to assess suicide risk and do not have staff with specialized training to deal with suicidal individuals" instead of a psychiatric setting specifically designed to be safe for suicidal patients [2].

Approximately 75% of inpatient hospital suicide attempts occurred by hanging in a bathroom, a bedroom, or a closet, and 20% resulted from jumping from the building. A 2008 study found that doors and wardrobe cabinets accounted for 41% of the anchor points when hanging was the method of self-harm [1]. The most frequent methods of self-harm in healthcare environments were hanging, jumping, cutting with a sharp object, intentional drug overdose, or strangulation [2]. Everyday objects that are commonly found in most patient rooms can be used by patients to harm themselves or others. Readily available items in EDs include nurse call system bell cords, bandages, sheets, restraint belts, plastic bags, elastic tubing, and oxygen tubing [4,5].

Designated treatment areas for psychiatric patients should be designed as if every patient poses a safety risk despite preliminary screens as they have proved unreliable [1]. Potential missteps may be avoided if the ED physician maintains some doubt when a suicidal patient minimizes or denies self-injurious behavior. Patients and staff in the ED should expect to feel safe and protected from harm. The ED environment represents a significant safety risk in that it may provide ample opportunities for patients to successfully harm themselves or others. Reasonable efforts to minimize the risk of harm using best practice design and construction should be considered. Psychiatric treatment areas should be designed to maximize both patient and staff safety, and designed in accordance with state and local fire and building codes as outlined in the National Association of Psychiatric Health Systems "Design Guide for the Built Environment of Behavioral Health Facilities" [6]. It was Louis Sullivan who in 1898 said that "form ever follows function," but healthcare design may significantly lag behind form due to the ever-evolving technology and the changing needs of a busy ED [1]. Collective experience has yielded some success in appropriate design of behavioral healthcare environments, and are presented here in this chapter.

Behavioral Emergencies for the Emergency Physician, ed. Leslie S. Zun, Lara G. Chepenik, and Mary Nan S. Mallory. Published by Cambridge University Press. © Cambridge University Press 2013.

Environment

Several important questions exist when designing space in EDs to care for psychiatric emergencies. A reference on specific products and vendors can be found in the Mental Health Environment of Care Checklist prepared by the VAH National Center for Patient Safety, Department of Veterans Affairs [7]. When considering products and facility structure the following are specific design recommendations to consider:

- Could a patient be hurt by any aspect of the environment? A critical eye should always be applied to minimizing potential physical hazards in every aspect of the overall design. Avoid selecting systems and materials that yield sharp edges, provide ligature points, or can be made into weapons.
- Could a patient harm someone else? Select abuse-resistant materials, furnishings, and fixtures. Always consider whether a structure or object selected could be weaponized. Inspect everything with this key principle in mind.
- Can staff easily navigate the environment to get to a patient in need of assistance? Address design needs for disabled and geriatric patients who may require the use of portable lifts. Avoid ceiling-mounted lift systems which can pose a ligature risk.
- Is it possible to maintain patient privacy in this environment? Consideration should be applied to design a space that strives to promote safety, privacy, and dignity for both males and females.
- Does the environment promote recovery? The treatment area should be designed to promote collaboration among care providers, and should allow for both enhanced patient and staff visibility in patient care areas.

Patient volume in the ED is unpredictable. Therefore it is prudent to prepare for surges by designing the space to be effective for both medical and psychiatric patients. Consider creating treatment rooms that function as "swing" rooms, capable of managing the patient with multiple diagnoses in the same setting, or quickly altered for either medical patients or psychiatric patients. Evaluate how to eliminate or secure any items that potentiate risk of hanging or any object which could be "weaponized." A "swing room" may be designed by installing a locked head-wall containing all electrical outlets and medical gases. Additional supplies can be stored outside of the room in a rolling locked cart which could be brought into the room for a medical patient as needed. Alternatively, consider creating an alcove in a patient room which is designed to contain all necessary equipment, monitors, and supplies which could be secured or locked away by a simple rolling door similar in design to a garage door.

Additional environmental considerations include the following:

- Elevation: If the patient room is located above ground level, jumping out of a window is always a concern. Reducing grade elevations and securing all windows are important considerations [8].

- Confidentiality: Chart rooms and staff areas should be located where confidential conversations can occur without being overheard by non-clinical staff, patients, or visitors [1,6].
- Medications: Medication rooms should be secured with an electromagnetic locked door and an automated medication system should be used [1,6,8,9].
- Comfort: Efforts should be made to make patient care areas look as attractive and residential as possible [6].
- Engineering controls: Locate areas for control of water, electric, and HVAC systems outside of the patient rooms, preferably in an outside corridor with locked access [1,6,8,9].
- Computers: Computers should be shielded from patients and their families to prevent the unauthorized viewing of patient records [6,8,9].
- Housekeeping: Locate service areas such as trash rooms and clean and soiled utility rooms so they are accessible from both the unit and the service corridor to minimize the need for non-patient care staff from entering patient rooms while they are occupied. Plan the housekeeping storage area with enough space to lock away carts and all cleaning materials when left unattended [1,6,8,9].
- Nurse call: Traditional nurse call systems for psychiatric patients are not required in rooms or bathrooms [6]. However, "swing rooms" will need to have a nurse call system installed in such a way that it can be locked away or dismantled [6,8,9].
- Comfort: Whenever possible, avoid an "institutional" look.

Significant safety risks exist when treating psychiatric patients in the ED. Patients present with unknown risks to staff or self, and many patients are aggressive and threatening to staff, and may requiring immediate intervention. Because of the potential for sudden danger, care areas are considered a Level 5 in terms of safety concern (Table 47.1) [6]. The level of necessary precaution depends on the staff's knowledge of the patient and the amount of overall supervision of the patient. When designing an ED (Level 5), consider the following safety features:

- Security: Facility security must be available when requested by ED staff to provide standby assistance or intervention for the patient who presents as a danger to themselves or others, who is potentially violent, agitated, or impulsive. The space should be accessible and designed for security or sitters to directly observe patients.
- Panic alarms: If security is not immediately available in the psychiatric area, the installation of a "panic" button system or portable duress devices will allow staff to discretely request assistance in a potentially threatening situation [6].
- Metal detectors – Facilities may want to consider using metal detectors that are free-standing or hand-held to screen patients for weapons upon entering the ED. If metal detectors are used, a protocol should be developed for the management of patients who screen positive and for patients who possess contraband [10].

Table 47.1. Levels of risk

- Level 1 – Staff and Service areas such as housekeeping closets. These areas should comply with all applicable codes and regulations and should be locked at all times.
- Level 2 – Corridors, counseling rooms, and interview rooms. Patients are typically not left alone in these supervised areas for prolonged periods of time. All unattended rooms should be kept locked at all times to prevent unauthorized/unsupervised patients from entering. Counseling rooms or interview rooms should have a "classroom" type lockset which requires a key to lock/unlock the outer handle but the inside handle is always free to allow for staff to exit.
- Level 3 – Lounges and Activity Rooms. Patients typically spend time with minimal supervision.
- Level 4 – Patient rooms. Patients spend a great deal of time alone with minimal or no supervision.
- Level 5 – Emergency Departments, admissions rooms, examinations rooms, and seclusion rooms. Staff typically interact with newly admitted patients and assess risk in admission and examination rooms. Violent or high-risk patients who are agitated or psychotic may be designated to a seclusion room for safety.

- Patient belongings: It is necessary to incorporate adequate storage space for both patient and visitor belongings to minimize the risk of accessing dangerous items [6,8,9].

When designing space to care for psychiatric patients in the ED, it is essential to consider all building products and materials to ensure a safe environment. The follow are specific design recommendations to consider:

Floors

- Vinyl flooring material meeting a class A rating is preferred [6,8,9].
- Because psychiatric patients may occasionally urinate on the floor, consider seamless epoxy flooring with integral cove base or sheet vinyl flooring with integral cove base. Avoid patterns or color combinations that may morph into visual misperceptions or "objects" by the patient [6].
- Avoid using metal strips that can be removed by patients and used as weapons [6,8,9].

Walls

- Walls should be constructed of impact-resistant gypsum board over 3/4 inch plywood on a minimum of 20 gauge metal studs spaced at 16 inches to center with a polyurethane resin type finish [6,8,9].
- All edges and corners should be protected by corner guards.
- The preferred paint finish should be an eggshell finish because of easy repair and low cost of renewing or changing colors. In general, warm colors and earth-tones are recommended.
- If wall padding is desired, a Kevlar-faced product or heavy vinyl material with 1 1/2 inch thick foam backing may be considered [6,8,9].

Ceiling

- A solid non-accessible gypsum board ceiling is preferred to prevent the patient from escaping from a lay-in type of ceiling. Brackets potentiate a significant risk of hanging and should be avoided [6,8,9].

Electrical

- All electrical outlets located in a patient room should be tamper resistant and located on separate Ground Fault Circuit Interrupters (GFCIs). The outlet breakers should be placed outside of the direct patient care area to allow for access without entering the patient rooms. Electrical cover plates for switches and receptacles should be made of polycarbonate materials that are secured with tamper-resistant screws [1,9].
- All electrical circuits with power plugs near water sources must be protected by GFCI receptacles. One GFCI-equipped receptacle will provide protection for an entire circuit [1,9].
- Consider installing additional wiring to accommodate Wi-Fi and wireless hubs.

Heating, ventilation, and air conditioning (HVAC)

- HVAC grills should be fully recessed and tamper-resistant with S-shaped air passageways to reduce escape risk by crawling through the vents. When possible, locate individual room HVAC equipment (fan/coil units) in a location away from the patient rooms where they can be serviced without entering the patient room. When designing new construction, use radiant heating and cooling systems designed to reduce need for mechanical devices in the patient rooms [6,8,9].
- Vents should be flush with the wall or ceiling and should be installed with tamper-proof screws and mounts [6,8,9].

Water

- Shut-off valves should be located in corridor walls where they can be reached from the corridor by opening a locked access door, and not from patient rooms [6,8,9].
- Water temperature should be controlled to not exceed 110 degrees F [6,8,9].

Sealants

- Tamper-resistant sealants are generally suitable for supervised areas, while pick proof sealants are generally unsuitable for unsupervised areas. Tamper-resistant sealants are generally flexible, abrasion resistant, and highly tenacious. They are usually based on urethane or silicone sealant technology. Pick-proof sealants are generally hard, inflexible and extremely durable and are generally based on epoxy technology. Pick-proof sealants are generally not suitable for active joints, due to their hardness [9].

- Recognize that patients will ingest anything that may be harmful. Accordingly, nonlaminated glazing should never be used. Laminated glazing should wholly resist breakage and retain broken glass in a manner that prevents dislodging from the interlayer [9].

Windows

- Natural light is therapeutic for both patients and staff and has been associated with reduced length of stay (by as much as 7 days, with women having a more favorable response than men) and more favorable treatment outcomes [1].
- Both exterior and interior windows provide an opportunity for a patient to escape. Thus, it is critical to consider the design of the entire window, together with the installation in wall openings [6,8,9].
- Patients may attempt to cut themselves or use objects in their environment to harm others. Laminated glazing can prevent access to broken glass, even if they are retained on the interlayer [6,8,9].
- All glazing should be safety glass. The glazing should pass "The Dade County hurricane test, ASTM E1886 and ASTM E1996 as alternative impact tests" [2]. If wire glass is required by code, install 1/4" polycarbonate type glazing on the side to which the patient has access [6,8,9].
- All glazing exposed to patients should be polycarbonate. Attention to the amount of recess in mounting frames will decrease the risk that an impact to the center of the window will cause it to flex out of the frame. If replacing existing glass with polycarbonate is not possible, application of a window film may suffice but may become scratched or defaced by patients [6].
- Windows with sash, frame, and glazing need to be capable of withstanding up to ten 2,000 foot-pound impact loads from a 1 foot diameter impact object without breach or breakage [9].
- Exterior windows should be either fixed windows or units equipped with sash control devices that limit the opening and can be governed to 4 inches or less [6,8,9].
- Window covering hardware
  - Window covering material or hardware should not be accessible to the patient. One option would be electronically controlled blinds or shades behind polycarbonate [6,8,9].
  - Care should be taken to assure that any exposed devices designed to control the tilt of the blinds does not create a potential ligature attachment point [6,8,9].
  - Roller shades, specifically manufactured for use in psychiatric hospitals, are comprised of enclosed security roller boxes and security fasteners with cordless operation and locking devices that resist tampering by patients [6,8,9].
  - If curtain tracks are used they must be flush mounted tightly to the ceiling and lack cords. A minimum

number of hook tabs should be used to limit the amount of weight that can be supported if the fabric is bunched together [6,8,9].
  - View windows to corridors in doors or as sidelights should be constructed of polycarbonate. If wire glass is required by code, a layer of polycarbonate on each side of the wire glass will increase its strength [6,9].

Bathrooms

Bathrooms represent areas of increased risk as patients are often left alone and unsupervised.

- Toilets
  - Wall surfaces must be flush with toilets to avoid gaps that can become ligature points [8].
  - Toilets should be floor mounted with back outlets and water supply [6,8,9].
  - Movable seats provide attachment points for ligatures: Toilet fixtures with built-in integral seats are preferred [6,8,9].
  - The ideal flush valve should be recessed in the wall and activated by a push button or motion sensor. If impractical, the flush valve should be enclosed within stainless steel or plastic with a sloped top that uses a push button activator for the valve [6,8,9].
- Lavatory
  - Whenever possible, lavatories should be constructed of a solid surface material with an integral sink. All piping below the sink should be concealed behind a panel fastened with tamper-resistant screws, accessible only to maintenance staff. Faucets should be simple sensor activated. Water should be no warmer than a preset temperature mix of 110 degrees F [6,8,9].
  - Single knob mixing valves that provide minimal opportunity for tying anything around are preferred [6,8,9].
- Grab bars, towel hooks, clothing hooks
  - Grab bars, as required for certain rooms, should be fixed to the wall with a welded horizontal plate on the bottom of the bar to prevent using these bars as anchor points.
  - Clothing or towel hooks should be designed to collapse when a weight above 4 lbs is applied [6,8,9].
- Bathroom mirror: If a mirror is installed in a bathroom it should be constructed of reflective polycarbonate with a stainless steel frame and firmly anchored to the wall with tamper-proof screws. No shelf should be a part of this frame assembly [6,8,9].
- Toilet paper dispenser: Fully recessed stainless steel toilet paper holders have been widely used for years. However, some facilities feel this creates an infection control problem because the users have to handle the entire roll [6,8,9]. One acceptable model is a recessed toilet paper dispenser

designed with a soft foam type spindle [6]. Other alternatives include a toilet paper hold that pivots down when vertical pressure is applied [6,8,9].

- Soap dispensers and paper towel dispensers
  - Accessories such as soap dispensers and paper towel dispensers should be installed in a recessed manner [6,8,9].
  - If not recessed, the dispenser should be constructed with a slope top and be wall mounted to prevent it from being used as an anchor point [6,8,9].
  - Paper towel tri-fold dispensers may be acceptable if covered with heavy duty secure covers [6].
  - Provide sealant bedding bead at the perimeter of surface-mounted units to prevent gaps between the unit and the wall. If possible locate soap dispensers and towel dispensers where drips are confined to a counter to minimize liquid on the floor which represents a fall hazard [6,8,9].

Doors

- Continuous hinges are preferred in patient areas because of the need to minimize possible attachment points and reduce hanging risks. Barrel type hinges are preferred because they are available with a sloped top edge, also referred to as a "hospital tip." Geared type continuous hinges are also recommended as they have a closed sloped top and continuous gears that resist ligature attachment [6,8,9].
- Integral system doors may be constructed with a nearly flush push plate on the outside that releases the continuous latch bar and a tapered pull handle that releases the latch bar from the other side. A recessed pull handle is necessary on the push side to aid in closing the door. This assembly resists upward, downward, and transverse attachment. The over the door attachment may be needed to discourage ligature tying. This product is available with an "emergency release hinge" [6,8,9].
- For restricted psychiatric area access, all exit and nearby stairway doors must be locked at all times. Exit doors may be locked with electromagnetic locks that are connected to alarm systems. Card readers or keypads adjacent to the door are also commonly used to provide access for staff and visitors [6,8,9].
- Patient doors to corridors should swing without creating blind spots or alcoves, discouraging patients from barricading themselves in their room. If this is impossible to accomplish with remodeling or new construction, consider the following options:
  - A wicket-type door can be constructed so that a portion of the center of the door is cut and hinged to swing into the corridor. This hinged panel is mounted on a continuous hinge and secured with a deadbolt lock [6,8,9].
  - If space is available, a separate narrow (18–24 inches) door that swings into the corridor can be mounted in

the same frame as the main door in a "double egress" configuration. Another option is to use a mullion, a vertical structural element which divides adjacent window units, between the two leafs [6,8,9].
  - Patient room doors should be hung using a continuous hinge. Closers are generally not required. If necessary, parallel arm security rated closers mounted on the corridor side of the door is recommended [6,8,9].
  - Pressure sensitive alarms may be installed at the door head to prevent its use as a ligature support [6,8,9].
  - Antiligature type door handles with a magnetic latch are recommended [9].
  - Locksets are often used for ligature attachment (pulling down or up and transverse: over the top of the door and fastened to either handle). All patient access areas should use antiligature locksets [6,8,9].
- Latch systems commonly used to prevent ligature attachment are as follows:
  - A lever handle lockset can effectively deal with vertical pressure but is susceptible to transverse attachment. This lever type is Americans with Disabilities (ADA) compliant [6,8,9].
  - Crescent handle locksets use a top pivoted handle and thumb turn, which are ligature resistant. However, its operation is not intuitive and confusing for patients and staff. This handle may also be ADA compliant [6,8,9].
  - A push-pull handle lockset installed with both handles pointing down resists pulling down, and to some extent, the transverse attachment. This type of lockset is also ADA compliant [6,8,9].
  - Conical knobs with flutes have been shown to resist up and down pressure and to some extent transverse attachment, but these devices are not ADA compliant [6,8,9].

Furniture and decoration

- Furniture selection should be done with care to assure that any furniture used will withstand abuse, resist being disassembled, and does not encourage hiding contraband [6,8,9].
- Furniture should be sturdy, easily cleaned and reupholstered, and as heavy as possible to minimize the risk of becoming projectiles.
- Furniture may also be built-in or securely anchored in place to prevent stacking or barricading of doors.
- If movable seating is required, consider using lightweight polypropylene chairs that resist breaking into sharp pieces.
- All upholstery and foam used in furniture and mattresses should have flame spread ratings that comply with the requirements of NFPA 1010 Life Safety Code, Section 10.3 [6,8,9].

- All pictures and art work mounted on walls should have polycarbonate type glazing and heavy frames should be screwed to the walls with a minimum of one tamper-resistant screw per side. Care should be taken to reduce the opportunity to attach ligatures to the frame. Joints should be beveled to slope away from the wall and the joint at the top should be sealed with a pick-resistant sealant.
- Murals have been very effective and add interest to corridors and day rooms. It is usually a good idea to cover them with at least two coats of a clear sealer for protection [6].
- TV sets in patient rooms provide entertainment and reduce boredom. They should not be mounted on walls using brackets because of a potential hanging risk. All cords and cables should be as short as possible [6,8,9].
  - If TV sets are installed they should be built into the walls.
  - Manufactured covers with sloped tops are available to fit a variety of TV set sizes.
  - For maximum safety, the electrical outlet and cable TV outlet should be located inside the cover to keep wires and cables away from patients.
- Cabinets: All cabinet pulls should either be the recessed type or the under the door "no handle" type [6,8,9].
- Shelves: A stainless steel suicide resistant shelf is available [6,8,9].
- Mirrors
  - Observation mirrors (convex mirrors) should be installed in corridors, seclusion rooms, and other locations to assist with patient observation and to eliminate blind spots. These mirrors should be made of a minimum 1/4 inch thick polycarbonate filled with high-density foam, and have a heavy metal frame that fits tightly to the wall and ceiling. The perimeter should be sealed with pick-resistant caulking [1].
  - Radius-edge stainless steel framed security mirrors are preferred for wall mounted mirrors and the reflective surface may be polycarbonate, tempered glass, stainless steel, or chrome plated steel [9].
- Light fixtures
  - Light fixtures and bulbs represent a major security threat. Therefore, care should be taken to assure that they are safely constructed [6,8,9].
  - Light fixtures should be security type fixtures. Glass components should not be used with any fixture. Neither incandescent light bulbs nor fluorescent tubes should ever be accessible to patients [6,8,9]. If light fixtures can be reached by patients or are located in areas not readily observed by staff, the fixture must be the tamper-resistant type or have minimum 1/4" thick polycarbonate prismatic lenses firmly secured with tamper-resistant screws [6,8,9].
  - Dimmable lights can be installed to promote rest without compromising patient visibility [9].

- Use of table lamps or desk lamps in patient areas should be avoided. If used in a non-patient area, they should be anchored in place. The bulb should be shatterproof and power cords should be shortened [6,8,9].
  - Consider installation of motion detectors for corridor light fixtures for nighttime use. This would alert the staff whenever a patient leaves his or her room at night if the corridor lights are dimmed [6,8,9].
- Trash cans
  - Trash cans should never be located in a patient room.
  - In addition, plastic trash can liners should not be allowed in any patient access space. Breathable paper liners are recommended [6].

Communication systems and telephones

- Cordless or wall mounted telephones or hands-free recessed wall mounted phone systems are preferable to prevent ligature risk from cords [6,8,9].
- Telephones located in corridors or common spaces should have a stainless steel case securely wall mounted with a non-removable shielded cord of minimal length (14 inches maximum) [6,8,9].
- Use of a public address system for regular paging or staff communications should be avoided [6].

Signage

- Signage systems should be fastened with tamper-proof fasteners. Double stick tape and Velcro are not acceptable means of attachments [6,8,9].
- Room signs should be either painted on the door or made from a flexible material that is applied with a non-toxic adhesive [6,8,9].

Fire alarms and sprinklers

- All fire alarm pull stations and fire extinguisher cabinets should be locked. Fire sprinklers should be selected to have institutional heads that will break away under a 50 pound load. Units should drop approximately one inch from the ceiling to minimize ligature risk [6,8,9].

Noise reduction

- Patient behavior is generally improved in areas of reduced noise levels. Whenever possible, maximize design to keep the area quiet from the noise of the main ED.
- Sound absorbing materials are softer and more porous than sound reflective material and may pose a challenge for infection control measures [3].

Infection control

- Alcohol-based gels and foams may be consumed by patients and therefore should not be accessible to patients at any time [6,8,9].

- Seamless floors that are chemically or heat welded can reduce staining.
- Avoid curtains in rooms as they pose both a contamination risk as well as a safety risk.
- Walls should be painted with washable paint.

Conclusion

The Emergency Psychiatric Service is inherently one of high risk and acuity. Patients, staff, and visitors share this risk. As self-injurious behaviors and violence in the ED remain a growing public health concern, the need to prevent and manage these concerns is apparent, but often limited by space. The physical construct of a properly designed Emergency Psychiatry Service will accommodate the necessary environmental modifications allowing for a multidisciplinary staff to safely perform assessments in a timely and efficient manner. The ideal model would have the Emergency Psychiatric Service physically contiguous with the medical ED.

References

1. Sine D, Hunt J. Following the evidence toward better design. Some patterns of what works in behavioral healthcare environments are emerging. *Behav Healthc* 2009;**29**:45–7.

2. Joint Commission. Sentinel Alert. *A Follow-up Report on Preventing Suicide: Focus on Medical/Surgical Units and the ED*. Issue 46, November 17, 2010. Available at: http://www.jointcommission.org/assets/1/18/SEA_46.pdf (Accessed August 10, 2012).

3. Cheng I C, Hu F C, Tseng M C. Inpatient suicide in a general hospital. *Gen Hosp Psychiatry* 2009;**31**:110–15.

4. Suominen K, Isometsa E, Heila H, Lonngvist J, Henriksson M. General hospital suicides - a psychological autopsy study in Finland. *Gen Hosp Psychiatry* 2002;**24**:412–41.

5. Bostwick J M, Rackley S J. Completed suicide in medical/surgical patients: who is at risk? *Curr Psychiatr Rep* 2007;**9**:242–6.

6. Sine D M, Hunt J M. *Design Guide for the Built Environment of Behavioral Health Facilities*. Distributed by the National Association of Psychiatric Health Systems. edition 4.3. May 31, 2011.

7. Department of Veterans Affairs. *Mental Health Environment of Care Checklist*. Irving, TX: VHA National Center for Patient Safety; Version 06-27-2011.

8. Mental Health Facilities. *Design Guide*. Washington, DC: Department of Veterans Affairs, Office of Construction & Facilities Management; December, 2010.

9. New York State Office of Mental Health. *Patient Safety Standards Materials and Systems Guidelines*, (5th Edition). Albany, NY: OMH; January 31, 2011.

10. Joint Commission. *Accreditation Program: Behavioral Health Care*. National Patient Safety Goals. Available at: http://www.jointcommission.org/assets/1/6/2011_NPSGs_PSYCHIATRICC.pdf (Accessed January 1, 2011).

Chapter 48

Legal issues in the care of psychiatric patients

Susan Stefan

Introduction

Most medical care is provided to patients who willingly seek treatment. Compared to other healthcare settings, emergency departments (EDs) see a disproportionate number of patients who arrive in stressed, frightened, confused, combative, intoxicated, delusional, delirious, demented, or semi-conscious states. In addition, EDs are one of the few health-care settings where patients arrive involuntarily. Many of these patients' perceptions of the source and solution of their problems differ – sometimes drastically – from the diagnoses and recommendations of ED staff. Some of those patients are in psychiatric crisis or have psychiatric issues which may complicate the assessment of their medical needs.

The needs of people in psychiatric crisis are often in tension with the ED staff's mission to rapidly assess, diagnose, provide stabilizing treatment, and either discharge or transfer the patient to an observation or inpatient unit. In the case of patients presenting in obvious psychiatric crisis, the task of disposition is intertwined with a legally mandated determination of whether the individual needs to be detained because he or she is a danger to self or others.

Assessment and stabilization of psychiatric crisis, or of the medical needs of a patient with a serious psychiatric disability, are best achieved in a calm, reassuring environment, with patience and time to build trust and establish a connection with the patient. Few EDs can fill this need [1–7]. Some ED staff try hard and even heroically. These efforts are appreciated by many patients, who may be unaccustomed to being treated with respect and concern. Other staff are frankly hostile or adversarial to psychiatric patients. Psychiatric patients may be seen as malingering or potentially violent [1,2,5–8]. ED staff overwhelmed with injury and death can become angry at having to treat self-inflicted injuries. And the specter of legal liability shadows many ED encounters with psychiatric patients. Most liability concerns are exaggerated and impede good patient treatment.

This chapter summarizes the unique legal issues that arise in the assessment and treatment of psychiatric patients in ED settings. While ED staff are not lawyers and should not be expected to be conversant with state and federal law, it is helpful

to be sufficiently aware of legal issues to recognize a potential problem when it arises, to check the hospital policy or consult with hospital counsel, or at least be aware of potential legal implications of various courses of action. It is also helpful to be aware of myths and misunderstandings with regard to legal liability that may undermine the quality of patient care [5,8,9]. These myths equate psychiatric difficulties with danger-ousness or incompetence, and may lead to assumptions that a person presenting for psychiatric reasons cannot meaningfully participate in disposition decisions, and will likely need inpa-tient care, or that medical complaints are simply a manifesta-tion of psychiatric disability. Fear of liability translates to a reluctance to discharge psychiatric patients, and a determina-tion to hold the patient as long as necessary to find an inpatient bed, which can be counterproductive, unnecessarily tie up needed resources, lead to escalation and frustration, and pro-vide no benefit to the patient.

This chapter will begin with a brief overview of the structure of the relevant U.S. law. It will then set out legal issues unique to psychiatric patients in EDs: limitations on duration of both involuntary and voluntary detention; systemic challenges to ED conditions and the settlements they have generated; issues related to disability discrimination; limitations on restraint and seclusion; the standard of care and potential malpractice issues; and Health Insurance Portability and Accountability Act (HIPAA) and confidentiality requirements. The chapter ends with a brief discussion of strategies to avoid nursing home "dumping" of behaviorally difficult patients in the ED. Other important legal issues, including Emergency Medical Treatment and Active Labor laws (EMTALA), interactions with the police, and potentially incompetent patients wishing to leave against medical advice, are covered in detail in other chapters in this book.

Brief survey of the legal system

There are two sources of law in the United States. Federal laws apply across the country, and state laws apply only in the individual state. Both federal and state laws can be divided into constitutional, statutory, and regulatory law. With minor

Behavioral Emergencies for the Emergency Physician, ed. Leslie S. Zun, Lara G. Chepenik, and Mary Nan S. Mallory. Published by Cambridge University Press. © Cambridge University Press 2013.

exceptions, federal constitutional law only applies to state and county hospitals and employees. By contrast, federal statutory and regulatory laws tend to be part of the Medicare/Medicaid program and therefore apply to all hospitals that accept Medicare and Medicaid reimbursement.

State laws obviously vary from state to state. It is difficult to underscore just how great the variance can be: some states, such as Maine, essentially immunize all decisions by ED physicians, whether the decision is to discharge or commit the patient. Different states have different lengths of time that a person with a psychiatric presentation can be held in an ED before and after filing statutorily mandated detention documentation; some states have no time limits at all. Federal laws and regulations addressing patients' rights, such as HIPAA and restraint regulations, often specify that state law will govern if it imposes stricter standards than the federal law. In some states, such as Massachusetts, state regulations govern hospital conduct as to confidentiality and restraint and seclusion.

Malpractice is governed by state law. Professional standards also underpin various aspects of federal constitutional litigation. There are a variety of sources of professional standards. The law provides one such source, e.g., the duty to report child abuse is a duty created by either case law or statute in many states. In each state, the nuances of such a duty may be different; hospital policy should capture the state's particular formulation. Courts are divided about whether certification standards of the Joint Commission or standards promulgated by professional associations amount to professional standards recognized by the law. Standards developed by national or state public health authorities such as the Surgeon General or the Centers for Disease Control and Prevention are considered more persuasive as sources of professional standards [10]. Finally, of course, courts require expert witnesses to opine on the content of professional standards; it is a basic rule of law that professional standards cannot be proven without expert testimony.

In general, the law creates broad duties, and the contours of these duties are filled in by professional and clinical standards. For example, the law prohibits involuntary civil commitment of an individual unless he or she is mentally ill, and as a result of that mental illness, dangerous to himself or herself or others. In determining whether an individual is mentally ill, a professional relies on professional materials such as the Diagnostic and Statistical Manual of Mental Disorders, 5th Edition (DSM-IV) and clinical literature, as well as his or her own training and experience. Importantly, the professional also relies on the patient's specific reports, words, and actions; information from collateral sources; a sufficient physical examination to rule out medical causes for the patient's symptoms; and, sometimes, brief testing instruments such as the mini-mental status exam.

Emergency department professionals should guard against assumptions that litigation brought by people with psychiatric disabilities revolves primarily around bad outcomes following discharge, and can best be avoided by detaining and admitting the patient to inpatient care. While litigation following adverse outcomes certainly receives a great deal of publicity, those cases are far from the only claims arising from care of psychiatric patients in EDs. A substantial amount of litigation is brought relating to the use of force, including force by security guards or restraint by hospital staff. Sometimes these restraints involve patients who arrived behaving calmly but become agitated after waiting for many hours [11]. Sometimes the restraints involve patients who were calm but refused to remove their clothing [12]. Other litigation involves injury or death because ED staff wrongly assumed a patient's medical complaints to be psychiatric in origin as described in the Discrimination through stereotyping section later in this chapter.

Almost all cases brought against EDs by people with psychiatric disabilities are won by defendants. However, litigation is enormously stressful and expensive for all concerned, and many of these cases are preventable. Prevention involves three steps: reducing unnecessary involuntary detentions, expediting disposition of patients who truly must be detained, and treating patients with true respect and concern.

The lessons of this chapter can be summarized briefly. EDs must ensure that involuntary detentions are not based on fear of liability or on the relative ease of writing an involuntary petition compared to the hard work of a good community discharge plan or truly voluntary hospitalization. If patients really do need inpatient care, ED processes should ensure that the disposition takes place as quickly as possible. The best preventive strategy of all, however, is a front-end investment of time, patience and respect, listening to the patient and creating a trusting connection [1,9]. This increases the chances of a better healthcare outcome, and reduces the chances that time will be spent later in documenting restraint or departure against medical advice, or searching for an eloped patient, or explaining decisions to an investigating body. Finally, in the rare event of litigation, the hospital's version of an event will depend almost entirely on the story told by the documentation, including videotapes.

Limitation on duration of ED detention

Many problems in EDs involving patients' agitation or escalation arise because of increasing delays in EDs, which fall disproportionately on patients with psychiatric disabilities, who experience waits that are almost twice as long as medical patients [13]. Yet, the law places limits on both the length of time that psychiatric patients may be detained and on the substantive reasons for involuntary detention. As the research and case law discussed in greater detail below reflects, EDs often fail to comply with these limitations, especially limitations on the length of time that patients can be involuntarily detained [2,3,5,6,7,14].

Limitations on involuntary detention: substantive criteria

Federal and state constitutions, as well as some state statutes, place limitations on involuntary detention and treatment. Federal constitutional limitations apply only in cases where the involuntary detention or treatment is considered to be a result of government, or "state," action. Most courts have held that the actions of private hospitals and physicians who involuntarily detain patients pursuant to state statutes do not ordinarily constitute state action [15, 16].

There are some exceptions to this general rule. If the private physicians work jointly with state employees in detaining an individual, the detention may constitute state action [17]. If state employees pressure or strongly influence the private actors in their decision to involuntarily detain an individual, it may amount to state action [18,19]. If the patient is held at a county facility that has contracted with private entities to provide psychiatric evaluations, those private entities may be considered sufficiently entwined with the state government for their actions to be considered state actions [20]. Cases also suggest that the employment of off-duty police or security guards denominated "special police" with arrest powers may be sufficient for their actions to constitute state action, and to make the hospital responsible for violation of the patient's constitutional rights [21].

Even if involuntary detention is considered state action, it is generally difficult for individual plaintiffs with psychiatric disabilities to prove that their constitutional rights have been violated. The constitutional standard is easy for defendants to meet: detaining physicians must simply adhere to the substantive standards and procedures of their profession [20,22]. However, on occasion, plaintiffs have won substantial damage awards when involuntarily detention or treatment in EDs was not supported by documented observation or findings of dangerousness [23], or when there was no evidence that the committing physician performed an examination at all [18,24].

Limitations on involuntary detention by private hospitals and physicians are imposed by state tort law. An individual who is unlawfully held in an ED has an action for false imprisonment; an individual who is treated against his will or restrained in an ED has an action for battery. It is also difficult for plaintiffs to win these cases. Some states have passed legislation that limits the liability of ED physicians for discharging psychiatric patients, or limits the ability of patients to sue any provider of emergency medical services, including EDs. Occasionally, plaintiffs win these tort cases, almost always because defendants have not complied with the requirements of the state commitment law [25,26].

In the case of Marion v. LaFargue, a jury awarded a plaintiff a million dollars after the ED evaluating doctor testified that even if there was only a small risk of harm, the Hippocratic Oath required that a patient be involuntarily committed, and that he would not sit in the same room with the plaintiff because his "inappropriate dialogue" (the patient's statements that there was "a government conspiracy to kill the poor") made the doctor concerned that "this patient is indeed very dangerous." [23]. The judge reduced the jury award to $188,000; the plaintiff requested a second jury trial on damages, and ultimately received $115,000 [27].

As a practical matter, both constitutional law and tort law fundamentally concur on certain essential points. The fact that a patient needs treatment is insufficient to justify involuntary detention or treatment. As a general matter, adults who are not under guardianship and who do not pose a risk of serious harm to themselves or others in the near future may not be held against their will. Occasionally, a legally competent patient will be clinically determined to lack capacity at a particular point in time (e.g., due to severe intoxication). The legal issues involved are complex and are described in a different chapter (Chapter 44, Assessing capacity, involuntary assessment, and leaving against medical advice). Finally, courts support a public policy of treating psychiatric patients in community settings (see The Americans with Disabilities Act section, below)

Limitations on involuntary detention: duration of detention

State constitutions and statutes sometimes, but not always, impose time limits on the duration that an individual can be detained involuntarily in an ED. These time limits are generally divided into three categories: the time between arrival and assessment by a mental health professional or physician (generally different time limitations, with less time for the former than the latter); the time between arrival or assessment and completing a legally mandated petition for involuntary detention; and the total time in the ED. In some states (e.g., New York, Massachusetts) there are different time limits for initial assessment in a psychiatric emergency and for stays in adjacent extended observation/crisis stabilization units. Some states have statutes or regulations limiting the amount of time a voluntary patient who has not yet been psychiatrically evaluated may be held (e.g., Ky., Me., Md., Mass., Mo., NY, Pa. Wa.) In the few cases covering this situation, courts have held that the law permits people to be detained briefly for a reasonable period in order for them to be evaluated: "briefly" and "a reasonable period" have been considered to be several hours, although each case has to be evaluated on an individual basis [28, 29].

It is illegal to involuntarily detain all patients who arrive voluntarily seeking psychiatric help. On the other hand, some of these patients clearly do need to be detained pending evaluation. The best policy is one recognizing the right of patients to leave in general, and creating exceptions for those evaluated by a trained and experienced triage nurse according to specifically defined standards to be currently mentally ill and dangerous or obviously lacking capacity from their mental or medical illness AND presenting an emergency situation (See Chapter 3). It is extremely important to underscore that a person may be seriously mentally ill and still have the capacity to decide to leave the emergency department. Of course, patients who arrive on a legally authorized detention by police or mental health professionals must be held until evaluation, but state statutes may specify a time frame in which that must take place.

After an evaluation takes place, some states limit the amount of time that a patient may be held in an ED pending disposition. In New York, although a statute limited stays at psychiatric emergency services to 24 hours, patient stays routinely exceeded that limitation. Litigation was brought regarding these delays, and a settlement was entered with specific mechanisms to ensure that patients would not exceed the statutory limit (see Emergency department conditions and treatment section, below).

Limitations on voluntary detention: ED boarding and legal limitations

"In other situations, my voice is valued, but not in the hospital. You have even less of a voice in the ER. People with physical problems seem to be more important. Their needs take precedence over yours. If you're there over 48 hours, you're just a burden. You can't even assert you want something to eat, or need your medicine" [2].

"Boarding" patients is a term subject to several definitions, but generally means holding a patient after the necessary diagnosis and referral have been accomplished because no inpatient bed is available. Often boarding goes on for days, tying up bed space needed by new patients and causing staff to become frustrated, as reflected above; occasionally boarding continues for weeks. During this time, a patient whose psychiatric condition was considered sufficiently acute to need inpatient psychiatric care may receive no psychiatric treatment whatsoever other than medication [2,3,6,7,14]. Sometimes suicidality or other conditions such as acute intoxication subside or resolve themselves; it is important to reassess initial recommendations for inpatient admission in the context of the patient's evolving condition. As the hours wear on, the patient may also begin to be more agitated, not because of mental illness but simply from prolonged waiting. The staff, who have no power over the delays, also may become frustrated with the situation and the patient. This kind of situation sometimes leads to seclusion restraint, and injuries.

Advocates for people with psychiatric disabilities are increasingly seeing ED boarding as a symptom of a larger systemic failure. In Rhode Island, the Mental Health Advocate brought litigation against the Rhode Island Department of Mental Health over the boarding of psychiatric patients in EDs, alleging that the Department failed to ensure that EDs complied with patients' rights provisions under Rhode Island law, including the right to privacy and dignity, individualized treatment plans, to wear one's clothes, and to be given reasonable access to telephones to make telephone calls [14]. Although this litigation was resolved before trial, responsible emergency providers and administrators have increasingly begun to pose the question of whether they should be treating boarding patients awaiting a bed as psychiatric inpatients [3].

Emergency department conditions and treatment: systemic cases

Litigation involving individuals far outnumbers systemic challenges to the conditions in EDs as a whole. Nevertheless, there have been several cases challenging the conditions which people endure as they await evaluation and care in EDs. Most of these cases have been brought in the State of New York; this is not coincidence, as will be seen below.

The first known litigation involving systemic relief for individuals subject to psychiatric evaluations in EDs was the Lizotte case, brought by the New York Civil Liberties Union over the conditions and treatment of patients in New York City psychiatric EDs. Plaintiffs filed a class action on behalf of people who "had been or might be forcibly detained" in a psychiatric emergency facility operated by defendants "without being provided a bed in an appropriate facility" [30]. The plaintiffs sought "at least minimally adequate care and treatment" for people who waited for days for an inpatient bed, and to end defendants' indiscriminate use of physical restraints, including shackling waiting psychiatric patients to wheelchairs and gurneys. They challenged the lack of privacy and opportunity for hygiene, the fact that bright lights were kept on twenty-four hours a day, and the days-long delays which made all of these conditions unbearable.

The settlement of the Lizotte case resulted in an agreement to hold patients no more than 24 hours in an ED after the determination that inpatient care was necessary, and to afford prompt medical clearance, if necessary, for admission. Patients who stayed overnight were also to receive hygiene items and have dimmed lights [30].

At the same time that the Lizotte case was settling, another putative class action was brought in Northern New York against a private hospital alleging that its ED staff routinely detained and committed patients on the basis of their past psychiatric history rather than their current condition [31]. Although the class was not certified, the attorney in Marion v. LaFargue brought a later class action making similar allegations, Monaco v. Stone, and that class was certified [32].

The plaintiffs in the Monaco case named both City and State defendants and the case involved several different allegations. For purposes of this chapter, the relevant claims were that the conduct and practice of psychiatric evaluations, including those done in EDs, did not conform to professional standards, because the evaluators based involuntary detention decisions on their opinions that the patient needed treatment rather than the required statutory standard of dangerousness. In addition, even if they did conform to professional standards, they could not meet constitutional due process requirements because there was no showing that the methods used resulted in a reasonable degree of accuracy. Because evaluators did not use evidence-based risk factors in determining dangerousness, their evaluations did not, could not, and were never intended to evaluate the individual's potential for dangerousness.

The City defendants settled, agreeing to use a form requiring evaluators to specifically obtain information that is clinically relevant to dangerousness, including information pertinent to both risk and protective factors. The settlement also required that evaluating physicians receive training on how to evaluate dangerousness, and the requirements of the involuntary commitment statute [33]. The state defendants fought the charges, and initially won when the district court found that the plaintiff could not succeed in his constitutional claims unless the mental health evaluations were so inadequate that they "shock[ed] the conscience" rather than the "falls below professional standards" test [34]. A year and a half later, however, the Second Circuit held that falling below professional standards in performing a civil commitment met the "shocks the conscience" standard, and explicitly questioned the district court's decision in Monaco v. Hogan [35] (discussed in Section IV). After that holding, plaintiffs in Monaco amended their complaint to add Americans with Disabilities Act claims based on stereotyping [36].

During this time, the improvements wrought by the *Lizotte* agreement began to crumble at one New York City hospital, King's County Hospital Center. At King's County's CPEP (psychiatric ED), patients waited *an average* of 27 hours, and problems were reported with overcrowding, people sleeping on floors, inadequate psychiatric evaluations, and use of force, among other issues [37]. In 2007, a wide-ranging complaint (*Hirschfeld Case*) was filed in federal court against King's County Hospital's psychiatric ED and psychiatric units, by, among other groups, the New York Civil Liberties Union, which had brought *Lizotte* [38]. Shortly thereafter, the Department of Justice began its own investigation of the hospital. The death of Esmin Green, who died after waiting 24 hours in the King's County ED and whose prone body was seen on video being nudged by the toe of a security guard, occurred during the ongoing litigation, an investigation by the Department of Justice investigation, and licensure problems with the Office of Mental Health in New York. Ms. Green's death, and the discovery that staff had tampered with her records, made national news. The Department of Justice ultimately filed its own lawsuit against King's County Hospital, charging that the hospital's ED violated the constitutional rights of people who sought care there.

Eventually, the New York City Health and Hospital Corporation settled both lawsuits [39]. The settlement agreements reflect some current best practice ideas in psychiatric emergency medicine. For example, the Hirschfeld settlement addressed length of stay concerns in numerous ways. In addition to agreeing to achieve a specific length of stay[1], the settlement contains numerous provisions that will help to support reducing patient lengths of stay.

First, the agreement contains a requirement that senior ED staff be notified by email when any patient has occupied an ED bed for 18 hours, and by telephone, at whatever hour of the day or night, if any patient exceeds the statutory limit of 24 hours (the "Step-Up Protocol"). The email notification form contains specific information regarding existing barriers to disposition in the specific patient's case. A copy of the email is also sent to the legal counsel of the New York Health and Hospital Corporation.

The agreement also obligates the hospital to discharge patients 24 hours a day, and to expand admission hours for crisis beds to 12 hours a day, seven days a week. The Hospital also agreed to develop policies to respect the rights of nondangerous patients to leave the hospital.

Because many extended stays are the results of delays related to admission, the agreement seeks to ensure that only those patients who truly need inpatient care are admitted. An admission rate exceeding 45% in any given quarter triggers detailed review and analysis. King's County Hospital reduced its average length of stay from 27 hours to 9 hours by the time the case was settled.

Another part of the Hirschfeld case involved overuse of restraint and seclusion. The Hospital committed to a goal of eliminating the use of restraint, eliminated the use of seclusion, and agreed to reduce to the maximum extent possible the use of STAT medications. The Hospital also hired peer counselors (see Chapter 4) for both its ED and its inpatient unit, and agreed to develop policies to ensure that patients with developmental disabilities received appropriate assessments.

Other cases have also addressed systemic issues in crisis care for people with psychiatric disabilities by requiring community psychiatric crisis services as a remedy. Recognizing that the problem of inappropriate use of institutional beds was tied to inadequate community crisis services and overuse of EDs, the U.S. Department of Justice brought suit or joined existing litigation in several states where ED crises had made national news, including Georgia, North Carolina, and Delaware [4,40,41]. In settling these cases, the Department of Justice has required each of these States to develop statewide community crisis systems, including mobile crisis units, ACT teams, and community crisis beds, as part of a remedy for violations of the integration mandate of the Americans with Disabilities Act (see below).

The Americans with Disabilities Act and Section 504 of the Rehabilitation Act

The Americans with Disabilities Act ("ADA") and its statutory cousin, Section 504 of the Rehabilitation Act of 1973, prohibit discrimination on the basis of disability. Although ED staff tend to be unfamiliar with these laws, all hospitals are subject to them, and the number of cases brought against hospitals for discriminatory treatment of patients with psychiatric disabilities is increasing. As noted above, plaintiffs in the Monaco v. Hogan case have just added an ADA claim to their class action on the basis of stereotyping [36]. The ADA's integration mandate, which prohibits unnecessary segregation of people with disabilities in institutional settings, also has been used to require the development of community crisis services [40,41].

---

[1] The agreement requires that the mean length of stay plus two standard deviations may not exceed 20.5 hours. The purpose of this formula is to reduce the number of outlier extended stays, which could not have been achieved by simply averaging all lengths of stay.

Discrimination through stereotyping

"When I told [the ED doctor] I had caught the person embezzling, I think he thought I was delusional and grandiose. This is a crime that happens regularly and apparently he didn't see me as capable of reading a bank statement and putting two and two together." (Maryland Disability Law Center 2008)

Sometimes the account of a psychiatric patient in the ED about his or her circumstances will be highly unlikely on its face. But the failure to credit relatively ordinary information without even trying to corroborate it is not only bad practice; it may be discriminatory if the disbelief is based on the fact that the patient has been diagnosed with mental illness.

The case of Bolmer v. Oliveira arose because a series of state and private mental health professionals (including an ED physician and psychiatrist) refused to believe a psychiatric patient who claimed he had a sexual relationship with his case manager [35]. Instead, he was diagnosed with "erotomania," and involuntarily detained by ED staff. Only upon arrival at an inpatient unit did staff's questions about his relationship reveal that he had saved many text messages corroborating his story. Upon reading the text messages, Mr. Bolmer was quickly discharged from the hospital, and brought suit.

Bolmer charged state defendants with violating his constitutional rights and with discriminating against him under the ADA because they engaged in "stereotyping Mr. Bolmer as an unreliable individual who manifested delusions because of his diagnosed mental illness." He charged the private ED defendants with discriminating against him under Section 504 of the Rehabilitation Act by stereotyping him, and also made several state law claims.

The district court, in a decision affirmed by the Second Circuit, held that defendants violated Mr. Bolmer's rights under the ADA if their stereotyping resulted in substituting general impressions of people with psychiatric disabilities (e.g., "they are delusional, therefore, he is delusional") for an adequate evaluation of the patient ("is Brett Bolmer delusional?"). However, Mr. Bolmer's claim against private ED defendants under Section 504 of the Rehabilitation Act failed because of differences between the two statutes.

It is hardly controversial that the ADA prohibits discrimination based on stereotyping. The application of this principle to mental health evaluations simply underscores a long-standing, basic professional standard that mental health evaluations must be individualized. Professional caution is advised. In one recent survey, psychiatrists held *more* negative stereotypes about people with psychiatric symptoms than members of the general population [8]. Harmful stereotyping is manifested in a variety of concrete circumstances in the setting of an emergency evaluation. The next three sections of this chapter discuss three potential sources of harm caused by stereotyping. First, the assumption that the medical complaints of psychiatric patients are actually manifestations of psychiatric problems. The second and third sections describe the consequences of classic stereotypes of dangerousness leading to blanket search policies applicable to psychiatric patients but not to any other kind of patient and to the overuse of security guards in dealings with psychiatric patients, including escorts, restraint, seclusion, and monitoring.

The case law, legislative history of the ADA, and patient surveys reflect that ED staff often treat medical complaints of people with mental illness as though they are psychiatric in origin, sometimes with fatal results [5,42–44]. As one survey respondent reported:

I had a pain in my abdomen. Once the [ED] doctor found out I was in [a psychiatric hospital] for an eating disorder, she blamed the pain on eating food. The next day I found out I had a cyst in my ovary. They thought it was pain from refeeding syndrome. They didn't believe it was real pain. The doctor didn't listen about my pain and didn't run any tests besides blood work [2].

Research also supports the failure to diagnose and treat psychiatric patients' medical problems [45]. Ironically, when patients diagnosed with mental illness seek *psychiatric* care, it is often delayed by unnecessary medical tests; but when they seek *medical* care, their symptoms are often assumed to be psychiatric in nature. This is not to say that patients never fabricate medical complaints or somatize. But medical patients do this as well as psychiatric patients, and they are, in general, suspected less quickly. The fact that psychiatric patients die, on average, twenty years before the rest of the population is well known and is a public health concern. There are clearly many reasons for this, but misidentification of medical problems as psychiatric problems may be one of them. As recommended by a panel of experts, hospitals should conduct trainings and "[a]n important component of the training should be addressing the doctor's own stereotypes about people with psychiatric disabilities, and how these stereotypes interfere with good medical practice" [5].

Cases challenging mandatory clothing removal for psychiatric patients

"I said I just want to sit and talk to someone for fifteen minutes and my anxiety will wear off. I won't be anxious anymore. The nurse said you're suicidal. Take your clothes off" [2].

Many EDs have different clothing removal requirements for medical patients than for psychiatric patients. Some have blanket policies requiring all patients presenting for psychiatric reasons to change from their street clothing into hospital johnnies. The rationale given for implementing these policies varies, from concern about contraband to making elopement more difficult. However, in creating these policies, few EDs consider the substantial portion of people with psychiatric disabilities, especially women, whose conditions arise from or are related to histories of sexual abuse. For these women, removal of clothing may raise anxiety levels, especially when they are given hospital johnnies that are thin or too small, leaving them feeling vulnerable and frightened. Some patients refuse to remove their clothing for these reasons. If the refusal leads to a physical restraint by security guards of a previously calm patient to remove the patient's clothing, the hospital and physician ordering the restraint is at risk of violating federal and state laws regarding restraints (see below).

In Massachusetts, the Department of Public Health and the Department of Mental Health, in conjunction with an extremely wide array of stakeholders from emergency medicine, psychiatry, hospitals, private psychiatric facilities, nursing, insurance, advocates, and consumers, developed a licensing policy regarding clothing removal in EDs. The policy states that medical and psychiatric patients should be treated alike in terms of requests for clothing removal, and that hospitals should rescind all clothing removal policies that apply solely to patients seeking psychiatric treatment or who had psychiatric histories. It recognizes that clinicians may have legitimate reasons to request clothing removal, and can do so; and that patients had the right to refuse to remove their clothing, and must be informed of that right if they refuse to remove their clothing. It recognizes that forcible removal of clothing is a physical restraint, and can only be justified by "compelling clinical information indicating imminent risk to self or others" [46].

Litigation and administrative actions regarding the use of restraint and seclusion

"I got tired of lying on the bed. They told me I have to stay in the room. I felt like I was in jail, and I hadn't done nothing. I became not compliant with them. They put you in restraints because you won't stay in the bed" [2].

The systemic litigation in *Lizotte, Rubenstein,* and both the *Hirschfeld* and Department of Justice cases against the New York City Health and Hospital Corporation all cited overuse and misuse of restraint and seclusion by EDs. Restraint in EDs is one of the foremost complaints of patients, especially because (unlike on hospital wards) it is usually accomplished by uniformed security guards. Reducing the use of restraint and seclusion is a priority for the Joint Commission, the National Association of State Mental Health Program Directors, the Center for Medicare and Medicaid Services (CMS), the United States Department of Justice, and advocates for people with psychiatric disabilities all over the country.

All hospitals participating in the Medicare/Medicaid program agree to a set of rules ("conditions of participation" or "COPs") including rules relating to patients' rights, found in the Code of Federal Regulations at 42 C.F.R. 482.13. These conditions of participation contain substantial limitations on the use of restraint and seclusion by hospitals, including EDs, as well as training and reporting requirements, 42 C.F.R. 482.13(e) and (f). Numerous allegations of violations of these rules have been investigated and substantiated by the CMS and its assignees (usually the state licensing authority for the hospital), and many of them involve restraint immediately resulting from the refusal of a patient to remove his or her clothes. For example,

the records of a hospital in North Carolina involved a patient who had been cooperative upon arrival, but who became "upset at request to drop pants at check-in." The patient informed staff he had a history of being raped in prison. Upon refusal, he was restrained forcibly. The restraint resulted in the patient having a broken tooth, facial bruises, and a fractured finger. The CMS review found that the standard requiring restraint to be used only when less restrictive measures have been found to be ineffective was violated [47].

Physical and mechanical restraint

Although mechanical restraints, using ties or straps, are what most people associate with the term "restraint," it also applies to physical restraint, when a patient is held down or immobilized by another person. The definition of restraint is "any manual method, physical or mechanical device, material or equipment that immobilizes or reduces the ability of the patient to move his or her arms, legs, body, or head freely," 42 CFR 482.13(e)(1)(i)(A). In EDs, physical restraints are most often used by security guards, who hold patients down for various involuntary procedures, from clothing removal to blood draws to involuntary catheterization. None of these is permissible under federal regulations unless it is the only means to ensure the immediate physical safety of the patient, staff or others, 42 C.F.R. 482.13(e), and less restrictive interventions have been determined to be ineffective. In addition, these restraints must be ordered, documented, and justified by a physician. In practical terms, this means that a patient cannot be physically restrained to forcibly remove his or her clothes if he or she is calm. Even if ED staff suspects the patient may be carrying contraband, less restrictive interventions are usually available to ensure that the patient does not use the contraband, such as one-to-one "sitters," often used if the patient is suspected of being suicidal in any event. Of course, there is no prohibition against asking a patient to remove his or her clothing. But physical restraint to strip a patient must meet federal regulatory standards on restraint.

"Escorts" by security guards of unwilling patients who are trying to leave their gurney or the hospital are also physical restraints, with the requisite documentation requirements, if the security guard lays hands on the patient. Helping a patient hold steady for a medical procedure is not considered a restraint (assuming the patient has consented to the procedure), 42 CFR 482.13(e)(1)(i)(C).

Many EDs use a variety of mechanical devices, most commonly cloth or leather restraints, in addition to physical restraints. These are subject to the same standards and regulations as mechanical restraints. Some patients arrive with police restraints, such as handcuffs or spit masks. To reduce the chances of asphyxiation, which has caused several restraint-related deaths, many hospital policies require these to be removed, unless the patient remains in police custody with a police officer present at all times. The better clinical practice for patients who spit or bite is for staff to wear bite gloves, masks, or clear face shields.

Chemical restraint

Chemical restraint is defined as "a drug or medication when it is used as a restriction to manage the patient's behavior or restrict the patient's freedom of movement and is not a standard treatment or dosage for the patient's condition." A CMS Surveyor's Manual adds that "if the overall effect of a drug or medication, or combination of drugs or medications, is to reduce the patient's ability to effectively or appropriately interact with the world around the patient, then the drug or medication is *not* being used as a standard treatment or dosage for the patient's condition" [48] (emphasis in original). Thus, when a medication results in the patient being knocked out, or asleep, or unable to be effectively interviewed, it must be recorded as a chemical restraint. Many patients who arrive at the ED in extremely agitated states are medicated. Because the ED staff cannot always know the source of the patient's agitation, his or her previous drug ingestion, or medication allergies, there is inherent risk in using medication as a restraint that should be balanced with the risk of not medicating an extremely agitated patient once less restrictive means have been unsuccessful.

Although anecdotal evidence suggests that chemical restraints are not always properly recorded as such, there appear to have been relatively few complaints and investigations on this issue compared with complaints relating to physical or mechanical restraints.

Medical malpractice and psychiatric patients in the ED

ED physicians may assume that malpractice claims associated with psychiatric patients in the ED stem primarily from improvident discharges of patients who later cause harm to themselves or others. In fact, a multi-year survey of the case law and jury verdicts shows a wide range of types of cases and a great predominance of defense verdicts [5]. A substantial proportion of malpractice cases challenge the patient's involuntary detention (with actions for false imprisonment); involuntary treatment or clothing removal (action for battery), or failure to provide informed consent. In Barker v. Netcare Corp., a voluntary psychiatric patient who was upset after being raped, left the hospital against medical advice. The nurse called the on-call doctor, who told her to call the police. Although no one at the hospital filled out involuntary detention papers required by statute, the police brought the woman back. The nurse called the doctor again, because the patient was agitated and combative. He ordered involuntary sedation and restraint by telephone. She was sent home in the morning. As the appellate opinion upholding the award of $150,000 stated: "Dr. Basobas never met Barker until the trial" [25].

One common misunderstanding about tort actions following the discharge of a patient is the belief that the crux of these actions is the discharge itself. Instead, it is the negligent or insufficiently documented evaluation that led to the discharge. In other words, ED physicians and psychiatrists are not liable for bad outcomes, but only for negligent evaluations that produce foreseeably bad outcomes. Courts also assume that evaluating physicians have a right to rely on their patients' responses: in one case, the court found that the plaintiff was also negligent because there was "evidence he was not completely truthful or forthcoming in his statements to ... the emergency room physician" and because he failed to keep the mental health appointment made for him the next day [49].

In all of these tort cases, it is generally only in extraordinary circumstances – absence of documentation, errors or contradictions in documentation, or clearly insufficient or improperly motivated evaluations – that plaintiffs prevail. In the Barker v. Netcare case, the defendants were denied immunity because they failed to fill out *any* paperwork at any time before involuntarily detaining the plaintiff. Courts have considerable sympathy for the burdens of ED practice and begin with an assumption of professionalism and regularity regardless of the claim. Courts are also clear about the balancing of rights and safety that must take place when evaluating psychiatric patients, and generally defer to well-documented decisions. Most courts understand that no discharge decision is entirely without risk, and that physicians must be protected if the public policy benefits of taking these risks are to be preserved. A court's observation many years ago has become a standard cited by many courts:

"The prediction of the future course of a mental illness is a professional judgment of high responsibility and in some instances it involves a measure of calculated risk. If liability were imposed on the physician or the State each time the prediction of future course of mental disease was wrong, few releases would ever be made and the hope of recovery and rehabilitations of a vast number of patients would be impeded and frustrated. This is one of the medical and public risks which must be taken on balance, even though it may sometimes result in injury to the patient and others" [50].

This language has been quoted many times by courts across the country in finding that mental health professionals are not liable for the actions of their psychiatric patients, if they display good judgment and documentation [51–53]. In another case, the court refused to find that a mental health provider could have predicted that his patient would become violent, despite the presence of certain risk factors, stating:

"Our conclusions [that the injuries were unforeseeable] are further supported by public policy concerns. A court must "evaluate [the plaintiff's] allegations in light of the goal of treatment, recovery and rehabilitation of those afflicted with a mental disease, defect or disorder." [Citation omitted]. Imposing liability on a psychiatrist in an outpatient, short-term care setting for the actions of a patient that were at most based on risk factors and not foreseeability would have an adverse effect on psychiatric care. It would encourage psychiatrists and other mental health providers to return to paternalistic practices, such as involuntary commitment, to protect themselves against possible medical malpractice" [52].

While the setting in this last case was not an ED, the analysis reflects a common perspective of courts. The future actions of people with psychiatric disabilities are hard to predict, and public policy favors community-based treatment for them. This policy cannot be effectuated without protection from liability for evaluating mental health professionals who seek to implement it. In many states this protection has been written into statutory law in the form of immunity from negligence actions for mental health professionals' commitment and discharge decisions.

HIPAA and confidentiality

"The doctor ran up and down the hallway telling everyone I couldn't have pain meds" [54].

"Female staff said she was mad a patient had returned to [**] . . . I thought it was unprofessional to say this out loud" [54].

"Nurses were making jokes about a patient [who was suicidal], saying he was stupid because he only shot himself in the shoulder" [5].

The requirements of patient confidentiality are often conflated with the requirements imposed by HIPAA, but they are not necessarily the same. While ethical requirements of patient care and confidentiality would preclude the comments overheard by patients who are quoted above, HIPAA does not prevent healthcare providers discussing the treatment of a patient in a busy ED hallway, even if there is a possibility of being overheard, although it does require that these conversations take place in lowered voices [55].

HIPAA also covers areas generally not considered to be part of confidentiality. For example, it provides a right for patients to have access to and copy their records, with very few exceptions. This right applies to ED records. Hospitals may not charge for "records review" although they may recoup reasonable copying charges. Denying a patient access to records is one of the three most commonly investigated issues by the Office of Civil Rights. Patients also have a right to ask to correct their records under HIPAA, which is not generally thought of as pertaining to confidentiality.

Patients presenting for psychiatric reasons to EDs rarely complain about HIPAA, but surveys of these individuals commonly found complaints about violations of patient confidentiality. Patients seeking psychiatric help are sensitive and feel stigmatized, and many are upset at the degree to which the confidentiality of patient information is violated in the ED, especially when they overhear ED staff complaining about psychiatric patients.

Nursing homes and "dumping"

In the past decade, complaints have increased that nursing homes "dump" behaviorally problematic residents by bringing them to EDs for psychiatric or medical evaluations, and then refusing to take the residents back. This practice is, for the most part, illegal, but the rights that exist to prevent it are time-sensitive, and ED social workers must act quickly to protect the patient.

Although Medicaid no longer pays nursing homes to hold beds for patients who are hospitalized, it still requires nursing homes to notify patients of their bed-hold policies in writing (42 U.S.C. 1396R(c)(2)(A) and (B)). Nursing homes are not required to permit patients to pay to hold their beds, but if they do, both bed-day limits and the charges must be clearly reflected in the written policy. In addition, even if patients exceed any bed-hold days, they have the right to be admitted to the first available semi-private bed at the nursing home (42 U.S.C. 1396R(c)(2)(D)(iii)). If the patient is being discharged due to the expected length of stay in the hospital, the patient has a right to notice of the proposed discharge, and to appeal the discharge, and the bed must be held pending the appeal. When a nursing home brings a patient to the ED, the ED may consider a protocol whereby an ED social worker immediately inquires whether the resident's bed is being held for him, and asks for a written copy of any decision involving discharge, including the reason for any exception to the 30-day notice rule (see below) as well as the nursing home's bed-hold policy. If the bed is being held, and the patient is being considered for hospital admission, the social worker should talk to the patient's family and inpatient unit about the possibility of paying to hold the bed, and about any bed-hold day limit.

If the nursing home states that the bed will not be held, this should be regarded as a discharge or transfer. A Medicare/Medicaid patient has a right not to be discharged or transferred without notice, and may appeal any discharge or transfer to an impartial reviewer called a quality improvement organization (call 1–800-MEDICARE for contact information in your state). The written notice provided by the nursing home is generally supposed to be thirty days, but nursing homes attempting to dump a patient at the ED will generally invoke one of two exceptions: the patient has urgent medical needs, or the patient is dangerous to the health and safety of other individuals in the facility. The nursing home is required to hold the patient's bed pending appeal. Most importantly, even if the nursing home has the right to discharge a resident for being dangerous, it cannot do so by refusing to readmit the resident after a hospitalization, but must readmit the resident and then take the necessary steps to transfer or discharge the resident [56,57].

The hospital should consider an in-service by legal services or an advocacy program for the elderly to both better understand the rights of nursing home patients brought to the ED and to create the relationships with legal services organizations that will enable family members to enforce those rights.

Conclusion

When a focus group of people with serious psychiatric disabilities were asked, "How would you change the way EDs treat people with psychiatric disabilities?" this is what they said:

"It takes someone with the ability to work with frightened people. The conditions of the ED create fear."

"I would like for people to stop looking and talking about me like I don't know what's going on."

"Understand that mental patients have a heart – it's okay to treat them as a person"[2].

Although this chapter has been about law, the apparently paradoxical truth is that the doctors who concentrate on caring for their patients and worry least about liability are the least likely to be sued, while the doctors most concerned about liability are more likely to be sued [5,9].

Worrying about liability may be adversarial; doctors who are completely allied with the patient and dedicated to his or her care are more easily forgiven their mistakes. This is particularly true with patients who are in emotional crisis: patience, respect, and listening are not only an important aspect of treatment, but an essential precondition for it.

References

1. Gilbert S. Psychiatric crash cart: treatments for the emergency department. *Adv Emerg Nurs J* 2009;31:298–308.

2. Maryland Disability Law Center and the Center for Public Representation. *Maryland Citizens in Psychiatric Crisis: A Report*. Baltimore: Maryland Disability Law Center; 2008.

3. Jayaram G, Triplett, D. Quality improvement of psychiatric care: challenges of emergency psychiatry. *Am J Psychiatry* 2008;165:1256–60.

4. Judd A, Miller A. *Mental Patient Backlog Jams ER,"* Atlanta Journal-Constitution, Nov. 28, 2007. Available at: www.gmhcn.org/files/Articles/AJC_response_Mentalpatient backlogjamser.html. (last visited September 30, 2011)

5. Stefan S. *Emergency Department Treatment of the Psychiatric Patient: Policy Issues and Legal Requirements*. New York: Oxford University Press; 2006.

6. U.S. Department of Health and Human Services. Office of Disability, Aging and Long-Term Care Policy. *A Literature Review: Psychiatric Boarding*. Available at: www.aspe.hhs.gov/daltcp/reports/2008/PsyBdLR.htm (Accessed October 2008).

7. U.S. Department of Health and Human Services. Office of Disability, Aging and Long-Term Care Policy. *Psychiatric Boarding Interview Summary*. Available at: www.aspe.hhs.gov/daltcp/reports/2009/PsyBdInt.htm (Accessed January 2009).

8. Nordt C, Rossler W, Lauber C. Attitudes of mental health professionals towards people with schizophrenia and major depression. *Schizophr Bull* 2006;32:709–14.

9. Mossman D. Defensive medicine: can it increase your malpractice risk? *Curr Psychiatry* 2008. Available at: www.currentpsychiatry.com/pdf/0812/0812CP_Malpractice.pdf.

10. Bragdon v. Abbott. 524 U.S. 624 (1998).

11. Jouthe v. City of New York.2009 U.S. Dist.LEXIS 18163 (E.D.N.Y. March 10, 2009).

12. Sampson v.BIDMC. No. 06-10973DPW (D.Mass. complaint filed August 4, 2006). Available at: www.centerforpublicrep.org/images/stories/docs/sampson-israel.pdf (Accessed September 30, 2011).

13. Committee on the Future of Emergency Care in the United States Health System. *Hospital-based Emergency Care: At the Breaking Point*. Washington, DC: The National Academies Press; 2007.

14. Hanlon P. *Advocate Files Lawsuit Against Rhode Island*. Available at: www.nepsy.com/leading/0712_ne_RI_advocate.html. (Accessed August 16, 2011).

15. Rockwell v. Cape Cod Hospital. 26 F.3d 254 (1st Cir.1994).

16. Scott v. Hern. 216 F.3d 897 (10th Cir.2000).

17. Tewksbury v. Dowling. 169 F.Supp. 103 (E.D.N.Y. 2001).

18. Ruhlmann v. Ulster County. 234 F. Supp.2d 140 (N.D.N.Y.2002).

19. Palaimo v. Lutz. 837 F.Supp. 55 (N.D. N.Y.1993).

20. Jensen v. Lane County. 222 F.3d 570 (9th Cir.2000).

21. Payton v. Rush Presbyterian St. Lukes Medical Center. 184 F.3d 623 (7th Cir. 1999).

22. Rodriguez v. City of New York. 72 F.3d1051 (2nd Cir. 1995).

23. Marion v. LaFargue. 2004 U.S.Dist. LEXIS 2601 (E.D.N.Y. Feb. 23, 2004).

24. Riffe v. Armstrong. 477 S.E.2d 535 (W.Va.1996).

25. Barker v. Netcare Corp. 147 Ohio App.3d 1 (2001).

26. James v. City of Wilkes-Barre. 2011 U.S. Dist.LEXIS 90575 (M.D.Pa. August 15, 2011).

27. Marion v. LaFargue. 2005 U.S.Dist. LEXIS 11682 (S.D.N.Y. June 15, 2005).

28. Benn v. Universal Health System. 371 F.3d 165 (3rd Cir.2004).

29. In re C.W. , 147 Wn.2d 259 (2002).

30. Lizotte v. New York City Health and Hospital Corporation. 1992 U.S.Dist. LEXIS 10976 (S.D.N.Y. July 16, 1992).

31. Rubenstein v. Benedictine Hospital. 790 F.Supp. 396 (N.D.N.Y. 1992).

32. Monaco v. Stone. 81 F.R.D. 50 (E.D. N.Y.1999).

33. Monaco v. Carpinello. 2007 U.S.Dist. LEXIS 28990 (E.D.N.Y. April 19, 2007).

34. Monaco v. Stone. 576 F.Supp.2d 335 (E.D.N.Y.2008).

35. Bolmer v. Oliveira. 594 F.3d 134 (2nd Cir.2010).

36. Monaco v. Hogan. 2010 U.S.Dist.LEXIS 131546 (E.D.N.Y. Dec. 10, 2010).

37. New York City Health and Hospitals Corporation. Press release. *With Major Reforms in Place, HHC Reaches Settlement Agreement to Resolve Lawsuit Against Kings County Hospital Program*, January 8, 2010. Available at: www.nyc.gov/html/hhc/html/pressroom/press-release-20100108.shtml (Accessed September 28, 2011).

38. Hirschfeld v. New York Health and Hospital Corporation. No. 1:07-cv-0819 (E.D.N.Y. complaint filed May 2, 2007). Available at www.nyclu.org/files/releases/KCHCcomplaint.pdf (Accessed Sept. 28, 2011).

39. Hirschfeld v. New York Health and Hospital Corporation. No. 1:07-cv-0819-KAM (E.D.N.Y. settlement filed Jan. 8, 2010). Available at: www.nyclu.org/files/releases/KCHCSettlement_1.8.10.pdf (Accessed September 28, 2011).

40. United States v. Delaware. Settlement agreement. Available at: www.justice.gov/crt/about/spl/documents/DE_settlement_7-6-11.pdf (Accessed October 1, 2011).

41. United States v. Georgia. Settlement agreement. Available at: www.justice.gov/crt/about/spl/documents/georgia/US_v_Georgia_ADAorder_10-2-10.pdf (Accessed October 1, 2011).

42. Jackson v. E. Bay Hospital. 246 F.3d 1248 (9th Cir. 2001).

43. Kauffman v. Frantz. 2010 U.S.Dist. LEXIS 29036 (E.D.Pa. March 26, 2010)

44. Baber v. Hospital Corp. of America. 977 F.2d 872 (4th Cir. 1992).

45. Felker B, Yazel JJ, Short D. Mortality and medical comorbidity among psychiatric patients: a review. *Psychiatr Serv* 1996;**47**:1356–63.

46. Massachusetts Executive Office of Health and Human Services, Department of Public Health. *Treatment of Individuals with Behavioral Health Issues in Hospital Emergency Departments.* Circular Letter DHCQ 08–07–495 (July 8, 2008).

47. Department of Health and Human Services, Center for Medicare and Medicaid Services. Statement of deficiency, Broughton Hospital, Event ID RMTM11, Survey Completed August 5, 2005.

48. Center for Medicaid and Medicare Services. State Operations Manual, Appendix A, Survey Protocol, Regulations and Interpretive Guidelines for Hospitals. Available at: www.cms.gov/manuals/downloads/som107ap_a_hospitals.pdf (Accessed 2009).

49. Sheron v. Lutheran Medical Center. 18 P.3d 796 (Colo.App. 2001).

50. Taig v. State. 19 A.D.2d 182 (N.Y.1963).

51. Cerbelli v. City of New York. 600 F. Supp.2d 405 (E.D.N.Y.2008).

52. Williamson v.Liptzin. 141 N.C.App. 1 (2000).

53. Durney v. Terk. 42 A.D. 3d 335 (N.Y.2007).

54. Hospital Survey of Psychiatric Patient Experiences in Emergency Departments (2009).

55. Department of Health and Human Services. Office of Civil Rights, Health Information Privacy, Frequently Asked Questions. Available at: www.hhs.gov/ocr/privacy/hipaa/faq/smaller_providers_and_businesses/196.html (Accessed September 27, 2011).

56. Kindred Nursing Centers West LLC v. California Health and Human Services Agency. 2005 WL 1460714 (Cal.App. 2005).

57. Smith v. Chattanooga Medical Investors. 62 S.W.3d 178 (Tenn.App. 2001).

Chapter 49

Law enforcement and emergency psychiatry

Daryl Knox

Introduction

"22-year-old African-American male brought in by the Sheriff's office. Individual has a history of mental illness. Currently experiencing paranoid delusions. Believes his mother is trying to poison him. He is not consuming sufficient food or liquids due to his paranoid delusions. Becoming increasingly aggressive at home. Sleeps in a closet and does not go outside. Is noncompliant with current medications. Admits to auditory hallucinations but cannot provide details."

"56-year-old Hispanic female brought in by police department officer who found patient in front of an elementary school, yelling, cursing at students, very delusional, disorganized, and paranoid."

"48-year-old White male brought in by police officers from a personal care home where patient was breaking and throwing things, disorganized, and disruptive behavior."

These vignettes, actually taken from the intake board of a Psychiatric Emergency Service (PES), illustrate that law enforcement personnel are routinely involved with patients who present to emergency departments (EDs) and specialized PES settings. Receiving facilities and their staff should endeavor to do all they can to expedite the process of patient hand-off and facilitate the law enforcement officer's return to their primary duty of protecting the community. It is important for physicians and clinicians working in emergency medical settings to understand the role of law enforcement in the mental health system, the history surrounding this relationship, and how law enforcement's involvement with mentally ill persons fits into the broader context of public health and safety.

This chapter will explore the benefits of embracing (rather than marginalizing) this law enforcement ED/PES partnership and identify strategies to facilitate the intake process to ensure positive outcomes for the patient as well as the public health and safety of the community. The chapter will also review the historical development of this relationship, examine some of the barriers to care and perceptions in regards to criminalization of the emergency treatment of the mentally ill, and outline innovative programs and initiatives that have leveraged this partnership to provide system efficiencies and better mental health outcomes.

Regardless of one's philosophical view or ethical stance regarding a patient's autonomy in the choice of whether to seek or not to seek psychiatric treatment, the fact is that when it comes to the care of the severe and persistently mentally ill patient population, the criminal justice system plays a key role within the emergency mental healthcare delivery system. The healthcare–justice system interface runs the gamut from the apprehension by police of a patient on a mental health warrant or hold, which mandates an evaluation by a physician or mental health professional, to the ordering and deliberation of a competency or sanity evaluation by a magistrate or judge. The types of law enforcement personnel involved varies by jurisdiction, community, and purpose, ranging from city police officers, county sheriffs, constables, school district or university police, airport police, and in some instances Department of Home Land Security officers. Perhaps more than any other aspect of medicine, ED physicians and psychiatric emergency service psychiatrists interface routinely with law enforcement officers as they escort patients to these settings for various types of evaluation and treatment.

Jails and mental health treatment

Increasingly prisons and jails are becoming primary providers of mental health care as community mental health resources are inadequately funded to intervene and treat the growing number of people needing mental health care [1]. Before the deinstitutionalization movement in the early 1950s state hospitals were large and provided the much needed custodial care for the severe and persistently mentally ill (SPMI) population. With the advent of first-generation antipsychotic medications, e.g., chlorpromazine, and their ability to quell psychotic symptoms, thousands of these patients were discharged from state institutions to communities that were and still are ill-equipped or funded to provide the resources necessary for these patients to maintain an adequate level of functioning and integration.

Jail diversion

As those with mental health disorders are abandoned by overwhelmed families and become homeless, they come to the

Behavioral Emergencies for the Emergency Physician, ed. Leslie S. Zun, Lara G. Chepenik, and Mary Nan S. Mallory. Published by Cambridge University Press. © Cambridge University Press 2013.

attention of law enforcement officers for mainly misdemeanor behaviors of public loitering, public urination, and trespassing. With community mental health resources shrinking or lacking altogether, law enforcement officers have few options other than to take these individuals to jail [2]. It is estimated that the "prevalence of serious mental illness in jails ranges from 7% to 16% and compared with the general population men with mental illness are four times more likely to be incarcerated and women with mental illness are more than eight times more likely to be incarcerated" [3].

Inadequate funding, overwhelmed outpatient mental health systems, and a lack of psychiatric inpatient beds additionally contribute to the incarceration of undertreated mentally ill patients. Numerous programs and partnerships have developed between mental health programs and police aimed at diverting the mentally ill into treatment rather than inappropriate incarcerations. Law enforcement agencies have become proactive in creating programs within their departments and in partnership with local mental health systems to educate officers about mental illness, divert patients from jail incarceration to mental health treatment, and decrease use of crisis emergency services [4,5].

Law enforcement initiatives

Law enforcement interactions with the mentally ill in our communities have existed for many years. Some jurisdictions developed Mental Health Deputy programs whereby some officers in local sheriff or municipal police departments completed various amounts of mental health training to receive the designation of Mental Health Deputy. These officers respond to mental health dispatch calls and transports of patients to local EDs or crisis centers for evaluation. Lamb et al. [2] discuss the common law principles that underlie this police responsibility to those with mental illness, having both power and authority to protect the safety and welfare of the community, and *parens patriae* obligations to protect individuals with disabilities.

More recently, training about mental illness, diagnosis, and treatments along with de-escalation techniques have come to be considered mandatory training for new cadets in many police departments. Usually these courses are given in partnership with mental health professionals aimed at educating officers on how to recognize the signs of mental illness and how to access local mental health resources.

Also, many of the Mental Health Deputy Programs have evolved into dedicated Crisis Intervention Training (CIT) for police officers [6]. Also known as Crisis Intervention Response Teams (CIRT), officers are paired with mental health professionals who respond to police dispatch calls where there is an identified or suspected mental health issue. These teams are familiar with mental health treatment resources in the community and may be able to de-escalate the situation at the scene and refer the patient and/or family to appropriate community mental health treatment resources. When the situation is more acute these teams will escort the patient to the nearest hospital ED or PES. CIRT may also work in conjunction with mobile crisis teams, operated by the mental health centers, which travel to the patient's environment, intervene, and link patients to outpatient mental health and other services.

One particularly innovative program initiated by the City of Houston (Texas) Police Department (HPD) in partnership with the local community mental health center (MHMRA of Harris County) is the Chronic Consumer Stabilization Initiative (CCSI). By auditing dispatch calls to HPD that were mental health related, the top 30 mentally ill utilizers of the dispatch system were identified. Mental health case managers were assigned to intervene, establish rapport, and connect patients with mental health services in hopes of decreasing police interactions. The outcomes included a significant drop in the usage of crisis services and hospitalizations along with a drop in the number of police dispatch calls involving these patients [7].

The roles and realities of law enforcement

The role of the emergency physician in the ED or PES is to evaluate a patient's mental and physical condition, treat and make an appropriate clinical disposition to either discharge with or without outpatient follow-up or admit for inpatient psychiatric treatment. The role of law enforcement is to ensure public safety and in the case of the *involuntary* mentally ill patient, provide transport to an appropriate setting for a mental health evaluation. With regard to the community interface with those with mental illness, the latter presents the greatest challenge to officers.

Escorting a mentally ill patient into the medical treatment environment of the ED or PES can be a daunting, unfamiliar, and time-consuming task for the officer. When there is no collaborative professional partnership that exists, mentally ill patients can often end up in jail because the booking procedure is often less time consuming than the PES/ED process, allowing the officer return to their primary duty of protecting the public and maintaining the public safety net [2]. As officers encounter obstacles such as prolonged wait times or refusal of patients by clinicians, they may become disillusioned and mistrustful of the healthcare system responsible for treatment. In extreme cases, these admission delays may result in officers resenting or avoiding their safety net role with the mentally ill.

Most interactions between law enforcement officers and the ED and PES physicians will revolve around the involuntary commitment process. In many states only law enforcement officials are authorized by the state's mental health code to apprehend and involuntarily transport persons exhibiting unusual behavior indicative of an underlying mental illness for evaluation.

Police-applied restraints

Often patients will present to an ED or psychiatric emergency service in the custody of an officer for an evaluation of behaviors that are indicative of a mental illness. These patients may come to the attention of the law enforcement officer who encounters these individuals while on routine patrol as they are exhibiting odd behaviors, or from family members or the general public who may call the officers out of concern that the odd behavior may be due to a mental disorder. More often than not these individuals are quite agitated due to the underlying psychiatric illness and/or the effects of illicit drug use and may present in handcuffs or other types of restraints that have been applied by law enforcement.

This presentation of patients in police restraints creates a dilemma for the clinicians as many of the restraints used by law enforcement, e.g., handcuffs and hog-tie (hobble) restraints, are considered inappropriate by hospital quality oversight agencies like the Center for Medicare and Medicaid Services CMS [8], The Joint Commission (TJC), state regulators, and the policies of the hospital for the ED or the PES, and for good reason as the hog-tie restraints have been associated with severe injury and death [9] and many police departments have policies against their use.

What about those instances where the patient is not calm on arrival to the hospital, is still agitated and aggressive, with a potential for violence? A difficult-to-identify overlap of time may occur between the point at which police custody ends and hospital treatment begins. Law enforcement officers, unlike hospital staffs, are less regulated and restricted in the types of restraint they can use, and instead are expected to use their training to protect the patient as well as themselves and others by applying best judgment. If the patient is given emergency medications by the physician while in police custody, does this mean the patient is now in ED/PES custody? What should be done with the handcuffs? When should police-applied restraints be removed and the patient placed in restraints appropriate for the hospital setting? What about the potential for injury to the patient, other patients and staff while trying to remove the police restraint and place hospital restraints?

Often officers are reluctant to remove the restraints immediately upon arrival to the hospital because of the patient's agitation and behavior during apprehension and transport. It is important for clinicians to respect the officer's reluctance and use de-escalation techniques to establish therapeutic rapport with the patient. Once rapport is established or if needed, hospital seclusion and restraint practices are implemented, and police-applied restraints are then removed. Hospital policy and protocols for patients in restraints, regardless of who applied the restraints, must be followed once the physician endorses their use. It is usually impractical and potentially unsafe to immediately remove one restraint type and apply another. Safety of the patient and staff must be primarily considered. Also the clinical staff, in transition with law enforcement personnel, must do all that is feasible to protect the dignity of the patient and keep the encounter as therapeutic as possible. For some patients, this may be their first encounter with treatment for a mental illness so clinicians must do all they can make this experience as therapeutic as possible so as to not deter the patient from seeking ongoing voluntary treatment once the crisis episode is resolved [10].

Embracing the interaction with law enforcement

Officers who bring patients to healthcare providers for assessment are a good source of information regarding a patient's behavior, the condition of the patient's home environment, and can convey valuable information from collateral resources such as family and neighbors which will meaningfully contribute to the physician's assessment accuracy and efficiency.

Just as with medical presentations, mental health presentations can evolve or stabilize in a short period of time. Care should be taken in communicating with an officer as to why a patient was escorted to the hospital, whom after the initial assessment, does not appear to have a behavioral health emergency. Even well-trained, experienced officers cannot be expected to operate at the level of a licensed mental health professional.

Officers are usually appreciative when a clinician takes the time to explain a disposition that is different from what the officer expected. Take the time to explain and communicate the clinical rationale as to why an escorted patient does not need admittion or why an involuntary commitment was not indicated. Officers may not understand that mental health patients do have a right to refuse necessary treatment as long as their decisional capacity is maintained.

Policies that prioritize the triage and assessment of patients brought in either voluntarily or involuntarily by law enforcement officers will expedite the hand-off of the patient, and return officers to their other primary duties. Where practical, providing a workspace for escorting officers to complete and submit their required documentation also improves law enforcement efficiency.

Inefficient use of law enforcement officers aside, scope-of-practice issues arise when police-escorted patients are turned away from free-standing psychiatric emergency services or psychiatric hospitals because of a perceived medical instability or chronic medical comorbidities. In as much as possible, a free-standing PES should have capability to recognize medical emergencies and differentiate them from non-emergent presentations of chronic medical conditions such as elevated blood pressure associated with chronic hypertension and hyperglycemia in a patient with diabetes. In addition to psychotropic medications, common medications for treating these conditions should be on their formulary. Where practical, medical protocols that outline the parameters for treatment of these conditions by the PES physician, when to contact medical consultants, and when to refer to a medical facility should be developed. These protocols can save time and money and avoid additional patient transport and law enforcement involvement. When a stand-alone PES lacks needed medical back-up, temporarily assuming responsibility for the patient, providing the limited medical assessment and care available, and arranging emergency transport by means of ambulance to the nearest treatment facility, not requesting police re-transport, is the safest and most appropriate plan for a patient deemed by PES staff to have an emergency medical condition.

Children

On occasion, children and adolescents are transported by law enforcement, usually school district security personnel, for assessment of a psychiatric or behavioral problem. Sometimes it is not possible to reach the parent or legal guardian to obtain the appropriate consent for treatment. Lack of parental approval should not be the sole basis for refusal to accept minors. The patient can be assessed to determine acuity and placed on one-to-one observation until parents or guardians can be reached or until child protective services staff can arrive. Unless an assessment is completed and a safe place has been established, officers should not be tasked with custody or transport of a minor simply because a legal guardian could not be contacted, particularly when a child appears to be in an acute psychiatric crisis. Emergency medication, restraints or seclusion would only be indicated in the most extreme circumstances for children where harm to themselves or others is imminent and less restrictive alternatives have failed.

Dementia/Intellectual Developmental Delay

Patients with dementia or intellectual developmental delay (IDD) are also presenting to EDs or psychiatric emergency services by law enforcement transport in growing numbers. Rapid triage is important for these patients who have not had the benefit of prehospital medical assessment and may have acute medical conditions contributing to the current behavior. Even if it becomes apparent that the primary issue is a social service one, for example a patient–caregiver conflict, ED or PES social service personnel should intervene to find the appropriate community resource for these patients. Finding safe dispositions for these patients is beyond the expertise of law enforcement officials.

Restarting or initiating pharmacologic treatment and the use of PES observation beds can mitigate the revolving door between crisis visits and hospitalization. PES/ED engagement with jail diversion initiatives may prevent inappropriate incarceration for those individuals whose criminal infractions are minor and directly attributable to their mental illness [1,3].

Many of the above strategies may seem impractical for EDs and PES, stretching already scarce resources even further. It is important for clinical leaders and administrators of EDs, emergency psychiatric services, and free-standing mental health treatment clinics and inpatient facilities to proactively collaborate with law enforcement, prehospital providers, and community leaders in the development of strategies to address their local problems with crisis mental health care. Lacking this, communities feel the strain on system resources, with the resultant overflow of mentally ill patients into jails instead of treatment.

Criminalization of mentall illness

Some could argue that involvement of law enforcement in the mental health treatment system stigmatizes mental health patients as criminals. State mental health codes may mandate the involvement of law enforcement in the apprehension of individuals with mental illness who are an apparent danger to themselves or others as a result of their illness, to allow for an evaluation by a physician or licensed mental health professional. The effects of this legal loss of autonomy are mitigated by efficient hand-offs between law enforcement and healthcare workers. Medical triage and psychiatric intake procedures should do all they can to protect the humanity and dignity of the patient. Law enforcement entities should train their officers on de-escalation techniques and other appropriate responses to distressed persons with mental illness. Use of unmarked police vehicles and creation of specialized mental health intervention teams without traditional uniforms can soften negative reactions to police involved in the commitment process. As law enforcement entities continue to collaborate with local mental health systems, EDs and other stakeholders in the care and treatment of those with mental illness, officers may come to be seen as treatment facilitators rather than treatment enforcers.

Summary

A coordinated interface between law enforcement officers and ED staff, physicians, and mental health clinicians is imperative. This relationship has existed for some time, stemming from the role of the police to protect the public safety as well as to protect the rights of people with mental illness and other disabling conditions. Jail can, unfortunately, become the expedient disposition for mentally ill patients encountered by law enforcement officers when adequate mental health resources and collaborations are lacking within the community.

In efforts to compassionately and effectively assist mental health patients, many police departments and local mental health systems have developed training programs, designated response teams, and intervention strategies to facilitate care for those in need of acute treatment. Emergency departments and psychiatric emergency services significantly impact both the system and the patient when the triage and psychiatric intake process for escorted patients is streamlined. Police escorts are simply that, and once a mentally ill patient has been delivered to an acute care facility, providers contribute to the safety of the public at large when they assume responsibility for patients so that law enforcement officers can resume a community presence to perform their primary role in public safety. Special circumstances, such as those encountered in patients with dementia or for unaccompanied children, present management challenges that are best handled with pre-arranged protocols and the assistance of social services. The ongoing supervision of patients awaiting treatment or placements, who are not under arrest, is beyond the scope of law enforcement.

Discussion

As cuts to mental health budgets continue to increase across the nation, EDs will encounter an ever-increasing volume of mentally ill patients seeking assistance and treatment. Emergency nurse and physician interactions with law enforcement will likely also increase. As with any partnership, questions regarding roles, boundaries, and responsibilities will emerge. ED and PES physicians must make preparations for an increase in census and develop collaborative and proactive approaches to care for patients escorted by law enforcement, rapidly assessing patients and facilitating the public safety role of officers back in the community. Needs exceeding limited resources spell crisis as the demand for psychiatric services increases in a system that, in many communities, is already overwhelmed. Leadership and collaborative initiatives, especially in the face of limited resources, are important to ensure that patients in crisis receive care, not incarceration.

References

1. Lamb HR, Weinberger LE. The shift of psychiatric inpatient care from hospitals to jails and prisons. *J Am Psychiatry Law* 2005;**4**:529–34.

2. Lamb HR, Weinberger LE, DeCuir WJ. The police and mental health. *Psychiatr Serv* 2002;**10**:1266–71.

3. Osher FC, Steadman HJ. Adapting evidence based practices for persons with mental illness involved with the criminal justice system. *Psychiatr Serv* 2007;**58**:1472–8.

4. Deane MW, Steadman HJ, Borum R, Veysey BM, Morrissey JP. Emerging partnerships between mental health and law enforcement. *Psychiatr Serv* 1999;**1**:99–101.

5. Steadman HJ, Osher FC, Robbins PC, Case B, Samuels S. Prevalence of serious mental illness among jail inmates. *Psychiatr Serv* 2009;**6**:761–5.

6. Hails J, Borum R. Police training and specialized approaches to respond to people with mental illness. *Crime Delinq* 2003;**1**:52–61.

7. MacLeod A, Pate M. CCSI Program. (unpublished presentation). Crisis Intervention Team International Conference; September 14, 2011; Virginia Beach, VA.

8. Federal Register. 482.13 Condition of participation: patients rights. December 2006: 7142 6–8.

9. Zun LS. A prospective study of the complication rate of use of patient restraint in the emergency department. *Emer Med J* 2003;**2**:119–24.

10. Berlin J. *Psychiatric Emergency Department: Where Treatment Should Begin.* Psychiatric News website. Available at: pn. psychiatryonline.org/ content/46/14/1.2.1 (Accessed September 4, 2011.)

Chapter 50

Research in emergency psychiatry

Ross A. Heller and Preeti Dalawari

Introduction

The top five most costly disorders for American health care are cancer, trauma, heart conditions, asthma, and mental health disorders [1,2]. Research funding for mental health and emergency psychiatry disorders significantly lags behind the other four problems [2].

Research into evaluation and treatment for emergency psychiatric patients is of extreme importance because of the current lack of data guiding treatment choice. Patients with an emergency psychiatric problem (as chief complaint) are estimated to represent up to 7% of all ED visits [1,3]. It has been reported that as many as 33% of all patients who visit the ED may have a mental disorder complaint [1,3]. Yet significant barriers and obstacles exist to scientists attempting to do research into evaluation and treatment for this varied patient population. This chapter will explore the various problems researchers face conducting emergency psychiatric research. A variety of issues which inhibit psychiatric emergency research have been identified.

The recruitment of patients into studies, proper consent of patients with psychiatric illnesses, a general lack of adequate funding of psychiatric emergency patient-related studies all have been identified as major problems which must be overcome to do research [3,4]. The issue of the reliability and therefore usefulness of studies performed has been found to be problematic in emergency psychiatric research [3,4]. Recommendations regarding methods and techniques to overcome the identified obstacles and barriers that currently exist will be presented to provide a path for researchers to do the work necessary to provide best practice treatments for this patient population.

Barriers and obstacles

There are special considerations for doing research in the emergency psychiatric patient population. A plethora of barriers and obstacles exist for those scientists attempting to conduct research into testing, treatment, and disposition of the psychiatric emergency patient population such as difficulty enrolling patients, problems with reliability of testing,

narrowness of enrollee populations, and others. D'Onofrio in 2010 reported the results of an National Institutes of Health (NIH) roundtable designed to advance research on psychiatric emergencies [3]. The group reported a "Paucity of well-designed, focused research on diagnostic testing, clinical decision making and treatments in the emergency setting" [3]. Barriers to psychiatric emergency research were examined. First, there are few experienced researchers in emergency medicine doing research in psychiatric emergencies. There is difficulty in conducting research in the "hectic and non-controlled environment" of the emergency department (ED), and there is a significant lack of funding for such research [3]. A lack of standardized definitions of "suicidal behavior" and other mental health terms also contribute to difficulties conducting this research. In addition, there is a lack of "validated" screening tools for patients with mental illness, thus patients can't be culled out before being treated and limiting their placement in studies.

Additional limitations include ED staff who have negative attitudes toward patients presenting with a mental illness and/or a psychiatric emergency. This can prevent recruitment of patients into a research project. Poorly designed outcome measures are present in many studies, so that the endpoint of treatment can be varied and unreliable. The ability to get consent presents a difficult barrier in research of mental health patients. Highly suicidal patients were routinely excluded from many trials. Subsequently, few diagnostic profiles exist to stratify mental health patients by risk [3].

Woodall et al. [4] examined the barriers to participation in mental health research by gender, ethnicity, and age in a review of 44 papers on psychiatric emergencies. They discovered the emergency psychiatric population is quite diverse but a diverse population of patients was not represented in the studies.

Black and other ethnic minority groups were reluctant to be part of any research project. For the black community, the infamous Tuskegee experiments in the 1930s engendered serious trust issues of medical research [5]. The black community also feels there is stigmata associated with mental health disease and "reject" their diagnosis. Many qualified candidates for studies refuse to participate arguing that they did not "have

Behavioral Emergencies for the Emergency Physician, ed. Leslie S. Zun, Lara G. Chepenik, and Mary Nan S. Mallory. Published by Cambridge University Press. © Cambridge University Press 2013.

the mental health problem" [4]. For other ethnic minorities, language barriers prevented proper communication about mental health diseases and treatment options [4]. For some ethnic groups, immigration issues and the fear of legal jeopardy from lack of proper identification or "status" may limit this group from agreeing to participate in mental health studies [4].

Analysis of recruitment of patients with dementia by investigators showed that the age of the patient is not itself associated with recruitment issues. Instead, this patient population often showed reluctance accepting their diagnosis of dementia. Because they did not believe they have dementia, they naturally refused to participate in studies [4]. The elderly also had transportation problems in getting to sites of treatment. Physical limitations requiring mobility assistance interfered with their ability to get to treatment or research centers. The elderly also do not wish to participate in activities that cause them fatigue [4].

Gender role issues for participation in research studies were also examined. One study found that males with depression were reluctant to be recruited into studies concerned that a negative social perception is attached to having the diagnosis of depression [4].

Woodall et al. concluded that in many of these patient populations a denial of illness allowed them to decrease their imagined stigmata associated with mental health disorders [4].

Barriers in pediatrics

The NIH reported in 1999 that more research was needed in child and adolescent psychiatric illnesses. Barriers for patient participation in research for this population exist and may be unique [6]. The Institute of Medicine identified that inadequate training of the providers who attempt to enroll the pediatric patients into research is one such barrier [6,7]. The report also detailed that a suboptimal environment for pediatric patients with a "lack of concern for the comfort of the patient and their family in ED settings" represent a barrier in this patient population. The issue of extended waiting times in the emergency room for pediatric psychiatric patients is a barrier to success [6,7].

Solutions to barriers

Strategies are necessary to overcome various barriers and obstacles to research and D'Onofrio and others have proposed some "fixes" [3,4]. Some methods to help prevent rejection by various populations were presented and the solutions seem quite simple. For example, transportation assistance can be made available for those patients who have problems getting to treatment. This assistance can be a cab, a car pool, a bus pass, or a medi-car.

Researchers should be trained to avoid using "buzzwords" that patient populations view negatively. Use of alternative words or phrases that are inviting to these populations may result in more favorable responses for participation in a research project.

Proper use of phrases might need to begin at the initial recruitment of patients seen as highly sensitized to the stigmata of having a mental health illness [3,4].

Those patients who do not use English as their primary language require the use of bilingual staff. This staff would need to be trained in the language of the research process and to avoid native words that cause a negative reaction and therefore a refusal of the patient to participate in the research process [3,4].

Patients with caregivers must have a recruitment approach that includes the caregivers in the consent process. This may require multiple discussions about the patient's disorder and the potential benefits of participation in a study [3,4].

Recruiters for the pediatric patient population who understand the impact wait times and comfort issues may have on the patient and their family can create a favorable environment in which to enroll this population [7].

Consent

Any medical research requires the consent of the patient, or a surrogate for the patient. Because research of neuropsychiatric disorders involves patients with illnesses that affect cognition, decision-making capacity, and awareness the consent process can pose interesting and potentially ethical challenges. While there is potential benefit to society from this type of research, special safeguards must be established when dealing with these "vulnerable" patients. Research may provide the greatest yield in treatment options from the study of the most ill of psychiatric patients or in those who suffer the most severe symptoms, problems with consent may limit participation of these patients in clinical trials.

There is much variation in the application and understanding of consent in emergency psychiatric research [8]. Brown reviewed studies in the spectrum of informed consent in emergency psychiatric research. Twelve studies were examined involving requirements of informed consent for studies using chemical sedation of agitated patients. The author reported that these studies had no uniform approach to dealing with the challenges involved in obtaining patient or caregiver consent. In slightly more than half of the studies an informed consent was attempted. The remainder of the studies made use of a waiver of consent, or an exception to informed consent. In some studies, no consent was obtained at all [8].

Brown's work showed that in treatment for agitation no uniformity or consensus existed for obtaining consent by patients or surrogates (if it was obtained at all). This study showed that several glaring defects for proper consent are present even in published studies. The consistent lack of an adequate description how an informed consent was obtained from agitated patients in dire need of urgent medication is additionally concerning [8]. Institutional Review Boards' requirements to assess consent lacked consistency. The definition of "capacity to consent" varied from study to study and the waiver of informed consent based on minimal risk exceeded the Food and Drug Administration final rule [9].

Determining decisional capacity of the patient is important to the physician. The patient's capacity may be relevant to a specific decision-making context, such as capacity to consent to treatment, capacity to consent to research participation, capacity to consent to hospitalization, and so forth [8,10]. A patient may have specific capacity but not global capacity (no impairments). Psychiatric diagnoses do not necessarily denote global incapacity as a patient may be depressed but still able to give consent. It is suggested that "consent" capacity may be the appropriate term to denote that a patient has the ability to understand information relevant to making an informed and voluntary decision to participate in treatments and research [8,10]. Competency is not the same as capacity. Competence is a legal status determined by a judge whereas capacity is a clinical status determined by a healthcare professional. Despite this distinction, the basis of informed consent in research stems from Applebaum and Roth's four legal standards to determine competence to consent [11]:

1. Evidencing a choice involves manifesting consent by cooperating appropriately in early procedures and giving responses to pertinent questions.
2. Factual understanding of the issues includes understanding the nature of participation versus nonparticipation, that he/she has a choice to make, available options and risks/benefits of these.
3. The individual must have decision-making capacity and good judgment (known as rational manipulation of information).
4. There should be an appreciation of the situation, which involves applying the information to one's own situation and appreciating the consequence of giving consent [11].

According to a 2006 review by Dunn et al. [12], there are 12 decisional capacity assessment instruments for research based on the Applebaum criteria, each with its own limitations and variation in reliability and validity. The question remains, how best to implement informed consent in those patients with impaired decisional capacity. One suggestion by Carpenter et al. found that an intensive educational intervention improved decisional capacity of schizophrenic participants to the level of their non-schizophrenic cohort control [13]. This type of model may be the type of answer needed to solve this vexing issue.

Funding concerns

The National Institute of Mental Health (NIMH) is the primary federal agency funding basic and clinical research for serious mental illness (SMI) disorders [3,5]. This list includes schizophrenia, depression, bipolar disorder, panic disorder, autism, and obsessive–compulsive disorder. The SMI disorders accounts for total direct costs of 6.2% of all healthcare expenditures or approximately 300 billion per year [2]. According to the National Survey on Drug Use and Health, in 2008, approximately 6% of all U.S. citizens 18 years of age or over have a SMI that results in functional impairment.[8] In jailed citizens of the United States, 16% of inmates have a SMI [2].

Funding for research into SMI was 1.49 billion in 2010 [2,14]. However, a report by the Treatment Advocacy Center depicts serious flaws in allotment of these monies. The report showed that while the budget for research at NIMH doubled from 1997 to 2002, approximately 75% of these awards went to research on issues other than SMI (drug and alcohol abuse, cigarette usage, and others). The Treatment Advocacy Center report stated the funding actually represented an 11% decrease of SMI research by NIMH during those years. The total research in how to improve treatment and quality of life for the SMI patients was only 5.8% of all NIMH awards [2]. Research funding in pediatric psychiatric disorders (which affect 13.1% of children ages 8–15) [7] is even more limited. Analysis of grant for research up to 2001 found only 6% dealing with depression in the pediatric primary care setting despite the fact that children and adolescents make up 26% of the total population of depressed patients [7]. Only 11 studies were funded by NIMH, consisting of less than half of one percent of the NIMH portfolio [2].

Future agenda

Downey and Zun studied the number of articles published on emergency psychiatric issues versus total number of articles published. Even though mental health disorders represent an enormous percentage of visits and cost in the emergency system, there is only a miniscule number of articles on the subject published [15]. In fact, mental health disorders constitute one of the five most costly conditions contributing to the cost of American health care [1,2]. Yet there is a lack of funding for research into this expensive and pervasive health problem. Future research efforts will depend on increases in funding for SMI at a rate comparable to that of the other most costly medical disorders.

The scarcity of evidence-based medicine in emergency psychiatry research allows for many opportunities of study. Suicide is the tenth leading case of death in the United States and the Emergency Department is the primary point of care for treatment of these patients. Funding of and research into suicide is necessary to provide measures and interventions which effectively reduce risk of suicide. For example appropriate screening tools and interventions need to be developed and validated. ED suicide registries may also be of benefit in a manner similar to tracking cancer risks and may further aid in standardization of definitions of terms [3,4]. Brown proposed a research agenda to examined structure, process, and outcomes [8]. Within the structure variations in clinical presentations and geographic differences could be studied. Process research would include factors that influence variation in response times, the availability of community resources, and the provision for emergency psychiatric care. Outcome research is needed to examine factors associated with client satisfaction and inpatient utilizations. Other opportunities for psychiatric research proposed include research into the management of agitation and delirium as well as novel interventions for delirium [3]. Post-traumatic stress disorder, and alcohol and drug abuse are additional areas of potential research important to emergency psychiatry practice [3]. Pediatric research into early diagnosis of mental illness in a uniform and cogent manner, the use of formal psychiatric evaluation, and with the community would also be beneficial [7].

Conclusion

With increasing numbers of patients requiring psychiatric services in the ED because of cuts in services elsewhere in the healthcare system, it is incumbent on ED physicians to do research on best treatments and plans of care for these patients in the ED. While there are barriers to doing this work, solutions are available to allow for this very important work. ED physicians must find pharmacologic and social service methods to treat our emergent psychiatric population to expedite their care and allow for admission, transfer, or discharge from the department. The current lack of a consistent and validated approach makes this an area of research quite fertile indeed.

References

1. Larkin GL, Claasen CA, Emond JA, et al. Trends in U.S emergency department visits for mental health conditions, 1992 to 2001. *Psychiatry Serv* 2005;**56**:671–7.

2. Torrey et al. *A Federal Failure in Psychiatric Research: Continuing NIMH Negligence in Funding Sufficient Research on Serious Mental Illness.* 2003 Treatment Advocacy Center. Available at: www.psychlaw.org/ (Accessed September 2011).

3. D'Onofrio G, Jauch E, Jagoda A, et al. NIH Roundtable on opportunities to advance research in neurologic and psychiatric emergencies. *Ann Emerg Med* 2010;**56**:551–64.

4. Woodall A, Morgan C, Sloan C, Howard L. Barriers to participation in mental health research. *BMC Psychiatry* 2010;**10**:103.

5. Thompson EE, Neighbors HW, Munday C, Jackson JS. Recruitment and retention of African American patients for clinical research. *J Consult Clin Psychol* 1996;**64**:861–7.

6. Institute of Medicine. *Emergency Care for Children: Growing Pains.* Washington, DC: National Academics Press; 2007.

7. Horowitz SM, Kelleher K, Boyce T, et al. Barriers to healthcare research for children and youth with psychosocial problems. *JAMA* 2002;**288**:1508–12.

8. Brown J. The spectrum of informed consent in emergency psychiatric research. *Ann Emerg Med* 2006;**47**:68–74.

9. National Institutes of Health. *National Institutes of Health Rule.* Available at: grants.nih.gov/grants/policy/ethic_research.htm (Accessed September 2011).

10. Sturman E. The capacity to consent to treatment and research: a review of standardized assessment tools. *Clin Psychol Rev* 2005;**25**:954–74.

11. Applebaum PS, Roth LH. Competency to consent to research. *Arch Gen Psychiatry* 1982;**39**:951–8.

12. Dunn LB, Nowrangi MA, Palmer BW, Jeste DV, Saks ER. Assessing decisional capacity for clinical research or treatment: a review of instruments. *Am J Psychiatry* 2006;**163**:1323–34.

13. Carpenter WT, Gold JM, Lahti AC, et al. Decisional capacity for informed consent in schizophrenia research. *Arch Gen Psychiatry* 2000;**57**:533–8.

14. Brown JF. Psychiatric emergency services: a review of the literature and a proposed research agenda. *Psychiatr Q* 2005;**76**:139–65.

15. Downey LA, Zun LS. Does the literature support the incidences? Submitted for publication 2011.

Chapter 51

Administration

Harvey L. Ruben and Lara G. Chepenik

Administration of emergency services for psychiatric patients typically resides with more than one person, and may include hospital business personnel, nurses and physicians with administrative duties, government agencies, and a board of directors. Despite the differences in training of the personnel involved, the shared goals of any administrator include matching available resources to the community's need and funding these resources. Estimating the number of patient visits to the emergency department (ED) for mental health problems, providing an appropriate setting and trained staff to process these patients, facilitating disposition from the emergency setting, measuring quality of performance, and securing financial support of these activities all constitute elements of this process.

Ideally, data and experience guide administrative decisions in the design and staffing of a new psychiatric service in an ED or facility dedicated to acute psychiatric patients. Unfortunately, as has been noted by colleagues, "If you have seen one psychiatric emergency service, you have seen one psychiatric emergency service." In other words, emergency psychiatric services frequently emerge unplanned as general ED resources become strained by psychiatric patients. What follows is one person's experience developing emergency psychiatric services both in a large academic hospital and in a private hospital. The remainder of the chapter provides an overview of major steps in development of emergency psychiatric services and available research to guide informed decisions around its design. Discussion of organization theory and management style are not included in this chapter but may be referenced elsewhere [1].

Part I: A Tale of Two Psychiatric ERs

Case example: dedicated psychiatric ED in an academic university hospital

A separate psychiatric emergency service, the Crisis Intervention Unit (CIU), was established as part of the Yale New Haven Hospital Emergency Department in 1982. Though its director had previous experience with emergency psychiatric services as the Chief of the Crisis Intervention Service at the Connecticut Mental Health Center, this new endeavor was a much larger undertaking and presented several unforeseen challenges. The early CIU was staffed primarily by psychiatry residents on a 24 hour/7 day per week basis, with the help of additional personnel. The CIU was initiated as a separate, locked unit within the ED of the Yale University New Haven Hospital. It contained six separate cubicles with doors, a small lobby and a nurses' station, much like any medical ER nurses' station, with a counter and a built-in desk. Behind the nurse's station, there was an office with a closed door for the residents and other professional staff. The ED administration set up the CIU and an architect, who had apparently never developed a psychiatric ED before, planned the facility. Problems arose immediately from beds placed too close to the wall, curtains hanging in the rooms and closed doors on patient rooms. Within the first several weeks, one patient punched a hole in the wall and another patient managed to set the curtain on fire with a lighter that he had hidden on his person. In addition, there were problems with the closed doors on patient rooms as this prevented direct observation of the patients (though it did provide some relief from noise, both for the patients and the staff). Another problem arose from the traditional nursing station counter, as patients were leaning on the counter, reaching over it, taking things, or disrupting the nursing staff while they were attempting to chart or do other activities.

We immediately had to make some changes to the physical plant. First, modification of the layout prevented the patient beds from directly abutting walls. In addition, we dispensed with the curtains in the rooms and developed a policy that the doors had to be open unless a staff person was in the room with the patient. Placement of a glass partition which sealed the space between the ceiling and the nursing station counter created privacy for the staff. Eventually, we had a door put at the end of the nurse's counter. This restricted the available room so that the patients could not wander in. Staffing consisted of a second year (PG2) Yale psychiatric resident and, on weekdays and occasionally weekend dayshifts, two psychiatric technicians. A social worker

Behavioral Emergencies for the Emergency Physician, ed. Leslie S. Zun, Lara G. Chepenik, and Mary Nan S. Mallory. Published by Cambridge University Press. © Cambridge University Press 2013.

and nursing staff completed the staff roster during the day; however, residents worked alone at night. As a result, the residents were overwhelmed within a short period of time. Not only were they managing the psychiatric needs of the patients, but they were also performing physical exams, drawing blood for laboratory tests and taking care of all other patient needs. After only a few weeks of this arrangement, and one unfortunate resident's experience admitting twelve people during an overnight shift, the Psychiatric Residents' Association of the Yale Department of Psychiatry was up in arms and demanded additional help or they would strike. Whether this would have happened or not remains unknown, but their persistence led to the addition of moonlighting psychiatric technicians hired from within the Yale Health System for overnight and weekend shifts. This arrangement started within two weeks of the residents' complaint. Having worked out these particular problems which had been unforeseen by the administration when planning the CIU, the unit began to function smoothly and effectively.

However, other unforeseen problems unrelated to patient care continued to arise. The CIU was located at a very back corner of the ED. Although it actually had a very small sign, non-psychiatric professional staff, patient families and medical students were often unable to find it. A larger sign was therefore obtained. Some found this location away from the mainstream ED activity a benefit since intrusion or interruption was rare and staff found they were basically left alone to do their work. The remote location also discouraged patient elopement and provided more opportunity to apprehend patients before they escaped from the hospital.

The CIU contained a common seating area with a television set where patients and visitors might congregate. Patients did not have television sets in their rooms, and it was believed this arrangement encouraged them to be out of their rooms, which was thought to be beneficial.

Over the years, increased patient demand caused both the staff and physical plant to expand, and the CIU is now a modern, specially designed unit with separate rooms for 12 patients and clinical personnel available to manage additional patient overflow in the main ER.

Case example: consultation model within a private hospital

The establishment of a psychiatric emergency facility at the Hospital of St. Raphael (HSR) was totally different from that at the Yale Health System. At Yale, there was a deliberate plan to establish a psychiatric ED. At HSR, the psychiatric ED evolved by default. Prior to staffing the ED at HSR with a psychiatrist, members of the inpatient psychiatric team performed consultations on those patients requiring psychiatric service. Coming to the ED to consult was very disruptive for the inpatient staff, and also caused extended wait times for patients. Initially a psychiatrist was hired on a 60% part-time basis to staff the psychiatry section of the ED, along with the help of a licensed clinical social worker (LCSW). Within a short time, a second highly skilled

bachelor of social work (BSW) with psychiatric experience was hired to enhance this service. The initial physical plant was a large four-bed partially enclosed space near the ambulance entrance of the ED. The beds were separated by curtains, and the nurse's station was a desk in the corner of the room. The professional staff had an office in a different part of the ED. Referrals from the ED increased as psychiatric consultation became more readily available. Ultimately, two additional beds were placed into this four-bed space, separated by screens. The room had no door. It did have a large entrance, and several patients eloped over a short period of time. One of them actually burst through a closed glass door before running away from the ED. As problems continued to occur with this makeshift psychiatric unit, it became clear that the volume of patients required additional staff and a better physical space. Initially, patients who arrived during the night were held in the ED until psychiatric consultants, social workers and psychiatrists could evaluate them the next morning. With the move towards the larger unit, additional staff was hired. The psychiatric director hired moonlighting Yale psychiatric residents along with a social worker to staff the evening shift. Eventually, a psychiatric advanced practice registered nurse (APRN) was also hired to work on the evening and/or night shift to provide additional clinical coverage.

The physical plant moved to a former eight-bed medical unit away from the ambulance entrance and a locked door was added for security. The eight beds were separated by curtains of the tear-away type so that the patients could not hurt themselves with the curtains. The nurses' station consisted of a rather long medical nurses' station on the wall opposite the patients' beds. The nurses, therefore, had line of sight of all the patients in the eight beds as long as the curtains remained open. Curtains were only closed by professional staff who needed privacy with patients. In addition to the small office in the medical unit that we had previously, an additional interview office located within this new facility provided space for staff to meet privately with patients. This space had a curtain, rather than a door, to increase staff safety should there be a problem. There was also a restroom and a shower, which did not have a locking door. The patients could only use these facilities if a staff person was waiting on the outside. Nurses reported to the head nurse of the ED and were drawn from the ED nursing pool. Therefore, ED nurses who had an interest in working with psychiatric patients staffed the unit. This worked fairly smoothly and the nursing staff coverage was reasonably adequate. Unfortunately, there were a number of different incidents that occurred that required intervention by the staff or by the ED security force. This included patients fighting, becoming quite agitated, or bothering other patients or visitors. The ED security staff would be called to supplement the professional staff in the unit when such an event occurred. Unfortunately, it might take them several minutes to arrive. Therefore, a uniformed security guard without a weapon was placed at a desk at the end of the nurses' station. This had an amazingly beneficial effect. Once the patients saw that there was a security guard facing them with line of sight to all of the beds, the disruptions and problems became far less. In addition, the security guard had a two-way radio so that he or she would radio immediately for assistance when any problem occurred. Within a very brief time, several security guards would arrive to help the professional staff. The staffing ultimately consisted of the psychiatry director, who worked weekdays from 8:00 AM until 1 PM. A psychiatry resident and two social workers worked on weekdays from 4:00 pm to midnight. A psychiatry resident and one or two social workers worked from 8:00 am until 8:00 PM on weekends with an APRN or resident covering the night shift from midnight to 8:00AM, depending on scheduling. With this complement of clinical staff and the presence of the security guard, the eight-bed unit functioned smoothly and efficiently.

There were two television monitors, one in front of each set of four beds, and the availability of television for the patients was quite helpful. The staff monitored the programming to ensure there were no violent shows or news that might disturb the patients. This room lacked a lobby, which discouraged gathering of groups of patients. However, on several occasions patients pulled chairs together in a corner of the room to sit and talk. This practice seemed to benefit the patients and became an accepted part of the emergency psychiatric service.

A change in the security policy arose after the occasional visitor brought some kind of contraband to a patient, such as cigarettes, lighters, or other objects which were not allowed. As a result, visitors were asked to secure their purses and other bags in a locked cupboard. People readily complied and contra-indicated items stopped appearing in patients' possession.

Ultimately, the hospital administration at HSR closed this separate psychiatric emergency department due to its cost, though it functioned well while open. Ironically, the psychiatric patients have since moved back to the original four-bed area within the main ED from which the undertaking to improve delivery of emergency psychiatric services started, and, as could be expected, many of the original problems have recurred.

Part II: Starting from Scratch

Determining need

Presently there are several means available to administrators to anticipate a community's need for emergency psychiatric services. In an established ED, data collected on patient visits by Current Procedural Terminology (CPT) or International Statistical Classification of Diseases and Related Health Problems (ICD-9) code, average length of stay (LOS) for patients with psychiatric codes, and revenue collections can begin to inform the number of beds and personnel necessary to meet current need.

In the absence of such data, need may be estimated based on incidence and prevalence of psychiatric illness combined with demographic information for a particular catchment area. On average, mental health disorders comprise 5–6.3% of ED visits [2, 3]. The National Institute of Mental Health also periodically publishes these data, and collection is ongoing [4, 5]. The Healthcare Cost and Utilization Project also provides information on ICD-9 codes, demographic data and expected payment

sources collected from federal, state and private resources, though there is a fee for this service (http://www.hcup-us.ahrq. gov/tech_assist/centdist.jsp). Additional considerations may be specific to the system providing emergency services. For example, some health care systems provide dedicated psychiatric emergency facilities primarily or exclusively for enrolled members. Therefore, hospitals outside of these systems might exclude participating members from estimates of the population in their catchment area.

In addition to the volume of patients expected to visit the psychiatric services in the ED, it is also helpful to know if specific populations exist in a given catchment area. This information usually depends on existent outpatient resources. Nursing homes, homeless shelters, residential facilities, community mental health centers, schools and forensic facilities may have mandatory referral policies which bring patients to the ED. The prevalence of these facilities will likely influence the demographic of patients referred for evaluation, and consequently the resources which the ED will be expected to provide. For example, individuals specifically requesting treatment of substance use disorders may be processed without evaluation by a licensed independent practitioner (LIP). Therefore, knowledge of the numbers of patients specifically requesting substance treatment can aid an administrator in decisions regarding logistics, personnel and space.

Logistics

Physical plant

The logistics in an ED essentially include patient arrival or referral to the ED, triage, evaluation and disposition. Many patients with mental health concerns come to EDs of their own volition. However, states also provide means to involuntarily transport and hold individuals with suspected psychiatric problems. This is one unique feature of patients referred to EDs for psychiatric evaluation, and will impact the facility and personnel accordingly. Facility design should account for arrival of patients by ambulance or police cruiser in addition to the usual pedestrian means of travel.

Identifying a mechanism to register and transport a patient in police custody may be particularly problematic in an ED without a dedicated emergency psychiatric facility. This process typically requires means to search the patient, secure their belongings, prevent against patient violence or elopement, and to do so while preserving a therapeutic setting. Special consideration of facility layout, hardware and décor is necessary to meet regulatory requirements for psychiatric facilities and avoid some of the difficulties described in the earlier case examples. Patients have been known to be extremely creative in their attempts to elope or harm themselves. To name just a few examples: they have climbed into the ceiling, quietly walked out with ambulance crews or visitors, and hung themselves from television monitors, doorknobs and curtains. If facility design accounts for the possibility every item in the psychiatric ED may serve as a potential means for patients to injure themselves or assault staff, thoughtful choices may limit these events. These choices will also likely affect choice of bed design, placement of patient rooms, and the location of nursing stations, offices and security personnel. Advance consideration of these challenges will help ensure adequate facility design and provision of appropriate support equipment such as metal detectors, secure storage, video monitors and secure interview rooms.

Extended ED stays may also impact facility decisions. Stays greater than 24 hours may increase patient demand to attend to general hygiene such as access to showers and means to change or launder clothes. Boredom may also become a problem, prompting some EDs to provide televisions, patient phones, playing cards or reading materials (though patients have been known to take the staples from magazines to cut themselves, so caution is advised). Patients who wish to socialize have been known to create impromptu groups on the floor or any available space, suggesting a designated area for such activity may be beneficial both to the patients and staff who might need to negotiate around them. Psychotic, manic, and demented patients can demonstrate restlessness which benefits from provision of a secure location to pace. Although these needs are best served by provision of additional space, a valuable ED resource, they are likely to reduce behavioral disturbance and warrant consideration in facility planning.

Triage

Typically, nursing staff triage patients based on acuity of their presenting problem. The expertise and training of the nurse performing this duty may vary dramatically in a general ED compared to a dedicated psychiatric ED. One challenge to performing an adequate triage assessment of psychiatric patients is the subjective nature of patients' complaints and limited objective means to verify their symptoms. Clinical observation typically constitutes the objective measure in these evaluations, which can lead to disagreement even among experts [6]. Survey of ED nursing staff reveals many nurses feel unsure of their ability to evaluate features of psychiatric illness such as suicidality, paranoia and intoxication [7]. In response to these challenges, some emergency rooms modified their triage process. Although discussed in more detail in the chapter on Triage, these changes might include adding mental health professionals (such as psychiatric nurses or social workers) or adoption of mental health screens [8, 9].

Vignette: Medicine vs. Psychiatry

A 53-year-old Caucasian woman with a history of schizophrenia and hypertension presented to the ED from her group home complaining she couldn't catch her breath. She was first evaluated by a physician in the medical ED. Because of a pre-existing policy, all patients 50 years of age and older need a physical exam prior to receiving a psychiatric exam. The patient appeared uncomfortable and kept her hand flat on her chest; however, she responded appropriately to questions and did not appear dyspneic. The woman's vital signs were all within normal limits; laboratory evaluation showed no signs of infection and her physical exam was unremarkable. Despite an absence of any history of anxiety and denial of any psychiatric

symptoms, she was referred to the psychiatric service for evaluation. The psychiatric nurse accepting the patient reviewed her laboratory results and discovered the patient had a positive d-dimer, consistent with the pulmonary embolism which was causing her symptoms.

This vignette illustrates the potential difficulty medical personnel may encounter when patients demonstrate symptoms consistent with either a psychiatric or non-psychiatric cause. Although one would hope the psychiatric clinician would have performed a similarly adequate evaluation for shortness of breath, resources for medical evaluation may be limited in a psychiatric emergency facility. It is also helpful to ensure the person with the most expertise in a medical specialty evaluates the patient's complaints. In some facilities a social worker might perform the psychiatric evaluation. A social worker lacks the medical training to adequately distinguish between a patient with anxiety and one with a life-threatening illness. Appropriate referral typically depends upon the skill of the triage nurse. This particular hospital's pre-existing policy helped ensure the patient received an exam in the medical ED.

Evaluation

The American Psychiatric Association provides a description of the components which comprise an appropriate emergency psychiatric assessment [10]. This recommended assessment includes an interview by a mental health practitioner, assessment of contributory medical conditions, determination of psychiatric and medical history including treatment, a targeted physical evaluation, detailed substance use history, information from collateral sources, and a treatment plan. This assessment includes many of the elements from the American Psychiatric Association guideline on Psychiatric Evaluation of Adults, which elaborates the details of recommended adult psychiatric evaluation [11]. Upon completion of this assessment, the LIP typically formulates a diagnosis and disposition for the patient.

Although these endpoints might be accepted by ED personnel, they may be inconsistent with patient expectations. Survey of consumers of emergency psychiatric services reveals a majority felt they received inadequate attention and treatment [12]. Since an average evaluation takes approximately 75 minutes, defined as the period from the beginning of the evaluation to a decision regarding disposition [13], the expectations of consumers are likely inconsistent with the typical resources provided by EDs. Fifty-eight percent of consumers identified relationship problems as their primary impetus for seeking emergency psychiatric care, compared to 5% who self-identified psychotic symptoms, 2% manic symptoms, and 25% depression/suicidality [14]. Since it is these latter criteria which often justify inpatient hospitalization, it may be consumers are seeking treatment other than inpatient hospitalization when coming for emergency psychiatric evaluation. These expectations may impact administrative decisions regarding choices of personnel and deliver model of care. The creation of dedicated observation rooms within the ED has been one response to patients who present with acute, but transient, stress [15, 16].

Vignette: Are psychiatrists the proprietors of communication

It was 8 am following the morning change of shift when one of the ED physicians requested assistance with a patient who had been found publically intoxicated and therefore brought to the ED per local regulation. Apparently the man engaged in a verbal altercation with one of the ED technicians, threatened the technician, and was now in restraints. The psychiatric service was consulted to determine whether the patient remained a danger to the ED personnel he threatened. Per the ED physician, the patient was not psychotic, had no history of psychiatric illness and was no longer intoxicated. It was a bit of a mystery why the ED attending didn't simply ask the man if he really planned to harm the technician, in which case the police should be called. When asked, the ED attending replied, "Where I used to work, psychiatry would do that."

But what exactly did "that" mean? Did it mean "talk to my patient about something difficult?" In this vignette, the patient lacked any psychiatric symptoms. Therefore, the psychiatrist had no particular expertise that enhanced his/her assessment of risk compared to the ED clinician. Still, the ED attending was uncomfortable speaking with the patient about his expression of emotion. It is possible the attending thought a psychiatrist had some means to absorb liability by the nature of his/her expertise. However, all physicians bear some responsibility to communicate with their patients, even regarding difficult or emotional matters. Congenial communication between ED and psychiatric clinicians may ease apparent disagreements over these issues. In this case, the psychiatrist relayed to the ED physician some appropriate questions to ask the patient and reassured him he possessed adequate training to conduct the interview. The ED physician appeared to accept this and resolved the matter himself.

Disposition

Should the ED clinician decide to refer a patient to outpatient mental health treatment, he/she will face several obstacles not encountered for referrals in other disciplines. Patients with insurance may face limited options for providers in their area. Despite increasing numbers of patients seeking mental health treatment, the number of psychiatrists in the U.S.A. remains unchanged [17, 18]. A 2002 survey of psychiatrists practicing in the U.S.A. demonstrated 85% of the group accepted new patient referrals; however this figure varied by insurance type and psychiatrist demographics. The largest group of psychiatrists accepted self-pay (77%), 65% accepted unmanaged private insurance, 63% accepted Medicare and 44% accepted Medicaid [19]. Of the 48% who participated in a managed care network, 75% accepted new patients. Nationally, the average range for days until a first appointment (after referral from an ED visit) is 29–40 days [20]. In a study of attempts to make an appointment with a new mental health provider (averaged over 9 cities and 322 clinics), research staff successfully scheduled appointments for 22% of the privately insured imaginary patients and 12% of those with Medicaid [21]. These figures suggest immediate outpatient

stabilization may be difficult for patients who do not already have psychiatric health care providers.

Government-funded community mental health centers typically treat patients who are uninsured or lack financial resources to pay for a private provider. These centers may offer walk-in hours or other flexible scheduling which facilitate referral from the ED. However, intake appointments at mental health clinics may be with a nurse or social worker, so there might be an additional delay until the patient meets with someone who can prescribe medications. ED staff that are alert to this delay may choose to provide medication prescriptions or referrals to primary care physicians to ensure patients receive suggested pharmacotherapy until their intake appointment with a new prescriber. Preparation of referral lists and relationships with outpatient providers or agencies to create a system for expedited referral from the ED may greatly increase the chance patients receive referrals to outpatient treatment in a timely manner. Additional practical support, such as taxi fare or tokens, may also be essential to successfully execute an anticipated discharge.

Referral to inpatient treatment typically involves pre-authorization from insurance companies. This procedure requires personnel trained to know which symptoms in a patients' presentation justify inpatient psychiatric hospitalization as initial refusal by an insurance company necessitates a lengthy review process between the ED psychiatrist and a physician representing the insurance company. Personnel must also be available to call various inpatient facilities to locate an appropriate inpatient bed. Finally, mechanisms need to exist to transport patients to outside facilities.

Personnel

There are two basic models for hospital based psychiatric emergency evaluations: the consultation model and independent psychiatric emergency setting (see Delivery Models of Psychiatry). In both models, however, the psychiatry department typically supplies the mental health personnel. Although this chapter provides a brief description of the different managerial and support staff positions, it primarily focuses on options for effectively staffing these two models. A number of other references are available for a more thorough discussion of personnel job descriptions [1, 22].

Management

Hospital presidents, vice presidents and boards of directors may make decisions regarding facility, policy and finance. However, they are typically removed from direct oversight of daily operations. The medical director, nursing director and middle management personnel hold responsibility for these latter duties.

The medical director for the department of psychiatry holds a doctorate of medicine and typically makes those policy decisions that define the department's mission and/or effects its implementation. This person holds final responsibility for management of clinical aspects for the department, compliance with regulatory measures, quality assurance and decisions regarding physician staff. The medical director may have a greater or lesser role in the hiring or policy decisions for non-physician LIPs, nurses or other staff. In addition, administration of policy decisions may be left to individual service managers (such as directors for the ED, consultation service, etc.) in organizations of sufficient size.

The director of nursing more typically maintains final responsibility for the non-physician mental health staff. However, depending on the size of the organization, the director of nursing may oversee various nurse managers who maintain responsibility for hiring and training of personnel. The director of nursing typically collaborates with the medical director and other middle management on quality assurance measures and liaison with other medical departments.

Consultation model

In this model, mental health personnel serve as consultants to the ED. The nursing staff triages patients with psychiatric complaints to an ED LIP, similarly to the procedure with any other patient. These patients may go to a designated area for psychiatric patients within the main ED; however, the ED nurses and LIPs perform evaluations, order and administer medications, and often complete the paperwork for involuntary commitment. ED clerks, nurses, or social workers file involuntary commitment paperwork, obtain pre-authorization from insurance companies, perform bed searches, fax evaluation materials and facilitate discharge from the ED.

Mental health consultants may consist of social workers, psychiatric nurses and LIPs (most commonly APRNs or physicians). Although a social worker without any specialized mental health training might assist patients with access to outpatient resources, including placement into substance treatment programs, one with a master's degree (MSW) possesses the skill to perform clinical interviews. Because an MSW receives training in mental health diagnoses, this person may also effectively gather collateral information from patients' friends, family and treaters, which will help diagnostic formulation and disposition planning. A LIP needs very specific information about a patient's recent behavior to formulate a risk assessment and potentially commit the patient involuntarily to a psychiatric facility. Although an LIP still needs to evaluate the patient to formulate his or her own clinical impression, the presence of trained support staff allows the LIP to evaluate a greater number of patients. A psychiatrist may be unnecessary in the consultation model, as the ED physician typically performs those duties reserved for M.D.s such as involuntary commitment and capacity evaluations. However, additional regulatory requirements may affect this decision (such as those governing training programs).

Mental health nurses may perform functions similar to those described for clinical social workers, with similar benefits to patient flow and decreased personnel costs. Benefits due to the presence of psychiatric nurses who performed mental health screens and assisted in triage include decreased time patients spend in the ED, facilitated discharge planning and access to outpatient resources, decreased security involvement and improved ED personnel satisfaction [7, 23–26].

Additional personnel may include security, technicians, substance counselors and religious ministers. Security and ED technicians hired through the hospital or ED may lack specialized training which allows them to work effectively with psychiatric patients. Psychiatric administrators may negotiate placing mental health workers or other trained personnel in these positions, or develop training programs to improve the care delivered to psychiatric patients within the ED. Religious ministers may function as crisis counselors; however, their duties are typically constrained to patient support, and do not extend to clinical evaluation.

Independent Psychiatric Emergency Room

The core personnel in a dedicated psychiatric emergency room includes security personnel, mental health workers, nurses and LIPs, all of whom typically receive specialty training in psychiatry. These facilities may function with a social worker, who has duties similar to those in a medical ED setting. Because a physician must be present or available to perform involuntary commitments, this will impact the decision to staff the facility full-time with an MD or with an APRN, using an MD only as a consultant for this task.

Either nurses or social workers perform screening evaluations, placement into substance or other specialized programs, and the clerical work necessary to arrange for inpatient hospitalization. Typically, one of the nurses liaises with referral sources such as police, mobile crisis teams and outpatient treatment centers. All personnel participate in patient restraint and should be trained accordingly.

Consideration for staffing the facility full-time will affect budget and physical plant decisions. Overnight shifts may require compensatory increases in salary, and there may be a shortage of key personnel or interpreter services during these times. Consideration for remote interviews or call rooms should minimize these potential difficulties. Decisions regarding the specialty make-up and numbers of staff are ideally based on preliminary research into the communities' mental health needs and subsequent measures of quality control. However, rough estimates for staff:patient ratios include 1 security officer, 1 nurse : 6 patients, and 1 mental health worker : 4–6 patients. The number of staff may increase if they also perform insurance pre-certification and arrange transportation. The number of LIPs needed depends on the number of patients processed through the ED as well as the length of time spent on interview, collection of collateral data and documentation. Assuming patient interviews in the ED last between 15 and 30 minutes, 10 minutes is spent on obtaining collateral information and another 20–45 minutes is spent on nursing orders and documentation, the total time a clinician spends on each psychiatric patient can last for 45–75 minutes. This estimate suggests a ratio of 1 clinician:patient/hour, though some of the data collection and interview may be performed by a mental health nurse or social worker, allowing an MD or APRN to evaluate a larger number of patients/hour.

Quality control

Hospitals might employ measures of quality control in order to assess standards of care, use of resources, and outcomes such as consumer satisfaction or personnel retention. Quality assurance describes the procedures implemented to improve quality control. In both cases, dissemination of the results of these efforts to ED personnel provides the education and means necessary to improve their system.

Regulatory agencies often influence the measures which hospitals use to assess standards of care. The Joint Commission on Accreditation of Healthcare Organizations (JHACO), local governments and insurance carriers regulate such activities as patient restraint, involuntary administration of medication, staff training, hand hygiene and required medical documentation (http://www.jointcommission.org/). Designated personnel, often a nurse manager and/or program director, collect this data for review by more senior administrators or mock inspectors prior to formal regulatory inspections. These mock inspections may help reduce staff anxiety around a formal inspection, in addition to providing useful data regarding compliance.

Quantification of resource use may inform decisions regarding budget development, purchasing and personnel. Although this might seem self-evident, the costs and resources required to deliver emergency psychiatric care may be combined with those of other departments, making it difficult to discern these numbers. This is especially true if the psychiatric ED is physically separate from a main ED but part of the same health system. Resources for shared costs may derive from a formula based on patient volume and insurance reimbursements. However, independent psychiatric EDs typically do not support themselves with insurance reimbursements alone. It may be helpful to know at the planning stage what additional financial support will be needed to cover these costs.

Time spent waiting to be evaluated and ED LOS constitute two measures that affect patient satisfaction, clinical outcome, and hospital resources. Patients associated extended time spent waiting to be seen in the ED with difficulty or inability receiving emergency treatment [27]. This delay may interfere with the therapeutic alliance between patient and staff as overcrowding in the ED contributes to frayed tempers for both parties. Extended wait times also associate with poorer compliance with outpatient referral [27–29]. For patients seeking mental health services, delay to evaluation may also limit available disposition options. Many outpatient resources will be unavailable after regular business hours for either consultation or scheduling. Residential facilities may be understaffed after hours and refuse to accept return of their residents from the ED until the morning. Shelters may fill early, and some inpatient treatment facilities only accept patient referrals during limited hours. These conditions may contribute to delay in patient discharge from the ED and increase in average LOS.

The Institute of Medicine and The Joint Commission identify timeliness and patient flow as primary measures of quality of care [30, 31]. Unfortunately, LOS appears to be increasing at a faster rate for psychiatric emergencies than for non-mental health related emergency complaints [32]. Extended LOS may be attributable to many factors, including wait for appropriate inpatient disposition, presence of suicidality, substance intoxication and lack of insurance [33–35]. Increased LOS can increase patient census as new patients continue to arrive in the ED. This consequently increases the use of hospital resources and staff, which impacts the financial burden for providing emergency psychiatric services. There may potentially be additional financial consequences if LOS becomes a measure of quality control affecting reimbursements as new federal regulations governing health care reimbursements may take such measures into account (http://www.healthcare.gov/law/full/). Though little data exists on increasing patient flow through psychiatric emergency settings, The Joint Commission published a study on the use of Toyota Production Principles to improve transfer of care between inpatient and outpatient services within a hospital system [36]. This study demonstrated effective reductions in wait times through identification of the steps in the transfer process and quantification of time delay added at each step. As with any quality control measure, collection of data, review of results, and subsequent education of staff will be critical to improving quality assurance for that hospital system.

Financial considerations

Reimbursements for emergency psychiatric visits come from a variety of sources including private insurance, government sponsored insurance (Medicaid and Medicare), government grants or budget allocation (for community mental health centers, Veterans Affairs), and managed care behavioral health systems (Kaiser Permanente, Veterans Affairs). Though the U.S. Department of Health and Human Services provides information regarding total costs for mental health services, this information lacks subcategorization (https://www.cms.gov/NationalHealthExpendData/). The most recent published summary on mental health expenditures that includes data on revenue source and type of organization receiving payment dates to 1986 [37]. This information pre-dates the Mental Health Parity Act of 1996 (P.L. 104–204), which modified caps on mental health expenditures. It also predates the relative explosion of pharmacotherapy options for mental health disorders that has increased the cost of delivering care [38]. Except for managed care facilities, the population requesting mental health treatment likely includes uninsured individuals, and those with Medicare and Medicaid, which reimburses only 25%–50% of that provided by private insurance [39]. Therefore, budget development should rely on estimates of anticipated need as well as insurance type in the target population.

Conclusion

The delivery of health care for psychiatric patients in an emergency setting is complex and continues to evolve. In particular, the effects The Affordable Care Act of 2010 will have on reimbursements or the structure of health care remains unknown. The proposed expansion of Medicaid may increase reimbursements to hospitals that currently treat uninsured individuals. However, the expense of maintaining a separate psychiatric emergency room may prove unfeasible, despite these potential increases in income, as such a facility creates redundancy in materials, staff and administration. Hospital systems which presently operate independent psychiatric EDs often do so at a financial loss [40]. However, they likely continue to do so because psychiatric EDs provide numerous benefits to patients, medical ED staff, and hospital mission or training goals. This may become increasingly difficult as The Affordable Care Act provides further disincentive to operate financially insolvent activities. However, much will depend on the measures used to compare cost vs. performance across different hospital systems. For example, will population served, presence of trainees, hospital size, non-profit status, or a host of other co-factors be taken into account when comparing hospital systems? Alternately, the new health care legislation may spur standardization of hospitals into a tiered system, much the same as the existent classification system used for trauma centers. In this model, a hospital receives a particular designation based on the presence of a stipulated minimum of services. Should this include emergency psychiatric care, there may be additional revenue streams to support such services.

Anticipation of the new health care legislation has already begun to modify the delivery of health care. Incorporation of electronic medical charting could facilitate the anticipated new data driven reimbursement system. Measures of quality control, as well as the health system's mission, may directly affect assignment of resources. The future challenge for health care administrators will certainly include understanding the tools to measure quality control and developing new measures as needs arise. Perhaps another expectation is the development and use of statistical models which predict high measures of clinical performance (and therefore higher reimbursements) with the minimal use of resources. Senior administrators in EDs will have to exercise their talents to manage these complexities, in addition to providing reassurance and education to personnel who may demonstrate resistance or anxiety over new expectations.

References

1. *Textbook of administrative psychiatry: new concepts for a changing behavioral health system.* 2nd ed. Talbott JA, Hales RE, Keill SL, editors. Washington, D.C., American Psychiatric Press, Inc., 2001.

2. Larkin GL, Claassen CA, Emond JA, Pelletier AJ, Camargo CA. Trends in U.S. emergency department visits for mental health conditions, 1992 to 2001. *Psychiatr Serv* 2005; **56**(6): 671–7.

3. Hazlett SB, McCarthy ML, Londner MS, Onyike CU. Epidemiology of adult psychiatric visits to US emergency departments. *Acad Emerg Med* 2004; **11**(2): 193–5.

4. Regier DA, Myers JK, Kramer M, Robins LN, Blazer DG, Hough RL, et al. The NIMH Epidemiologic Catchment Area program. Historical context, major objectives, and study population characteristics. *Arch Gen Psychiatry* 1984; **41**(10): 934–41.

5. Robins LN, Regier DA. *Psychiatric disorders in America-the epidemiologic catchment area study.* New York, The Free Press, 1991.

6. Way BB, Allen MH, Mumpower JL, Stewart TR, Banks SM. Interrater agreement among psychiatrist in psychiatric emergency assessments. *Am J Psychiatry* 1998; **155**(10): 1423–8.

7. Wand T, Happell B. The mental health nurse: contributing to improved outcomes for patients in the emergency department. *Accid Emerg Nurs* 2001; **9**(3): 166–76.

8. Bengelsdorf H, Levy LE, Emerson RL, Barile FA. A crisis triage rating scale. Brief dispositional assessment of patients at risk for hospitalization. *J Nerv Ment Dis* 1984; **172**(7): 424–30.

9. Smart D, Pollard C, Walpole B. Mental health triage in emergency medicine. *Aust N Z J Psychiatry* 1999; **33**(1): 57–66; discussion 7–9.

10. Allen MH, Forster P, Zealberg J, Currier GW. Report and recommendations regarding psychiatric emergency and crisis services. APA task force on psychiatric emergency services [Internet]. 2002.

11. Association AP. Practice guideline for psychiatric evaluation of adults. American Psychiatric Association. *Am J Psychiatry* 1995; **152**(11 Suppl): 63–80.

12. Allen MH, Carpenter D, Sheets JL, Miccio S, Ross R. What do consumers say they want and need during a psychiatric emergency? *J Psychiatr Pract* 2003; **9**(1): 39–58.

13. Chang G, Weiss AP, Orav EJ, Jones JA, Finn CT, Gitlin DF, et al. Hospital variability in emergency department length of stay for adult patients receiving psychiatric consultation: a prospective study. *Ann Emerg Med* 2011; **58**(2): 127–36 e1.

14. Allen MH, Currier GW, Hughes DH, Docherty JP, Carpenter D, Ross R. Treatment of behavioral emergencies: a summary of the expert consensus guidelines. *J Psychiatr Pract* 2003; **9**(1): 16–38.

15. Ianzito BM, Fine J, Sprague B, Pestana J. Overnight admission for psychiatric emergencies. *Hosp Community Psychiatry* 1978; **29**(11): 728–30.

16. Gillig PM, Hillard JR, Bell J, Combs HE, Martin C, Deddens JA. The psychiatric emergency service holding area: effect on utilization of inpatient resources. *Am J Psychiatry* 1989; **146**(3): 369–72.

17. Olfson M, Marcus SC, Druss B, Elinson L, Tanielian T, Pincus HA. National trends in the outpatient treatment of depression. *JAMA* 2002; **287**(2): 203–9.

18. Cooper RA. There's a shortage of specialists: is anyone listening? *Acad Med* 2002; **77**(8): 761–6.

19. Wilk JE, West JC, Narrow WE, Rae DS, Regier DA. Access to psychiatrists in the public sector and in managed health plans. *Psychiatr Serv* 2005; **56**(4): 408–10.

20. Reschovsky JD, Staiti AB. Access and quality: does rural America lag behind? *Health Aff (Millwood)* 2005; **24**(4): 1128–39.

21. Rhodes KV, Vieth TL, Kushner H, Levy H, Asplin BR. Referral without access:

for psychiatric services, wait for the beep. *Ann Emerg Med* 2009; **54**(2): 272–8.

22. Fauman BJ. Personnel: the psychiatric emergency care team. In: Barton G, Friedman R, editors. *Handbook of emergency psychiatry for clinical administrators.* New York, The Hawthorne Press, Inc., 1986.

23. Clarke DE, Hughes L, Brown AM, Motluk L. Psychiatric emergency nurses in the emergency department: the success of the Winnipeg, Canada experience. *J Emerg Nurs* 2005; **31**(4): 351–6.

24. McArthur M, Montgomery P. The experience of gatekeeping: a psychiatric nurse in an emergency department. *Issues Ment Health Nurs* 2004; **25**(5): 487–501.

25. Bristow DP, Herrick CA. Emergency department case management: the dyad team of nurse case manager and social worker improve discharge planning and patient and staff satisfaction while decreasing inappropriate admissions and costs: a literature review. *Lippincotts Case Manag* 2002; **7**(6): 243–51.

26. Vingilis E, Hartford K, Diaz K, Mitchell B, Velamoor R, Wedlake M, et al. Process and outcome evaluation of an emergency department intervention for persons with mental health concerns using a population health approach.

Adm Policy Ment Health 2007; **34**(2): 160–71.

27. Kennedy J, Rhodes K, Walls CA, Asplin BR. Access to emergency care: restricted by long waiting times and cost and coverage concerns. *Ann Emerg Med* 2004; **43**(5): 567–73.

28. Bindman AB, Grumbach K, Keane D, Rauch L, Luce JM. Consequences of queuing for care at a public hospital emergency department. *JAMA* 1991; **266**(8): 1091–6.

29. Sherman ML, DBarnum DD, Nyberg E, Buhman-Wiggs A. Predictors of preintake attrition in a rural community mental health center. *Psychological Services* 2008; **5**(4): 332–40.

30. Medicine Io. *Crossing the quality chasm: a new health system for the 21st century.* Washington, D.C., National Academy Press, 2001.

31. Leaders develop and implement plans to identify and mitigate impediments to efficient patient flow througout the hospital, Standard LD.04.03.11 (2008).

32. Slade EP, Dixon LB, Semmel S. Trends in the duration of emergency department visits, 2001–2006. *Psychiatr Serv* 2010; **61**(9): 878–84.

33. Breslow RE, Klinger BI, Erickson BJ. Time study of psychiatric emergency service evaluations. *Gen Hosp Psychiatry* 1997; **19**(1): 1–4.

34. Kropp S, Andreis C, te Wildt B, Reulbach U, Ohlmeier M, Auffarth I, et al. Psychiatric patients turnaround times in the emergency department. *Clin Pract Epidemiol Ment Health* 2005; **1**(27): 1–5.

35. Park JM, Park LT, Siefert CJ, Abraham ME, Fry CR, Silvert MS. Factors associated with extended length of stay for patients presenting to an urban psychiatric emergency service: a case-control study. *J Behav Health Serv Res* 2009; **36**(3): 300–8.

36. Young JQ, Wachter RM. Applying Toyota Production System principles to a psychiatric hospital: making transfers safer and more timely. *Jt Comm J Qual Patient Saf* 2009; **35**(9): 439–48.

37. Sunshine JH, Witkin MJ, Manderscheid RW, Atay J. Expenditures and sources of funds for mental health organizations: United States and each state, 1986. *Ment Health Stat Note* 1990; (193): 1–27.

38. Frank RG, Goldman HH, McGuire TG. Trends in mental health cost growth: an expanded role for management? *Health Aff (Millwood)* 2009; **28**(3): 649–59.

39. Chepenik LG, Hajdasz D. unpublished. 2011.

40. Chepenik LG, Hajdasz D, Powsner S. unpublished. 2011.

Index

Printed in the United States
by Bookmasters

Printed in the United States
By Bookmasters